Suicide Over the Life Cycle:

Risk Factors, Assessment, and
Treatment of Suicidal Patients

Suicide Over the Life Cycle:
Risk Factors, Assessment, and
Treatment of Suicidal Patients

Edited By

Susan J. Blumenthal, M.D., M.P.A.
Chief, Behavioral Medicine Program
National Institute of Mental Health
Rockville, Maryland
and
Clinical Associate Professor of Psychiatry
Georgetown University School of Medicine
Washington, D.C.

and

David J. Kupfer, M.D.
Professor and Chairman
Department of Psychiatry
University of Pittsburgh School of Medicine
Western Psychiatric Institute and Clinic
Pittsburgh, Pennsylvania

American
Psychiatric
Press, Inc.

Washington, DC
London, England

Copyright © 1990 American Psychiatric Press, Inc.

American Psychiatric Press, Inc.
1400 K St., N.W., Washington, DC 20005

ALL RIGHTS RESERVED
Manufactured in the United States of America
First Edition
93 92 91 90 4 3 2 1

The paper used in this publication meets the minimum requirements of the American National Standard for Information Sciences—Permanence of Paper for Printed Library Materials ANSI Z39.48-1984.   ∞

Library of Congress Cataloging-in-Publication Data

Suicide over the life cycle: risk factors, assessment, and treatment of suicidal patients/ edited by Susan J. Blumenthal and David J. Kupfer.
    p.   cm.
Includes bibliographical references.
ISBN 0-88048-307-5
    1. Suicidal behavior.   2. Suicidal behavior—Risk factors.   3. Suicidal behavior —Epidemiology.   I. Blumenthal, Susan J., 1952- .   II. Kupfer, David J., 1941-
    [DNLM: 1. Risk Factors.   2. Suicide—epidemiology.   3. Suicide—prevention & control.   4. Suicide, Attempted—psychology.   HV 6545 S94854]
RC569.S936   1990
362.2'8—dc20
DNLM/DLC
for Library of Congress   89-18368
                                                 CIP

British Cataloguing in Publication Data
A CIP record is available from the British Library

Contents

Contributors

Editors

Susan J. Blumenthal, M.D., M.P.A.
Chief, Behavioral Medicine Program
National Institute of Mental Health
Rockville, Maryland
        and
Clinical Associate Professor of Psychiatry
Georgetown University School of Medicine
Washington, DC

David J. Kupfer, M.D.
Professor and Chairman
Department of Psychiatry
University of Pittsburgh School of Medicine
Western Psychiatric Institute and Clinic
Pittsburgh, Pennsylvania

Kenneth S. Adam, M.D.
Professor of Psychiatry
McMaster University
Hamilton, Ontario, Canada

Jess Amchin, M.D.
Assistant Professor of Psychiatry
Director, Psychiatric Consultation-Liaison Program
Faculty Member, Law and Psychiatry Program
University of Pittsburgh School of Medicine
Western Psychiatric Institute and Clinic
Pittsburgh, Pennsylvania

Aaron T. Beck, M.D.
Professor of Psychiatry
University of Pennsylvania
Philadelphia, Pennsylvania

Donald W. Black, M.D.
Assistant Professor of Psychiatry
The University of Iowa Hospitals and Clinics
Psychiatric Hospital
Iowa City, Iowa

David A. Brent, M.D.
Associate Professor, Child Psychiatry
Director, STAR Center
University of Pittsburgh School of Medicine
Western Psychiatric Institute and Clinic
Pittsburgh, Pennsylvania

Martin Buda, M.D.
Clinical Instructor, Section of Psychiatric Epidemiology and Genetics
Department of Psychiatry
Harvard Medical School
Massachusetts Mental Health Center
Brockton, Massachusetts

Rene F. W. Diekstra, Ph.D.
Professor and Chairman
Department of Clinical and Health Psychology
University of Leiden
Leiden, West Netherlands

Brian B. Doyle, M.D.
Clinical Professor of Psychiatry and of Family and Community
    Medicine
Georgetown University School of Medicine
Washington, DC

Felton Earls, M.D.
Professor of Human Behavior and Development
Harvard School of Public Health
Boston, Massachusetts

Javier I. Escobar, M.D.
Professor of Psychiatry
University of Connecticut
Veterans Administration Medical Center
Newington, Connecticut

Daniel K. Flavin, M.D.
Assistant Clinical Professor of Psychiatry
New York Medical College
Medical/Scientific Officer, The National Council on Alcoholism, Inc.
Cornell Medical Center
White Plains, New York

Allen Frances, M.D.
Professor of Psychiatry
The New York Hospital
New York, New York

Richard J. Frances, M.D.
Vice-Chairman and Director of Residency Training
Department of Psychiatry and Mental Health Science
University of Medicine and Dentistry of New Jersey
Newark, New Jersey

John E. Franklin, Jr., M.D.
Assistant Professor of Psychiatry
Department of Psychiatry and Mental Health Science
University of Medicine and Dentistry of New Jersey
Newark, New Jersey

Minna Fyer, M.D.
Assistant Professor of Psychiatry
The New York Hospital
New York, New York

Mark J. Goldblatt, MBBCH
Instructor in Psychiatry, Harvard Medical School
Psychiatrist-in-Charge, Affective Disorders Inpatient Unit
McLean Hospital
Belmont, Massachusetts

Scott J. Goldsmith, M.D.
Director, Central Evaluation Services, Payne-Whitney Clinic
Instructor in Psychiatry
Cornell Medical Center
The New York Hospital
New York, New York

Madelyn S. Gould, Ph.D., M.P.H.
Assistant Professor of Clinical Social Sciences in Psychiatry and
   Public Health (Epidemiology)
College of Physicians and Surgeons of
   Columbia University
Department of Psychiatry
Division of Child Psychiatry
New York, New York

Robert L. Hendren, D.O.
Associate Professor of Psychiatry
Director, Division of Child and Adolescent Psychiatry
University of New Mexico School of Medicine
Medical Director, Children's Psychiatric Hospital
Albuquerque, New Mexico

Valerie F. Holmes, M.D.
Assistant Professor of Psychiatry
Department of Psychiatry and Behavioral Science
Health Sciences Center
State University of New York at Stony Brook
Stony Brook, New York

Lewis L. Judd, M.D.
Director, National Institute of Mental Health
Rockville, Maryland

Alvin Kahn, M.D.
Clinical Instructor in Psychiatry
Harvard Medical School
Beth Israel Hospital
Boston, Massachusetts

Seymour S. Kety, M.D.
Associate Director for Basic Research
National Institute of Mental Health
Bethesda, Maryland

David J. Kolko, Ph.D.
Associate Professor, Child Psychiatry
Director, Child and Parent Behavior Clinic
University of Pittsburgh School of Medicine
Western Psychiatric Institute and Clinic
Pittsburgh, Pennsylvania

Thomas B. Mackenzie, M.D.
Associate Professor of Psychiatry and Medicine
University of Minnesota Medical School
Minneapolis, Minnesota

Spero M. Manson, Ph.D.
Associate Professor of Psychiatry
University of Colorado Health Sciences Center
Director, National Center for American Indian and Alaska Native
    Mental Health Research
Denver, Colorado

Patrick W. O'Carroll, M.D., M.P.H.
Medical Epidemiologist
Center for Environmental Health and Injury Control
Centers for Disease Control
Public Health Service
U.S. Department of Health and Human Services
Atlanta, Georgia

Nancy J. Osgood, Ph.D.
Associate Professor of Gerontology and Sociology
Gerontology Program
Medical College of Virginia
Virginia Commonwealth University
Richmond, Virginia

Herbert Pardes, M.D.
Vice President for Health Sciences
Dean of the Faculty of Medicine
Professor and Chairman, Department of Psychiatry
College of Physicians and Surgeons of Columbia University
Director, New York State Psychiatric Institute
New York, New York

Michael K. Popkin, M.D.
Professor of Psychiatry and Medicine
University of Minnesota Medical School
Minneapolis, Minnesota

Charles L. Rich, M.D.
Professor of Psychiatry
Department of Psychiatry and Behavioral Science
Health Sciences Center
State University of New York at Stony Brook
Stony Brook, New York

Loren H. Roth, M.D., M.P.H.
Professor of Psychiatry
Vice-Chairman, Department of Psychiatry
Director, Law and Psychiatry Program
University of Pittsburgh School of Medicine
Western Psychiatric Institute and Clinic
Pittsburgh, Pennsylvania

Harvey L. Ruben, M.D., M.P.H.
Associate Clinical Professor
Department of Psychiatry
Yale University School of Medicine
New Haven, Connecticut

Alan F. Schatzberg, M.D.
Professor of Psychiatry
Harvard Medical School
Clinical Director, Massachusetts Mental Health Center
Consultant, McLean Hospital
Belmont, Massachusetts

Allan J. Schwartz, Ph.D.
Associate Professor of Psychiatry
School of Medicine and Dentistry
Chief, Mental Health Section
University Health Service
University of Rochester
Rochester, New York

Barbara Stanley, Ph.D.
Associate Professor, John Jay College of Criminal Justice, Department
    of Psychology, City University of New York
Department of Psychiatry
College of Physicians and Surgeons of Columbia University
New York State Psychiatric Institute
New York, New York

Michael Stanley, Ph.D.
Associate Professor
Departments of Psychiatry and Pharmacology
College of Physicians and Surgeons of Columbia University
Department of Neurochemistry
New York State Psychiatric Institute
New York, New York

Samuel Thielman, M.D., Ph.D.
Assistant Professor of Psychiatry
Department of Psychiatry and Health Behavior
Medical College of Georgia
Augusta, Georgia

Ming T. Tsuang, M.D., Ph.D., D.Sc.
Professor of Psychiatry and Director
Harvard Program in Psychiatric Epidemiology
Harvard Schools of Medicine and Public Health
Chief of Psychiatry, Brockton/West Roxbury Veterans Administration
    Medical Center
Brockton, Massachusetts

George E. Vaillant, M.D.
Raymond Sobel Professor of Psychiatry
Dartmouth Medical School
Hanover, New Hampshire

Marjorie E. Weishaar, Ph.D.
Clinical Assistant Professor
Department of Psychiatry and Human Behavior
Division of Biology and Medicine
Brown University
Providence, Rhode Island

Robert M. Wettstein, M.D.
Assistant Professor of Psychiatry
Co-Director, Law and Psychiatry Program
University of Pittsburgh School of Medicine
Western Psychiatric Institute and Clinic
Pittsburgh, Pennsylvania

Leighton C. Whitaker, Ph.D.
Director of Psychological Services
Swarthmore College
Swarthmore, Pennsylvania

Ronald M. Winchel, M.D.
Research Psychiatrist
Department of Psychiatry, College of Physicians and Surgeons of
    Columbia University
Department of Neurochemistry
New York State Psychiatric Institute
New York, New York

George Winokur, M.D.
The Paul W. Penningroth Professor and Head, Department of
    Psychiatry
College of Medicine
Psychiatric Hospital
The University of Iowa
Iowa City, Iowa

Acknowledgment

This volume, which deals with a comprehensive view of suicide across the life cycle, has received the support of and encouragement from many individuals, in addition to all the authors and coauthors of the various chapters. While several individuals aided in the preparation of this volume, an enormous debt is owed to Ms. Donna Donovan for her assistance and diligence in the preparation of the manuscript, the solving of many technical issues relating to the typing, and the preparation of figures and tables.

Foreword

A sharp upturn in rates of suicide among adolescents and young adults in the United States that began in the 1950s emerged as one of the highly visible and alarming public health trends of the 1980s. In fact, the clarity of those trends in adolescent suicide may have obscured for some the pervasiveness and persistence of suicide and suicidal behavior in all other age groups of the population.

During the past decade, many talented investigators responded energetically—and with some success—to demands for research focused specifically on the prevention of suicide among adolescents. However, following the lead of the National Institute of Mental Health (NIMH), most of the mental health research community chose to take a broader approach to this extraordinarily complex public health problem. The NIMH's strategy included stimulating a broad spectrum of basic and clinical research to determine the psychobiological risk factors for suicide and to test both psychosocial and psycho-pharmacologic treatment interventions. This position reflected lessons learned after decades of attempts to understand and prevent suicide through more limited approaches. Of equal importance is the NIMH's broad scientific program, which has made possible significant progress in the field's capacity to diagnose, treat, and, in many instances, prevent the psychiatric and substance abuse disorders so disproportionately represented in the life histories of those individuals who complete suicide.

The NIMH has long maintained a productive commitment to the study of suicide. In the late 1960s, growing public and professional concern about rising suicide rates had contributed to the creation of a Center for Studies of Suicide Prevention at the NIMH, to a growth spurt in the nascent field of "suicidology," and to a flurry of activity creating new suicide hotlines and suicide prevention centers. However, many of these interventions were not formally evaluated, so that the efficacy of these prevention strategies could not be determined. Thus suicide prevention, as it had been implemented in the 1960s and 1970s, came to be viewed with growing skepticism in some policy-making and scientific quarters during the 1980s.

In recent years, there has been a changing NIMH programmatic focus on suicide. The Center for Studies of Suicide Prevention evolved into the Center for Mental Health Emergencies and, later, into a Suicide Research Unit under the outstanding leadership of Dr. Susan Blumenthal. With her direction, the unit shifted the NIMH's research focus to emphasize the complex interaction of diagnostic, biological, and social variables contributing to suicidal behavior and fostered treatment studies incorporating psychosocial, pharmacologic, and environmental interventions. The unit underscored the importance of the early detection and treatment of psychiatric disorders, particularly the affective disorders, as a major suicide prevention strategy. Additionally, more than compensating for that refocusing has been a strengthening of the scientific foundation on which preventive strategies necessarily must be built.

In the early 1970s, a time when the efficacy of suicide prevention strategies was being increasingly scrutinized, mental health research was entering an era of unprecedented productivity. Advances in classification and diagnosis, in the tools and techniques of psychiatric epidemiology, and in the refinement of clinical practices were paralleled and invigorated by a virtual revolution in research on the fundamental biological and behavioral processes that underlie mental illness and healthy psychological development.

This broad strengthening of the mental health research base benefited the study of suicide and suicide prevention immensely. One significant development was the elucidation of the role of mental illness—particularly the affective disorders, alcoholism, and, among the younger generations, conduct disorders, depression, and drug abuse—as valid indicators of risk for suicide. Wide variations over the years in estimates of the proportion of suicides attributable to mental illness and substance abuse disorders have tended to undercut efforts to target clinical interventions to people with these disorders. But increasing diagnostic precision has helped to produce persuasive evidence that depressive disorders are implicated in as many as 60% of all suicides; that 15% of depressed patients will end their lives in suicide; and that among patients suffering from bipolar disorder, the suicide rate may be as high as 40%.

These data linking mood disorders and suicidal behavior strongly suggest that public and professional educational programs focused on encouraging recognition and appropriate treatment of the psychiatric disorders associated with suicide (e.g., the NIMH Depression Awareness, Recognition, and Treatment [D/ART] program and the American Psychiatric Association's Medical Interactive Workshops on Depression) may offer productive approaches to suicide prevention.

The research reported in this volume attests to the fact that our understanding of suicide risk factors is deepening. As reflected in the broad scope of treatment interventions described, it is clear that a more comprehensive understanding of such risk factors can greatly enhance capacities for clinical management and prevention of suicidal behaviors throughout the life span.

In developing this volume, Drs. Blumenthal and Kupfer, who themselves have made outstanding contributions to our knowledge about this public health problem, have obtained the participation of the key researchers and thinkers in the field of contemporary suicide research—indeed, in contemporary psychiatric research. Their life-cycle approach to understanding and treating suicidal behavior provides a unique and important perspective. My confidence in the continuing progress of the suicide research field is based in large measure on their work, as reported in this exemplary, comprehensive, and landmark volume.

Lewis L. Judd, M.D.
Director
National Institute of Mental Health

Preface

Suicide—it is the tragic and untimely loss of human life, all the more devastating and perplexing because it represents a volitional act. Why some people turn against themselves—what psychological, biological, and social factors contribute to the wish to stop living—remains a mystery, although one that is being increasingly deciphered through systematic research investigations.

Suicide is a complex human behavior. There is no *one* reason why an individual chooses to end his or her life. Most people who commit suicide have seen a health care professional in the week to month prior to the act. Therefore, the clinician has an important opportunity and responsibility to assess suicidal people, to provide appropriate treatment, and to intervene to prevent these needless tragedies. Unfortunately, many medical practitioners do not have the necessary knowledge about who is at risk or know what to do when confronted with suicidal patients in their practice. Additionally, once a suicide has occurred, many clinicians are not informed about their professional and legal responsibilities.

This volume is aimed at filling these major gaps in our understanding about suicide by integrating and translating current research knowledge about suicidal behavior as it occurs over the life cycle into a comprehensive and contemporary guide to assessment, intervention, and treatment strategies that the clinician can apply with suicidal patients and their families.

Since the major purpose of this volume is to assist the health care professional to improve the day-to-day assessment and management of suicidal patients based on knowledge from scientific advances, the chapters are authored both by prominent psychiatric researchers and by clinicians who share these perspectives. The contributors to this volume have sought to combine the most current scientific information about psychological, biological, social, and genetic-familial risk factors for suicide with state-of-the-art assessment and treatment approaches that can be used with patients over the life cycle.

We have divided these contributions into four sections: 1) risk factors for suicide; 2) techniques for assessment and management of suicidal patients over the life cycle; 3) special issues; and 4) a synopsis of many of the topics raised in this volume. The aim of each of these sections is to provide a comprehensive view of the current state of knowledge about suicidal behavior and to describe prevention and intervention strategies for suicidal patients targeted to specific stages of the life cycle.

First, in Chapter 1, Drs. George Vaillant and Susan Blumenthal provide an important developmental perspective for understanding suicide over the life cycle. In examining suicide risk and life-span development, they conclude that while the interaction between predisposing risk factors, immediate risk factors, protective factors, and precipitants is complex, the delineation of the relative contributions of specific risk factors at different stages of the life cycle offers a most promising approach for future research. This chapter serves as an introduction to the volume and as a conceptual framework for the chapters that follow.

The eight chapters in Section 1 review the risk factors for suicide. The chapter on the epidemiology of suicide, by Drs. Martin Buda and Ming Tsuang, reviews current epidemiologic information on suicide and examines how this information relates to the prevention of premature deaths and the treatment of specific psychiatric illnesses often associated with suicide attempts. The chapter covers sociodemographic factors influencing the rates of suicide in the general population and risk factors for patients with major psychiatric disorders. The next chapter, by Dr. Kenneth Adam, is concerned with the environmental, psychosocial, and psychoanalytic aspects of suicidal behavior. In a most comprehensive manner, Dr. Adam demonstrates how the social environment impacts on suicidal behavior and how suicide represents an act with important social consequences. He also reviews the role of psychosocial factors in the causal chain of events leading to suicide and shows how both social and environmental factors may act as predisposing factors, as precipitating factors, and as contributing factors in suicidal behavior both from a macrosocial view as well as an ecological perspective.

The biological component to suicidal behavior is thoroughly discussed in the chapter by Drs. Ronald Winchel, Barbara Stanley, and Michael Stanley. These authors extensively review possible biological correlates of suicidal behavior—including altered serotonergic metabolism in individuals who have completed suicide and those with a history of aggressive behavior—and suggest how these important discoveries may lead to improvements in the identification of those at risk. They conclude their chapter by describing the implications of these findings for current clinical practice and treatment approaches.

The chapter on genetic factors and suicide, by Dr. Seymour Kety, reviews the current state of knowledge about genetic factors and how they might contribute to our understanding of suicide in relationship to specific psychiatric illnesses as well as whether genetic and familial factors influence suicidal behavior independent of psychiatric disorders. The author points out how well the problem of suicide illustrates the need to ascertain the very crucial and important interactions between genetic factors and environmental influences. Drs. Donald Black and George Winokur, in their chapter, direct the reader's attention to the important topic of the relationship between suicide and specific psychiatric diagnoses. After systematically reviewing what is currently known about selected psychiatric disorders (e.g., affective disorders, alcoholism, schizophrenia) and their association with suicidal behavior over the life cycle, they reaffirm the important point that psychiatric diagnosis is perhaps the most significant alerting signal for the clinician. Furthermore, because most patients who commit suicide suffer from major psychiatric illness, assessing suicidal risk in these patients is always a mandatory clinical step.

The next risk factor to be explored is the impact of personality on suicide, discussed in the chapter by Drs. Scott Goldsmith, Minna Fyer, and Allen Frances. The authors review nosologic and methodological issues relating to personality traits and disorders and suggest how these factors may directly interact with suicidal behavior. They also describe the implications of these findings for the evaluation and treatment of suicidal patients and conclude that personality traits, particularly aggression and impulsivity, and borderline and antisocial personality disorders, are essential to identify in suicidal patients because they often require specialized treatment approaches.

The chapter by Drs. Daniel Flavin, John Franklin, and Richard Frances focuses on substance abuse and suicidal behavior. In this chapter, the authors explore how the use of alcohol and other psychoactive substances increases individuals' risk for suicide and other forms of self-destructive behavior. These issues are discussed in terms of a diagnosis of alcoholism or substance abuse as well as in terms of how substance use generally affects suicidal behavior and suicide rates. A case study illustrates the need to consider in such patients prior attempts, frequency of intoxication, presence and severity of comorbid psychiatric disorders, other drug use, level of patient insight, and loss and quality of social support systems.

The final chapter in this section, by Drs. Thomas Mackenzie and Michael Popkin, deals with the relationship of medical illness and suicide. While it has been well accepted that medical illness is an important risk for suicide, the authors provide significant new and useful information defining how the presence of particular physical disorders (e.g., cancer, Huntington's chorea, AIDS, or head trauma) can result in an increased risk of suicide.

Section 2 focuses on strategies for assessment and management of suicidal patients at different stages of the life span. Specific evaluation and treatment interventions are discussed for children and adolescents, college students, adults, and elderly people. The first chapter in this section, by Dr. Robert Hendren, provides the clinician with useful techniques for interviewing suicidal patients of different ages. Such interviewing principles for individuals who have demonstrated suicidal behavior are discussed using a developmental approach, with suggestions about how specific risk factors for each age group can be evaluated. The author provides examples of age-specific interviewing techniques for use with children and adolescents, as well as with adults and the elderly. He emphasizes the need to adapt one's interviewing style to the patient's position in the life cycle to ensure accurate assessment of suicide potential.

The second chapter in this section, by Drs. David Brent and David Kolko, deals specifically with the assessment and treatment of children and adolescents at risk for suicide. After reviewing the epidemiology and associated risk factors for youth suicide and suicidal behavior, including a delineation of the contribution of specific stresses, psychiatric disorders, medical disease, and personality factors, the authors describe how this knowledge can be incorporated into clinical interventions for young people. They also review the indications for psychiatric treatment and its potential effectiveness in diminishing risk for subsequent suicidal behavior in young people. Developmental issues in late adolescence and young adulthood are the emphasis of the chapter on suicide among college students by Drs. Allan Schwartz and Leighton Whitaker. They review the epidemiology of suicide on campuses and focus on assessment, treatment, and community interventions for college students. Contrary to popular lore, suicide rates among university students are lower than the general population rates for this age group. The authors emphasize that opportunities for suicide prevention on campus exist in two complementary areas: modification of structural aspects of the university environment that stimulate suicidality and identification of students at risk for suicidal behavior.

The assessment and treatment of suicidal behavior in older individuals are reviewed in the chapter by Drs. Nancy Osgood and Samuel Thielman. Suicide rates for older Americans rose in the 1980s. The authors discuss pertinent life-cycle issues for the aged that impact on patient evaluation. They also provide specific indications for interventions that are best suited to this population in a variety of ambulatory and institutional settings. This chapter is essential reading for clinicians dealing with older individuals. In the chapter by Dr. Brian Doyle, which focuses on crisis management of the suicidal patient, in a variety of clinical settings, key elements of crisis management with suicidal persons are presented. Specific interventions are described, including the establishment and maintenance of the doctor-patient relationship, evaluation of lethality, and the implementation of a treatment plan. Dr. Doyle raises important points about caring for acutely suicidal patients that represent a challenge for the clinician in all treatment settings.

The next four chapters focus on specific treatment interventions: somatic treatment, psychodynamic psychotherapy, cognitive approaches, and community interventions. The chapter by Drs. Mark Goldblatt and Alan Schatzberg deals with assessment and somatic treatments for adult suicidal patients. These authors stress an organized approach to treating the underlying psychiatric disorder with both psychotherapeutic interventions and adequate doses of appropriate psychotropic medications. The use of serotonin reuptake blockers for suicidal alcoholic and depressed patients is emphasized, as well as the considered use of neuroleptics for individuals with schizophrenia, borderline personality disorders, and psychotic depression. Psychodynamic explanations of suicide and treatment approaches with suicidal patients are discussed in the chapter by Dr. Alvin Kahn. An overview of principles of psychodynamic psychotherapy as they relate to understanding suicidal behavior over the life cycle is provided, including a section on countertransference. The next chapter in this section, by Drs. Marjorie Weishaar and Aaron Beck, is concerned specifically with cognitive approaches to understanding and treating suicidal behavior. The authors present a clear introduction to behavioral treatments and cognitive therapy techniques that can be used as effective interventions for suicidal behavior. This chapter provides an interesting link between hopelessness (a major component in the profile of suicidal persons) and a treatment intervention designed to deal specifically with the cognitive distortions associated with suicidal behavior. The last chapter in this section, by Dr. Patrick O'Carroll, is concerned with community strategies for suicide prevention and intervention and presents the Centers for Disease Control (CDC) plan for the prevention and containment of suicide clusters. Specific recommendations for communities are provided to deal with these crisis situations effectively. The clinician's role in developing and implementing such a program is highlighted.

Section 3 deals with special issues that have not been specifically covered in the first two sections. The first of these topics, suicide clusters and media exposure, is fully developed by Dr. Madelyn Gould. In her chapter, Dr. Gould discusses suicide clusters, the mechanisms of contagion, the pros and cons of media exposure, and how clinicians can deal with these concerns in their community. A set of guidelines for interaction with the media on this issue is provided. The subsequent chapter, authored by Dr. Rene Diekstra, is concerned with international perspectives on the epidemiology and prevention of suicide. In this chapter, our attention is focused on cross-cultural differences in suicide in various countries across the world. Additionally, an international perspective on recommendations for suicide prevention in the areas of surveillance, clinical research, and community programs is provided.

The importance of understanding suicide in minority groups is emphasized in the chapter by Drs. Felton Earls, Javier Escobar, and Spero Manson. These authors specifically examine the epidemiologic and cultural perspectives of suicide in three minority groups across different strata of American society. Recommendations are provided for interventions that are culturally sensitive. Specifically, they emphasize the need to target educational and prevention strategies to high-risk populations, particularly toward young males in all three groups.

The next series of chapters in Section 3 deal with issues directly affecting the clinician. The chapter by Drs. Valerie Holmes and Charles Rich is directly concerned with suicide among physicians. The authors examine what is currently known about suicide among both non-mental health medical practitioners and psychiatrists, providing information on the rates of suicide in specific medical specialties. The authors describe the similarities and differences between suicide in physicians and the general population and conclude with specific recommendations for particular high-risk physician groups. They also emphasize the need to monitor changing patterns of medical specialty susceptibility. The chapter by Dr. Harvey Ruben discusses how to survive a suicide in your own clinical practice. He provides a sensitive, practical guide to dealing with the multiple critical issues that arise when a patient commits suicide. This chapter represents a vital contribution to the clinician's knowledge base about this very disturbing issue. Additional pragmatic clinical information is offered in the next chapter by Drs. Jess Amchin, Robert Wettstein, and Loren Roth, which reviews the legal and ethical issues pertaining to suicide. The authors present a comprehensive survey of these important considerations and provide the clinician with suggestions about how to deal appropriately with these concerns in clinical practice. The final chapter in Section 3 focuses on public policy and research issues in youth suicide. Drs. Herbert Pardes and Susan Blumenthal use youth suicide as an example of how public policy can be effected for critical social and medical problems. The chapter provides an example of the kind of fruitful integration that can occur between a public policy perspective and a clinical research agenda.

In the last section, Dr. Susan Blumenthal provides a review and condensation of the entire volume. In this synopsis, the author provides models for understanding suicidal behavior and summarizes what is known about risk factors for suicide in both adolescent and adult populations. The aim of this overview is to summarize for the reader the different domains of risk factors and to translate this knowledge into practical considerations for the clinician about the assessment and treatment of suicidal patients. It also provides the reader with a distillation of the contents of this volume when time does not permit a more detailed reading. The reader is encouraged to turn to other chapters in this book for comprehensive coverage of the topics covered in this synopsis chapter.

In the final chapter, we close with the hope that this volume will contribute to the illumination of new research frontiers and provide you, the reader, with the necessary knowledge and skills to prevent this tragic loss of life in your practice.

Susan J. Blumenthal, M.D., M.P.A.
David J. Kupfer, M.D.

Chapter 1

Introduction:
Suicide Over the Life Cycle—
Risk Factors and Life-Span
Development

George E. Vaillant, M.D.
Susan J. Blumenthal, M.D., M.P.A.

THIS BOOK EXAMINES what is known about risk factors, assessment, and treatment of suicidal behavior at different stages of the life cycle. Chapters in this volume will approach suicide from many other vantage points than development, but in constructing a conceptual framework for the multiaxial causation of suicide, developmental stage certainly needs to be one of the organizing axes.

One of the most basic facts about suicide in the United States is that its risk increases as a function of age (see Figure 1). Completed suicide is extremely rare in children under the age of 12; becomes more common after puberty, with its incidence increasing in each of the adolescent years; and reaches a peak among youth at age 23. However, the highest rates of suicide are among elderly men (Shaffer et al. 1988). Although secular changes over the past 30 years have resulted in a tripling of the rate of suicide among young adults, 80-year-olds are still twice as likely to commit suicide as 20-year-olds. Why?

In examining the ways in which adult development may affect suicide risk, univariate answers will not be possible because, throughout the adult life span, there are many fluctuating and competing risk and protective factors that affect suicide. Usually, suicide results from the unlikely convergence of multiple predisposing and immediate risk factors, and these risk factors must come together in

1

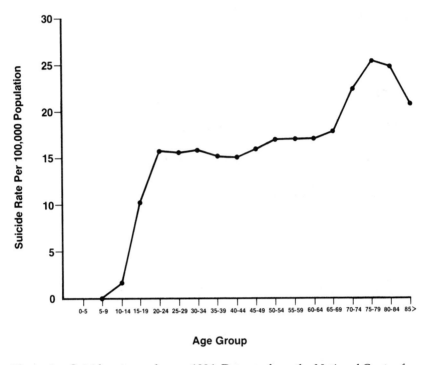

Figure 1. Suicide rates and age—1986. Data are from the National Center for Health Statistics, Vital Statistics of the United States.

the absence of multiple protective factors (Blumenthal 1988). People may move in and out of suicidal crises at different points over their lifetime as a result of disruptions in the homeostasis between these risk and protective factors. However, little knowledge exists to clarify whether suicide is the same phenomenon in childhood as it is in old age or whether it has a different meaning and set of risk factors across the life span. In part, our lack of understanding can be attributed to the dearth of prospective, longitudinal research on this public health problem. The chapters in this volume, using a cross-sectional approach, strongly suggest that suicidal behavior throughout the life cycle is on a continuum: similar risk factors appear to operate across the various stages of the life span but their contributory weights differ. Correspondingly, particular protective factors appear to impact differently at various stages of development.

Additionally, temporal trends—including age, period, and cohort effects and their interactions—are known to impact on the epidemiology of medical and psychiatric disorders. Klerman and Weissman (1989) described how these effects appear to influence suicide rates, particularly in shifting higher rates in recent years to young people.

Age effects are observed when the occurrence or frequency of an illness varies with age. Period effects occur when the rates of a syndrome or disease vary with the time period, usually months or years (e.g., the effects of unemployment on the suicide rates). Cohort effects refer to changes in the rate of illness among persons who share some temporal experience (usually the year or decade of their birth), and these effects are often sustained throughout the cohort's lifetime. Additionally, age-period interactions can occur when the period effect changes with age-related vulnerability, observed in the increase of substance abuse among young people in recent years (Klerman and Weissman 1989; O'Malley et al. 1984). These temporal effects may help explain the changes in suicide statistics over the past several decades, particularly the increased suicide rates for youth. Higher rates of depression, bipolar disorder, suicide, and substance abuse for the baby boom generation have also paralleled important temporal, social, and economic events, including changes in family structure, shifts in gender roles, age of entrance into the work force, age of marriage, increased access to lethal weapons, and the effects of increased media exposure on violence (Klerman and Weissman 1989).

Additionally, the size of a birth cohort may "shape its destiny" (Klerman and Weissman 1989). Such a model posits that a large birth cohort may result in increased competition for scarce resources, resulting in higher unemployment, lower earnings, and decreased access to educational opportunities. These factors may help explain the higher rates of depression and suicide in the baby boom cohort (Holinger et al. 1987; Klerman and Weissman 1989). Cohorts born since World War II have been healthier and were raised during a time of economic prosperity. Nonetheless, there has still been a rise in the rates of suicide, depression, conduct disorder, substance abuse, and homicide in these groups. Yet the explanations encompassed by the effects described above are not sufficient to explain why particular individuals end their life by suicide. In all likelihood, these environmental influences interact with individual genetic and biologic vulnerability (Klerman and Weissman 1989).

In developing a complete model for suicide across the life cycle, other chapters in this volume will discuss many contributory risk factors, relatively unaffected by developmental changes, that this introductory chapter will not address. On the one hand, genes, race, and gender do not change throughout the life span. On the other hand, many effects of historical and secular changes (e.g., ever-increasing handgun availability in the United States and the protective effects of reducing carbon monoxide content of domestic coal gas in England) are not predictably affected by a developmental model.

In addition, there are two important protective factors for suicide that are outside the scope of this introduction. First, the availability of active clinical and social intervention is relatively independent of development from age 15 to 85, although for certain age groups (children, adolescents, and the elderly) there are often barriers to obtaining treatment (e.g., lack of financial resources, access to transportation,and knowledge of appropriate resources). Second, there is hope (Beck et al. 1985). *Hope*, like *love*, is a most important word ignored by psychoanalysts, social scientists, and biologic psychiatrists alike. We know that "hopelessness" can identify up to 91% of future completed suicides (Beck et al. 1985; Weishaar and Beck, this volume), but we know little of hope's determinants, operational definition, and biologic correlates, or even why hope should be so important to suicide prevention. In the future, study of the development and biology of hope and the modification of hopelessness throughout the life span merits our attention.

In organizing risk factors for suicide, it is helpful to assign them to five overlapping domains, as shown in Figure 2 (Blumenthal 1988). This chapter will examine how four of these domains—psychosocial milieu, biologic vulnerability, psychiatric disorder, and personality—

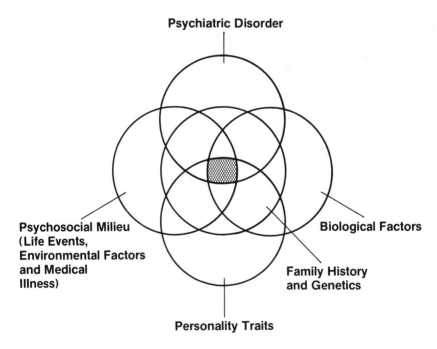

Figure 2. Overlap model for suicide risk (five domains). This figure is adapted with permission from Blumenthal and Kupfer 1986.

are affected by adult development. How the fifth domain, genetic vulnerability, changes over the adult life span and interacts with environmental influences still remains uncharted territory. However, studies have demonstrated that for both adult and adolescent suicide attempters and completers, there are important genetic and familial influences (Kety, this volume; Pfeffer 1989).

PSYCHOSOCIAL MILIEU

Stressful life events, depression, physical illness, and loss, even when they occur together, rarely result in a completed suicide if the social support system is vigorously maintained (Havens 1965). Thus social support, or as Alvin Kahn (this volume) poetically reminds us, the fact that "other lives have twined themselves with mine," is perhaps the single most important protective factor (aside from the appropriate treatment of associated psychiatric disorders) in suicide prevention. Throughout Erikson's (1963) model of life-span development, "the human personality, in principle, develops according to steps predetermined in the growing person's readiness to be driven toward, to be aware of, and to interact with a widening social radius" (p. 270). As adults mature, their social network usually becomes more resilient. In counterpoint, it is at the time when everyone in the environment of a potentially suicidal person seems to be moving away that the risk of completed suicide may peak. It is during the individuation and leaving home period, ages 15 to 25, and again in old age that individuals are at particular risk of losing important loves and caretakers faster than they can be replaced.

It is also in adolescence and again in old age when cultural permission for suicide is highest. The fluid identity of adolescence promotes susceptibility to "contagious" and "romantic" suicide (Gould, this volume). Erikson (1963) discussed how role confusion during this stage of development may result in an apparent loss of identity, resulting in over-identification with heroes, cliques, or crowds. This mechanism of a young person projecting his or her own "diffused ego image on another and by seeing it thus reflected and gradually clarified" may underlie imitative or cluster suicides: the phenomenon whereby one youngster's suicide in a school or community triggers subsequent suicides in other vulnerable youth.

As individuals grow old, membership, both literally and metaphorically, in Hemlock societies becomes increasingly culturally syntonic. Indeed, among the very elderly, as the mythic death of Socrates and the actual death of Sigmund Freud illustrate, self-willed suicide can be an act of reflective choice rather than of unreasoned impulse.

Additionally, another important risk factor, medical illness, appears to have a differential impact on suicidality across the life cycle. Medical illness is associated with as many as 50% of adult completed suicides (Mackenzie and Popkin, this volume) and contributes more prominently in late life. Few studies of completed suicide in children and adolescents have been undertaken, but evidence suggests that medical illness does not play as significant a role. Juvenile diabetes and epilepsy combined with the use of phenobarbital for its treatment have been associated with some suicides in adolescents (Brent and Kolko, this volume). Shafii et al. (1988) found that 48% of the adolescent suicide victims in their study had a history of some form of physical disorder such as asthma, allergies, seizures, or congenital birth defects. However, this finding was also true of the control group and therefore was not statistically significant. In contrast, suicides in the elderly are often associated with the presence of medical illness, particularly cancer, musculoskeletal disorders, and gastrointestinal illnesses. One medical illness that appears to bridge risk between adolescence and adulthood is acquired immuno deficiency syndrome (AIDS), a disease that affects young adults more frequently than older people. A recent report found a 36 times greater incidence of suicide among AIDS victims than in the general population (Marzuk et al. 1988). People with AIDS have a high incidence of depression and cognitive impairments associated with AIDS-related dementia. Importantly, AIDS patients may suffer the humiliation of having an illness that is not well accepted by our society, and the protective buffer of cohesive social supports may be absent for many AIDS victims.

How can the differences in the importance of specific risk factors for suicide across the life cycle be explained? One hypothesis suggests that the impact of a particular risk factor such as presence of a medical illness depends on the co-occurrence of other risk factors for suicide and the extent to which protective factors buffer the risk (Blumenthal 1988). For example, the risk factor, medical illness, may have less impact in childhood and adolescence because medically ill youngsters generally have cohesive social supports, including concerned parents and health care professionals. Hope for future improvement is also greater. Additionally, the incidence of associated psychiatric disorders such as depression is lower in this age group than in adulthood. In the elderly, however, medical illness may contribute significantly to risk because of the convergence of multiple risk factors, including decreased social supports, more interpersonal losses, cognitive impairments associated with aging, the use of certain medications affecting mood and judgment, hopelessness about the future, and the loss of dignity that may accompany growing older or having a terminal illness.

Biologic Vulnerability

Biology governs development. As discussed earlier, completed suicide is a rare phenomenon in childhood and early adolescence, but increases dramatically in late adolescence and young adulthood, with the preponderance of suicidal deaths occurring among the elderly. These differences in rates of suicide across the life span may, in part, be attributable to biologic factors. Biology drives the child willy-nilly to the cognitive and executive skills whereby adolescent suicide can be effective. The increasing cognitive capacity of adolescents to appreciate the future and to develop and carry out a plan may also play an important role in the sharp increase of successful suicides as adolescents mature. Interestingly, young adolescents with an IQ greater than 130 have a higher rate of suicide (Shaffer 1974). Therefore, intellectual precocity may override the potentially protective effects of cognitive immaturity. Additionally, developmentally, adolescence is a time of tremendous biologic and psychological change for young people. It is also a time when the risk factors of access to drugs, handguns, and alcohol are introduced, when certain psychiatric disorders such as depression may have their onset, and when the chances of humiliation and sexual abuse peak. Risk is magnified further because protective cognitive strategies about how to control such dangers are still at a minimum and impulsive, risk-taking behaviors are more common. Then, 40 years later, biology relentlessly inflicts the loss of sight, mobility, and autonomy, which enhances hopelessness and thereby suicide. In old age, where the suicide rate is almost two times greater than the general population, cognitive capacities may decline because of impairments associated with medical illness, Alzheimer's disease, and depression. At the end of the life span, biologic aging of the brain also increases the likelihood of dementia and organic psychosis, important suicide risk factors that impair judgment, and impulsivity, and may produce concurrent depression.

Psychiatric Disorder

Very few people take their lives without concomitant psychiatric disorder, and the prevalence of these illnesses change dramatically across the life span (Black and Winokur, this volume). Studies of both adult and adolescent completed suicides reveal that more than 90% of suicide victims suffered from one or more psychiatric illness (Barraclough et al. 1974; Dorpat and Ripley 1960; Hagnell and Rorsman 1980; Robins 1981; Shafii et al. 1988; Shaffer et al. 1988). There are four broad psychiatric disorders that put individuals at particular risk for suicide: affective disorders, conduct disorders, schizophrenia, and organic mental disorders (Black and Winokur, this volume). Recent studies suggest that panic disorder patients also have an increased risk of suicidal behavior (Weissman et al. 1989). The comorbidity of these syndromes with particular personality traits (including impulsivity and aggressivity) and with substance abuse appears to increase risk across the life cycle (Blumenthal, this volume). Adolescents who kill themselves tend to manifest depression and conduct disorders where the affective component is often only recognized in retrospect (Brent and Kolko, this volume). In a general population study of suicide, Rich et al. (1986) found that the psychiatric diagnosis associated with suicide changed with age. Under the age of 30, suicides were more frequently associated with antisocial personality disorder and substance abuse. In persons over the age of 30, suicides were more frequently associated with affective disorders. Between ages 20 and 30, schizophrenic patients and patients with bipolar affective disorder are perhaps the highest risk group for suicide; between ages 30 and 50, suicide peaks among the affective disorders. It is in old age, with its heightened risk of both organic brain damage and psychotic affective disorder, that the risk of suicide is at its peak (see Osgood and Thielman, this volume).

However, as Weinberger (1987) and Adams and Lyons (1982) have underscored, the four disorders can be in part a reflection of developmental stage. If one examines the dominant psychopathology that accompanies the *onset* of Huntington's chorea, Wilson's disease, and metachromatic leukodystrophy, there is a tendency for the result to be conduct disorder if genetic penetrance first occurs between ages 10 and 20, schizophreniform disorders if onset is between ages 20 and 30, major depressive disorder if onset is between ages 30 and 50, and dementia if after age 50. In other words, psychiatric disorder per se may be more important than subtype in the genesis of suicide.

Although it is easy to understand why the pathophysiology of dementia is associated with advanced age, our understanding of the transformation of conduct disorder to schizophreniform-like illnesses to affective disorder is speculative. However, as Weinberger (1987) suggested in his review, there is evidence for actual brain development until age 30, not only in terms of increasing complexity of synaptic and dendritic development but also in terms of increasing myelinization (Yakovlev and LeCours 1967). There are also, as yet, poorly understood changes in the activity of the major neurotransmitters over the adult life span. For example, brain serotonin metabolism, thought to be implicated in suicide risk and related to increased impulsivity and aggressivity (Mann et al. 1986; Winchel et al., this volume) is believed to change in predictable fashion during adult life (Wong et al. 1984). The parkinsonian symptoms produced by haloperidol are different at age 18 than at age 65. Additionally, differences across the life span in biologic rhythms, including sleep and menstrual cycle function, may impact on psychological state and on the expression of psychiatric disorder. Thus the brain changes in adult life and so may its neurobiologic contributions to suicide risk.

PERSONALITY

The degree to which personality changes over the life span is debatable. On the one hand, there is the theoretical evidence offered by popular writers on adult development (e.g., Erikson 1963; Sheehy 1976), and there are the obvious differences in personality that make it so hard for parents and grandparents to identify with adolescents and vice versa.

In *Childhood and Society*, Erikson (1963) described the tasks that must be negotiated during the eight stages of human development and delineated the essential strengths that successful resolution of these crises imparts at each life stage:

basic trust versus basic mistrust: drive and hope
autonomy versus shame and doubt: self-control and willpower
initiative versus guilt: direction and purpose
industry versus inferiority: method and competence
identity versus role confusion: devotion and fidelity
intimacy versus isolation: affiliation and love
generativity versus stagnation: production and care
ego integrity versus despair: renunciation and wisdom

Hypothetically, according to this developmental theory, failure to negotiate the challenge of each stage successfully may render the individual more vulnerable to suicidal behavior. Conversely, successful resolution of these passages may result in the establishment of enduring personality strengths and individual resiliency.

On the other hand, as investigators like McCrae and Costa (1984) have shown, efforts to prove such popular theories of adult development or even to document the lawful stages of Eriksonian development have not been easy. Since the truth probably lies somewhere between these competing viewpoints, it makes sense to consider the interactions between adult development and personality that might affect suicide risk over the life span.

To the extent that maturation decreases impulsivity and allows increasing tolerance and mastery of anger without an individual turning it violently against the self, suicide risk will diminish. Studies of the elderly without organic brain damage suggest that, with advanced age, hostility *and* impulsivity *and* depression may all appear muted (Neugarten 1977). With development from adolescence to mid-life comes increasing patience and the capacity to tolerate both hostile and sad feelings. Even the self-defeating, passive aggression of an adolescent can evolve into selfless but self-enhancing altruism in mid-life.

This protective effect of maturity is enhanced by the fact that one's sense of personal control is probably greatest between the ages of 30 and 50 (Neugarten 1977). However, with more advanced age, the sense of personal controllability decreases with the onset of medical illnesses, the awareness of mortality, and the loss of significant others, perhaps canceling the diminution in risk resulting from the declining morbidity of personality disorders.

It also behooves us to pay attention to how personality development across the life span can strengthen social networks. It is the very personality variables that attenuate and mitigate depression, impulsivity, and hostility that also enhance potentially supportive new relationships. As has been suggested elsewhere (Vaillant 1977), ego strength can be defined by one's dominant choice of defense mechanisms. In adolescence, the defenses of projection, hypochondriasis, schizoid fantasy, acting out, and turning against the self (i.e., passive aggression and masochism) are common. Although each of these defenses serves to bind conflict, these defenses repel other people. Over time, however, these mechanisms may be replaced by suppression (stoicism), altruism (empathy), sublimation, humor, and anticipation (planful rehearsal of affect). Such mechanisms become increasingly more common as adolescents mature.

For example, at 30 Beethoven was an angry, impulsive, and depressed man who, in the face of chronic illness (deafness) and the resulting loss of control, wrote that he was very close to suicide. Had young Beethoven, as an isolated, dysthmic musician killed himself, his psychological autopsy would have made perfect sense. In late mid-life, Beethoven's chronic illness (i.e., his deafness) was still more severe. But over time both this irascible musician's social network and his ego's coping skills had become ever stronger. When totally deaf, he put to music Schiller's *Ode to Joy* (e.g., "Be embraced all ye millions, with a kiss for all the world"), and there was little evidence that Beethoven was still suicidal.

Yet as stated in the introduction, biology, psychiatric disorder, social supports, and personality are interlocking domains. Organic brain damage, from the ravages of advanced age, drives the maturation of ego defenses in the reverse direction, increases personality disorder, shatters social supports, and increases suicidal risk.

The three facets of personality that are most closely associated with increased risk of suicide are hostility, impulsivity, and depression, with its associated retroflexed rage (Goldsmith et al., this volume). Turning against the self is an ego defense mechanism often associated with the personality of suicidal individuals and has been described as an underlying mechanism of self-destruction (Freud 1917). Additionally, shame and guilt, essential components of humiliation, are important emotions in precipitating suicidal behavior.

The simplest exogenous way to increase all of these personality risk factors—depression, hostility, impulsivity, and shame—is by alcohol and hypnotic substance abuse. The prevalence of alcoholism and hypnotic drug dependence increases steadily from age 15 until about 45 and then declines. The risk of suicide from alcoholism also goes up with advancing age. However, this correlation probably has more to do with the natural history of the disorder of alcoholism than it does with development per se. As alcoholism progresses, it destroys three factors known to protect against suicide. By means of guilty and angry outbursts, chronic alcoholism destroys social supports. Progressive alcoholism destroys brain cells and intellectual function. It also ravages health, bringing with it a high incidence of medical complications that increase risk for suicide (Flavin et al., this volume). Finally, chronic alcoholism undermines personal control. Indeed, as alcoholism progresses, social networks are so diminished and self-efficacy and self-esteem so impaired that clinicians often mistakenly blame the *resulting* secondary affective disorder for *causing* the alcohol abuse and eventual suicide.

Young suicidal adults, especially young adults from chaotic homes, have hostility, impulsivity, and depression as their most salient personality traits (Shafii et al. 1988). But why? Is the reason why a disruptive childhood is associated with an increased risk of future suicide due to the lack of stable internalized object relations? Is early object loss a predisposing risk factor to suicide, as Adam suggests in his chapter? Or is the chapter by Seymour Kety correct? Is suicide the result of the penetrance of a genetic curse? Is the individual's disturbed childhood and early object loss simply one more reflection that his or her biologic relatives suffered themselves from suicide, alcoholism, affective disorder, and antisocial personality? We must await adequate cross-fostering studies to separate the effect of genes from environment in suicide risk before we know the answer to this developmental riddle.

We wondered at the beginning of this chapter why the rates of suicide increase with age. One explanation for higher rates of completed suicide across the life span may be related to the increased contribution of the major risk factors. The incidence of affective disorders, alcoholism, substance abuse, loss of social supports, humiliating life experiences, and hopelessness appear to increase with age.

Additionally, genetic and biologic factors may play a greater role later in life as environmental influences trigger genetic expression of vulnerability for suicidal behavior. The incidence of major risk factors for suicide, including depression and substance abuse, has been increasing since World War II. In fact, changing environmental factors (e.g., geographic mobility with its loss of attachments, social anomie, increasing urbanization, and changes in family structure) interacting with genetic liability probably have played a role in shifting in recent years the increased rates of both depression and suicide to younger age groups (Klerman and Weissman 1989). The chapters that follow address what is known about risk factors, assessment, and treatment strategies for suicidal patients throughout the life span. It is the task of future research to delineate the relative contributions of risk factors for suicide at different stages of the life cycle and to specify further gene-environment interactions in determining suicide risk. The chapters in this volume review our best knowledge about suicide across the life span.

In summary, the interaction between predisposing risk factors, immediate risk factors, protective factors, and precipitants is complex. The study of adult development from ages 15 to 85 is only one of the possible ways of understanding the complex and intricate interrelationships that can lead to that irrevocable, but fortunately rare, interaction in which a completed suicide occurs.

References

Adams RD, Lyons G: Neurology of Hereditary Metabolic Diseases of Children. New York, McGraw-Hill, 1982, pp 5–6, 376–381

Barraclough B, Bunch J, Nelson B, et al: A hundred cases of suicide: clinical aspects. Br J Psychiatry 125:355–373, 1974

Beck AT, Steer RA, Kovacs M, et al: Hopelessness and eventual suicide: a 10-year prospective study of patients hospitalized with suicidal ideation. Am J Psychiatry 142:559–563, 1985

Blumenthal SJ: Suicide: a guide to risk factors, assessment, and treatment of suicidal patients. Med Clin North Am 72:937–971, 1988

Blumenthal SJ, Kupfer DJ: Generalizable treatment strategies for suicidal behavior. Ann NY Acad Sci 487:327–340, 1986

Dorpat T, Ripley H: A study of suicide in the Seattle area. Compr Psychiatry 1:349–359, 1960

Erikson E: Childhood and Society, 2nd Edition. New York, WW Norton, 1963

Freud S: Mourning and melancholia, in The Standard Edition of the Complete Psychological Works of Sigmund Freud, Vol 14. Translated and edited by Strachey J. London, Hogarth Press, 1917

Hagnell O, Rorsman B: Suicide in the Lundby study: a controlled prospective investigation of stressful life events. Neuropsychobiology 6:319–332, 1980

Havens LL: The anatomy of a suicide. N Engl J Med 272:401–406, 1965

Holinger PC, Offer D, Ostrov E: Suicide and homicide in the United States: an epidemiologic study of violent death, population changes, and the potential for prediction. Am J Psychiatry 144:215–219, 1987

Klerman GL, Weissman MM: Increasing rates of depression. JAMA 261:2229–2235, 1989

Mann JJ, Mcbride PA, Stanley M: Postmortem monoamine receptor and enzyme studies in suicide. Ann NY Acad Sci 487:114–121, 1986

Marzuk PM, Tierney H, Tardiff K, et al: Increased risk of suicide in persons with AIDS. JAMA 259:1333–1337, 1988

McCrae RR, Costa PT: Emerging Lives, Enduring Dispositions. Boston, Little, Brown, 1984

Neugarten BL: Personality and aging, in The Handbook of the Psychology of Aging. Edited by Birren JE, Schaie KW. New York, Van Nostrand Reinhold, 1977, pp 626–649

O'Malley PM, Bachman JG, Johnston LD: Period, age and cohort effects in substance use among American youth, 1976–1982. Am J Public Health 74:682–688, 1984

Pfeffer CR: Life stress and family risk factors for youth fatal and nonfatal suicidal behavior, in Suicide Among Youth: Perspectives on Risk and Prevention. Edited by Pfeffer CR. Washington, DC, American Psychiatric Press, 1989, pp 143–164

Rich CL, Young D, Flowler RC: San Diego suicide study: young versus old subjects. Arch Gen Psychiatry 43:557–582, 1986

Robins E: The Final Months: A Study of the Lives of 134 Persons Who Committed Suicide. New York, Oxford University Press, 1981

Shaffer D: Suicide in childhood and early adolescence. J Child Psychol Psychiatry 15:275–291, 1974

Shaffer D, Garland A, Gould M, et al: Preventing teenage suicide: a critical review. J Am Acad Child Adolesc Psychiatry 27:675–687, 1988

Shafii M, Steltz-Lenarsky J, McCue Derrick A, et al: Comorbidity of mental disorders in the post-mortem diagnosis of completed suicide in children and adolescents. J Affective Disord 15:227–233, 1988

Sheehy G: Passages: Predictable Crises of Adult Life. New York, Dutton, 1976

Vaillant GE: Adaptation to Life. Boston, Little, Brown, 1977

Weinberger DR: Implications of normal brain development for the pathogenesis of schizophrenia. Arch Gen Psychiatry 44:660–669, 1987

Weissman MM, Klerman GL, Markowitz JS, et al: Suicidal ideation and suicide attempts in panic disorder and attacks. N Engl J Med 321:1209–1214, 1989.

Wong DF, Wagner HN Jr, Dannals RF, et al: Effects of age on dopamine and serotonin receptors measured by positron tomography in the living human brain. Science 226:1393–1396, 1984

Yakovlev PI, LeCours AIR: The myelogenetic cycles of regional maturation of the brain, in Regional Development of the Brain in Early Life. Edited by Minkowski A. Oxford, Blackwell Scientific Publications, 1967, pp 3–70

Risk Factors for Suicide

Chapter 2

The Epidemiology of Suicide: Implications for Clinical Practice

Martin Buda, M.D.
Ming T. Tsuang, M.D., Ph.D., D.Sc.

THE PURPOSE OF this chapter is to review epidemiologic information on suicide and to examine how this information relates to the prevention of premature deaths by suicide and to the treatment of psychiatric illness. We introduce our discussion with a presentation of suicide rates and trends in the general population, considering several variables such as age, gender, race, and marital status. The recent shift in high suicide rates toward younger age groups is discussed. In addition, consideration is also given to other sociodemographic factors and geographic differences in rates of suicide. The remainder of the chapter focuses on the epidemiology of suicide and the determination of risk factors for various psychiatric disorders, including depression, alcoholism, schizophrenia, neurosis, and personality disorder. In addition, readers are made aware of possible suicide risk factors that may occur in the relatives of these psychiatric patients. Finally, strategies for applying this knowledge about risk factors for patients and their relatives in clinical practice are presented.

The authors thank Jerome Fleming, M.D., for assistance in the preparation of this chapter. The work involved in the writing of this chapter was supported in part by funds from the Veterans Administration Medical Merit Review Grant (M.T.T.).

EPIDEMIOLOGY OF SUICIDE

The study of the distribution of suicide in a population allows for the establishment of general associations between suicide and the characteristics of individuals who kill themselves. For instance, variables such as age, gender, marital status, religious affiliations, and occupational status can be examined. Suicide rates obtained from epidemiologic studies of the general population supply public health officials with the necessary information to set up programs of prevention among high-risk groups and to establish centers in those areas where the problems are most severe (Monk 1975). In a study of mortality occurring in England and Wales, Sainsbury (1986b) found that suicide accounted for approximately 1% of all deaths. In addition, suicide was found to be more common in the elderly, but was also cited as the fourth leading cause of death among 15- to 34-year-olds. The overall suicide rate was about 9/100,000, the rate being higher for males (12) than for females (8). In the United States, the overall suicide rate per 100,000 is higher, 12.7 in 1987. Suicide is the eighth leading cause of death for the general population and is the third leading cause of death in ages 15 to 24 in the United States. During the past century, the rate in the United States has averaged 12.5/100,000. A high rate of 17.4 observed during the depression in 1932 was seen to dip to a low of 9.8 in 1957, rose steadily to a peak of 13.3 in 1977, and then dipped to a rate of 12.7 in 1987 (Cross and Hirschfeld 1985; National Center for Health Statistics 1987). This trend is represented by suicide rates in the United States for the years 1957 through 1987 (Figure 1).

Age and Suicide

When the relationship between age and suicide is examined over the past 2 decades, it is seen that the percentage of deaths due to suicides by persons 15 to 25 years of age has increased, while the percentage of total suicide deaths by persons over 44 years of age has decreased. In fact, in 1970 the median age of persons who died by suicide was 47.2; by 1980 it was 39.9 (Rosenberg et al. 1987). Figure 2 presents age-specific suicides as a percentage of total suicides described in 5-year age groups, for the census years 1970 and 1987. This figure illustrates the shift toward younger age groups in 1987 compared to 1970. As can be seen, the rates of suicide in the younger age categories (20–24, 25–29, 30–34) are substantially lower in 1970 when compared to those of 1987. On the other hand, the trend is just the opposite for older age groups (45–49, 50–54, 55–59), where the rates of suicide are much higher for 1970 compared to 1987. Suicide rates have increased most dramatically over time in the 15- to 24-year-old group. This is shown

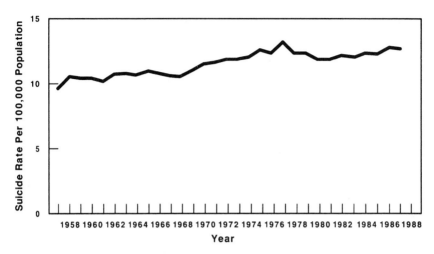

Figure 1. Suicide rates per 100,000 in the general population in the United States, 1957–1987. Data are from the National Center for Health Statistics, Vital Statistics of the United States.

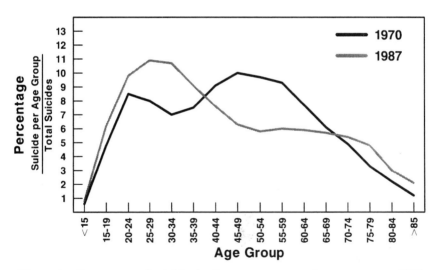

Figure 2. Percentage of suicides by 5-year age groups for census years 1970 and 1987. Data are from the National Center for Health Statistics, Vital Statistics of the United States.

in Figure 3, which presents the rates for the 15- to 24-year-old group compared to the rates for all ages for the years 1900 through 1987. In 1978, the rate in the younger age group exceeded the rate for all persons for the first time. In their epidemiologic report on this group, Rosenberg et al. pointed out that from 1950 to 1980 rates for suicide

among white males aged 15 to 19 increased by 305%; among 20- to
24-year-old males, the rate increased by 196%.

Gender and Suicide

Suicide rates have been shown to be higher in men than they are in
women. The fluctuation of suicide rates over time in males is also
greater when compared to females. This is illustrated in Figure 4,
which presents suicide rates in the United States for men and women
for the years 1900 through 1987. When the interaction of age and
gender is examined, it is interesting to note that the *ratio* of male-to-
female suicide for persons 15 to 19 years old has gone from a low point
of 0.7:1 in 1911 (males lower rate than females) to a reversed ratio of
4.7:1 (males in excess) in 1980. However, females make three times as
many attempts as males within this age group. This is illustrated in
Table 1, where the ratio of male-to-female suicides within the 15–19
year age bracket is presented for certain years between 1876 and 1987.
Additionally, when methods of suicide are examined by gender, there
seem to be clear differences. Males chose violent means (e.g., firearms, explosives, hanging) to commit suicide more frequently than
females, who chose nonviolent means (e.g., drug overdose). This is
illustrated in Figure 5, which shows the method of suicide based on
1987 data. As noted in the figure, the most frequent method of suicide
was firearms and the least frequent was gases and vapors.

The relationship of age and sex to changing rates of suicide over
time is illustrated by the data presented in Table 2. This table shows

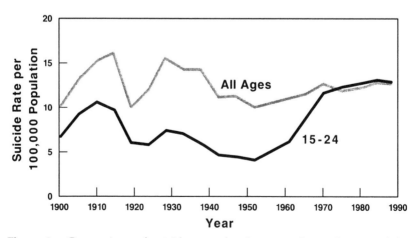

Figure 3. Comparison of suicide rates for the general population and for
persons 15 to 24 years old in the United States, 1900–1987. Data are from the
National Center for Health Statistics, Vital Statistics of the United States.

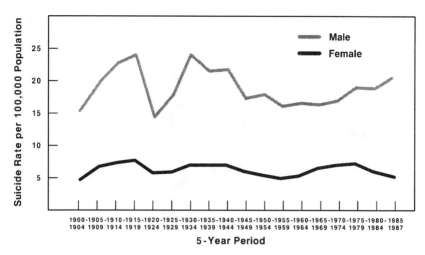

Figure 4. Suicide rates in the United States for men and women, 1900–1987 (5-year averages). Data are from the U.S. Bureau of the Census, Vital Statistics Rates in the United States, 1947 and 1968, and the National Center for Health Statistics, Vital Statistics of the United States, 1960 to 1987.

Table 1. Ratio of male-to-female suicide rates for certain years between 1876 and 1987 for 15- to 19-year-olds

Year	Ratio
1876–1885[b]	2.2
1897–1901[a]	1.2
1911[c]	0.7
1931[c]	1.4
1940[d]	1.6
1950[d]	1.8
1960[d]	3.4
1970[d]	3.2
1980[d]	4.7
1983[d]	4.4
1985[d]	4.3
1986[d]	4.3
1987[d]	3.9

[a]Bailey (1903).
[b]Miner (1922).
[c]Dublin and Bunzel (1933).
[d]National Center for Health Statistics.

the percentage of change in suicide rates by age group and sex between 1950 and 1987. The single most striking change in rates was the percentage of increase for males in both the 15- to 24-year-old group and in the 25- to 34-year-old group, and the consistent decrease

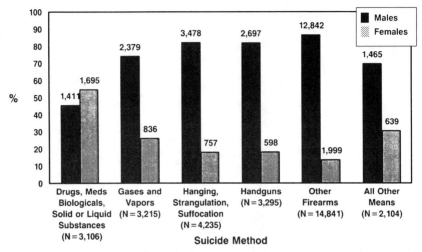

Figure 5. Number and percentages of suicide method by gender, United States rates 1987. Data are from the National Center for Health Statistics, Vital Statistics of the United States.

Table 2. Percentage of change between 1950 and 1987 for suicide rates by age group and sex

Age Group	Change (%)	
	Males	Females
15–24	228	65
25–34	85	20
35–44	8	− 4
45–54	− 26	− 14
55–64	− 39	− 22
65–74	− 31	− 29
75–84	− 2	− 14

in rates observed in the older age groups (over age 44), for both males and females (National Center for Health Statistics 1952, 1989). From the table, there is a 228% increase in suicide rates between 1950 and 1987 for males, age 15 to 24, and a 65% increase for females in the same age group.

Noting the shift in rates to increased suicide among younger populations, questions have arisen about the determinants of these epidemiologic trends in suicidal behavior. Hellon and Solomon (1980) studied changes among the young in rates for suicide in Alberta, Canada, between 1951 and 1977. They found that the significant increase in suicides among younger people as compared to the older groups was more than might be explained by population shifts. In a second article, Solomon and Hellon (1980) concluded that once a cohort of 15- to 19-year-olds had a high suicide rate, the group continued to exhibit an increased rate as that group aged. Other studies with similar conclusions have been published analyzing United States vital statistics (Murphy and Wetzel 1980) and rates among Australians (Goldney and Katsikitis 1983). However, Holinger and Offer (1982) proposed a different explanation that relates changes in the adolescent population, changes in the proportion of adolescents in the United States population, and adolescent suicide. Based on this theory, the proportion of adolescent suicide increases or decreases in relation to the proportion of adolescents in the general population.

Other Demographic Factors

Within the general population, further demographic factors need to be mentioned. These include race, marital status, religion, employment status, and seasonal variation. Suicide rates for whites are approximately twice those for nonwhites. In 1987, the suicide rate per 100,000 in caucasians was 13.7, whereas in noncaucasians it was 6.9. The relationship of race and age is presented in Figure 6, where we see suicide rates per 100,000 for 10-year age groups based on statistics for 1987 compiled from data from the National Center for Health Statis-

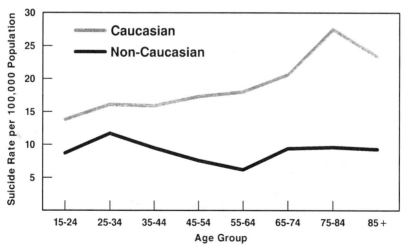

Figure 6. United States suicide rates for caucasians and noncaucasians by age group, sexes combined. Data are from the National Center for Health Statistics, Vital Statistics of the United States, 1987.

tics. As can be seen from the figure, the ratio of suicide in whites to nonwhites changes substantially across age categories. The ratio is smallest for the age groups 15 to 24 and 25 to 34 and largest for those over 75 years of age.

Suicide is more common in persons who are single, separated, divorced, or widowed. Married couples with children are at reduced risk for suicide, and, according to Durkheim (1966), this risk decreases further with increased numbers of children. The loss of a spouse increases risk, the risk for suicide being greater during the first year after the loss, and extending for 4 years thereafter (MacMahon and Pugh 1965). Figure 7 shows the suicide rate per 100,000 by marital status and age group. As seen in the figure, there are many age groups in which the suicide rates for widowed and divorced men are more than four times those of married men. In women there are some age groups in which the suicide rate runs three to four times higher in the widowed and divorced than in those married.

Rates vary by religious affiliations, being generally higher among Protestants than among Catholics and Jews (Durkheim 1966). Templer and Veleber (1980) reported an inverse relationship between the percentage of a state's Catholic population and its suicide rate. In one study reporting suicide rates in New York City, rates per 100,000 were found to be highest among Protestants (31.4) and lowest among Catholics (10.9), with Jews having a rate of 15.5 (Cross and Hirschfeld

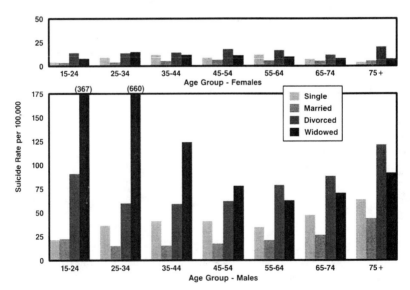

Figure 7. 1985 United States suicide rates per 100,000 population by marital status and age group. Data are from the National Center for Health Statistics, Vital Statistics of the United States and U.S. Bureau of the Census, 1985.

1985). Such data, of course, are limited by the fact that religious affiliation is not generally mentioned on death certificates.

Economic conditions and national suicide rates have been studied by MacMahon et al. (1963). They found that the two correspond closely, especially in the white male population. Suicide rates appeared to increase during troublesome economic times and economic depression and decrease during times of prosperity. Boor (1980) compared unemployment rates with suicide rates in eight countries: the United States, Canada, Sweden, France, Great Britain, Germany, Italy, and Japan. This study showed that suicide rate and unemployment correlated positively in all countries except Italy and Great Britain, and also found these relationships to hold true for both men and women. This latter finding is in disagreement with earlier studies that reveal higher rates for men than for women during adverse economic stress; it may reflect the fact that more women have been employed or have been entering professions. In general, empirical studies have shown that the unemployment rate among those who commit suicide is greater than 50%.

It is also interesting to note that the distribution of suicide within the United States differs substantially by geographic region. The mountain region has the highest overall rate per 100,000 of 17.6, where Nevada ranks number one. The middle Atlantic region, which includes New Jersey (the state with the lowest rate of 7.5) has the lowest overall suicide risk of the nine geographic regions in the United States. Differences have been attributed to the sex, age, and racial makeup of the various regions.

Suicide rates show a seasonal relationship as well. They seem to increase in the fall, and during April and May. December often has the lowest rate of suicide, which is contradictory to the belief that rates are higher during the holiday season.

SUICIDE IN PSYCHIATRIC POPULATIONS

Death by suicide has long been of concern to psychiatrists. Thus the early detection of suicidal individuals is of major importance. To identify the potentially suicidal patient, the clinician must evaluate the patient presenting with psychiatric symptoms within the framework of diagnostic, demographic, and social factors. This can be accomplished in part by evaluating specific risk factors, such as those outlined in the assessment summaries provided in other chapters in this volume (Hendren; Blumenthal, this volume). The meaningfulness of such an evaluation becomes apparent when these risk factors are seen in the light of the epidemiologic data as presented. It is through this process that those individuals with greater vulnerability for self-destructive behavior may be screened from those with low potential for suicide.

Approximately 95% of patients who complete suicide have a psychiatric disturbance. Between 45% and 70% of such patients, depending on the study, may carry a diagnosis of affective disorder such as major depression or bipolar illness (Barraclough et al. 1974; Dorpat and Ripley 1960; Robins et al. 1959a; Sainsbury 1986a). According to Murphy (1986), 25% had a diagnosis of alcoholism; the remaining cases carried a diagnosis of schizophrenia, neurosis, or personality disorder.

In a previously reported study on suicide risk among 200 schizophrenic, 100 manic, and 225 depressive patients (Tsuang 1978), the number of observed suicides in the study sample was compared to that expected based on the general population. Increased risk of suicide was found in all psychiatric groups except female schizophrenics. Death by suicide was particularly pronounced in male patients with affective disorders shortly following discharge from the hospital. The major finding of this study was that suicide was an important factor in the long-term outcome of both schizophrenia and primary affective disorders, and that suicides seem to cluster in the period shortly after discharge.

In addition to the above analysis of suicide risk in the typical groups of those with schizophrenia, mania, and depression, the rate of suicide in 94 cases of "other psychotics" (schizoaffective disorder, schizophreniform disorder, and atypical psychotic disorder) was also examined (Buda et al. 1988). Death by suicide in this group was in excess of what would be expected in the general population, a finding that was not only statistically significant, but important because this group represented a different set of patients. Although they presented with features of schizophrenia or affective psychoses, these patients failed to meet DSM-III (American Psychiatric Association 1980) criteria for schizophrenia, bipolar disorder, or major depression and fell into the "other" psychoses category. In fact, the diagnoses for these patients using DSM-III criteria were defined by exclusion from such categories, yet related to them by shared features (e.g., features of schizophrenia and affective disorder coexisting). Attempts to refine adequately the diagnosis of individuals in the atypical group have implications for the treatment and prevention of suicide. For instance, decreased risk of death by suicide has been demonstrated if these patients are treated with electroconvulsive therapy (Tsuang et al. 1979). This study suggests that such patients may respond to treatment in a similar way to those with affective disorder when these two groups are compared with the general population. These results seem to indicate that atypical patients appear to behave more like patients with affective disorders in terms of suicide experience. Given, however, the lack of clear nosologic definition for this group and the paucity of data available that specifically address this "other" category on suicide, we will not discuss it separately below. The point that such a group was identified in our work by its high risk for suicide needs emphasis and requires more research into the variables that relate to that risk.

To understand the relationship of psychiatric disorder and suicide, specific disorders must be examined. The following presents a clinical description of depression, alcoholism, schizophrenia, and personality disorders and neuroses and the way in which suicide relates to these illnesses.

Depression

Estimates of the lifetime prevalence of major affective disorder in the general population range from 6.1% to 9.5% (Robins et al. 1984). Studies that have followed cohorts of depressed patients over time have shown that 15% of depressed patients kill themselves (Sainsbury 1986a). Having conducted psychiatric autopsies by interviewing families and the treating physicians of suicide victims and by examining their records, Barraclough et al. (1974) concluded that about 64% of persons who kill themselves suffer from a major uncomplicated affective illness. When alcoholism was the primary diagnosis and coexisted with depression, the figure increased to 77%. There are also those studies that assess suicide attempters (Kiev 1976) and conclude that the majority of serious attempters, as opposed to less serious ones (defined below), meet criteria for major affective disorders.

The presenting picture may be quite similar for a depressed patient who goes on to commit suicide and one who does not. Each may meet criteria for a major affective disorder and present with such complaints as insomnia, weight loss, change in appetite, low interest in usual activities, social withdrawal, agitation, impaired concentration, and feelings of hopelessness. The severity of such symptoms may be greater in suicidal patients. According to Barraclough and Pallis (1975), symptoms such as insomnia, self-neglect, and memory impairment tend to be more prominent in high-risk patients. Pessimism and hopelessness about future prospects are greater (Beck 1963; Minkoff et al. 1973). Suicide attempts are classified as serious (marked medical seriousness of the attempt, lethal method of attempt, secretiveness, and preparation to prevent discovery) and less serious (lack of a major psychiatric diagnosis, presence of personality disorder, impulsivity, use of less lethal means, and less secrecy about the attempt). Serious attempters correlate highly with those patients having a psychiatric presentation of major depression or bipolar illness (Bagley 1973; Clayton 1985; Kiev 1976). Barraclough (Barraclough and Pallis 1975; Barraclough et al. 1974) found that those who completed suicide had made attempts 10 times more often than living depressive patients and that the course of depression was often longer in those who completed suicide than in controls. Factors that relate to increased risk are being over age 45; male; white; single, widowed, divorced, or separated; and unemployed. Most are situated higher socioeconomically and, according to Clayton (1985), may be of higher intelligence or accomplishment. The perception of losses and other stresses (economic, social, financial) may be greater, depending on a background of achievement.

Clearly, the largest proportion of psychiatric patients who kill themselves are the affectively disturbed. Several studies showed that a major proportion of these were under the care of a physician when they killed themselves (Clayton 1985; Robins et al. 1959a, 1959b). According to Murphy (1975), 82% of patients who committed suicide saw their physician within 6 months; 53% within 1 month. These studies indicated that at least two-thirds of these patients directly and specifically made their suicidal intention known to physicians, family members, or friends. The family or personal physician was the person most often consulted, but in about 25% of the cases a psychiatrist was seen. Often the patient was prescribed barbiturates,benzodiazepines, other sleeping medicines, tranquilizers, or antidepressants in an attempt to treat insomnia or anxiety symptomatically. These medications were then often used in the suicide. Sometimes antidepressants were prescribed to be taken in low, nontherapeutic dosages, but dispensed in quantities that proved lethal when used in the suicide. Clayton (1985) concluded that many of these patients were being treated symptomatically for insomnia and agitation without appropriate regard for the serious depressive state or syndrome that these symptoms represented. The fact that many such patients, especially men, had never seen a psychiatrist underscores the point that attention to these issues is a problem in general health care assessment and not solely a psychiatric one. It also makes clearer the fact that many of these deaths could probably have been prevented, if the illness was recognized, the risk appreciated, and the care given appropriate.

Alcoholism

According to the Epidemiologic Catchment Area (ECA) study (Robins et al. 1984), alcoholism, including alcohol dependency and episodic habitual drinking, afflicts more than 10% of the population. As a class, alcoholic patients are at markedly increased risk for other medical problems, such as cirrhosis, esophagitis, other gastrointestinal bleeding, ulcers, breast cancer, depression, and other neurologic damage. The lifetime risk of suicide in alcoholism is similar to major affective disorder and is estimated to be around 15% (Murphy 1986). Approximately three-quarters of alcoholic patients who commit suicide also suffer from major depression (Barraclough et al. 1974; Dorpat and Ripley 1960; Robins et al. 1959a). In his review of the literature, Murphy (1986) indicates that following depression, alcoholism carries with it the highest risk for suicide. The suicide rate associated with alcoholism is 75 to 85 times greater than that found in the general population. Male alcoholic patients are six times more likely than women alcoholic patients to commit suicide. Men are more likely than women to have an underlying antisocial personality disorder. Dysthymic disorder was more often present in women alcoholic patients.

When suicide does occur, it tends to happen after a mean duration of 20 years of drinking (Murphy 1986), between the ages of 30 and 60 years; the mean age of alcoholic suicide victims is about 47 years. Explanations for this include the higher probability of earlier mortality from other alcohol-related illnesses or accidents so that fewer alcoholic patients reach old age. Those who do reach old age are more likely to have benefited from treatment and are more likely to have remained abstinent; few alcoholic patients kill themselves during periods of abstinence (Murphy 1986; Flavin et al., this volume). Most data appear to indicate that alcoholic patients, like other psychiatric patients, are at increased risk for suicide following discharge from hospital treatment. The fact that most are actively drinking, hopeless, or discouraged over their failure to stop drinking may also play a role. Personality difficulties may also contribute: many are without social supports, drop out of treatment, and further isolate themselves prior to suicide. In addition, alcoholism can create marked psychosocial and economic disruptions so that alcoholic patients in their middle years are especially vulnerable. Related to this is the fact that most alcoholic suicide victims are unmarried or divorced. Those described as sensitive, nervous, ambitious, and worried are especially prone to suicide. In fact, Berglund (1984) found that 18% of such suicide victims had a peptic ulcer.

As mentioned above, losses play a substantial role in the suicides of alcoholic patients. In a study of 31 alcoholic suicide victims, Murphy and Robins (1967) observed that 50% had experienced a loss in a significant relationship in the year preceding the suicide, compared to fewer than 20% of depressed persons who took their lives. Even more striking was the finding that 33% of the alcoholic patients had experienced a close personal loss within 6 weeks of the suicide. These investigators repeated the study with another group of 50 alcoholic suicide victims with almost the same results; 26% had experienced an interpersonal loss within 6 weeks of their death (Murphy et al. 1979).

It is beyond the scope of this chapter to consider extensive premorbid and personality factors that relate to alcoholism and to suicide within that group (see Flavin et al., this volume; Goldsmith et al., this volume). However, the serious social, financial, and occupational losses that usually accompany this disorder devastate an already handicapped individual. Often a person beginning to acknowledge a drinking problem will present to a physician for help, not infrequently for other alcohol-related medical problems such as an ulcer, blackout, or esophagitis. The evaluating physician may focus on the medical problems or chief complaint of the patient and not attend to the underlying alcoholism. Sometimes, only emergency care is given, such as after an accident, and follow-up is neglected. The clinician's sensitivity to the dimension that these difficulties assume for an individual patient mandates an equally broad inquiry into the effects of alcoholism on the patient's world, including the patient's relationships and social life and the presence of depression and/or suicidality. The clinician's early attention to patterns of substance use in his or her patients, especially in younger persons at risk who utilize alcohol or drugs to cope with stress (e.g., professionals, executives, those in high-pressure and competitive jobs), might well pay dividends in decreasing the suicide rate in this group.

Schizophrenia

According to Roy (1986), 10% of individuals with schizophrenia die from suicide. Epidemiologic studies have been concerned with those characteristics that tend to differentiate a schizophrenic patient who commits suicide from one who does not. Schizophrenia, as opposed to the major affective psychoses, tends to occur earlier in life. Males appear to be at greater risk for suicide than females and are affected at a younger age. They also tend to be unmarried. Additionally, each exacerbation of the illness often leaves the patient more emotionally handicapped. Most schizophrenic patients are in a depressive state, rather than an intensely psychotic state, when they commit suicide (Drake et al. 1985). Furthermore, antipsychotic medicines that are used in the treatment of schizophrenia carry with them a substantial risk for side effects, including involuntary movement disorders that at times can incapacitate a patient. Recurring decompensations frequently require repeated hospitalizations. Often patients are left jobless, without prospects for employment, inadequately understood, unaccepted in their family and community, and hopeless about their future. Suicide frequently occurs following hospitalization, although not necessarily after the first or index admission.

In previous studies, schizophrenic patients who committed suicide were found to do so in the first few years of their follow-up (Tsuang 1978). Methods chosen by males tended more often to be violent (e.g., shooting, jumping, stabbing); women chose less violent means (e.g., drug overdoses). There is often a previous attempt for both males and females. According to Shaffer et al. (1974), the number of previous attempts was the most important risk factor associated with suicides in schizophrenia.

Drake et al. (1985) described most of the schizophrenic patients who committed suicide in their study as having been better educated and often at the beginning of a career when they became ill. Many had jobs, were in school, and functioned reasonably well prior to the onset of the illness. For these patients, awareness of the devastating implications of their illness, the dashing of hopes for the future intensified by the repeated needs for hospitalization, and a decreased ability to function normally in society may make living intolerable. Often financial, social, and family disintegration accompany their illness. Virkkunen (1976) found that more schizophrenic suicide victims than schizophrenic controls eventually "gave up." They no longer asked for support or attention and became negative in their attitude toward treatment and indifferent toward staff and personnel. The postdischarge period was especially critical in that the structure of the inpatient setting gives way on discharge to joblessness and lack of social supports. For the schizophrenic patient already wary about future prospects, these stresses may tip the balance toward suicide.

Personality Disorder and Neurosis

According to Miles (1977), approximately 5% of psychiatric patients who die by suicide carry a diagnosis of personality disorder or neurosis. He describes such categorization as problematic for several reasons. Several patients who committed suicide, diagnosed as "neurotic" in this study, were discovered on review of their records to have been more seriously disturbed; some more properly should have been diagnosed as psychotic. Additionally, at the time these studies were conducted, many varied disorders were considered under the single rubric of neurosis or personality disorder. Given that the numbers of suicides in these studies were small, comparisons and statistical evaluation within this group are difficult. Nevertheless, Miles concluded that this group is at greater risk for suicide than the general population. In his review of the data, he indicated that two diagnoses—psychopathic (sociopathic) personality disorder and depressive neurosis (reactive depression, dysthymic disorder)—disproportionately accounted for that increased risk. He also found that other uncomplicated neuroses, such as obsessional neuroses and hysteria, are not especially vulnerable to suicide. Topp (1979) reported a higher rate of suicide among prison inmates than among the general population. In his review of some of these cases, it was unclear whether the mental state of the patient shortly before the suicide involved a more complicating set of circumstances, such as coexisting depression. (Depression is a common accompanying feature of many personality disorders, anxiety conditions, drug abuse, and alcoholism.)

Relatives of Suicides

We have shown that the incidence of suicide is significantly greater among patients with affective disorders and schizophrenia than in the general population (Tsuang 1978). We have also shown that the risk of both schizophrenia and affective disorders are significantly higher among the relatives of schizophrenic and manic-depressive patients, respectively (Tsuang et al. 1980). These results suggest that the rate of suicide in relatives of psychiatric patients is higher than expected. Genetic and familial factors in suicide are discussed by Kety (this volume). Data on suicides from twin studies have shown that concordance rates in monozygotic pairs are significantly higher than in dizygotic pairs (Juel-Nielsen and Videbech 1970). In a review of the literature, data were pooled from a number of studies to obtain 149 sets of twins in which at least one twin had committed suicide. In nine cases, the co-twin had also committed suicide. All of these occurred in identical twin pairs. Similar indications of a genetic factor in suicide come from findings of American-Danish adoption studies, where suicide in relatives of adoptees who had committed suicide occurred mainly in biologic relatives (Kety 1983; Schulsinger et al. 1979).

In another study that further examines the genetic contribution to suicide, the risk of suicide among the first-degree relatives of 195 schizophrenic and 315 manic-depressive patients (Tsuang 1983) was analyzed. The findings demonstrated a higher risk of suicide among relatives of psychiatric patients in comparison with relatives of surgical controls. Male relatives had a higher risk of suicide than female relatives. When suicide risk in the relatives was analyzed according to the presence or absence of suicides in patients, relatives of patients who had committed suicide showed significantly higher risk of suicide than the remaining relatives. This risk of suicide was particularly high in male relatives of the patients with affective disorders, especially unipolar depression.

Because relatives of schizophrenic and manic-depressive patients are at a higher risk for suicide than the general population, and especially because relatives of those psychiatric patients who commit suicide may be even more significantly at risk, clinicians should pay closer attention to family history as part of general assessment. Other family members at risk might be identified with such screening measures and encouraged to seek help.

DISCUSSION

In this chapter, epidemiologic studies of suicide in the general population and in relationship to specific psychiatric disorders have been presented. The point has been underscored that adequate patient assessment can be achieved only if important epidemiologic variables are understood as part of the background against which suicide occurs. The data have shown that 94% of patients who go on to kill themselves suffer from a major treatable psychiatric illness (Robins et al. 1959b; Sainsbury 1986a).

Successful treatment derives from correct diagnosis. The recognition of major psychiatric syndromes is made clearer by defined inclusionary and exclusionary criteria, such as found in DSM-III-R (American Psychiatric Association 1987). An understanding of the patient's psychiatric diagnosis leads next to treatment considerations, the first of which might be whether or not to hospitalize. Since epidemiologic data derived from population studies indicate probable risks for suicide and as such do not predict the specific patients who will kill themselves, intervention decisions become a matter of the clinician's informed judgment based on an understanding of risk factors. The clinician must ask "which patient is at significant risk for suicide?"

Although it is helpful at times to list specific risk factors, the careful evaluation of a patient depends on that particular patient's presentation and mental state, which together will dictate treatment directions, especially in crisis settings (see Blumenthal, this volume). Of the many factors that can be considered in determining suicide risk, the first consideration needs to be diagnostic. Treatment decisions, including hospitalization, follow from the results of evaluation establishing the likelihood of illness and judgment about its seriousness, severity, impairment, and risk of harm.

CONCLUSION

In this chapter, we have presented a detailed discussion of the epidemiologic studies of suicide and how they relate to psychiatric disorders. However, the task of predicting who is at risk for suicide remains a difficult one. In a prospective study of suicide predictors in

4,800 patients who were consecutively admitted to inpatient psychiatric services at a Veterans Administration Hospital, Pokorny (1983) found that even though there were some positive correlations between baseline measures and subsequent suicides or attempts, these factors were unsuccessful in identifying specific subjects who would later commit suicide. For the prevention of suicide and premature death in psychiatric patients, attention must be paid specifically to those individuals who are at the highest risk of committing suicide. In this case, it is a matter of identifying those persons having the most risk factors for suicide and not a matter of the prediction of suicide (Pokorny 1983).

However, the above statements on suicide prediction should not diminish the importance of continued epidemiologic research. Some predictors and risk factors associated with suicide are more important than others. Age, sex, race, and psychiatric diagnosis have been shown to be important variables in determining suicide risk. At the present time, the best procedure for preventing suicide is for clinicians to use combined information from statistical studies about suicide and from the patient's clinical presentation. Strengthening linkages between epidemiology and clinical practice should contribute to improving both the care of suicidal patients and future research studies.

REFERENCES

American Psychiatric Association: Diagnostic and Statistical Manual of Mental Disorders, 3rd Edition. Washington, DC, American Psychiatric Association, 1980

American Psychiatric Association: Diagnostic and Statistical Manual of Mental Disorders, 3rd Edition, Revised. Washington, DC, American Psychiatric Association, 1987

Bagley C: Social policy and the prevention of suicidal behaviour. British Journal of Social Work 3:473–495, 1973

Bailey WB: Suicide in the United States, 1897–1901. Yale Review 12:70–89, 1903

Barraclough BM, Pallis D: Depression followed by suicide: a comparison of depressed suicides with living depressives.Psychol Med 5:55–61, 1975

Barraclough BM, Bunch J, Nelson P, et al: A hundred cases of suicide: clinical aspects. Br J Psychiatry 125:355–373, 1974

Beck A: Thinking and depression. Arch Gen Psychiatry 9:324–333, 1963

Berglund M: Suicide in alcoholism: a prospective study of 88 suicides; I: the multidimensional diagnosis at first admission. Arch Gen Psychiatry 41:888–891, 1984

Boor M: Relationship between unemployment rates and suicide rates in eight countries: 1962–1967. Psychol Rep 47:1095–1101, 1980

Buda M, Tsuang MT, Fleming JA: Causes of death in DSM-III schizophrenics and other psychotics (atypical group): a comparison with the general population. Arch Gen Psychiatry 45:283–285, 1988

Clayton PJ: Suicide. Psychiatr Clin North Am 8:203–214, 1985

Cross CK, Hirschfeld RMA: Epidemiology of disorders in adulthood: suicide, in Psychiatry, Vol 3. Edited by Michels R, Cavenar J, Brodie HKH, et al. Philadelphia, JB Lippincott, 1985, pp 1–15

Dorpat TL, Ripley HS: A study of suicide in the Seattle area. Compr Psychiatry 1:349–359, 1960

Drake RE, Gates C, Whitaker A, et al: Suicide among schizophrenics: a review. Compr Psychiatry 26:90–100, 1985

Dublin LI, Bunzel B: To Be, or Not To Be: A Study of Suicide. New York, Smith and Haas, 1933

Durkheim E: Suicide: A Study in Sociology. Translated by Spalding JA, Simpson G. New York, Free Press, 1966

Goldney RD, Katsikitis M: Cohort analysis of suicide rates in Australia. Arch Gen Psychiatry 40:71–74, 1983

Hellon CP, Solomon MI: Suicide and age in Alberta, Canada, 1951 to 1977: the changing profile. Arch Gen Psychiatry 37:505–510, 1980

Holinger PC, Offer D: Prediction of adolescent suicide: a population model. Am J Psychiatry 139:302–307, 1982

Juel-Nielson N, Videbech T: A twin study of suicide. Acta Genet Med Gemellol (Roma) 19:307–310, 1970

Kety SS: Observations on genetic and environmental influences in the etiology of mental disorder from studies on adoptees and their relatives, in Genetics of Neurological and Psychiatric Disorders. Edited by Kety SS, Rowland LP, Sidman RL, Matthyse SW. New York, Raven, 1983

Kiev A: Cluster analysis profiles of suicide attempters. Am J Psychiatry 133:150–153, 1976

MacMahon B, Pugh TF: Suicide in the widowed. Am J Epidemiol 81:23–31, 1965

MacMahon B, Johnson S, Pugh TF: Relation of suicide rates to social conditions: evidence from U.S. vital statistics. Public Health Rep 78:285–293, 1963

Miles P: Conditions predisposing to suicide: a review. J Nerv Ment Dis 164:231–246, 1977

Miner JR: Suicide and its relation to climatic and other factors. American Journal of Hygiene Monograph Series 2, 1922

Minkoff K, Bergman E, Beck A, et al: Hopelessness, depression, and attempted suicide. Am J Psychiatry 130:455–459, 1973

Monk M: Epidemiology, in A Handbook for the Study of Suicide. Edited by Perlin S. New York, Oxford University Press, 1975

Murphy GE: The physician's responsibility for suicide, II: errors of omission. Ann Intern Med 82:305–309, 1975

Murphy GE: Suicide in alcoholism, in Suicide. Edited by Roy A. Baltimore, Williams & Wilkins, 1986, pp 89–96

Murphy GE, Robins E: Social factors in suicide. JAMA 199:303–308, 1967

Murphy GE, Wetzel RD: Suicide risk by birth cohort in the United States, 1949–1974. Arch Gen Psychiatry 37:519–523, 1980

National Center for Health Statistics: Standardized micro-data transcripts, data on vital events, detailed mortality tapes. Hyattsville, MD, Health Resources Administration, 1970, 1980, 1987

National Center for Health Statistics: Vital Statistics of the United States: 1970, Vol 2, Mortality, Part A, Tables I-26, (DHEW Pub No HRA-75-1101). Rockville MD, 1974

National Center for Health Statistics: Vital Statistics of the United States: 1987, Deaths for Selected Causes, Tables 290, 292, Rockville, MD, 1989

Pokorny AD: Prediction of suicide in psychiatric patients: report of a prospective study. Arch Gen Psychiatry 40:249–257, 1983

Robins E, Gassner S, Kayes J, et al: The communication of suicidal intent: a study of 134 consecutive cases of successful (completed) suicide. Am J Psychiatry 115:724–733, 1959a

Robins E, Murphy G, Wilkinson R, et al: Some clinical consideration in the prevention of suicide based on a study of 134 successful suicides. Am J Public Health 49:888–899, 1959b

Robins LN, Helzer JE, Weissman MM, et al: Lifetime prevalence of specific psychiatric disorders in three sites. Arch Gen Psychiatry 41:949–958, 1984

Rosenberg ML, Smith JC, Davidson LE, et al: The emergence of youth suicide: an epidemiologic analysis and public health perspective. Annu Rev Public Health 8:417–440, 1987

Roy A: Suicide in schizophrenia, in Suicide. Edited by Roy A. Baltimore, Williams & Wilkins, 1986, pp 97–112

Sainsbury P: Depression, suicide, and suicide prevention, in Suicide. Edited by Roy A. Baltimore, Williams & Wilkins, 1986a, pp 73–88

Sainsbury P: The epidemiology of suicide, in Suicide. Edited by Roy A. Baltimore, Williams & Wilkins, 1986b, pp 17–40

Schulsinger F, Kety SS, Rosenthal D, et al: A family study of suicide, in Origin, Prevention, and Treatment of Affective Disorders. Edited by Schou M, Stromgren E. New York, Academic, 1979, pp 277–287

Shaffer J, Perlin S, Schmidt C, et al: The prediction of suicide in schizophrenia. J Nerv Ment Dis 159:349–355, 1974

Solomon MI, Hellon CP: Suicide and age in Alberta, Canada, 1951 to 1977: cohort analysis. Arch Gen Psychiatry 37:511–513, 1980

Templer DI, Veleber DM: Suicide rate and religion within the United States. Psychol Rep 47:898, 1980

Topp DO: Suicide in prison. Br J Psychiatry 134:24–27, 1979

Tsuang MT: Suicide in schizophrenics, manics, depressives, and surgical controls: a comparison with general population suicide mortality. Arch Gen Psychiatry 35:153–155, 1978

Tsuang MT: Risk of suicide in the relatives of schizophrenics, manics, depressives, and controls. J Clin Psychiatry 44:396–400, 1983

Tsuang MT, Dempsy GM, Fleming JA: Can ECT prevent premature death and suicide in schizoaffective patients? J Affective Disord 1:167–171, 1979

Tsuang MT, Winokur G, Crowe RR: Morbidity risks of schizophrenia and affective disorders among first degree relatives of patients with schizophrenia, mania, depression and surgical conditions. Br J Psychiatry 137:497–504, 1980

U.S. Department of Commerce, Bureau of the Census: Marital status and living arrangements: March 1985, population characteristics series p-20, No. 410, 1987

Virkkunen M: Attitude to psychiatric treatment before suicide in schizophrenia and paranoid psychoses. Br J Psychiatry 128:47–49, 1976

Chapter 3

Environmental, Psychosocial, and Psychoanalytic Aspects of Suicidal Behavior

Kenneth S. Adam, M.D.

THE NOTION THAT the social environment impacts on suicidal behavior over the life cycle and that suicide is an act with important social consequences are constant features of the literature on suicide. However, the precise role of social factors in the causal chain of events leading to suicide has been and continues to be a controversial matter. Historical and cultural accounts of suicide are divided between those that describe suicide as a venerated response to social humiliation, military defeat, or a realistic assessment of life travails and those that describe it as an act of madness or perversity (Rosen 1971). Prevailing views about human nature heavily color these accounts, as evidenced by the highly idealized descriptions of suicide from the writers of the classical period of Greek and Roman civilization, and the pervasive moral views of suicide that predominated the Christian writings of the Middle Ages. The trends toward secularization and demystification of our understanding of human behavior, which began during the 18th century, saw a preoccupation with the topic of suicide and an ongoing debate over whether it was best understood as an individual's response to social and economic forces or the result of insanity whose origins lay in brain pathology (Maris 1969).

Systematic studies of the social variables in suicide can be dichotomized between the macrosocial point of view, as expressed in sociological and ecological studies that have examined the association between suicide rates, suicidal behavior, and various social conditions, and the microsocial point of view, as exemplified by psychiatric and psychoanalytic studies that have tried to show how the immediate social environment impinges on the individual and is incorporated within the person to produce a vulnerable personality. In its most extreme position, the macrosocial view would suggest that all individuals are equally vulnerable to suicide given sufficient exposure to social stress, whereas the extreme microsocial view would suggest that only those specifically vulnerable will respond to social stress by suicidal behavior.

A contemporary understanding of the role of social and environmental factors would suggest that suicidal behavior, like most psychiatric illnesses and behavioral disorders, is best understood as being multi-determined and the result of an interaction between the more basic causal factors that render the individual susceptible, and those that interact with this susceptibility to produce symptoms, illness, or symptomatic behavior.

In keeping such a complex model, this chapter will demonstrate that social and environmental factors may act in three main ways to produce suicidal behavior: 1) as predisposing factors producing a more or less specific vulnerability; 2) as precipitating factors to trigger suicidal activity in previously predisposed individuals, whether or not this vulnerability is socially determined or otherwise; or 3) as contributing factors increasing the exposure of the individual in more general ways to the other predisposing or precipitating conditions.

In this chapter, a general summary of the macrosocial findings from social and ecological studies of suicide will be presented, followed by a more detailed examination of the microsocial environment from the point of view of the family and immediate social network to show how they have been implicated in suicidal behavior. In each of these cases, the limitations of the evidence will be summarized, whether it appears to act to predispose to suicidal behavior, to precipitate it, or to serve as a more general contributing agent. Where possible, evidence of social factors that appear protective in each of these categories will be discussed. Finally, this chapter will review some of the more important theories that have attempted to conceptualize these variables in a more comprehensive way.

SOCIOLOGICAL STUDIES

Suicide has long been of interest to sociologists who, following the pioneering work of Durkheim (1952), have been interested in explaining the association between suicide rates and the social characteristics of large populations. It was well known throughout the 19th century that suicide rates increased during periods of economic depression and decreased in times of war, and that suicide tended to co-vary with crime rates and to vary inversely with homicide rates. It was also common knowledge that suicide rates were higher in some countries than others and that within these countries certain groups were at greater risk than others. Protestants had higher rates for suicide than Catholics or Jews, city-dwellers than country-dwellers, and professional and liberal occupation groups had higher rates than the chronically poor. Similarly, men, the elderly, and the unmarried, widowed, and divorced were all overrepresented.

Durkheim's landmark work *Le Suicide*, which was first published in 1897, was based on a comparison of the crude suicide rates of a number of European countries and the United States with a number of these social variables in an attempt to arrive at some generalizations about society as a whole (Durkheim 1952). In this sense it is as much a study of sociological method as it is a study of suicide, as the title "Suicide: A Study in Sociology" implies. Observing that suicide appeared to vary inversely with the degree of integration of the individual into religious, domestic, and political society, he arrived at a basic hypothesis encompassing all of these: "Suicide varies inversely with the degree of integration of the social groups of which the individual forms a part" (p. 209).

He described four types of suicide categorized according to the degree to which the individual was integrated with and regulated by society. "Egoistic" suicide occurred when excessive individuation or insufficient integration into society led to life weariness and depression. "Altruistic" suicide, by contrast, occurred when there was insufficient individuation and excessive integration into society and led the individual to see his or her social group as more important than the self. The samurai ritual of hara-kiri and the ancient Indian practice of suttee where the widow "chooses" to die on her husband's funeral pyre are examples of this type. "Anomic" suicide occurs where the individuals feel they have been abandoned by a society that no longer provides them with the regulation that they need. Such suicides were felt to occur during periods of abrupt social change, such as those that follow economic recession, unemployment, or divorce, where the collective order of the individual's life is disturbed. "Fatalistic" suicide, the last type, occurs when the individual's life is subject to excessive social regulation beyond his or her choice or control so that the individual despairs of any life of his or her own. Slaves, prisoners, and those trapped in premature or unwanted marriages fall into this category.

Although Durkheim (1952) recognized that individual factors might be implicated in the antecedents to suicide, he felt these to be constant in all societies and therefore not sufficient to explain variations in the "social suicide rate." "The causes of death are outside rather than within us, and are effective only if we venture into their sphere of activity" (p. 43).

Later sociologists following Durkheim, while confirming many of his general findings, have attempted to refine these and to take more account of the way in which social variables impact on the individual. Henry and Short (1954), for example, while substantiating Durkheim's findings on the relationship of suicide rates to business cycles in general, found that suicide increased more during periods of economic depression than it decreased in periods of prosperity and that these relationships impacted more strongly on men than on women. According to their model, which combined Durkheim's concepts with a social-psychological view of aggression, the external restraints imposed by society that produce frustration and aggression interact with the internal restraints (psychological) of the individual. The balance of these forces of internal and external restraint determines whether aggression will be expressed outwardly in homicide, or inwardly in suicide. Gibbs and Martin (1964) extended Durkheim's hypothesis to examine role functioning in society, concluding that it was the degree of the individual's "status integration" that governed vulnerability to suicide. According to this theory, the more integrated individuals in a society are into their occupational roles, the higher their status integration and the lower their suicide risk.

More recent sociological studies have moved away from the investigation of static variables such as occupational status and social status, to examine the dynamics of social change in relation to suicide. Breed (1963) and Maris (1975), for example, established that suicide is more directly related to loss of social status and downward mobility than to social status in itself. Maris (1969) cautioned against the dangers of the ecological fallacy in which the characteristics of a society are used to explain individual behavior, noting that attributes of groups are not necessarily applicable to individuals or subsets of individuals within these groups.

In an attempt to overcome some of the difficulties involved in the more traditional sociological studies of suicide based exclusively on suicide rates in large populations, clinical researchers have designed more detailed ecological studies of the social environment of suicidal individuals.

ECOLOGICAL STUDIES

Ecological Studies of Completed Suicide

One of the most frequently cited of the ecological studies of completed suicide is that of Sainsbury (1955), who combined a sociological study of 28 boroughs in London, England, in which the social characteristics of the boroughs and their suicide rates were compared, with an epidemiologic study of 409 suicides in North London around the same period of time. The boroughs with the highest rates of suicide were characterized by high numbers of boarding homes and hotels with a transient population, and those with the lowest rates had a high proportion of family dwellings. The suicide victims from North London were more likely than the general population to be living alone and to be old, unemployed, widowed or divorced, or separated from their spouses. He concluded that suicide rates were significantly correlated with social disorganization, social isolation, and social mobility.

In a correlational analysis of suicide in Edinburgh, McCulloch et al. (1967) found high suicide rates to be associated with overcrowding, areas with many tenement houses and fewer owner-occupied houses, and high rates of juvenile delinquency, truancy, and children placed in foster care. Rates for attempted suicide and divorce were also extremely high in these areas. These researchers suggested that there might be two socially distinguishable groups of suicide, one consisting of relatively old persons, who were often divorced or widowed and living alone, and another consisting of younger persons living in overcrowded conditions with grossly disturbed family settings and high rates of juvenile delinquency and self-injurious behavior.

Lester (1970) attempted to replicate these findings in the United States in a study of suicide in Buffalo, New York, and found that, while completed suicide was common in areas where there was a high proportion of old, widowed, divorced, and relatively educated individuals, it was not associated with overcrowding, dilapidated housing, or juvenile delinquency as was the case in Edinburgh. Comparison of the two studies is complicated by the fact that the criteria for the social variables under study may not have been compared and the racial characteristics of the two countries may have affected the findings. Of the 16 census tracts constituting the inner city of Buffalo, which were characterized by dilapidated accommodations and overcrowding, 8 also had high proportions of black residents who at that time (1958–1962) had considerably lower suicide rates than whites.

In a study of suicide in Chicago, Maris (1969) found those community areas with high suicide rates to have twice as much substandard housing as those with low rates but, in contrast to the Sainsbury study, he found residential mobility almost the same in both groups, and the population density was lower. He found two types of areas within the high suicide rate group. One, which he called the "gold coast area," was characterized by a high proportion of older individuals with high educational levels, high percentages of white-collar workers with medium income, low unemployment, and only moderate levels of substandard housing. These areas had a low percentage of blacks and high residential mobility. The other area, the "skid row area," was characterized by a lower percentage of older persons, lower educational attainment, and fewer white-collar workers. The areas with the lowest suicide rates were in the suburban areas at the periphery of the city, with elderly populations, medium educational level, high incomes, low-density high-quality housing, and a low percentage of blacks. (A second area, which included three of the six lowest suicide areas, was characterized by a high percentage of blacks.) While some of the other low suicide areas had many adverse social characteristics such as low income, high unemployment, high density of population, substandard housing, and high residential mobility, the high percentage of blacks in these regions was felt to have moderated their suicide rates. Maris hypothesized that the stronger relational systems of black families, generally younger populations, and higher externally directed aggression, acted as protective factors.

In two Canadian studies, Sakinofsky and Roberts (1985), compared the suicide rates of 10 Canadian provinces on a number of demographic, cultural, and social variables. They showed that low provincial suicide rates were related to the stability of residence, intact families, or single-parent families and the existence of "companionship." High provincial suicide rates, on the other hand, were associated with nonfamily households, divorce, alcoholism, and couples with no children. In a further longitudinal investigation, the authors compared two groups of five provinces according to whether there was a high or low percentage of change in the suicide rates across the decades from 1969–1971 to 1971–1981. Increases in rates for males during these years paralleled increases in alcoholism, crimes of rape, and the proportion of nonfamily households; low suicide rates were linked to social stability. Unfavorable economic changes leading to decreased social integration, affecting some provinces more than others, appeared to be responsible.

Ecological Studies of Attempted Suicide

Ecological studies of attempted suicide are more recent than those on completed suicide, and these have been concerned with comparing the social characteristics of high attempted-suicide areas with those of low attempted-suicide areas. In some cases, the findings for attempted suicide have been compared with similar data on completed suicide within the same city, and some have complemented their findings with a more direct study of social variables in smaller samples of actual cases. While many of these studies have employed relatively straightforward distributional analyses, others have employed more sophisticated multivariate techniques in their investigations. Although the studies differ considerably from one another in their details, there is general agreement that attempted suicide, like completed suicide, is associated with poor living circumstances and other indices of social disorganization.

One of the earliest of these is a study by Schmid and Van Arsdol (1955), who analyzed the pattern of attempted suicide within Seattle, Washington, and found positive correlations in both the place of occurrence of the act and the place of residence between rates of attempted suicide and suicide. Central city areas had the highest rates and the suburban residential areas of the city had the lowest rates. Kessel (1965) examined the self-poisoning rates in the 23 wards of Edinburgh and found that those wards with highest rates were in the older central areas with overcrowded tenements. The highest rates of all occurred in the heart of the areas where the majority of the hostels and lodging houses of the city were found. In Bristol, England, Morgan et al. (1975) found attempted suicide to be represented in all electoral wards of the city but found the central area had morbidity rates 2.8 times that of the city as a whole. Socioeconomic correlates found in these areas were overcrowding, lack of exclusive domestic amenities, and a high proportion of foreign-born residents, marital breakdown, unemployment, and legal and social difficulties. These results were very similar to the Edinburgh findings, with the exception that no correlation was found between the proportion of persons living alone nor with the type of accommodation. Similar findings regarding the centripetal distribution of attempted suicide have also been reported by Termansen (1972) for Vancouver, Canada, Jarvis et al. (1982) for London, Canada, and Koller and Cotgrove (1976) for Hobart, Australia. Several studies have shown that these patterns exist even when age and sex are standardized (Buglass et al. 1970; Jarvis et al. 1976; Kreitman 1977).

Buglass and Duffy (1978) employed multivariate analysis to examine the relationship between both completed suicide and attempted suicide and a set of 98 social indicators in Edinburgh. They found that while the central areas of the city had high rates for both forms of behavior, two of the areas with the highest rates for attempted suicide were located at the very edge of the city. Areas with high rates for both suicide and parasuicide (attempted suicide) had low property values, high rates for mental hospital admissions, poor housing, and a high proportion of divorced residents. The two peripheral areas where attempted suicide was common but suicide rare were similar in social class and overcrowding to the central area, but they had different population structures. Whereas the central district had a high proportion of elderly, these areas had high proportions of children under the age of 15, more working women with a child under the age of 5, and low proportions of widowed and single adults. Unemployment, poverty, and juvenile delinquency were prominent. The only item that strongly correlated with suicide alone was that of single-person households.

In a study of attempted suicide in the city of London, Ontario, Canada, Jarvis et al. (1982) took special care to identify all possible cases of attempted suicide from a wide range of sources—including hospitals, institutions, agencies, and private physicians—occurring over a period of 2 years. Cases were located geographically according to their usual place of residence rather than the address immediately preceding the suicidal act to correct for the overrepresentation of suicidal behavior in areas with institutional settings. They found the rates for self-injury based on usual address were highest in the center of the city and decreased with distance from the center. The central area contained the poorer, more socially disorganized areas, and the suburban districts had the higher socioeconomic areas. Multivariate analysis of the key social variables showed that areas with high density of housing and single-person households were strongly associated with self-injury, even when socioeconomic, family status, and mobility were controlled. Low socioeconomic status was also related to self-injury, even when other variables were controlled, although the relationship here was less consistent than that for living arrangements.

Ecological studies have in general confirmed that the relationships between adverse social and economic conditions and suicidal behavior that were identified by sociologists in large populations hold true in the more focused study of urban social geography. Poverty, transience, poor living circumstances, and other indices of social disorganization are striking features of the areas containing the highest numbers of suicidal individuals, whereas higher socioeconomic status, residential stability, and other indices of social integration are features of low suicide areas. Although these adverse conditions are most likely to be found in central city areas, the studies of Buglass and Duffy (1978) and Maris (1969) show that a unique population structure may sometimes override geographical and social considerations.

The fact that the same social geography and social conditions are generally found in studies of both attempted and completed suicides argues against these being distinctly different behaviors, as has been suggested by some authors (Linehan 1986; Stengel et al. 1958). It may well be that differences in the age, sex, and diagnostic distributions noted in the two groups when viewed cross-sectionally simply reflect the differing impact of social variables on men and women at different points of the life cycle in a group with a common vulnerability. The effects of social disorganization, for example, may well be more severe in old age, when social and economic alternatives are less readily available than early on, and they may have a greater impact on men and women. Women tend to value and maintain familial and inter-personal networks more than men, and this may buffer them from the effects of social change to a greater extent.

Social Isolation

Although the various measures of social disorganization mentioned above have been convincingly related to suicidal behavior, it has been argued that it is the social isolation they lead to that is most directly causal (Stengel 1964). Trout (1980) pointed out that Durkheim's (1952) categories of anomic and egoistic suicide are characterized by a lack of social ties and that both in their extremes lead to social isolation. In his Chicago study, Maris (1969) examined a random selection of the coroners' records of a group of older white males who had committed suicide and found a high percentage of them had been physically isolated and living alone at the time of their death or socially isolated and detached from friends, dependents, and relatives. Often no relative had appeared at the inquest into their deaths and those who did had had no contact with them for some time. In several cases the only informants were their landlords. While his general findings supported Durkheim's social integration hypothesis, he felt that this was largely related to the cohesiveness of social relationships. "Generally, the more 'significant others,' the lower the suicide rate" (Durkheim 1952, p. 15). Giddens (1971) suggested that the principal variable linking the psychological with social views of suicide is the isolation of the suicidal individual from significant relationships on which the individual is dependent. A number of studies would appear to support this point of view.

Maris (1981) compared the social behavior of a group of suicides with groups of attempted suicides and natural deaths. In contrast to the other groups, the suicides participated less in social organizations, were often friendless, and showed a progressive deterioration of interpersonal relationships leading to a state of total social isolation. Reece (1967) described chronic social isolation as one of the most striking features differentiating school-age suicide victims from their peers, and Seiden (1969) found social isolation was a major prodromal sign in college suicides whom he described as "terribly shy, virtually friendless individuals, alienated from all but the most minimal social interactions" (p. 35). Murphy and Robins (1967), while identifying alcoholism and depressive disorder as major correlates of 134 suicides, found that a significantly higher percentage of these lived alone than in the general population.

The question of whether social isolation is more strongly associated with completed suicide than attempted suicide has been raised by some authors. Stengel et al. (1958), for example, found that social isolation was a feature of between 22.6% and 38.2% of the three groups of attempted suicides they studied in London, England, whereas, it figured in 42.7% of cases of completed suicide. Even more striking was their finding that most of those making suicide attempts did so in such a way as to appeal to others in the social environment, whereas they rarely found any indication of this in completed suicides.

One possible interpretation of these findings is that while many attempted suicides are in difficulty with their social environment, they are nonetheless actively engaged with it, whereas completed suicides have reached a more profound degree of social isolation, with more complete alienation from the social environment.

Marital Status

One of the more consistent findings in the literature on suicidal behavior is the strong correlation it has with marital status (Buda and Tsuang, this volume). Single, separated, divorced, and widowed individuals are almost always overrepresented in studies of completed and attempted suicide, and marriage appears to exert a strongly protective effect, a feature that Durkheim (1952) termed the "co-efficient of preservation." In his Chicago study, for example, Maris (1969) found that the suicide rate for those who were married was lower than that for those who were never married, widowed, or divorced, in that order. While widowhood and divorce were associated with suicide in females, the effect was not as marked as in the males. The presence of children added to the protective factor of marriage—a finding reported by Durkheim and confirmed by Maris.

An exception to this general rule on the protective effect of marriage is that early marriage tends to have an aggravating influence on suicide. Dublin (1963) noted that the rates for suicide were higher for married persons than for single persons under the age of 24. Petzel and Cline (1978) have shown that the suicide rate in the United States, for married 15- to 19-year-olds of both sexes is around 1.5 times the rate for unmarried peers. Bancroft et al. (1975) and Kreitman and Schreiber (1979) both noted that teenage wives are at greater risk than single persons for attempted suicide. Maris (1969) has speculated that this may be because younger married couples are often less emotionally developed and are more likely to be mismatched than older married couples. Hawton (1986) suggested that teenage marriages often represent an escape from unsupportive backgrounds and that those marriages are likely to encounter difficulties. Mattson et al. (1967) reported several of the female adolescents in their series to have been pregnant at the time of their suicide attempt, but neither pregnancy nor fear of pregnancy has been found to be significant variables by others (Hawton 1986).

Unemployment

The effects of unemployment on suicidal behavior, although frequently cited, are more difficult to assess because of both inconsistencies in the research findings and the complex interrelationships that employment has with so many other variables, both social and individual, that impinge on suicidal behavior. An extensive review by Platt (1984) found fairly consistent evidence indicating that more attempted suicides are unemployed than among the general population, and that attempted suicide rates are higher among the unemployed than the employed. On the whole, increased duration of unemployment is associated with increased risk, although there are exceptions to this rule.

Studies that have compared suicide rates across geographic areas have produced no consistent evidence of a relationship between unemployment and completed suicide, although individual longitudinal studies comparing employment history over time with suicide rates have confirmed that completed suicides generally have higher rates of unemployment, job instability, and occupational problems than nonsuicides (Platt 1984). Shepherd and Barraclough (1980), for example, examined the work records of 75 suicides and compared them to 150 matched controls. Completed suicides showed more sickness, more unemployment, and more job instability overall.

The direct association of unemployment as a precipitant to either attempted suicide or completed suicide is weak. Platt (1984) reviewed 17 studies in which unemployment or related socioeconomic factors were cited between 2% and 47% of the time as precipitating events, with a wide spread of figures in between. He concluded that "the surprising overall impression is of the relative *unimportance* of unemployment or related socio-economic factors as major precipitants of para-suicide" (p. 106). A study by Platt and Dyer (1987) found that hopelessness, as rated by the Beck Hopelessness Scale (Beck et al. 1974), was significantly higher among the unemployed group. If, as they pointed out, hopelessness increases the risk of suicidal behavior without affecting the degree of suicidal intent, then unemployment may be a stronger risk factor than has generally been recognized.

Studies that have looked at the temporal relationship between unemployment and suicide within defined geographic areas have shown somewhat inconsistent results. In the United States, where the suicide rate was highest during the Great Depression, most studies have found a positive association between increased unemployment and suicide, although some have reported negative findings (Platt 1985). In the United Kingdom, several studies have found a significant association between suicide and unemployment, although this does not hold for all time periods. Kreitman and Platt (1976), for example, reported a significant correlation between the male unemployment rate and the total male suicide rate overall during the years of 1955 to 1980, but this did not hold when smaller time periods were considered. They attributed this to the overriding effect of decreasing the carbon monoxide content of domestic coal gas during this time, which decreased suicide rates after 1962. Goldney and Burvill (1980) reported that during the 1960s in Australia, when the country was experiencing a time of great prosperity, male suicide rates rose to the high levels of the 1930s; during the 1970s, when unemployment rates were second only to the 1930s, there was a progressive fall in suicide rates.

In their study of the suicide rates in the various provinces of Canada, Sakinofsky and Roberts (1985) found that, while the general finding of high unemployment with high suicide held, the maritime provinces, which have traditionally had high levels of unemployment, have always had the lowest suicide rates in the country. They suggested that those areas that have long-standing high unemployment may have greater cultural acceptance and tolerance for it and are less stigmatized by it. By contrast, the sharp rise in suicide rates in Alberta and Saskatchewan in recent years may be linked to a sudden and unacceptable change in an area where employment has traditionally been high.

There are a number of ways in which unemployment may be causally implicated in suicidal behavior. Unemployment may adversely affect self-esteem, provoke depressive reactions, and increase hopelessness; it may also lead to family tension, marital friction, and alcoholism, all of which may increase the individual's alienation from family and friends. On the other hand, personality disorder, alcoholism, drug abuse, and psychiatric illness, all of which are strongly correlated with suicidal behavior, may lead to unemployment. Furthermore, major social changes that affect employment are likely to have other important social consequences that may be more directly related to suicidal behavior. Cormier and Klerman (1985) undertook an analysis of economic fluctuations and suicide rates in the province of Quebec for three different time periods over a period of 30 years. They found a clear positive association between unemployment and suicide for both men and women during the period of 1966 to 1981, a weaker one for the entire period of 1950 to 1981, and a low association for the period of 1950 to 1965. They also found there had been a 381% increase in the divorce rate from 1969 to 1978 and an increase in the female labor force from 32.6% in 1966 to 47% in 1981, both of which they suggested may have changed patterns of social integration and contributed to the increase in suicide rates.

PSYCHOSOCIAL FACTORS PREDISPOSING TO SUICIDAL BEHAVIOR

Early Loss and Suicidal Behavior

Psychoanalytic hypotheses concerning the role of early loss in the etiology of depression and suicide (Abraham 1924; Bowlby 1951; Freud 1917/1957) have generated an extensive literature over the years. Since 1941, when Palmer published his findings on the high incidence of death or absence of a parent or sibling in the backgrounds of 25 serious attempted suicides, more than 30 studies have appeared examining the role of parental loss in suicidal adults (Adam et al. 1978, 1982a, 1982b; Batchelor and Napier 1953; Birtchnell 1970; Bruhn 1962; Crook and Raskin 1975; Dorpat et al. 1965; Farberow 1950; Flood and Seager 1968; Gay and Tonge 1967; Goldney 1981; Greer 1964, 1966; Greer and Gunn 1966; Greer et al. 1966; Hill 1969; Koller and Castanos 1968; Levi et al. 1966; Lukianowicz 1972; McConaghy et al. 1966; Morgan et al. 1975; Moss and Hamilton 1956; Oliver et al. 1971; Paffenbarger and Asnes 1966; Paffenbarger et al. 1969; Palmer 1941; Reitman 1942; Roy 1984; Simon 1950; Stengel et al. 1958; Walton 1958; Werry and Pedder 1976). Twenty of these studies have used case-control design inquiring about the incidence of parental loss in suicidal patients and various control populations. Most have studied patients making suicide attempts, although a few have included patients making suicidal threats, and a small minority (only six studies) have been concerned with completed suicides. A majority have studied consecutive admissions to general hospitals for suicide attempts but several have considered special groups of patients such as psychiatric inpatients, hospitalized depressive patients, or women only. In general, the referral biases of these study groups have been poorly described, and most have included patients with all degrees of severity, although some have restricted themselves to the study of serious attempted suicide.

Many questions can be raised about the methodology of the studies (Munro and Griffiths 1969). To begin with, definitions of what constitutes "parental loss" have not been consistent, with some studies restricting their criteria to permanent parental loss by death, divorce, or separation and others including separations from parents for other reasons or for briefer periods of time. Adult reports about childhood experiences have been shown to be unreliable as to detail, although key events such as the death of the parent and definitive breakup of the parental marriage have been shown to be reported with high reliability (Barraclough and Bunch 1973; Finlay-Jones et al. 1981; Wolkind and Coleman 1983). Data on these matters obtained from case notes and coroners' reports are particularly likely to be unreliable, unless one can be assured the questions of interest are well defined and pursued with vigor by the original interviewer; this assurance is seldom found. This poses particular problems for the study of completed suicide because one is necessarily forced to rely on existing medical records and coroners' records for data unless careful information is sought from surviving family members, a step that has been taken in only one study of completed suicide. Only 10 of the 20 control studies of attempted suicide reviewed used structured research interviews to obtain their data; the others relied on existing case records.

The question of what should constitute an adequate comparison group in studies of this type is also a difficult one. The use of psychiatric patients as controls has been criticized because deficiencies in the early family environment have been reported in many psychiatric disorders, and it has been suggested that this could confound the results (Gregory 1966a, 1966b; Tennant et al. 1980). Although it has been argued that general medical patients and general practice patients likely constitute a more valid control group than psychiatric patients, significant differences in the incidence of parental deprivation between suicidal patients and *all* of these control groups have been found. Greer et al. (1966) used two control groups, one consisting of nonsuicidal patients and another of nonpsychiatric medical and surgical patients, and found the same incidence of loss or absence of parents in both and both to be significantly less in attempted suicide patients. Koller and Castanos (1968) similarly found no differences in the incidence of parental loss in three different control groups: nonsuicidal psychiatric patients, nonsuicidal general hospital patients, and nonsuicidal general population subjects. Significant differences were found between all of these control groups and the suicidal subjects.

Almost all of the studies have selected nonsuicidal subjects for their comparison groups, although it is not always clear just what is meant by this. Most do not specify whether the controls were "nonsuicidal" at the time of the study or whether a lifetime history of suicidal behavior was considered. Even when this has been done, there is the possibility that some of the control populations may have harbored individuals with suicidal predisposition as yet not expressed in overt suicidal behavior. One study that systematically inquired about suicidal ideation as well as suicide attempts found that 18% of general practice control subjects had a significant degree of suicidal ideation, although none had made suicide attempts (Adam et al. 1980).

Despite these methodological differences, support for the notion that early parental loss is associated with later suicidal behavior is strong and consistent. Nearly all of the 20 control studies of attempted suicide have found a higher incidence of parental loss in suicidal patients than controls, although these differences did not always reach statistical significance, possibly because of difficulties with their control samples. McConaghy et al. (1966), for example, do not appear to have screened their control subjects for a history of suicidal behavior, which may have affected the findings. Goldney (1981) compared the 110 attempted suicides in his study to only 25 controls, making adequate statistical comparison questionable. Crook and Raskin (1975) found parental divorce or separation before the age of 12 to be significantly greater in attempted suicides than in controls, but not parental death. The report contains little detailed data, and description of the methodology is extremely sketchy.

Although there appears to be a wide variation in the incidence of parental loss in these studies, ranging from a low of 10% to a high of 77%, close examination suggests that methodological differences account for much of the variation. In general, studies using very broad definitions of parental loss, such as those that include parental strife (Walton 1958) or any separation from a parent for more than 3 months (McConaghy et al. 1966), tend to report high figures; those using very restrictive definitions, such as parental death only, tend to report lower figures. Similarly, studies that limit the age period under consideration to the earliest years of childhood report relatively low figures for parental loss; those extending the age period under consideration to the late teens or early adulthood years tend to report higher figures. Adam (1982) reviewed only those studies restricting the definition of parental loss to permanent loss of one or both parents prior to the ages of 15 to 18 and found greater consistency. The incidence of permanent loss of parents ranged from 32% to 47% in various samples of consecutive attempted suicides, with figures for control groups ranging from 15% to 27%.

Other variables known to affect the incidence of parental loss in such studies are social class and changing patterns of mortality and marital breakdown (Brown and Harris 1978; Crook and Eliot 1980;

Dennehy 1966; Gregory 1958, 1966a, 1966b; Tennant and Bebbington 1978). Gregory (1966b) noted that mortality rates have steadily declined throughout this century (excepting wartime) and divorce rates have increased so that any study sample containing an older age distribution is more likely to have experienced the death of a parent in childhood than parental divorce or separation. This may explain why the two studies that report the highest incidence of early parental death and the lowest incidence of parental divorce or separation are both from the early 1950s (Batchelor and Napier 1953; Farberow 1950). Since 1967, all studies have reported parental divorce or separation to be at least as frequent or in excess of losses from parental death.

Another variable that affects the proportion of losses from various causes in these studies is the age of the subject at the time of parental loss. Families are more likely to break up early on from the divorce or separation of parents than from the death of a parent simply in the nature of things, and this will foster an overrepresentation of losses from divorce or separation in the early years of life. Studies that have examined for parental loss only in the earlier years of childhood are likely to show a predominance of loss from divorce and separation, and those examining parental loss throughout the later years of childhood are more likely to include losses from parental death. One study (Adam et al. 1982b) examining parental loss from birth until the age of 25 and then for smaller age periods in between found two peaks for loss: one for the period from 0 to 5 years of age, where losses from divorce or separation predominated, and a second peak from 17 to 20 years of age, where losses from parental death predominated. Furthermore, as attempted suicide samples tend to have a younger age distribution than completed suicides, they can be expected to have a higher frequency of early parental divorce or separation than studies of completed suicide. This observation is nicely borne out in the study by Dorpat et al. (1965), where a younger sample of attempted suicides was compared to an older sample of successful suicides. While both were found to have a high incidence of broken homes, the predominant cause of the broken home in the attempted suicides was divorce or separation of parents whereas that of the successful suicides was from parental death. The authors interpreted these findings as an indication that the more severe types of loss (parental death) led to a more severe type of suicidal behavior (completed suicide), a conclusion that may, in fact, be erroneous.

Another variable that has been repeatedly examined in these studies with extremely inconsistent results is the sex of the lost parent. Paternal losses have been found to be in excess of maternal losses in a number of studies (Adam et al. 1982a, 1982b; Batchelor and Napier 1953; Hill 1969; McConaghy et al. 1966; Moss and Hamilton

1956; Paffenbarger et al. 1969). Others have reported loss of both parents to stand out over single parent loss (Bruhn 1962; Dorpat et al. 1965; Greer 1964, 1966; Oliver et al. 1971). Koller and Castanos (1968) found loss of the mother significantly higher in attempted suicides than in controls. A number of factors confuse this issue. Many of the studies do not clearly differentiate whether they were referring to losses caused by death of a parent or losses from other reasons, and, where divorce is concerned, it is often extremely difficult to ascertain the extent to which the noncustodial parent is in fact "lost" to the child. In the case of parental death, the surviving parent also may be "lost" through prolonged grief or disruption of the home. Moreover, none of these address the question of what effects these events had on the care given to the child.

Anterospective Studies of Attempted Suicide

Although all of the above studies have examined the incidence of parental loss in samples of attempted suicides, two studies, while collecting data retrospectively, have taken an anterospective *view* of the problem, selecting subjects with a history of parental loss and examining them for the incidence of suicidal behavior. Gay and Tonge (1967) compared on a number of social and psychiatric variables a sample of 136 psychiatric referrals with a history of parental loss before age 15 with 358 patients not reporting such experiences. Of the loss group, 30% reported making suicide attempts compared to 19% of the controls.

In a more focused study, Adam et al. (1982a) interviewed three groups of university students referred to a student health service: one group with a history of parental death before age 17, a second with a history of parental separation or divorce, and a third (the controls) with intact families. All were randomly assigned to a blind interview that inquired in detail about suicidal ideation and behavior. Nearly half (47%) of the parental loss group were found to have suicidal ideation, compared to 13% from intact homes. Furthermore, of the 17 who had made suicide attempts, 14 had a history of early parental loss. Differences were highly significant in both cases.

Parental Loss and Completed Suicide

Studies of completed suicide are fewer than those of attempted suicides, presumably because of the greater difficulty in accessing information about the early childhood of these persons. None offers conclusive evidence for or against a role for parental loss, and most have serious methodological problems. Flood and Seager's (1968) study, which found no difference in the incidence of broken homes between former inpatients who had killed themselves and two comparison groups of inpatients who did not, involved a review of case notes written when the patients were under psychiatric care earlier and in which the recording of data regarding parental deaths, divorces, and separations may not have been reliable. Indeed, the authors acknowledged that when no specific note of such events was found, it was assumed that the subject's childhood had been "normal." The sole criterion for selecting comparison patients was that they were alive, and they noted that both control groups contained significant numbers of patients who had made suicide attempts. No actual figures for "broken homes" are given in the article and although the authors noted that the suicide group had a slightly higher number of patients with broken homes, they state that "this did not approach statistical significance" (p. 449).

Paffenbarger and colleagues (Paffenbarger and Asnes 1966; Paffenbarger et al. 1969) studied the case records of 381 college students who had attended university 15 to 40 years before and who eventually committed suicide. Significantly more of the suicidal students had lost their fathers from death or separation by the time of college case taking than among living students matched from the same college year. There is no indication in these studies whether such information was routinely inquired about at the time the original history was taken or how diligently it was recorded.

Bunch et al. (1971) examined a sample of 75 consecutive suicides and acquired data on parental deaths and their dates from interviews with relatives, cross-checked from the official death register. Subjects whose informants had wrongly identified the parental death were excluded. These were compared to 150 living subjects matched for age group, sex, marital status, and residence drawn from two general practices. No significant differences were found in the proportion of suicides and controls bereaved of a parent before the age of 16. No attention was given to loss or absence of parents for other reasons.

Dorpat et al. (1965) compared 114 consecutive completed suicides with 121 subjects who attempted suicide and found both to have experienced a high incidence of parental loss (50% and 63.9%, respectively), they did not compare these samples with nonsuicidal controls. Furthermore, the authors reported that they were unable to get information on the early family background of 22% of the attempted suicides and 8% of the suicides.

Roy (1984) compared 13 manic-depressive patients who had committed suicide with a sample of 13 manic-depressive patients who did not and found a high incidence of permanent separation from parents (54%) compared to controls (8%). This study does not specify the time period of early life under consideration, and the sample is extremely small.

Quality of Parental Care and Suicidal Behavior

Although there would appear to be little doubt from this examination of the evidence that parental deprivation in childhood plays some role as a causal agent in suicidal behavior, the nearly exclusive attention given to the role of permanent parental loss as an etiologic variable has been criticized. Munro (1965) drew attention to the obvious fact that many persons appear to experience the breakup of a home without developing serious psychiatric illness, and others have pointed out that a variety of moderating variables may act to attenuate the harmful consequences of such events. The presence of substitute parents, siblings, and other extended family and community supports may all decrease the emotional impact of loss on the child, just as separation from siblings, relocation from familiar surroundings, and multiple changes of care takers may make the effects more severe (Birtchnell 1974; Nelson 1982; Rutter 1972; Tennant et al. 1980).

Considering the importance of such moderating factors, it is surprising how little attention they have been given in studies of the early family environment of suicidal individuals. Equally surprising is the relative paucity of data on the quality of the early home environment in those subjects not experiencing the actual disruption of the home from a major loss.

Greer (1964) examined the family environment subsequent to the breakup of the home and found no differences between attempted suicides and controls in the numbers reared by the remaining parent, by other persons, or in an orphanage, findings replicated by Koller and Castanos (1968). In a second study (Greer et al. 1966), however, nonpsychiatric controls from broken homes were more likely to have lived with the remaining parent than either attempted suicides or nonsuicidal psychiatric controls. Neither study evaluated the quality of the family environment in any detail.

A number of other authors have pointed to the frequency with which the early family environment is disturbed, quite apart from the definitive breakup of the home. Greer (1964) found that while 51.8% of the attempted suicides had experienced parental loss, an additional 13.6% came from "otherwise disturbed homes." A high degree of marital strife, marital disharmony, and disturbed relationships with parents has also been reported by others (Batchelor and Napier 1953; Bruhn 1962; Walton 1958). In a study of suicidal adolescents, Haider (1968) concluded that only 12.5% of her sample came from "normal" families. Werry and Pedder (1976) noted that only 36% of attempted suicides compared to 83% of controls came from intact, conflict-free homes, and only 25% of their attempted suicides reported "good relations" with their parents.

Several more recent studies have examined the long-term quality of early parental care in suicidal patients more systematically. Using a standardized scale of perceived childhood stress, Goldney (1981) found that, in addition to reporting a broken home more frequently, attempted suicides were more likely to report that their parents had often quarreled, that they had frequent disagreements with their parents, and that they perceived their parents' characters negatively. In another study (Goldney 1985), the Parental Bonding Instrument (PBI), a standardized measure of parental care, was administered to 43 young women who had taken drug overdoses and compared to nonsuicidal community health clinic patients. Suicidal subjects scored significantly less than controls on measures of maternal and paternal care and significantly higher on measures of maternal and paternal overprotection. Silove et al. (1987), also using the PBI, found fewer early adverse experiences among attempted suicides than in the Goldney study, with no significant differences between subjects and controls on parental care, although paternal overprotection was found higher. However, a complex measure combining affectionless and controlling parents with recent interpersonal stress did differentiate the two.

Ross et al. (1983) examined a group of 266 nonpsychiatric subjects for the presence of suicidal ideation and compared the suicidal ideators with the others on a standard measure of parental rearing patterns. Results showed that those with suicidal ideation had significantly higher scores on parental rejection, guilt engendering, and favoring of siblings. In addition, fathers were more often rated as abusive, depriving, and punitive than the fathers of controls.

Adam et al. (1982b) made a detailed inquiry into the family backgrounds of attempted suicides and nonsuicidal general practice controls. Losses and separation from parents were recorded, and the quality of the overall family environment was rated according to standardized criteria. While more than half of the attempted suicide sample experienced parental loss by the age of 25 compared to only 22% of the controls, 92% were rated as having had an unstable or chaotic early family environment compared to 40% of the controls. Moreover, the percentage of suicidal subjects in the most severe "chaotic" category was much higher (45%) compared to the controls (21%).

Furthermore, the severity of suicidal activity was found to be correlated with the severity of the early family disturbance. Of the attempted suicides rated as having chaotic family backgrounds, 75%

were multiple attempters in contrast to 55% of those rated unstable and 44% of the stable group. Of particular interest was the finding that 18% of the control subjects, all of whom had been screened for attempted suicide, were found to have suicidal ideation. Of this small subgroup of controls, only 8% of subjects who had stable homes were rated as having suicidal ideation, compared to 23% of those with unstable homes and 83% of those with chaotic homes. Indeed, taking both attempted suicides and control subjects together, 95% of all subjects having a chaotic early family environment had suicidal ideation compared to 62% of those rated unstable and 20% of those rated stable.

These general findings were confirmed in another study examining suicidal behavior in university students with a history of parental loss (Adam et al. 1982a). In this study, too, suicidal ideation and suicidal behavior were particularly prominent in those patients experiencing early parental loss when this resulted in long-term disruption of family stability. Taken together, both findings suggested strongly that, while parental loss is significantly associated with suicidal behavior, it is at best a crude indicator of more general and pervasive inadequacies and discontinuities in the childhood environment.

Family Environment of Suicidal Children and Adolescents

Studies of suicidal children and adolescents bear scrutiny as the family influences of interest are closer to hand, although this very proximity can make the distinction between predisposing and precipitating events more difficult to assess. In general, they support the notion that pervasive and long-standing family disturbances are associated with suicidal behavior and that these disturbances involve a variety of deficiencies in parental care beyond simply the loss or absence of parents.

As in the case of some of the adult studies, studies in children that have focused on parental loss as an isolated variable have produced equivocal and misleading findings. Roughly half of most samples of suicidal adolescents or children appear to have experienced permanent loss of parental figures, but so have many other psychiatrically disturbed children. When these children have been used for comparison purposes, differences have sometimes been negligible. Mattson et al. (1967) found that only half of all children and adolescents presenting as emergency cases had intact families, but found no significant differences between those with suicidal behavior and those without. Stanley and Barter (1970) found parental loss before the age of 12 to be greater in suicidal adolescent inpatients than other psychiatrically ill adolescents, but no differences for losses after age 12.

Garfinkel et al. (1982), on the other hand, found more than half of 505 children and adolescents presenting to a pediatric hospital following a suicide attempt had a history of "parental absence" in contrast to 16% of nonsuicidal controls.

Other studies have found, as in the adult studies, that quite apart from parental loss there is almost always evidence of serious deficiencies in parenting. In a clinical study of 64 suicidal children and adolescents, Haider (1968) noted that while half her sample were living in broken homes with only one parent or in an institutional environment, the majority of others came from homes disorganized in other ways, such as frequent marital strife, parental alcoholism, or the presence of a problem relative in the home. Topol and Reznikoff (1982) found serious family problems of all sorts to be greater in suicidal than in nonsuicidal hospitalized adolescents or in normal coping adolescents, and their families were least like "the physician's view of a well-adjusted family." In a study of 16 preschool children who had made suicide attempts, Rosenthal and Rosenthal (1984) found that while the families of suicidal children had the same incidence of divorce and parental death as a comparison group of children with serious behavioral problems, the suicidal children had been subject to more direct child abuse and neglect. This study and that of Green (1978), who found the incidence of self-destructive behavior including suicidal ideation and self-mutilation dramatically higher among battered children than among those who were neglected or normal, suggest that the direct experience of physical abuse may be an underrated predisposing variable.

Less direct forms of parental unavailability have been implicated in younger children as well. Pfeffer and colleagues (Pfeffer 1981; Pfeffer et al. 1979) found no differences in the incidence of parental separations or absent fathers in latency-age children admitted with suicidal behavior when they were compared with nonsuicidal children. However, there was a significantly higher percentage of depression in their mothers. In a study comparing 16 adolescents with severe depression who had made suicide attempts with 18 severely depressed adolescents who had not, Friedman et al. (1984) found that a family history of chronic illness, either physical or psychiatric, was the main variable differentiating the two groups. Other authors, in less rigorous studies, have also referred to the emotional neglect experienced by some suicidal children whose parents, while physically present, were emotionally unavailable (Glaser 1965; Gould 1965; Sabbath 1969; Schrut 1964). Cohen-Sandler et al. (1982a, 1982b) looked at the impact of a variety of family-related life events across the life span of suicidal children. Comparing latency-age children with suicidal behavior to two comparison groups of depressed nonsuicidal children and nonsuicidal children with other psychiatric illness, they found that the suicidal children had experienced family-related events to a greater degree than both comparison groups and that they had experienced increasing amounts of these stresses as they matured.

Two studies that have examined families of suicidal children directly are of interest. Williams and Lyons (1976) compared the family interactions of families with a suicidal adolescent member with those of six families containing a normal adolescent. Direct observation of family interactions around a task-centered family interview showed significantly more indications of family dysfunction in families with a suicidal member than in the nonsuicidal families. They were less effective in communicating, showed more conflictual interaction and hostile affect, and more fragmented and disorderly speech. Tishler and McKenry (1982) had the parents of suicidal adolescents and the parents of children who presented to the emergency room with minor injuries fill out a number of questionnaires measuring self-esteem, depression, anxiety, alcohol abuse, and suicidal ideation. While there were no major differences in the numbers of either group that came from single-parent families, the parents of suicidal adolescents had considerably more psychiatric symptomatology. Excessive alcohol use was significantly higher in both parents of suicidal adolescents. Fathers were found to have lower self-esteem and more evidence of depression and the mothers more suicidal ideation and anxiety than control parents.

A study of Hawton et al. (1982) provided some further support for the notion that the degree of family instability and the severity of suicidal activity may be directly correlated. In this study of suicidal adolescents, those with higher suicidal intent had experienced significantly more severe family disturbance and had poorer communication with their parents than those with less severe suicidal intent at initial presentation. Moreover, they were more likely to make a repeat suicide attempt within a year than were other groups.

Taken as a whole, these studies argue strongly and consistently for the importance of social and environmental factors in predisposing to suicidal ideation, suicide attempts, and completed suicide. Of all the factors explored, disturbances in the early family environment stand out as most likely to be causal. While much attention has been given to the role of parental loss, particularly in the early studies, it is by no means the only deficiency in parental care that has been implicated, nor may it be the most important. Rutter (1985) pointed out that the ultimate effects of adverse experiences in childhood are dependent on a number of interacting variables, including the inherent resiliency of the child and the presence or absence of alternative caretakers and helpful siblings. While systematic studies of the role of these protective factors have lagged behind those that have studied adverse experiences in suicidal patients, the available evidence suggests that they are often missing. Indeed, in the few studies that have looked in detail at the quality of the early family environment prior to and subsequent to parental loss in suicidal patients, the resiliency of the families in the nonsuicidal subjects who had experienced loss was a striking and significant finding (Adam et al. 1982a, 1982b).

Although the focus of this review has been on examining the evidence linking such experiences specifically to suicidal behavior, they may well contribute to some of the more enduring personality traits described in suicidal patients. Personality studies of attempted-suicides have repeatedly pointed to immaturity, impulsivity, and hostility in interpersonal relationships and a number of these studies have shown that these difficulties are both long-standing and extend over broad categories of relationships (Eastwood et al. 1972; Farmer and Creed 1986; Pallis and Birtchnell 1977; Philip 1970; Weissman et al. 1973). These characteristics would seem almost certain to contribute to the absence of supportive relationships, which has previously been noted in these patients, and over time may be one of the principal reasons for the social isolation so often seen in completed suicides. Indeed, it seems likely that personality variables, particularly those that affect potentially supportive key relationships, are the principal agents mediating between the earlier predisposing events and the later social and life events that so often precipitate suicidal actions.

CURRENT SOCIAL ENVIRONMENT AND PRECIPITATING EVENTS

Interpersonal Events in Attempted Suicide

Clinical studies of attempted suicide over the life cycle have repeatedly pointed to the importance of interpersonal conflict as an antecedent event in suicide attempts (Adams 1985; Goldney and Burvill 1980; Stengel 1964; Weissman 1974). Greer (1966), for example, found 35% of attempted suicides to have experienced the actual recent disruption of a close interpersonal relationship compared to 16% of nonsuicidal controls and 8% of normal controls. Much higher percentages, between 50% and 80%, are reported when quarrels, threatened separations, and other types of interpersonal conflict are included (Adam 1982; Adam et al. 1978; Lukianowicz 1972; Morgan et al. 1975; Oliver et al. 1971). In adults, lovers, spouses, or other family members are most often involved, but other significant persons such as nursing staff and psychotherapists have also been mentioned (Maltsberger and Buie 1974; Modestin 1987). In a detailed study of the 2 days preceding self-poisoning in 103 cases, Fieldsend and Lowenstein

(1981) found interpersonal events with "key persons" had occurred in 58% of cases and in a further 11% of cases with a "non-key person." Quarreling was the most common event, followed by separation, infidelity, and "other acts."

Similar findings have been reported in children and adolescents where conflict with parents, siblings, peers, boyfriends, and girlfriends have been widely found as key events preceding suicidal actions (Hawton et al. 1982; Mattson et al. 1967; Stanley and Barter 1970; Tishler et al. 1981). To cite one example, Garfinkel and Golombek (1983) studied 505 suicidal adolescents and found conflict with parents, siblings, and opposite-sexed friends to be the precipitating event in 75% of cases, and school-related problems, problems with the law, and abuse or severe neglect, all of which carry implications for interpersonal conflict, in others. Such events are extremely common as precipitating events leading to psychiatric referral in children generally, and studies comparing suicidal children and adolescents to other disturbed children and adolescents have not always found significant differences (Pfeffer et al. 1979; Stanley and Barter 1970).

Several clinical studies have suggested that the family conflict that precedes suicidal behavior may involve not only profound rejection and intense hostility directed to the suicidal member but sometimes direct death wishes as well. Rosenbaum and Richman (1970) conducted family interviews with the families of 35 attempted suicides and found that the majority expressed feelings of being fed up with the patient and that implicit or explicit suggestions that they would be better off dead occurred with "unexpected frequency." Sabbath (1969) described three cases of "expendable" adolescents whose parents unmistakably conveyed their desire to be rid of the child, one of whom subsequently killed himself. Similar findings have been reported by others (Gould 1965; Glaser 1965; Stone 1973).

Interpersonal Events and Completed Suicide

Data about the events leading up to completed suicide over the life cycle are more fragmentary because information about the final period must usually be reconstructed from the reports of others, and this information may not be readily available due to the relative social isolation of many suicides at the time of their deaths and the reluctance of informants to give complete information for a variety of reasons. Suicide notes are found only in a fraction of cases, and these may not reflect a full or accurate account of the reasons for the act. Coroners' reports, unless they make use of psychological autopsy techniques, often obscure the account rather than clarify it. Yet, taken together, they suggest that the events preceding suicide are often similar to those described in studies of attempted suicide. Robins' (1981) account of the detailed case histories of his well-known diagnostic study of 134 suicides, for example, is replete with accounts of difficulties in close relationships prior to the final suicidal act. While the extensive evidence linking social isolation to completed suicide suggests that the final suicidal act may be less closely linked to interpersonal conflict and disappointment than in attempted suicide, more careful studies suggest that this may be more apparent than real.

Conroy and Smith (1983) conducted a detailed study of 19 patients who committed suicide during psychiatric hospitalization, collecting information from case notes, letters, other communications, and the reports of psychological autopsies conducted following the patient's death. In 18 of the 19 cases they reported a significant "family loss" issue such as estrangement from family members, death or illness of significant others, or divorce or separation issues between the patient or spouse. In five cases, most of whom were chronic patients, the loss or threatened loss seemed to be that of a powerful institutional attachment, and the suicide appeared to have occurred at a point when discharge plans or talk of transfer to another hospital was in progress. A number of similar studies have noted the relationship between conflict with family members or with hospital staff and difficulties around discharge plans in suicide among psychiatric patients. Hankoff (1980) has shown that suicide in hospitalized patients is more likely to occur during periods of staff disorganization and staff demoralization, when staff are likely to be less tolerant and resilient in their handling of difficult patients. In a case review of 10 patients who killed themselves, Yarden (1974) noted that relations between the patients and their social environment, including family and caretakers, were grossly unfavorable in every case. Maltsberger and Buie (1974) pointed to the dangers that countertransference hostility poses in the psychotherapeutic management of suicidal patients who tend to be difficult and demanding and who tend to provoke rejection. Modestin (1987) reported on a small series of inpatient suicides where countertransference issues had led to serious failure in therapeutic judgment, which contributed to the patient's suicide. His investigations, which involved the review of clinical records of 149 patient suicides, found clear evidence of these countertransference difficulties in only 6% of cases, but he suggested this is likely to be a low figure.

Shafii et al. (1985) conducted a psychological autopsy of 20 children and adolescents, aged 12 to 19 years, who had committed suicide and a matched control group selected from the victims' friends. Compared to the controls, suicides showed more antisocial behavior, alcohol and drug abuse, and previous suicidal behavior, and significantly more had been exposed to a sibling's or friend's attempted suicide or completed suicide, parental emotional problems, and parental absence or physical or emotional abusiveness. In their case note review of psychiatric patients who subsequently killed themselves, Flood and Seager (1968) reported that there were twice as many patients in the suicide group having had a marked degree of disturbed hospital relationships than in either of their two control groups. More of the suicidal patients discharged themselves against advice, and hospital notes suggested they were often considered overdemanding and uncooperative by nursing staff. The direct collusion of spouses or other persons who, through direct hostility or neglect, appear to have wished the patient dead has also been reported (Miller 1979; Rubinstein and Winston 1976).

A considerable body of evidence would seem to indicate that the interpersonal difficulties that precede suicidal behavior are not merely the result of transient conflict but are part of more pervasive and long-standing difficulties with relationships. While the higher incidence of single, divorced, and separated persons among those who make suicide attempts or who kill themselves may be taken as presumptive evidence of this, a number of studies have addressed the issue more directly. Adam et al. (1980) found 47% of attempted suicides were rated as having chaotic interpersonal relationships at the time of their interview in contrast to 7% of controls; only 10% had stable current relationships. These difficulties were often long-standing. Moreover, 28% saw no hope of change, 32% felt that their current relationship was likely to fail, and 41% felt it was certain to fail.

Using a standardized social interaction scale to measure the availability and perceived adequacy of social bonds, Hart and Williams (1987) compared the interpersonal network of 52 attempted suicides with 52 matched nonsuicidal psychiatric patients. Two visual analogue scales allowed the patients to self-rate their degree of satisfaction with their interpersonal network and the strength of their desire to live. The social interaction interview and the visual analogue scales were administered within 48 hours of the suicide attempt and again 6 weeks later; the visual analogue scales were also given at weekly intervals in between. The attempted suicides' scores showed them to have a significantly more limited interpersonal network, which extended across a wide spectrum of interpersonal bonds. They reported significantly less satisfaction and a lower degree of perceived adequacy on their self-ratings of their relationships, indicating they were aware of the deficits and troubled by them. Over the 6-week period, attempted suicides showed some improvement in their perceptions of the adequacy of relationships, although the actual availability of the interpersonal bonds and the observer-rated adequacy of their general interpersonal contacts did not change. Control subjects showed little change in their ratings over the 6-week period. Whether these effects in the attempted suicides were because of a less pessimistic outlook associated with improvement in their mood or because the relationships had altered in response to the suicide attempt is impossible to discern from their data.

The absence of supportive relationships in suicidal patients, while implied in many studies, has been specifically reported by a number of other authors. Cohen-Sandler et al. (1982b) noted that repeat suicide attempts are more frequent in suicidal children discharged from the hospital who were not returned home. Topol and Reznikoff (1982) reported suicidal adolescents far less likely to have a close confidant than either nonsuicidal hospitalized adolescents or nonhospitalized coping adolescents. Slater and Depue (1981) reported that lack of confidant social support was one of the main factors differentiating suicidal depressive patients from nonsuicidal depressive patients and felt it confirmed the idea that the presence of social support may buffer against the impact of life-threatening events.

Similar findings have been reported in completed suicides. In a study of 75 suicides, Bunch (1972) found that significantly more suicides were bereaved of a parent in the 5 years before their suicide than were matched general population controls. Maternal bereavement, in particular, stood out, and single male suicides were more often bereaved of mothers than other suicides, suggesting that unmarried men who maintain more dependent relationships on their mothers may be more vulnerable to that particular loss. As with other studies on suicide, vulnerability was also related to divorce and separation; intact marriage appeared to be protective.

Life Events in Suicidal Behavior

Several studies using life events scales have shown life events generally to be increased preceding suicide attempts. Paykel et al. (1975) found attempted suicides to have experienced four times as many life events in the 6 months prior to their suicide attempt than general population controls in the 6 months prior to their interviews, and twice as many life events as depressive patients before the onset of their depression. The rate for life events among the attempted suicides was elevated throughout the whole 6-month period, but reached a peak in the month before the suicide attempt when one-third of all events had occurred. More of these events were classified as undesirable than in either of the other two groups.

Cochrane and Robertson (1975) came to similar conclusions in their study of 100 male attempted suicides. A standardized life events inventory showed they experienced far more life stress in the year preceding their attempt than did a comparison group of general practice patients. More of the events were negative and beyond the patient's control. A cluster of events associated with interpersonal relationships such as quarrels, fights, and sexual problems were particularly prominent in the attempted suicide group.

Studying 47 male patients admitted following a suicide attempt, Luscomb et al. (1980), using a life change inventory, did not find suicide attempters to differ from nonsuicidal psychiatric patients in the levels of stress experienced during the year preceding hospital admission. Older patients, however, reported three times as much stress and more exit events than did older controls, and the middle-aged group experienced more exits than did younger patients. Methodological problems make this study somewhat harder than others to assess. The attempted suicide group were slightly younger than controls, and they contained a higher ratio of married persons (51%) than is usually found among groups of attempted suicides. The use of psychiatric patients as controls may have also lessened differences between the two groups, although the authors claimed these to be a more valid control group than general practice patients.

Isherwood et al. (1982) compared 150 attemped suicides, 100 drivers injured in automobile accidents, and 200 matched general population controls. Patients were compared on a schedule of recent life events, and a discriminate function analysis was applied to the data. Excessive amounts of life events stress were found strongly associated with attempted suicide but not with either accident or control subjects.

Hagnell and Rorsman (1980) examined the records of 28 of the 3,563 persons in a prospective psychiatric cohort (the Loudby study) who had killed themselves during the course of the study, comparing them to normal controls and subjects who died natural deaths. Almost all were considered to have been psychiatrically ill at the time of their suicides, and significantly more suicides than controls had experienced undesirable events (e.g., a blow to self-esteem, object loss) in the week prior to their deaths. In the year prior to their deaths, significantly more had experienced occupational problems, changes in residence, and object loss.

Interaction of Early Predisposing Events With Later Precipitating Events

If the early family disturbances noted above indeed predispose to later relationship difficulties and if these in turn are directly linked in the causal chain of suicidal behavior, then one would expect to find a significant interaction between the two. A number of studies have investigated this with somewhat mixed results.

Bruhn (1962) found both the incidence of broken homes in childhood and absence or death of a family member in the year prior to admission to be significantly elevated in suicide attempters than in psychiatric outpatient controls. A significant interaction was noted between the history of a broken home and more recent household instability. Of the attempted suicides with broken homes, 66% also had recent absence or death of family members compared to 42% of attempted suicides with no broken home.

Greer (1964) reported that subjects with parental loss were significantly more likely to have experienced recent disruption of a close interpersonal relationship than controls (44% versus 26%), but this was not the case for those with intact homes. Levi et al. (1966) compared 40 patients hospitalized for attempted suicide with 40 matched patients with suicidal urges or thoughts and a control group of 40 nonsuicidal patients. Inquiry was made into childhood history of separations of more than 6 months' duration prior to age 17 from parents, parental surrogates, or siblings. Antecedent separations, defined as actual disruption of a close interpersonal relationship within 1 year of admission or a suicide attempt, were also considered. Childhood separations were significantly more frequent in attempted suicides than in controls, but not significantly more frequent than in the suicidal ideation group. Attempted suicides had more separation per patient than in either of the two other groups. Attempted suicides also had significantly more reports of antecedent separations than controls, although once again differences between suicide attempters and the suicidal ideation group were not significant (attempted suicides 60%, suicidal ideation 50%, controls 30%). A significant interaction was found between *early* childhood separation (before age 7) and antecedent separation when controls and suicide attempters were compared, but not overall. However, when all 120 patients were pooled, a highly significant interaction between childhood separation and antecedent separation was found.

These findings are difficult to place in perspective because of a number of methodological problems. The inclusion of separations from siblings or schooling and camp separations in the inclusion criteria for early childhood separation may have diluted the figures in this study. Moreover, the criteria for antecedent separation in this study (as the investigators pointed out) are problematic. Separations occurring over a 12-month period may have included events too remote from the suicide attempt to have been clinically significant (the sharp increase in life events during the month preceding a suicide attempt has already been mentioned). Moreover, the exclusion of threatened separation may have ruled out important experiences that other workers have repeatedly implicated as precipitants to attempted suicide. The authors reported that 7 of the 16 attempted suicides in their study *not* classified as having "antecedent separation" did in fact report the recent threat of loss of an important person, and the inclusion of these would clearly have affected their results on interaction. Inclusion of these would have increased the number of antecedent events involving interpersonal difficulties from 61% to 77% in the attempted suicide group. Unfortunately, the authors did not report figures on threatened separations in the other two groups.

Stein et al. (1974) conducted a similar study comparing childhood and antecedent separations in both black and white attempted suicide patients using nonsuicidal controls for comparison. They used identical criteria for defining both childhood and antecedent separation as in the earlier study (Levi et al. 1966) and found very similar results. White and black attempted suicides of both sexes had more childhood separations than controls, although among blacks the findings were statistically significant only for females. Antecedent separations were greater in attempted suicides than controls for all groups except black females, although a trend was found for them as well. All the attempted suicides showed a trend toward a greater incidence of patients with both childhood and antecedent separations, but no significant interactions were found between early childhood separation and separations experienced later in life. However, as in the previous study, when the total population of whites (both attempted suicides and controls) was considered, significant interaction was found between antecedent and childhood separations. This was not found for either of the black populations.

While this study would appear to confirm the overall results of the previous study by Levi et al. (1966), it contains the same faults in study design—namely criteria for childhood separation are rather broad and those for antecedent separations rather narrow. Furthermore, neither study addresses the quality of the childhood experience, or the experiences prior to and following separation, and the effects of these later on in life. While the authors of this study noted that they inquired about threatened separations, they did not include these in their analysis of antecedent separations.

Lester and Beck (1976) collected data on both early loss and recent interpersonal loss as part of a larger study of 246 attempted suicides interviewed within 48 hours after admission to the hospital. Their criteria defined early loss as any permanent separation from mother or father before the age of 15. Interpersonal loss (real, threatened, or imagined) and interpersonal friction with parents, children, spouses, and lovers were all inquired about for the 6 months preceding admission to the hospital. They found an association between permanent separation and the experience of recent loss for females but not for males and not for interpersonal friction or marital breakdown. In females, the loss of both parents before age 10 appeared to bear a stronger relationship than later losses. The report of this study is extremely sketchy and it contains little raw data to support its conclusions. No descriptions of the sample referral bias are given and no control population was used.

Silove et al. (1987) compared 43 attempted suicides from three general hospitals to 42 general practice patients from the same areas. Separations from parents of more than 6 months before age 16 were considered. Subjects completed the PBI and items from a life event inventory, which inquired about major conflict and separations from significant others in the previous year. Attempted suicides rated their fathers as more overprotective than did controls, and there was a trend to rate them as uncaring as well. Mothers were rated as somewhat uncaring and excessively protective, but the differences were not significant. The rates for early parental separations were almost identical for attempted suicides and controls, but the rates for recent interpersonal stress were significantly higher (77% versus 33%). More of the attempted suicide patients than controls had both early loss and recent interpersonal stressors and more had exposure to at least one neglectful and controlling parent, as well as stressors prior to admission. Of the attempted suicides, 47% reported one form of adversity in their families of origin in addition to a recent interpersonal stressor. A pattern of early exposure to neglectful and overprotective parenting followed by recent conflict or separations in adulthood was found to discriminate most clearly between the attempted suicide and control groups.

Social Variables and Psychiatric Illness

The prevalence of psychiatric illness in suicidal patients is such a prominent feature that suicidal behavior has been characterized by some authorities simply as a symptom of mental illness (Barraclough et al. 1974; Clayton 1985; Murphy 1987). This relationship of psychiatric disorder and suicide is explored in Black and Winokur's chapter, this volume. Yet those few studies that have compared psychiatric patients who exhibit suicidal behavior with those who do not suggest that the same early family, social, and personality variables may differentiate between suicidal and nonsuicidal patients as between suicidal and nonsuicidal controls generally. The most extensive body of data is that which compares suicidal depressive patients with nonsuicidal depressive patients. This section will examine the impact of psychosocial factors on suicide risk in psychiatrically ill persons.

Parental Loss in Suicidal Depressive Patients

Six studies have been reported comparing the early family environment of suicidal depressive patients to nonsuicidal depressive patients. Four of these have examined the incidence of early parental loss and two have looked at the quality of early family environment in more detail. Walton (1958) compared 60 depressed inpatients who had made suicide attempts or serious threats to 163 depressed inpatients with no history of suicide threats or behavior. He found an incidence of parental deprivation in 76.6% of the suicidal subjects compared with only 19.6% of controls. Hill (1969) compared 469 depressed inpatients who had made suicide attempts with a total of 1,483 nonsuicidal depressed inpatients, examining for the incidence of parental death before the age of 15. The death of a father between the ages of 10 and 14 in males was found significantly greater in the suicidal depressed inpatients than in the controls but differences were not significant for maternal deaths or for female patients. Crook and Raskin (1975) compared 115 depressed patients with 115 nonsuicidal depressed inpatients and 285 normal controls for the incidence of separation from one or both natural parents because of parental death, divorce, or separation before the age of 12. No differences were found between the two groups in the incidence of parental death up to age 12, although parental divorce and separation were significantly greater. Roy (1984) compared 13 manic-depressive patients who had killed themselves with a control group of 13 manic-depressive patients who were living and found that the incidence of early parental loss, which included death or permanent separation from parents, was 54% in the suicidal patients and only 8% in the controls. The small number of patients in this study has previously been noted.

Kosky et al. (1986) compared 147 depressed children under the age of 15 who scored positively for suicidal ideation with 481 depressed children without suicidal ideation on a number of demographic and clinical variables. There were no differences in the numbers coming from broken homes, but the suicidal ideation group showed significantly more disturbance of child-father relationships, child-sibling relationships, persistent discordant intrafamilial relationships, and persecution and discrimination (including child abuse). The two groups did not differ significantly on psychiatric symptoms as rated by a symptom checklist. Friedman et al. (1984) compared 16 highly suicidal depressed adolescents with 18 adolescents who were equally depressed by DSM-III criteria (American Psychiatric Association 1980) and Research Diagnostic Criteria (RDC) (Spitzer et al. 1978) but who were not suicidal and found that the suicidal adolescents had experienced significantly more chronic illness in their parents (both physical and psychiatric) before the age of

14. Psychiatric illness had not only occurred more frequently in these parents but had occurred earlier in the child's life. Of the mothers of the attempted suicides' families, 50% had chronic illness before the patient was age 14. Additionally, these families were more likely to have had psychiatric illness in both parents.

Social and Interpersonal Variables in Suicidal Depressed Patients

Paykel and Dienelt (1971) followed 189 depressed patients after discharge from the hospital and compared the 13 of these who had made a suicide attempt during the ensuing 10 months with the others. The suicidal depressed patients were found to be significantly younger, to have a previous history of suicide attempts, and to show evidence of underlying personality disturbance with persistent overt hostility. Their depressions were felt to be of the neurotic rather than the endogenous type. Birtchnell and Alarcon (1971) compared a group of patients making suicide attempts with a control group of nonsuicidal depressed outpatients. They found that while the attempted suicides were equally depressed, the depressive episode during which they had attemped suicide had occurred following an acute conflict with a significant other with whom the attempter had had an intensely hostile and ambivalent relationship. In a similar study, Weissman et al. (1973) compared 29 women referred because of attempted suicide with a control group of 29 women referred with acute depression but no attempted suicide. As with the previous study, they found no difference in the degree of depression on standardized scales between the two groups, but those who had attempted suicide had made more previous attempted suicides, more often had impaired work records, and had histories of drug abuse and criminal convictions. Furthermore, they showed significantly more overt hostility, demandingness, and interpersonal friction than the nonsuicidal depressed patients and reported more arguments with family members, friends, and dates. Barraclough and Pallis (1975) found depressive suicides more likely than living depressed patients referred to the hospital to be unmarried, to be living alone, and to have made a previous suicide attempt.

While all these studies have described the personality difficulties in terms of traits, two studies used DSM-III Axis II diagnostic criteria. Friedman et al. (1983) studied a group of 53 adolescents and young adults consecutively admitted to a unit specializing in the treatment of depression. Those patients with the DSM-III Axis II diagnosis of borderline personality disorder as well as an Axis I diagnosis of depression had a significantly higher incidence of attempted suicide than depressed patients with no Axis II diagnosis or Axis II diagnosis other than borderline personality disorder. Additionally, the patients made more seriously lethal suicide attempts. A smaller study by the same research group that compared depressed adolescents who were highly suicidal with equally depressed nonsuicidal adolescents found no differences in the incidence of Axis II diagnosis of borderline personality disorder (Friedman et al. 1984). Although the authors made no comment on the inconsistency of their findings, a number of methodological issues may have contributed to their negative findings in the second study. For one thing, the validity of DSM-III criteria and RDC for personality diagnosis is questionable in a sample so young (average age, 16), as the authors pointed out, and for another, their criteria for selecting their nonsuicidal control sample are unclear. While their control subjects reported no history of suicide attempts and were not considered to be "immediate" suicide risks on the basis of their current communications, the extent to which they had ever experienced suicidal ideation is not reported. All these subjects were entering an age period when suicidal behavior increases sharply (15 to 24 years) and differences between the two groups might well diminish over time. It is important to note that their other study sample was, on average, 5 years older.

Social and Interpersonal Variables in Alcoholic Patients Who Commit Suicide

Next to affective disorder, alcoholism is the most frequent recorded diagnosis among completed suicides, and here too the evidence suggests that social and interpersonal variables are strongly implicated (see Flavin et al., this volume). Murphy and Robins (1967) compared 60 suicides who had suffered from affective disorder and 31 who had a diagnosis of alcoholism to general population data on a number of social and interpersonal variables. The alcoholic suicides are more often divorced, separated, or living alone than the general population, whereas those with affective disorders differed only in terms of living alone. Of the alcoholic suicides, 32% experienced disruption of affectional relationships within 6 weeks of their suicide, and 48% within the past year. Several others were faced with impending threats of loss, imminent financial crises, or serious medical diagnoses, and only seven were employed. In a second study, Murphy et al. (1979) examined the case records of 48 alcoholic suicides and interviewed the nearest available relatives of the victim. Half of the subjects had experienced loss of a close affectional relationship within 12 months of their suicide, and 26% had experienced a loss within 6 weeks. The definition of "loss" in this study, as in the first, included only interpersonal disruptions that had *actually* occurred; the authors noted that an even larger number of impending events (e.g., threatened rejections, threats of separation and divorce, and serious physical illness) were recorded. Self-reports of comparable experiences in a matched group of living alcoholic patients showed significantly fewer incidences of affectional loss within 6 weeks of the interview, but not within a year.

Virkkunen (1971) and Lonnqvist and Achte (1971) did not find evidence of recent loss preceding suicide in their studies of alcoholic patients, but Murphy et al. (1979) pointed to substantial difficulties in the methodology of these studies that cast doubt on their findings.

Social and Interpersonal Variables in Suicidal Members of Other Diagnostic Groups

Systematic data comparing suicidal with nonsuicidal members of other diagnostic groups are not as extensive, but the role of interpersonal conflict, social isolation, recent life events, loss, and a family history of suicide have been shown in various studies to distinguish psychiatric patients who commit suicide from those who do not (Borg and Stahl 1982; Roy 1985). The importance of hallucinated commands as a precipitant to suicide in schizophrenic patients is often pointed to, although their actual occurrence would appear to be relatively rare, while the social variables shared by other suicidal patients are relatively common (Breier and Astrachan 1984; Roy 1982). In Roy's study, only 2 of 30 chronic schizophrenic patients who committed suicide had hallucinated commands or persecutory delusions as part of their clinical picture, but 90% of them were unmarried, 80% were unemployed, and 46.6% were living alone. Similarly, none of the 20 schizophrenic patients who killed themselves described by Breier and Astrachan (1984) showed evidence of hallucinatory commands to kill themselves, although most had never been married. The most common significant life event preceding their suicides was being told that they could no longer return home.

It seems clear that, while psychosocial, biologic, and psychiatric factors all contribute to the etiology of suicidal behavior, there are a number of ways in which they can be fitted into the causal chain (Blumenthal, this volume). Early psychosocial and environmental influences may act as primary predisposing factors leading to a specific vulnerability to suicidal behavior, either alone or in association with other related personality variables, such as low self-esteem, a proneness to dysphoric states, poor impulse control, and interpersonal hostility. Later psychosocial events may act as precipitating factors, either through their specific interactions with the personality-sensitive vulnerabilities mentioned above or more generally through their effects on adaptational capacities or the precipitation of syndromal psychiatric illness. Psychiatric or physical illness, on the other hand, may act in a general way as a contributing factor by increasing the individual's exposure to social or environmental stressors (whether early or late), or it may act more directly on the individual's capacity to cope with psychosocial stress through its effect on the brain, ego capacities, or social support systems. The effects of chronic physical illness and acute or chronic alcohol intake are two examples of contributing factors that may act in this way. It must also be borne in mind that early psychosocial and environmental influences have been implicated in the etiologic chains of many of the psychiatric illnesses that intercorrelate with suicidal behavior—such as depression, alcoholism, borderline personality disorder, and other personality disorders—and these may, in part, represent different but closely interrelated outcomes of these influences (Blumenthal and Kupfer 1986).

In view of the weight of evidence pointing to psychosocial stressors in both the early and later histories of suicidal patients, a strong case can be made for assigning them a primary role in a causal model for suicidal behavior and regarding the other factors as contributing agents, bearing in mind that each category of factor may, at one time, play a predisposing role and, at another time, a contributing role. While such a matrix model that allocates different causal components according to whether their effects predispose, precipitate, or contribute to the outcome of interest is useful in conceptualizing interactions between variables, it does not help us to understand why they should interact as they do. A number of theories that contribute to our understanding of this have been advanced.

PSYCHOANALYTIC CONTRIBUTIONS

Psychoanalytic writers have been concerned with understanding suicide within the framework of the individual examining the intrapsychic forces that could give rise to suicidal behavior, the unconscious fantasies expressed by it, and the developmental conditions out of which it may spring. Earlier psychoanalytic theory was primarily concerned with the role of instinctual forces and the mechanisms by which these become subverted into suicidal impulses. More recent psychoanalytic writing has concerned itself with the effects of critical childhood experiences on ego structures, the development of object relations, and the self. Considering the importance of the subject and the centrality of the issues to psychoanalytic theory, it is surprising how little attention it has been given in recent years by psychoanalysts. Key articles dealing with the specific subject of suicide have appeared only episodically, with most references to suicidal dynamics and theory appearing in general theoretical works or in case studies. Most of the psychoanalytic studies appear based on experience with severely depressed patients or those with major characterologic disturbances in the borderline spectrum, with much less psychoanalytic attention given to lower-risk patients with milder disturbances, who form the bulk of those presenting with attempted suicide (Maltsberger and Buie 1980).

Traditional Psychoanalytic Theory

The classical psychoanalytic theory of suicide derives directly from Freud's (1917/1957) influential paper, "Mourning and Melancholia," in which he outlined the psychodynamic mechanisms in severe depression. Freud had been intrigued for many years by the fact that the "extraordinarily powerful life instinct" could be overcome and felt the answer lay in understanding the extremes of self-deprecation and self-torment found in melancholics (Friedman 1967). He hypothesized that, while the loss of the loved object was an experience that could ordinarily be coped with through the process of mourning, in certain predisposed individuals (those who had made "narcissistic object choices"), this experience was intolerable and produced rage that could be of murderous proportions. In an attempt to preserve the loved object, its mental representation is internalized (identification) and becomes a part of the individual's own ego. The angry reproaches previously felt toward the disappointing loved object are then expressed as self-reproaches and, when the anger is sufficiently intense, the attack on the internalized loved object contained in the ego results in suicide.

Although Freud did not dwell in this paper on the developmental traumata that might lead to "narcissistic object choice," other writers (Abraham 1924; Menninger 1933; Zilboorg 1936) felt that "oral fixation" as a result of an earlier experience of loss or frustration was responsible and that it was a regression to the phase of "oral sadism" that accounted for the murderous aggression. Other traditional psychoanalytic writers, observing that many suicidal patients had fantasies of rejoining or joining an idealized internal object, suggested that the erotic or libidinal aspects of oral regressions were as important in some suicidal patients as the aggressive aspects. Hendrick (1940) and Friedlander (1940) published case reports of patients with strong suicidal impulses, which they felt were motivated primarily by libidinal rather than aggressive wishes. While the suicide attempts of their patients were clearly a response to threatened loss of a loved object, these authors proposed that their patients' actions were associated with pleasurable rather than aggressive fantasies. Hendricks' patient, for example, appeared motivated by a wish to join a dead relative with whom she was strongly identified. Friedlander's patient experienced pleasurable fantasies at the thought of getting revenge on a disapproving mother and brother whom she hoped would feel sorry if she died. Although Friedlander's patient made repeated suicide attempts, he showed little of the guilt and self-reproach described by Freud. Menninger (1933, 1938) felt that every suicide entailed three distinct elements: the wish to kill, which had its basis in the death instinct; the wish to be killed, which arose out of the superego in response to a need for punishment; and the wish to die, arising from a more fundamental desire to return to the womb. While these formulations represent a restatement of Freud's original views on suicide in depressed patients, Menninger extended these by emphasizing the primary role of the death instinct, which had been speculatively advanced by Freud.

In a psychoanalytically inspired study of 100 attempted suicides, Hendin (1963) described a number of fantasies that seem to underly the patient's suicidal actions. Although in many patients the traditional depressive dynamics of suicide as anger turned inward or death seen as self-punishment were present, other patients appeared to have the fantasy of death as a reunion with a loved object or as a rebirth, and others yet appeared to be gaining a sense of omnipotent mastery over their situation through taking control of their deaths. In an essay on this theme, Morse (1973) suggested that the common element in all suicidal fantasy is a gratification of a wish in relation to a loved object and that the main condition leading to suicide is a disturbance in reality testing, which allows the individual to believe he or she will live after death and experience the "after pleasure" of the suicidal action and its effects on others.

Object Relations Approaches

Melanie Klein (1935) pointed out that while she agreed with Freud's assertion that suicide represented an attack on an internalized object, this attack was directed primarily at the bad part of the object and was motivated by a wish to preserve the good internal object, which was a valued part of the self. Like Menninger, Klein saw the origins of the aggression arising from the death instinct and the fear that one's aggression could annihilate a good object. Guntrip (1968) made a distinction between depressive suicide, where the driving force is aggression and hatred redirected toward the self from the hated and loved object, and schizoid suicide, where the individual, facing the loss of self, longs for death as a fantasied pathway to rebirth.

Several American authors, using object relations concepts derived from the theories of Margaret Mahler (1968), have conceptualized the developmental problem in suicidal patients as a failure to negotiate the transition from the symbiotic phase of development, where mental representations of the infant self and mother are undifferentiated, to the rapprochement subphase of separation individuation, where self and object representations are differentiated. The end result of this failure is a tendency to become involved in relationships later in life where individuals are treated as parts of the self rather than as unique. This situation, called "symbiotic object choice," is equated by Asch (1980) with Freud's concept of narcissistic object choice. Asch, like Klein, sees the primary goal of suicidal behavior as getting rid of bad internal objects, but differs from her in viewing the principal aim of this as fusion with the symbiotic mother of infancy. Masterson (1976, 1983) used Mahlerian concepts to explain suicidal behavior in borderline patients. Richman (1978) applied these concepts in understanding family dynamics in suicidal patients. Maltsberger (1986), using a self psychology framework, has described suicidal patients as individuals who have failed to develop stable self-regulatory structures. They remain overly reliant on self objects to comfort them and, in the face of abandonment, are vulnerable to crises of "aloneness, self-contempt and murderous rage (p. 3)," which may lead to suicidal behavior.

Maltsberger and Buie (1980), summarizing contemporary psychoanalytic views, stated "suicide is a phenomena of disturbed internalization, an effort to cope with hostile introjects, and to cope with the absence of comforting inner presence is necessary for stability and mental quiet" (pp. 61–62).

Interpersonal Aspects of Suicidal Behavior

While most psychoanalytic attention has been directed at the delineation of the intrapsychic mechanisms leading to suicide, less attention has been given by psychoanalysts to the interpersonal aspects of suicidal behavior and the theoretical implications of the current interpersonal crisis that often precipitates it. This is not to say that psychoanalytic writers have failed to observe these interactions. Menninger (1933) pointed out that attacking oneself may be a very effective means of hurting another person. Zilboorg (1936) emphasized the importance of spite as a motivation in suicide, mentioning that such patients do not necessarily exhibit depressive symptoms although they may be sadistic. Friedlander (1940), in her case study, pointed out that the central issue with her patient did not involve an intrapsychic conflict, but an external one motivated by the wish to cause concern in his mother and brother. Asch (1980) stated that many suicides become understandable if one assumes as a constant the fantasy of two people being involved, pointing out that aggressiveness toward fate and the family remains a major element in all suicides. He described a specific fantasy in which the suicidal individual responds to object loss by trying to enlist the significant other to act as an actual or imagined persecutor to whom he can succumb as a passive victim. While Asch pointed to the essential dyadic nature of this interaction, referring to it as a sadomasochistic relationship, he described the mechanism in terms of intrapsychic defenses of projection and displacement. Similar views on the dyadic nature of suicidal acts have been advanced by Hale (1985).

In a study of suicidal adolescents in psychoanalytic treatment, Friedman et al. (1972) noted that all their patients had markedly ambivalent relationships with their mothers and that the ongoing relationship of the patients to their "original" objects seemed to be a major determination in their suicidal behavior. However, they restrict their theoretical formulations to the traditional psychoanalytic views regarding narcissistic object choice and the suicide attempt as an attack on an internalized object.

Adam (1982, 1986) suggested that attachment theory, which conceptualizes the attachment bond as a goal-directed system involving reciprocal interaction between the child and mother, might be a more useful conceptual model for understanding both the earlier and later interactional aspects of suicidal behavior. The work of John Bowlby (1951) and followers has shown that human infants regularly respond with distress to even brief separations from primary caretakers during early childhood and that a number of forms of insecure and anxious attachment result from various deficiencies in parental care. Further research has shown that these patterns persist over time (Ainsworth 1985; Main et al. 1985; Weiss 1982). Although systematic research into adult attachment is just beginning, there is good reason to believe that attachment pathology may be at the root of much of the interpersonal and behavioral disturbance observed in adults with severe personality disturbance (West and Sheldon 1987). Adam suggests that such individuals are not only more prone to form insecure relationships, but are unduly sensitive to threats to their continuity, reacting strongly with the activation of separation and abandonment anxiety, of which suicidal ideation and behavior may be an important component. Suicide attempts can be seen in this light as active attachment behaviors serving the functions of signaling distress to others in the social environment, punishing them for rejection, and coercing them into reconstituting a vitally needed bond. Repeated failure to form stable attachments, which is made more likely by associated personality difficulties and excessive demands on attachment figures, may lead to the extreme social isolation and alienation that is such a large part of the social context of completed suicide. He suggested a general model for suicidal behavior, which places the early discontinuities and deficiencies of parental care as predisposing factors, the current threats to attachment figures as precipitating factors, and associated mental illness and alcohol and drug abuse as contributing factors allowing pathologic attachments to be more readily unmasked (Adam 1982, 1986).

Direct support for this hypothesis is found in a study of suicidal preschool children who were noted to exhibit patterns of pathologic attachment (Rosenthal and Rosenthal 1984) and suicidal adults whose behavior in the acute suicidal crisis strongly resembled that of children following brief separations (Adam and Adam 1978). Further support comes from animal studies, which have shown that self-injurious behavior is a response to a number of biologic and social variables, including stressful life events, interference with sexual bonding, and isolation and confinement (Jones et al. 1979). Jones and Barraclough (1978) pointed to striking similarities between the affective state and social situation preceding suicidal acts in humans and those in animal self-injury, suggesting they may be homologous behaviors.

Other Theoretical Perspectives

Hendin (1964, 1969) combined the intensive study of individuals with cultural studies in an attempt to explain group differences in suicidal vulnerability. In one such study he examined suicidal patients and nonsuicidal controls using hypnosis, dream study, and psychoanalytic interviewing techniques to explore suicidal fantasies and attitudes toward death in three Scandinavian countries. As well, he examined cultural attitudes toward aggression, competition, and dependence using literature, psychological testing, and personal impressions of the cultures. Differences between high suicide rates in Denmark and Sweden and the low rates in Norway were attributed to cultural differences in child-rearing patterns, particularly those involving the handling of aggression, guilt, and competition. He hypothesized that these differences lead to a greater sensitivity to loss and abandonment in the suicide-prone countries that was associated with later suicide attempts. A similar approach was used to explain differences between suicide in blacks and in whites in the United States and suicide in students (Hendin 1975).

In a small but ambitious work, Farber (1968) formulated a general theory of suicide in which a developmental-psychological model is integrated with social and cultural findings using *hope* as the central linking concept. According to this model, suicide vulnerability results when individuals with an impaired sense of competence encounter situational factors that threaten "acceptable life conditions" and lead to a loss of hope, which finds its expression in suicide. Faulty experiences with parental figures, such as those involving abandonment, disparagement, and guilt induction, are held to be responsible for damaging the individual sense of self-competence, and this personality deficit renders the individuals particularly sensitive to later blows to self-competence and a proneness to feel hopelessness and to use suicide as a way out of an unbearable life situation. The frequency of suicide within a given population is seen as a function of the extent to which it contains vulnerable individuals and the degree to which they are exposed to certain types of deprivation; both of these may be culture bound. Like Hendin (1964, 1969), Farber illustrated his contentions by comparisons between the different child-rearing practices in Denmark, which has a high suicide rate, and Norway, which has a low rate, and by various other cultural examples. His theoretical maxims are presented in a series of equations (e.g., suicide varies inversely with hope, inversely with a sense of competence, and directly with threat), and he ends with a general equation incorporating all the individual and social variables affecting the degree of hope within a given society.

Farber's (1968) model is ingenious in the comprehensiveness with which he takes into account many of the relevant social and psychological variables involved in suicide, and it probably deserves greater attention than it has received. This model, which conceptualizes suicide as the result of several causal agents, some of which may be essential but none of which in themselves is sufficient, is consistent with contemporary notions of causality. Unfortunately, the persuasiveness of his general argument is somewhat weakened by the evidence he marshals to support it, which tends to be impressionistic and unconvincing.

The central role Farber (1968) gives to hope as a protective factor against suicide has considerable support in more recent cognitive studies, which have shown that hopelessness is a stronger indicator of suicidal intent than depression itself (Beck et al. 1975, 1985). These findings have been replicated in a number of independent studies using the Beck Hopelessness Scale (Adam et al. 1980; Dyer and Kreitman 1984; Minkoff et al. 1973; Wetzel 1976; Wetzel et al. 1980).

IMPLICATIONS FOR TREATMENT

Many approaches to the problems of prevention, intervention, and treatment have been suggested in the literature, although clear demonstration of their effectiveness in reducing suicidal behavior has not yet been determined. While a detailed consideration of these issues is beyond the scope of this chapter, our knowledge of the social, environmental, and psychological variables associated with suicidal behavior point to some general considerations.

At the macrosocial level of prevention, any social measures that either decrease social disorganization and social isolation or increase social integration and the availability of social supports would be expected to have some effect on the incidence of suicidal behavior at the population level. The implementation of strategies to effect this, specifically targeted to suicidal individuals, is clearly unfeasible. However, the broader effects this might have on a wider range of behavioral and psychiatric disorders that interrelate with suicidal behavior makes it a legitimate social goal.

At the microsocial level, our knowledge of the importance of early family influences in the predisposition to suicidal vulnerability should lead us to encourage any preventive and interventive measures that support and sustain the family unit and decrease the extent to which children are exposed to parental unavailability, discontinuities in parental care, and child neglect and abuse. The recent advocacy of legal change to allow for custodial disputes to be resolved in the best interests of the child, and programs providing for counseling and support for families following bereavement are just two examples of such initiatives that could have longer-term effects. Although it can be argued that little can be done to mitigate against the devastating effects of long-standing family disturbances, such as many of these patients have been exposed to, an awareness of the effects these experiences may have in terms of the personality and interpersonal relationships should be taken into account in service planning and clinical work. Clinical services for patients presenting with suicide attempts should include evaluation of the social, familial, and interpersonal networks as a part of any overall assessment and treatment planning, and the organization of services should be structured as much as possible to provide continuity of care and ongoing support beyond the immediate suicidal crisis. Crisis intervention services attached to general hospital emergency departments, which can be structured to deal with such patients in both the immediate assessment, treatment, and follow-up phases of their management, are one example of how this may be achieved. Traditional psychiatric emergency services, which provide only immediate assessment and referral elsewhere for treatment, would seem ill suited for suicidal patients and probably contribute to the high drop-out rates that have been noted in outpatient referrals following suicide attempts (Goldney 1975).

The importance of the "significant other" in the acute suicidal crisis is often referred to, but direct involvement of the spouse, family, and social network in the evaluation process of psychiatric emergency services is by no means routine. The use of family therapy in the treatment of suicidal patients has been reported in the literature, and family-oriented crisis intervention services for dealing with these patients have been described (Adam et al. 1983; Alanen et al. 1981; Morrison and Collier 1969; Richman 1979). Although the effectiveness of such approaches has not been critically evaluated, Adam et al. (1983) have shown that the routine use of family assessment in the emergency department and family and couples therapy in follow-up treatment is feasible and increases treatment engagement.

In view of the long-standing nature of their associated interpersonal and social difficulties and the repetitiveness of suicidal behavior in some patients, it is not surprising that suicidal patients are often referred for individual psychotherapy. Psychotherapeutic approaches have been described from a number of theoretical frameworks, ranging from supportive (Kiev 1975; Lesse 1975) to cognitive (Kovacs et al. 1975; Weishaar and Beck, this volume) and insight-oriented approaches (Birtchnell 1983; Hendin 1981; Kahn, this volume; Mintz 1961). Moreover, issues related to the management of suicidal behavior are a feature of most standard psychotherapy textbooks (Basch 180; Fromm-Reichmann 1950) and a host of articles dealing with severely characterologically disturbed patients (Masterson 1976; Silver 1985). Evaluative data dealing specifically with the relative efficacy of the various approaches in dealing with suicidal behavior are lacking, although one clinical study of borderline patients supports the general clinical impression that, with successful engagement in intensive psychotherapeutic treatment, self-destructive actions decrease and become less problematic over time (Waldinger and Gunderson 1987). In addition, there would seem to be a good deal of agreement regarding the importance of certain technical procedures, such as therapist availability, the monitoring of suicidal risk, and countertransference issues (Blumenthal, this volume; Kahn 1982; Maltsberger and Buie 1974; 1980).

The establishment of 24-hour telephone hotlines, which have been a standard feature of the suicide prevention movement over the past 20 years, is based on an awareness of the importance of the immediate availability of social support for such patients. However, here, too, clear evidence of their effectiveness in preventing suicides is lacking (Bagley 1968; Bridge et al. 1977; Jennings et al. 1978). Special follow-up services providing intensive social support following suicide attempts would seem to make good sense, but the evidence that they decrease further suicidal behavior is conflicting and difficult to evaluate. Outcome studies that have demonstrated decreases in attempted suicide following special management are outnumbered by those that do not, but methodological problems in many of these studies make their conclusions open to question (Streiner and Adam 1987).

Termansen and Bywater (1975), for example, randomly allocated suicidal patients seen in an emergency department to four follow-up groups that provided a range of aftercare varying from no treatment to direct intensive contact by a mental health worker. At 12 weeks' follow-up, the direct contact group showed less role impairment and had made fewer suicide attempts than the other three groups. However, the poor rate of follow-up in some of the treatment groups makes the results impossible to evaluate. Welu (1977) allocated suicide attempters randomly to either routine service or a special outreach program that followed them intensively in their homes for 4 months. At the end of that period, the experimental group had made significantly fewer repeat attempts and were using less alcohol than other groups. A total of 20% of the original sample refused to participate in the study.

Four other special follow-up programs have reported no differences between patients receiving the program and those receiving routine treatment in the incidence of repeat suicide attempts, although they all have demonstrated other beneficial social and psychological effects. Buglass and McCulloch (1970) and Chowdhury et al. (1973) showed that suicidal patients receiving special intensive aftercare were more improved in their social circumstances than those receiving conventional care. Gibbons et al. (1978) showed that patients receiving intensive social work follow-up, including home visits, made greater changes in their social problems and were more satisfied with the service they had received than patients randomly allocated to psychiatric treatment or general practice care. Hawton et al. (1981) found treatment compliance better in patients assigned to domiciliary care compared to those in an outpatient follow-up program. Although none of these studies demonstrated any differences in the incidence of repetition of suicidal behavior, it must be borne in mind that all these studies followed their patients for relatively short periods of time, most under 6 months and only one for up to a year. Although this encompasses the period of greatest risk for repeated suicide attempts, it may well be that the small minority of frequent multiple attempters who contribute disproportionately to rates of repeated suicide over the short term are the very patients for whom brief therapy, however intensive, is least well suited (Ennis et al. 1985).

This chapter has demonstrated how psychosocial factors impact on suicide risk over the life cycle. Consideration of these variables in the formulation of interventions is an important part of suicide prevention efforts.

REFERENCES

Abraham K: A short study of the development of the libido, in Selected Papers on Psychoanalysis. Edited by Jones E. London, Hogarth Press, 1924

Adam G, Adams KS, Taylor G, et al: A family oriented crisis intervention service for attempted suicide, in Depression and Suicide: Proceedings of the XIth International Congress for Suicide Prevention, Paris, July 5–8, 1981. Edited by Soubrier JP, Vedrinne J. Elmsford, NY, Pergamon, 1983

Adam KS: Loss, suicide and attachment, in The Place of Attachment in Human Behaviour. Edited by Parkes CM, Stevenson-Hinde J. New York, Basic Books, 1982, pp 269–294

Adam KS: Attempted suicide. Psychiatr Clin North Am 8:183–201, 1985

Adam KS: Early family influences on suicidal behaviour. Ann NY Acad Sci 487:63–76, 1986

Adam KS, Adam G: Attachment theory and attempted suicide. Paper presented at the 15th Annual Congress of the Royal Australian and New Zealand College of Psychiatrists, Singapore, 1978

Adam K, Bianchi G, Hawker F, et al: Interpersonal factors in suicide attempts: a pilot study in Christchurch. Aust N Z J Psychiatry 12:59–63, 1978

Adam KS, Bouckoms A, Scarr G: Attempted suicide in Christchurch: a controlled study. Aust N Z J Psychiatry 14:305–314, 1980

Adam KS, Lohrenz JG, Harper D, et al: Early parental loss and suicidal ideation in university students. Can J Psychiatry 27:275–281, 1982a

Adam KS, Bouckoms A, Streiner D: Parental loss and family stability in attempted suicide. Arch Gen Psychiatry 39:1081–1085, 1982b

Ainsworth MD: Attachments across the life span. Bull NY Acad Med 61:792–812, 1985

Alanen Y, Rinne R, Paukkonen P: On family dynamics and family therapy in suicidal attempts. Crisis 2:20–26, 1981

American Psychiatric Association: Diagnostic and Statistical Manual of Mental Disorders, 3rd Edition. Washington, DC, American Psychiatric Association, 1980

Asch S: Suicide and the hidden executioner. International Review of Psychoanalysis 7:51–60, 1980

Bagley C: The evaluation of a suicide prevention scheme by an ecological method. Soc Sci Med 2:1–14, 1968

Bancroft JH, Skrimshire A, Reynolds F, et al: Self-poisoning and self-injury in the Oxford area: epidemiological aspects 1969–1973. British Journal of Preventative Social Medicine 29:170–177, 1975

Barraclough BM, Bunch J: Accuracy of dating parent deaths: recollected dates compared with death certificate dates. Br J Psychiatry 123:573–574, 1973

Barraclough B, Pallis D: Depression followed by suicide: a comparison of depressed suicides with living depressives. Psychol Med 5:55–61, 1975

Barraclough BM, Bunch J, Nelson B, et al: A hundred cases of suicide: clinical aspects. Br J Psychiatry 125:355–373, 1974

Basch MF: Doing Psychotherapy. New York, Basic Books, 1980

Batchelor IRC, Napier MB: Broken homes and attempted suicide. British Journal of Delinquency 4:99–108, 1953

Beck A, Weissman A, Lester D, et al: The measurement of pessimism: the hopelessness scale. J Consult Clin Psychol 42:861–865, 1974

Beck A, Kovacs M, Weissman A: Hopelessness and suicidal behavior: an overview. JAMA 234:1146–1149, 1975

Beck A, Steer RA, Kovacs M, et al: Hopelessness and eventual suicide: a 10-year prospective study of patients hospitalized with suicidal ideation. Am J Psychiatry 142:559–563, 1985

Birtchnell J: The relationship between attempted suicide, depression and parent death. Br J Psychiatry 116:307–313, 1970

Birtchnell J: Is there a scientifically acceptable alternative to the epidemiological study of familial factors in mental illness? Soc Sci Med 8:335–350, 1974

Birtchnell J: Psychotherapeutic considerations in the management of the suicidal patient. Am J Psychother 37:24–36, 1983

Birtchnell J, Alarcon J: The motivation and emotional state of 91 cases of attempted suicide. Br J Med Psychol 44:45–52, 1971

Blumenthal SJ, Kupfer DJ: Generalizable treatment strategies for suicidal behavior, in Psychobiology of Suicidal Behavior, Annals of the New York Academy of Sciences, Volume 487. Edited by Mann JJ, Stanley M. New York, New York Academy of Sciences, 1986, pp 327–340

Borg ES, Stahl M: Prediction of suicide: a prospective study of suicides and controls among psychiatric patients. Acta Psychiatr Scand 65:221–232, 1982

Bowlby J: Maternal Care and Mental Health. New York, Columbia University Press, 1951

Breed W: Occupational mobility and suicide among white males. American Sociology Review 28:179–188, 1963

Breier A, Astrachan B: Characterization of schizophrenic patients who commit suicide. Am J Psychiatry 141:206–209, 1984

Bridge TP, Potkin SG, Zung WW, et al: Suicide prevention centers: ecological study of effectiveness. J Nerv Ment Dis 164:18–24, 1977

Brown GW, Harris T: Social origins of depression: a study of psychiatric disorders in women. London, Tavistock, 1978

Bruhn JG: Broken homes among attempted suicides and psychiatric outpatients: a comparative study. Journal of Mental Science 108:772–779, 1962

Buglass D, Duffy JC: The ecological pattern of suicide and parasuicide in Edinburgh. Soc Sci Med 12:241–253, 1978

Buglass D, McCulloch JW: Further suicidal behaviour: the development and validation of predictive scales. Br J Psychiatry 116:483–491, 1970

Buglass D, Dugard P, Kreitman N: Multiple standardization of parasuicide ('attempted suicide') rates in Edinburgh. British Journal of Preventative Social Medicine 24:182–186, 1970

Bunch J: Recent bereavement in relation to suicide. J Psychosom Res 16:361–366, 1972

Bunch J, Barraclough B, Nelson B, et al: Early parental bereavement and suicide. Soc Psychiatry 6:200–202, 1971

Chowdhury N, Hicks RC, Kreitman N: Evaluation of an after-care service for parasuicide (attempted suicide) patients. Soc Psychiatry 8:67–81, 1973

Clayton P: Suicide. Psychiatr Clin North Am 8:203–214, 1985

Cochrane R, Robertson A: Stress in the lives of parasuicides. Soc Psychiatry 10:161–171, 1975

Cohen-Sandler R, Berman A, King R: A follow-up study of hospitalized suicidal children. J Am Acad Child Psychiatry 21:398–403, 1982a

Cohen-Sandler R, Berman AL, King RA: Life stress and symptomatology: determinants of suicidal behaviour in children. J Am Acad Child Psychiatry 21:178–186, 1982b

Conroy RW, Smith K: Family loss and hospital suicide. Suicide Life Threat Behav 13:179–194, 1983

Cormier HJ, Klerman GL: Unemployment and male-female labor force participation as determinants of changing suicide rates of males and females in Quebec. Soc Psychiatry 20:109–114, 1985

Crook T, Eliot J: Parental death during childhood and adult depression: a critical review of the literature. Psychol Bull 87:252–259, 1980

Crook T, Raskin A: Association of childhood parental loss with attempted suicide and depression. J Consult Clin Psychol 43:277, 1975

Dennehy CM: Childhood bereavement and psychiatric illness. Br J Psychiatry 112:1049–1069, 1966

Dorpat TL, Jackson JK, Ripley HS: Broken homes and attempted and completed suicide. Arch Gen Psychiatry 12:213–216, 1965

Dublin LI: Suicide: A Sociological and Statistical Study. New York, Ronald Press, 1963

Durkheim E: Suicide: A Study in Sociology. Translated by Spaulding JA, Simpson G. London, Routledge & Kegan Paul, 1952

Dyer J, Kreitman N: Hopelessness, depression and suicidal intent in para-suicide. Br J Psychiatry 144:127–133, 1984

Eastwood M, Hendeson H, Montgomery I: Personality and parasuicide: methodological problems. Med J Aust 1:170–175, 1972

Ennis J, Barnes R, Spenser H: Management of the repeatedly suicidal patient. Can J Psychiatry 30:535–538, 1985

Farber ML: Theory of Suicide. New York, Funk & Wagnalls, 1968

Farberow NL: Personality patterns of suicidal mental hospital patients. Genetic Psychology Monographs 42:3–79, 1950

Farmer R, Creed F: Hostility and deliberate self-poisoning. Br J Med Psychol 59:311–316, 1986

Fieldsend R, Lowenstein E: Quarrels, separations and infidelity in the two days preceding self-poisoning episodes. Br J Med Psychol 54:349–352, 1981

Finlay-Jones R, Scott R, Duncan-Jones P, et al: The reliability of reports of early separations. Aust N Z J Psychiatry 15:27–31, 1981

Flood RA, Seager CP: A retrospective examination of psychiatric case records of patients who subsequently committed suicide. Br J Psychiatry 114:443–450, 1968

Freud S: Mourning and melancholia (1917), in The Standard Edition of the Complete Psychological Works of Sigmund Freud, Vol 14. Translated and edited by Strachey J. London, Hogarth Press, 1957, pp 237–260

Friedlander K: On the "longing to die." Int J Psychoanal 21:416–426, 1940

Friedman M, Glasser M, Laufer E, et al: Attempted suicide and self-mutilation in adolescence: some observations from a psychoanalytic research project. Int J Psychoanal 53:179–183, 1972

Friedman P: On Suicide, With Particular Reference to Suicide Among Young Students. New York, International Universities Press, 1967

Friedman RC, Arnott M, Clarkin J, et al: History of suicidal behavior in depressed borderline inpatients. Am J Psychiatry 140:1023–1026, 1983

Friedman RC, Corn R, Hurt S, et al: Family history of illness in the seriously suicidal adolescent: a life-cycle approach. Am J Orthopsychiatry 54:390–397, 1984

Fromm-Reichmann F: Principles of Intensive Psychotherapy. Chicago, University of Chicago Press, 1950

Garfinkel BD, Golombek H: Suicidal behaviour in adolescence, in The Adolescent and Mood Disturbance. Edited by Golombek H, Garfinkel B. New York, International Universities Press, 1983, pp 189–217

Garfinkel BD, Froese A, Hood J: Suicide attempts in children and adolescents. Am J Psychiatry 139:1257–1261, 1982

Gay MJ, Tonge WL: The late effects of loss of parents in childhood. Br J Psychiatry 113:753–759, 1967

Gibbons JS, Butler J, Urwin P, et al: Evaluation of a social work service for self-poisoning patients. Br J Psychiatry 133:111–118, 1978

Gibbs J, Martin W: Status Integration and Suicide: A Sociological Study. Oregon, University of Oregon Press, 1964

Giddens A (ed): The Sociology of Suicide: A Selection of Readings. London, Frank Cass & Co, 1971

Glaser K: Attempted suicide in children and adolescents: psychodynamic observations. Am J Psychother 19:220–227, 1965

Goldney RD: Out-patient follow-up of those who have attempted suicide: fact of fantasy? Aust N Z J Psychiatry 9:111–113, 1975

Goldney RD: Parental loss and reported childhood stress in young women who attempt suicide. Acta Psychiatr Scand 64:34–49, 1981

Goldney RD: Parental representation in young women who attempt suicide. Acta Psychiatr Scand 72:230–232, 1985

Goldney RD, Burvill PW: Trends in suicidal behaviour and its management. Aust N Z J Psychiatry 14:1–15, 1980

Gould RE: Suicide problems in children and adolescents. Am J Psychother 19:228–246, 1965

Green AH: Self-destructive behavior in battered children. Am J Psychiatry 135:579–582, 1978

Greer S: The relationship between parental loss and attempted suicide: a control study. Br J Psychiatry 110:698–705, 1964

Greer S: Parental loss and attempted suicide: a further report. Br J Psychiatry 112:465–470, 1966

Greer S, Gunn JC: Attempted suicides from intact and broken parental homes. Br Med J 2:1355–1357, 1966

Greer S, Gunn JC, Koller KM: Aetiological factors in attempted suicide. Br Med J 2:1352–1355, 1966

Gregory I: Studies of parental deprivation in psychiatric patients. Am J Psychiatry 115:432–442, 1958

Gregory I: Retrospective data concerning childhood loss of a parent, I: actuarial estimates vs. recorded frequencies of orphanhood. Arch Gen Psychiatry 15:354–361, 1966a

Gregory I: Retrospective data concerning childhood loss of a parent, II: category of parental loss by decade of birth, diagnosis and MMPI. Arch Gen Psychiatry 15:362–367, 1966b

Guntrip H: Schizoid Phenomena, Object Relations and the Self (International Psycho-Analytical Library). London, Hogarth Press, 1968

Hagnell O, Rorsman B: Suicide in the Lundby study: a controlled prospective investigation of stressful life events. Neuropsychobiology 6:319–332, 1980

Haider I: Suicidal attempts in children and adolescents. Br J Psychiatry 114:1133–1134, 1968

Hale R: Suicide and the violent act. Bulletin of the British Association of Psychotherapy 16:13–24, 1985

Hankoff L: Suicidal behavior in the institutional setting. Journal of Psychiatric Treatment and Evaluation 2:19–24, 1980

Hart EE, Williams CL: Suicidal behaviour and interpersonal network. Crisis 8:112–124, 1987

Hawton K: Suicide and Attempted Suicide Among Children and Adolescents. Beverly Hills, Sage, 1986

Hawton K, Bancroft J, Catalan J, et al: Domiciliary and out-patient treatment of self-poisoning patients by medical and non-medical staff. Psychol Med 11:169–177, 1981

Hawton K, Osborn M, O'Grady J, et al: Classification of adolescents who take overdoses. Br J Psychiatry 140:124–131, 1982

Hendin H: The psychodynamics of suicide. J Nerv Ment Dis 136:236–244, 1963

Hendin H: Suicide and Scandinavia: A Psychoanalytic Study of Culture and Character. New York, Grune & Stratton, 1964

Hendin H: Black Suicide. New York, Basic Books, 1969

Hendin H: Growing up dead: student suicide. Am J Psychother 29:327–338, 1975

Hendin H: Psychotherapy and suicide. Am J Psychother 35:469–480, 1981

Hendrick I: Suicide as wish-fulfillment. Psychiatr Q 14:30–42, 1940

Henry AF, Short JF: Suicide and Homicide. Glencoe, IL, Free Press, 1954

Hill OW: The association of childhood bereavement with suicidal attempt in depressive illness. Br J Psychiatry 115:301–304, 1969

Isherwood J, Adam KS, Hornblow A: Life event stress, psychosocial factors, suicide attempts and auto-accident proclivity. J Psychosom Res 26:371–383, 1982

Jarvis GK, Ferrence RG, Johnson FG, et al: Sex and age patterns in self-injury. J Health Soc Behav 17:146–154, 1976

Jarvis GK, Ferrence RG, Whitehead PC, et al: The ecology of self-injury: a multivariate approach. Suicide Life Threat Behav 12:90–102, 1982

Jennings C, Barraclough BM, Moss JR: Have the Samaritans lowered the suicide rate? a controlled study. Psychol Med 8:413–422, 1978

Jones IH, Barraclough BM: Auto-mutilation in animals and its relevance to self-injury in man. Acta Psychiatr Scand 58:40–47, 1978

Jones IH, Congiu L, Stevenson J: A biological approach to two forms of human self-injury. J Nerv Ment Dis 167:74–78, 1979

Kahn A: The moment of truth: psychotherapy with the suicide patient, in Lifelines: Clinical Perspectives on Suicide. Edited by Bassuk E, Schoonover S, Gill A. New York, Plenum, 1982

Kessel N: Self-poisoning: part I. Br Med J 2:1336–1340, 1965

Kiev A: Psychotherapeutic strategies in the management of depressed and suicidal patients. Am J Psychother 29:345–354, 1975

Klein M: A contribution to the psychogenesis of manic depressive states (1935), in Contributions to Psycho-Analysis 1921–1945: Melanie Klein. London, Hogarth Press, 1968

Koller KM, Castanos JN: The influence of childhood parental deprivation in attempted suicide. Med J Aust 1:396–399, 1968

Koller KM, Cotgrove RCM: Social geography of suicidal behaviour in Hobart. Aust N Z J Psychiatry 10:237–242, 1976

Kosky R, Silburn S, Zubrick S: Symptomatic depression and suicidal ideation: a comparative study with 628 children. J Nerv Ment Dis 174:523–528, 1986

Kovacs M, Beck AT, Weissman A: The use of suicidal motives in the psychotherapy of attempted suicides. Am J Psychother 29:363–368, 1975

Kreitman N: Parasuicide. London, John Wiley, 1977

Kreitman N, Platt S: The coal gas story: United Kingdom suicide rates, 1960–71. British Journal of Preventative Social Medicine 30:86–93, 1976

Kreitman N, Schreiber M: Parasuicide in young Edinburgh women, 1968–1975. Psychol Med 9:469–479, 1979

Lesse S: The range of therapies in the treatment of severely depressed suicidal patients. Am J Psychother 29:308–326, 1975

Lester D: Social disorganization and completed suicide. Soc Psychiatry 5:175–176, 1970

Lester D, Beck AT: Early loss as a possible sensitizer to later loss in attempted suicide. Psychol Rep 39:121–122, 1976

Levi LD, Fales CH, Stein M, et al: Separation and attempted suicide. Arch Gen Psychiatry 15:158–164, 1966

Linehan M: Suicidal people: one population or two. Ann NY Acad Sci 487:16–33, 1986

Lonnqvist J, Achte KA: Excessive drinking in psychiatric patients who later committed suicide. Psychiatria Fennica 2:209–213, 1971

Lukianowicz N: Suicidal behaviour: an attempt to modify the environment. Br J Psychiatry 121:387–390, 1972

Luscomb RL, Clum GA, Patsiokas AT: Mediating factors in the relationship between life stress and suicide attempting. J Nerv Ment Dis 168:644–650, 1980

Mahler M: On Human Symbiosis and the Vicissitudes of Individuation, Vol 1: Infantile Psychosis. New York, International Universities Press, 1968

Main M, Kaplan N, Cassidy J: Security in infancy, childhood and adulthood: a move to the level of representation, in Growing Points of Attachment: Theory and Research. Edited by Bretherton I, Waters E. Chicago, University of Chicago Press, Monogr Soc Res Child Dev 50(1–2), 1985

Maltsberger J: Suicide Risk: The Formulation of Clinical Judgement. New York, New York University Press, 1986

Maltsberger JT, Buie D: Countertransference hate in the treatment of suicidal patients. Arch Gen Psychiatry 30:625–633, 1974

Maltsberger JT, Buie DH: The devices of suicide revenge, riddance, and rebirth. International Review of Psychoanalysis 7:61–72, 1980

Maris R: Suicide, status and mobility in Chicago. Social Forces 46:246–256, 1967

Maris R: Social Forces in Urban Suicide. Homewood, IL, Dorsey Press, 1969

Maris R: Sociology, in A Handbook for the Study of Suicide. Edited by Perlin S. New York, Oxford University Press, 1975, pp 93–112

Maris R: Pathways to Suicide: A Survey of Self-Destructive Behaviours. Baltimore, Johns Hopkins University Press, 1981

Masterson JF: Psychotherapy of the Borderline Adult: A Developmental Approach. New York, Brunner/Mazel, 1976

Masterson JF: Abandonment depression in borderline adolscents, in The Adolescent and Mood Disturbance. Edited by Golombek H, Garfinkel B. New York, International Universities Press, 1983, pp 135–144

Mattson A, Hawkins JW, Seese RS: Child psychiatric emergencies: clinical characteristics and follow-up results. Arch Gen Psychiatry 17:584–589, 1967

McConaghy N, Linane J, Buckle RC: Parental deprivation and attempted suicide. Med J Aust 1:866–892, 1966

McCulloch JW, Philip AE, Carstairs GM: The ecology of suicidal behaviour. Br J Psychiatry 113:313–319, 1967

Menninger KA: Psychoanalytic aspects of suicide. Int J Psychoanal 14:376–390, 1933

Menninger K: Man Against Himself. New York, Harcourt Brace World, 1938

Miller M: Cooperation of some wives in their husbands' suicides. Psychol Rep 44:39–42, 1979

Minkoff K, Bergman E, Beck AT, et al: Hopelessness, depression, and attempted suicide. Am J Psychiatry 130:455–459, 1973

Mintz R: Psychotherapy of the suicidal patient. Am J Psychother 15:348–367, 1961

Modestin J: Countertransference reactions contributing to completed suicide. Br J Med Psychol 60:379–385, 1987

Morgan HG, Pocock H, Pottle S: The urban distribution of non-fatal deliberate self-harm. Br J Psychiatry 126:319–328, 1975

Morrison GC, Collier JG: Family treatment approaches to suicidal children and adolescents. J Am Acad Child Psychiatry 8:140–153, 1969

Morse S: The after-pleasure of suicide. Br J Med Psychol 46:227–238, 1973

Moss LM, Hamilton DM: The psychotherapy of the suicidal patient. Am J Psychiatry 112:814–820, 1956

Munro A: Childhood parent loss in a psychiatrically normal population. British Journal of Preventative Social Medicine 19:69–79, 1965

Munro A, Griffiths AB: Some psychiatric non-sequelae of childhood bereavement. Br J Psychiatry 115:305–311, 1969

Murphy G: Suicide and attempted suicide, in Psychiatry, Vol I. Edited by Michels R, Cavenar J Jr. Philadelphia, JB Lippincott, 1987

Murphy GE, Robins E: Social factors in suicide. JAMA 199:303–308, 1967

Murphy G, Armstrong J, Hermeles S, et al: Suicide and alcoholism: interpersonal loss confirmed as predictor. Arch Gen Psychiatry 36:65–69, 1979

Nelson G: Parental death during childhood and adult depression: some additional data. Soc Psychiatry 17:37–42, 1982

Oliver RG, Kaminski Z, Tudor K, et al: The epidemiology of attempted suicide as seen in the casualty department, Alfred Hospital, Melbourne. Med J Aust 1:833–839, 1971

Paffenbarger RS, Asnes DP: Chronic disease in former college students, III: precursors of suicide in early and middle life. Am J Public Health 56:1026–1036, 1966

Paffenbarger RS, King SH, Wing A: Chronic disease in former college students, IV: characteristics in youth that predispose to suicide and accidental death in later life. Am J Public Health 59:900–908, 1969

Pallis D, Birtchnell J: Seriousness of suicide attempt in relation to personality. Br J Psychiatry 130:253–259, 1977

Palmer DM: Factors in suicidal attempts, a review of 25 consecutive cases. J Nerv Ment Dis 93:421–442, 1941

Paykel E, Dienelt M: Suicide attempts following acute depression. J Nerv Ment Dis 153:234–243, 1971

Paykel ES, Prusoff BA, Myers J: Suicide attempts and recent life events: a controlled comparison. Arch Gen Psychiatry 32:327–333, 1975

Petzel SV, Cline DW: Adolescent suicide: epidemiological and biological aspects. Adolesc Psychiatry 6:239–266, 1978

Pfeffer C: Suicidal behavior of children: a review with implications for research and practice. Am J Psychiatry 138:154–159, 1981

Pfeffer C, Conte H, Plutchik R, et al: Suicidal behavior in latency-age children: an empirical study. J Am Acad Child Psychiatry 18:679–692, 1979

Philip A: Traits, attitudes, and symptoms in a group of attempted suicides. Br J Psychiatry 116:475–482, 1970

Platt S: Unemployment and suicidal behaviour: a review of the literature. Soc Sci Med 19:93–115, 1984

Platt S, Dyer J: Psychological correlates of unemployment among male parasuicides in Edinburgh. Br J Psychiatry 151:27–32, 1987

Reece FD: School-age suicides: the educational parameters. Dissertation Abstracts International 27:2895–2896, 1967

Reitman F: On the predictability of suicide. Journal of Mental Science 88:580–582, 1942

Richman J: The family therapy of attempted suicide. Fam Process 18:131–142, 1979

Richman J: Symbiosis, empathy, suicidal behavior, and the family. Suicide Life Threat Behav 8:139–149, 1978

Robins E: The Final Months: A Study of the Lives of 134 Persons Who Committed Suicide. New York, Oxford University Press, 1981

Rosen G: History in the study of suicide. Psychol Med 1:267–285, 1971

Rosenbaum M, Richman J: Suicide: the role of hostility and death wishes from the family and significant others. Am J Psychiatry 126:1652–1655, 1970

Rosenthal PA, Rosenthal S: Suicidal behavior by preschool children. Am J Psychiatry 141:520–525, 1984

Ross MW, Clayer JR, Campbell RL: Parental rearing patterns and suicidal thoughts. Acta Psychiatr Scand 67:429–433, 1983

Roy A: Suicide in chronic schizophrenia. Br J Psychiatry 141:171–177, 1982

Roy A: Suicide in recurrent affective disorder patients. Can J Psychiatry 29:319–322, 1984

Roy A: Suicide and psychiatric patients. Psychiatr Clin North Am 8:227–241, 1985

Rubinstein M, Winston A: Suicide and the participation of others. Diseases of the Nervous System 37:534–536, 1976

Rutter M: Maternal Deprivation Reassessed. Harmondsworth, Middlesex, England, Penguin Books, 1972

Rutter M: Resilience in the face of adversity: protective factors and resistance to psychiatric disorders. Br J Psychiatry 147:598–611, 1985

Sabbath JC: The suicidal adolescent—the expendable child. J Am Acad Child Psychiatry 8:272–289, 1969

Sainsbury P: Suicide in London: an ecological study (Maudsley Monographs No 1). London, Chapman & Hall, 1955

Sakinofsky I, Roberts R: The ecology of suicide in Canada, 1971–81. Paper presented to Epidemiology and Community Psychiatry Section, World Psychiatric Association, Edinburgh, 1985

Schmid CF, Van Arsdol M: Completed and attempted suicides: a comparative analysis. American Sociology Review 20:273–283, 1955

Schrut A: Suicidal adolescents and children. JAMA 188:1103–1107, 1964

Seiden RH: Suicide Among Youth: A Review of the Literature 1900–1967, Supplement to the Bulletin of Suicidology (PHS Publ No 1971). Rockville, MD, National Institute of Mental Health, 1969, p 35

Shafii M, Carrigan S, Whittinghill JR: Psychological autopsy of completed suicide in children and adolescents. Am J Psychiatry 142:1061–1064, 1985

Shepherd DM, Barraclough BM: Work and suicide: an empirical investigation. Br J Psychiatry 136:469–478, 1980

Silove D, George G, Bhavani-Sankaram V: Parasuicide: interaction between inadequate parenting and recent interpersonal stress. Aust N Z J Psychiatry 21:221–228, 1987

Silver D: Psychodynamics and psychotherapeutic management of the self-destructive character-disordered patient. Psychiatr Clin North Am 8:357–375, 1985

Simon W: Attempted suicide among veterans. J Nerv Ment Dis 111:451–468, 1950

Slater J, Depue RA: The contribution of environmental events and social support to serious suicide attempts in primary depressive disorder. J Abnorm Psychol 90:275–285, 1981

Spitzer RL, Endicott J, Robins E: Research Diagnostic Criteria: rationale and reliability. Arch Gen Psychiatry 35:773–782, 1978

Stanley EJ, Barter JT: Adolescent suicidal behavior. Am J Orthopsychiatry 40:87–96, 1970

Stein M, Levy MT, Glasberg HM: Separations in black and white suicide attempters. Arch Gen Psychiatry 31:815–821, 1974

Stengel E: Suicide and Attempted Suicide. Harmondsworth, Middlesex, England, Penguin Books, 1964

Stengel E, Cook N, Kreeger RI: Attempted suicide: its social significance and effects (Maudsley monographs No 4). London, Oxford University Press, 1958

Stone MH: The parental factor in adolescent suicide. International Journal of Child Psychotherapy 2:163–201, 1973

Streiner DL, Adam KS: Evaluation of the effectiveness of suicide prevention programs: a methodological perspective. Suicide Life Threat Behav 17:93–106, 1987

Tennant C, Bebbington P: The social causation of depression: a critique of the work of Brown and his colleagues. Psychol Med 8:565–575, 1978

Tennant C, Bebbington P, Hurry J: Parental death in childhood and risk of adult depressive disorders: a review. Psychol Med 10:289–299, 1980

Termansen P: Suicide and attempted suicide in Vancouver. British Columbia Medical Journal 14:125–128, 1972

Termansen PE, Bywater C: S.A.F.E.R.: a follow-up service for attempted suicide in Vancouver. Canadian Psychiatric Association Journal 20:29–34, 1975

Tishler CL, McKenry PC: Parental negative self and adolescent suicide attempts. J Am Acad Child Psychiatry 21:404–408, 1982

Tishler CL, McKenry PC, Morgan KC: Adolescent suicide attempts: some significant factors. Suicide Life Threat Behav 11:86–92, 1981

Topol P, Reznikoff M: Perceived peer and family relationships, hopelessness and locus of control as factors in adolescent suicide attempts. Suicide Life Threat Behav 12:141–150, 1982

Trout DL: The role of social isolation in suicide. Suicide Life Threat Behav 10:10–23, 1980

Virkkunen M: Alcoholism and suicides in Helsinki. Psychiatria Fennica 2:201–207, 1971

Waldinger R, Gunderson J: Effective Psychotherapy With Borderline Patients. New York, Macmillan, 1987

Walton HJ: Suicidal behaviour in depressive illness: a study of aetiological factors in suicide. Journal of Mental Science 104:884–891, 1958

Weiss RS: Attachment in adult life, in The Place of Attachment in Human Behavior. Edited by Parkes CM, Stevenson-Hinde J. New York, Basic Books, 1982, pp 171–184

Weissman M: The epidemiology of suicide attempts, 1960–71. Arch Gen Psychiatry 30:737–746, 1974

Weissman M, Fox K, Klerman GL: Hostility and depression associated with suicide attempts. Am J Psychiatry 130:450–455, 1973

Welu T: A follow-up program for suicide attempters: evaluation of effectiveness. Suicide Life Threat Behav 7:17–30, 1977

Werry JS, Pedder J: Self-poisoning in Auckland. New Zealand Medical Journal 83:183–187, 1976

West M, Sheldon A: Attachment dynamic in adult life. Br J Psychiatry 150:408–409, 1987

Wetzel RD: Hopelessness, depression, and suicide intent. Arch Gen Psychiatry 33:1069–1073, 1976

Wetzel RD, Margulies T, David R, et al: Hopelessness, depression, and suicide intent. J Clin Psychiatry 41:159–160, 1980

Williams C, Lyons CM: Family interaction and adolescent suicidal behaviour: a preliminary investigation. Aust N Z J Psychiatry 10:243–252, 1976

Wolkind S, Coleman EZ: Adult psychiatric disorder and childhood experiences: the validity of retrospective data. Br J Psychiatry 143:188–191, 1983

Yarden PE: Observations on suicide in chronic schizophrenics. Compr Psychiatry 15:325–333, 1974

Zilboorg G: Differential diagnostic types of suicide. Archives of Neurology and Psychiatry 35:270–291, 1936

Chapter 4

Biochemical Aspects of Suicide

Ronald M. Winchel, M.D.
Barbara Stanley, Ph.D.
Michael Stanley, Ph.D.

T HE EXPLORATION OF a biologic component to suicidal behavior drew relatively little attention until recently. Although a few studies of brain biochemistry in suicide victims occurred more than 20 years ago (Bourne et al. 1968; Shaw et al. 1976), most research in this area has been conducted over the past decade (e.g., Asberg et al. 1976; Mann and Stanley 1986; Stanley and Mann 1988). Despite the fact that biochemical aspects of suicide have been addressed only recently, findings are promising in at least two ways: 1) possible improvements in identification of those at risk and 2) a reconceptualization of suicidal behavior, with possible ramifications for treatment of suicidal patients.

It is surprising that the biology of suicide has not received more attention, particularly in light of the dramatic growth in research examining the biologic basis of many other forms of mental illness and the increasing use of pharmacotherapy in psychiatry. Neuroleptics and antidepressants are in common use in clinical settings, and more novel pharmacologic approaches to mental illness are being explored

Supported in part by USPHS Grants MH42242 and MH41847 and by the Scottish Rite Schizophrenia Research Program and the Lowenstein Foundation.
    Portions of the material in this chapter have been presented at the following meetings: American College of Neuropsychopharmacology, December 1987; American Psychiatric Association, May 1987; and Biological Psychiatry, May 1989.

(e.g., pharmacologic treatment of eating disorders and obsessive-compulsive disorders). This inattention to the biology of suicide might be understandable if available means were successful in preventing suicide and identifying those at risk. However, this is not the case. Most efforts aimed at identifying the potentially suicidal individual have focused on demographic, psychosocial, and personality factors (Goldney 1982; Monk 1975; Perlin and Schmitt 1975). Although several of these factors have been found to be associated with suicide, these variables offer too weak a prediction to be of substantial clinical utility. Suicide risk indicators tend to overpredict suicide potential, and, consequently, many more patients are identified falsely as suicide risks (Pokorny 1983). Furthermore, currently available methods of identification and therapies do not seem to be very helpful in preventing suicide since the suicide rate has remained stable over the last several decades. Therefore an approach that examines suicide from a biochemical perspective offers the hope of improved identification of suicidal persons and the promise of new prevention strategies. In addition, a biochemical approach to suicide focuses directly on understanding the behavior itself instead of on other ways of conceptualizing suicide (e.g., as a symptom of affective illness or as a response to the social environment).

This chapter will present evidence suggesting that suicidal behavior should be viewed as a separate syndrome that occurs in the presence of psychiatric disturbances but that is not necessarily a symptom of these disturbances. The evidence for suicidal behavior being considered as a separate syndrome derives from three sources: 1) the lack of a reduction in the suicide rate despite new treatments for specific psychiatric disturbances; 2) the occurrence of suicide across a diversity of psychiatric diagnoses; and 3) biochemical findings suggesting abnormalities specific to suicidal behavior but not to a particular psychiatric diagnosis.

STABILITY OF SUICIDE RATES

The overall suicide rate in the United States has remained fairly stable over the last 50 years (National Center for Health Statistics 1984), with the rate hovering around 12 per 100,000. While this overall rate has maintained stability, the rates within various age groups have shifted. Specifically, suicide rates in the age group of 15 to 24 years have risen dramatically over the last three decades, and the rate for elderly males has shown a decline. This steady rate reinforces the notion that progress in suicide risk identification and in treatment techniques has not had a major impact on suicide rates.

This lack of impact on suicide rates is not limited to the psychologically oriented treatments. It also appears that the introduction of pharmacologic treatments for the major mental illnesses has not served to decrease the rate of suicide. Suicide rates from 1945 to 1985 have shown little change. The introduction of neuroleptics (e.g., chlorpromazine) in 1954 and antidepressants (e.g., imipramine) in 1959 did not lower the suicide rate during subsequent years. This lack of reduction is particularly striking in relation to the use of imipramine because suicide is often viewed as a sequela of depression. Yet the availability of an effective pharmacologic treatment for depression has not substantially reduced the number of suicides.

There are many possible reasons for this lack of impact, including incorrect identification of those at risk with the consequence of inadequate treatment. It is also possible that suicidal behavior is not amenable to treatment and that a certain number of people in the population are inexorably determined to commit suicide despite intervention efforts. Another possibility, which will be focused on in this chapter, is that traditional conceptualizations of suicidal behavior may be flawed. For most instances, suicidal behavior is viewed as a symptom of a major psychiatric disturbance (most often depression), and suicidal patients are treated for this primary disturbance. The rationale for this treatment approach is that treatment of the primary disturbance (depression) will result in the amelioration of suicidal behavior.

The conceptualization of suicidal behavior presented in this chapter is one of a syndrome existing typically in the presence of major psychiatric disturbances but distinct from these disorders. This alternative view is consistent with the way in which eating disorders are seen, that is, not necessarily as a symptom of another disorder such as depression but as a disturbance in and of itself.

DIAGNOSIS AND SUICIDE

Suicide and depression are commonly linked, and suicidal behavior is often seen as a symptom of depression. Clinically, it is often presumed that if a patient is suicidal then he or she must also be depressed. The way in which depression is defined varies from a severe major depression to the experience of depressive mood. The assumption of a strong link between suicide and depression is not surprising given that depression is by far the most common diagnosis of those who die by suicide (Barraclough et al. 1974; Robins 1981). However, it is misleading to look at the diagnostic rates associated with suicide in this manner because depression has a much higher incidence in the general population than other psychiatric diagnoses. When the proportion of people who commit suicide within other major diagnostic groups is examined, a different picture emerges. About the same percentage of schizophrenic patients commit suicide as do patients suffering from major depression and bipolar disorders (Tsuang 1978). These findings indicate that suicide may not be specific to any one major psychiatric disturbance. Thus viewing suicide as a symptom of one particular psychiatric disturbance may be unwarranted even though DSM-III-R (American Psychiatric Association 1987) lists suicidal ideation as a criterion for depression. It may be possible that suicidal behavior is a separate syndrome that occurs in a certain number of the mentally ill and, consequently, must be targeted and treated as a problem in and of itself, apart from the major psychiatric disorders.

In the past, it was not uncommon for researchers to explore biologic hypotheses related to specific psychiatric illnesses (e.g., depression and schizophrenia). In the course of one such study, a unique neurochemical finding was observed and related to a specific behavior (suicide) rather than to a psychiatric diagnosis. This study has set the tone for much of the subsequent research in the field of suicide.

In this study, Asberg et al. (1976) were conducting biologic investigations of depression, specifically exploring the role of serotonin (5-HT) in this disorder. During the course of their research, it was noticed that those patients who had either attempted or committed suicide appeared to have low levels of the 5-HT metabolite, 5-hydroxyindoleacetic acid (5-HIAA), in their cerebrospinal fluid (CSF). Indeed, this group's published findings indicated that there was a bimodal distribution for 5-HIAA levels, with those who had attempted or completed suicide falling within the low mode. Although this finding was not confined to depressed patients who were suicidal, it was the forerunner of future investigations into a possible biochemical substrate for suicide in other diagnostic groups.

Following the publication of the Asberg et al. (1976) article, several reports have not only confirmed this finding of a lower 5-HIAA CSF level in depressed suicide attempters but also have extended it to include persons suffering from psychiatric disorders other than depression.

CSF Studies of Suicide Attempters

Many of the studies that have explored the relationship between suicidal and related behavior (e.g., aggression) and biochemistry have relied on the measurement of 5-HIAA in the CSF. However, it is important to know the extent to which this measure accurately reflects the utilization of 5-HT in the brain. Several studies using indirect approaches to this question have been reported. In general, these studies involved the measurement of 5-HIAA and homovanillic acid (HVA), the major metabolite of dopamine, in patients with transected spinal cords and the comparison of these values with either a group in which the block is incomplete or a control group without spinal injury. The findings of these studies have been inconclusive (Ashby et al. 1976; Curzon et al. 1971; Post et al. 1973). In an attempt to directly assess the degree to which 5-HIAA in the CSF reflects brain levels of 5-HIAA, Stanley et al. (1985) measured 5-HIAA in the brain and CSF of the same individual in samples obtained at autopsy; they found that there was a significant positive correlation ($r = .78$) between CSF and brain 5-HIAA levels. These findings provide the best proof that CSF 5-HIAA does, in fact, reflect biogenic amine metabolism in the brain.

The Asberg et al. (1976) CSF study reporting low levels of 5-HIAA in depressed suicide attempters has served as the prototype for subsequent biochemical studies of suicidal behavior. In addition to studies that have reported low levels of 5-HIAA in the CSF of suicidal depressed patients, numerous other reports have shown similar findings for patients with schizophrenia and personality disorders (e.g., Stanley and Mann 1988).

Agren (1980) was among the first investigators to confirm that suicidal depressed patients had lower CSF levels of 5-HIAA than nonsuicidal depressed patients. Other confirmatory studies in depression include those by Van Praag (1982), Montgomery and Montgomery (1982), Palaniappan et al. (1983), Banki et al. (1984), and Perez de los Cobos et al. (1984).

It should be noted that not all studies that have examined CSF levels of 5-HIAA in suicidal patients with affective illness have reported significant decreases in this measure. For the most part, the failure to find decreased levels of CSF 5-HIAA can be attributed to those studies in which the diagnosis of bipolar disorder predominates (Berrettini et al. 1986; Roy-Byrne et al. 1983). Although it is well known that manic-depressive illness carries a particularly high risk of suicidal behavior (Jamison 1986), it has been suggested that a significant degree of serotonergic dysfunction may be directly related to the illness itself and therefore obscure any potential suicide–5-HT relationship (Goodwin 1986).

Schizophrenic patients have been identified as being at high risk for suicide (Miles 1977; Roy 1982; Tsuang 1978). Van Praag (1983) reported that 5-HIAA levels were significantly lower in schizophrenic patients who had attempted suicide in comparison to those who had never attempted suicide. These findings have subsequently been replicated by another research team (Ninan et al. 1984). However, two other groups have failed to observe a difference in CSF levels of 5-HIAA between schizophrenic suicide attempters and nonattempters (Pickar et al. 1986; Roy et al. 1985).

In addition to depression and schizophrenia, decreased levels of CSF 5-HIAA have also been reported for suicidal patients with personality disorders. Brown et al. (1979, 1982) reported that, in both antisocial and borderline personality disorder patients, it was possible to identify those who had a history of suicidal behavior on a group basis by the presence of lower concentrations of 5-HIAA in the suicide group. Traskman et al. (1981) obtained similar results in a group of patients with personality disorders compared to normal controls. Linnoila et al. (1983) found lower levels of 5-HIAA in the CSF of a group of violent prisoners who had attempted suicide.

Banki et al. (1986) noted that alcoholic patients who had made a suicide attempt had lower CSF levels of 5-HIAA than did alcoholic patients who had not attempted suicide. However, these findings must be viewed in the context that the effects of ethanol consumption on biogenic amine metabolism in humans are poorly understood and have not been studied extensively in alcoholic suicide attempters.

The CSF finding of decreased levels of the 5-HT metabolite 5-HIAA is consistent with postmortem studies that have reported decreased levels in either 5-HIAA or 5-HT itself in the brain. These observations suggest that suicide and suicidal behavior are largely independent of diagnostic boundaries, as is their correlation with serotonergic measures. Thus a review of the literature reveals numerous reports of decreased levels of 5-HIAA in the CSF of suicidal patients across psychiatric diagnoses, including depressive illness, personality disorders, schizophrenia, and alcoholism (Table 1).

Another area that relates both behaviorally and biochemically to the subject of suicide is violence. In a study conducted by Brown et al. (1982), a significant inverse correlation was observed between 5-HIAA and a history of aggressive behavior. Similarly, a study by Linnoila et al. (1983) found that violent criminals (murderers and those who attempted murder) who committed their crimes in an impulsive manner had significantly lower levels of 5-HIAA than those whose crimes were premeditated. It is interesting to note that within this group of violent individuals, several had made suicide attempts. Consistent with the findings listed above, that group had significantly lower levels of CSF 5-HIAA. Other criminal offenders with poor impulse control (e.g., arsonists) were also found to have lower levels of CSF 5-HIAA relative to other violent offenders and normal controls (Virkkunen et al. 1987).

Table 1. Cerebrospinal fluid (CSF) studies of suicide attempters

Study	Diagnosis	Findings
Asberg et al. (1976)	Depression	↓ CSF 5-HIAA
Brown et al. (1979)	Personality disorders	↓ CSF 5-HIAA
Agren (1980)	Depression	↓ CSF 5-HIAA
Banki (1981)	Depression	↓ CSF 5-HIAA
Traskman et al. (1981)	Depression and personality disorders	↓ CSF 5-HIAA
Ninan et al. (1984)	Schizophrenia	↑ CSF 5-HIAA
Banki et al. (1984)	Alcoholism	↓ CSF 5-HIAA
Van Praag (1983)	Schizophrenia	↓ CSF 5-HIAA
Banki et al. (1983)	Schizophrenia	↓ CSF 5-HIAA
Roy et al. (1985)	Schizophrenia	No significant difference in CSF 5-HIAA
Berrettini et al. (1986)	Bipolar disorder	No significant difference in CSF 5-HIAA
Secunda et al. (1986)	Depression	No significant difference in CSF 5-HIAA

Note. 5-HIAA = 5-hydroxyindoleacetic acid.

POSTMORTEM STUDIES OF SUICIDE VICTIMS

In concert with the studies of 5-HIAA in suicide attempters, a number of investigations have been conducted in suicide victims. In general, this series of postmortem studies measured biogenic amines and their metabolites in suicide victims compared with nonsuicide controls. Decreases in the levels of 5-HT and 5-HIAA have been the most consistent findings from these studies. In general, decreases were noted in the area of the brain stem (raphe nuclei) and in other subcortical nuclei, including the hypothalamus. Lloyd et al. (1974) measured 5-HT and 5-HIAA in raphe nuclei of five suicide victims and five controls and found no significant difference in 5-HIAA levels between the two groups. There was, however, a significant reduction in 5-HT levels for the suicide group. Pare et al. (1969) determined norepinephrine, dopamine, 5-HT, and 5-HIAA levels in suicide victims who died by carbon monoxide poisoning. They reported a significant reduction in brain-stem levels of 5-HT for the suicide group, but found no significant difference between the two groups for norepinephrine, dopamine, and 5-HIAA. Shaw et al. (1967) found lower brain-stem levels of 5-HT in the suicide victims compared with controls, a statistically significant difference. Korpi et al. (1986) reported significant decreases in the hypothalamic concentration of 5-HT of suicide victims compared with nonsuicide controls.

Other research has reported significant reductions in the levels of 5-HIAA in suicide victims. Bourne et al. (1968) measured norepinephrine, 5-HT, and 5-HIAA in the hindbrain and found significantly lower levels only for 5-HIAA. Beskow et al. (1976) measured dopamine, norepinephrine, 5-HT, and 5-HIAA in brain-stem areas of suicide victims and controls. They noted significant reductions in 5-HIAA levels for the suicide group. Changes in dopamine, norepinephrine, or their metabolites were either negative or inconsistent.

In general, the results obtained in these postmortem studies point to some alteration in 5-HT turnover. These findings, together with the more recent postmortem receptor studies described below and CSF studies in suicide attempters described previously, are internally consistent and mutually supportive of a link between 5-HT and suicidal behavior. It is appropriate, however, to add a note of caution concerning postmortem work in general and the early postmortem work in particular.

In many of the studies described above, factors such as death by overdose or carbon monoxide poisoning, extensive postmortem delay, and lack of age-matched control groups figure significantly in the interpretation of these findings. These variables may also account in part for the lack of uniformity of findings among the postmortem studies. In addition to these potential sources of error, the levels of monoamines and their metabolites are known to be influenced by factors such as diet (Muscettola et al. 1977), acute drug use (Banki et al. 1983), and alcohol use (McEntee and Mair 1978). Although it is possible to control for the acute influence of these factors in CSF studies, for obvious reasons this is not always the case in postmortem assessments (Table 2).

In an effort to minimize the impact of the aforementioned variables, several investigators decided to use receptor binding assays, which have been shown to be generally nonresponsive to acute influences (Peroutka and Snyder 1980). Binding studies have shown that changes in the number of sites (or their density) can be induced by either a sustained increase in transmitter following chronic exposure to a chemical agent, for example, antidepressants (Peroutka and Snyder 1980), or by a sustained reduction in the level of a particular amine, for example, by lesioning neurons (Brunello et al. 1982).

Table 2. Postmortem neurotransmitter and metabolite studies of completed suicides

Study	Findings
Shaw et al. (1967)	↓ Brain-stem 5-HT
Beskow et al. (1976)	↓ Brain-stem 5-HIAA
Bourne et al. (1968)	↓ Brain-stem 5-HIAA
Pare et al. (1969)	↓ Brain-stem 5-HT
Lloyd et al. (1974)	↓ Brain-stem 5-HT
Korpi et al. (1986)	↓ Hypothalamus 5-HT ↓ Nucleus accumbens 5-HIAA
Cochran et al. (1976)	No change in brain 5-HT
Stanley et al. (1983)	No change in 5-HIAA or 5-HT levels in frontal cortex
Crow et al. (1984)	No change in 5-HIAA or 5-HT levels in frontal cortex
Owen et al. (1983)	No change in 5-HIAA levels in frontal cortex

Note. 5-HT = serotonin; 5-HIAA = 5-hydroxyindoleacetic acid.

Assays of receptors that appear to be associated with pre- and post-synaptic 5-HT neurons have been developed (Brunello et al. 1982; Langer et al. 1980). Imipramine binding sites associated with presynaptic binding sites have been characterized in platelets and various regions of the brain (Langer et al. 1980; Rehavi et al. 1982).

The rationale for studying imipramine binding in suicide victims was derived in part from the clinical findings of Langer et al. (1980), who had reported significantly reduced B_{max} values in platelets of depressed patients compared to controls (Raisman et a. 1981). The combined association of imipramine binding with 5-HT function, as well as the significant reduction in binding density in depressed patients, suggested the possibility that alterations in imipramine binding might be present in suicide victims. To test this hypothesis, Stanley et al. (1982) determined imipramine binding in the brains of suicide victims and controls. Because of the problems previous research groups had encountered conducting postmortem studies, particular care was taken in selecting cases matched for age, gender, and postmortem delay for this study. The suicide victims died in a determined manner (e.g., gunshot wound, hanging, jumped from height), and the control group was similarly chosen to match for sudden and violent deaths. The findings indicated a significant reduction in the number of imipramine binding sites in frontal cortex with no difference in binding affinity (K_d). The results of this experiment are consistent with the accumulating evidence suggesting the involvement of 5-HT in suicide. Specifically, reduced imipramine binding (associated with presynaptic terminals) may indicate fewer functional serotonergic terminals, which may result in reduced 5-HT release and be in agreement with reports of reduced postmortem levels of 5-HT and 5-HIAA in suicides, as well as lower levels of 5-HIAA in the CSF of suicide attempters.

Since the completion of this study, several additional studies have measured imipramine binding either in suicide victims or in depressive persons who died from natural causes (Table 3). Paul et al. (1984) measured imipramine binding in hypothalamic membranes from suicides and controls. Imipramine binding was significantly lower (B_{max}) in the suicide victims compared with controls. This group also measured desipramine binding in the same samples and noted no significant difference between the suicide and control groups. The selective reduction in imipramine binding argued against the possibility that this finding could be attributed to a drug-induced effect. Perry et al. (1983) measured imipramine binding in the cortex and hippocampus of depressed individuals dying from nonsuicidal causes. They reported a significant reduction in imipramine binding in the depressive group relative to a nondepressed control group that had been well matched. Crow et al. (1984) also reported a significant decrease in imipramine binding in the cortex of suicide victims compared with controls. In contrast to the findings cited above, one study found an increase in imipramine binding in the brains of suicides compared with controls (Meyerson et al. 1982). Possible explanations offered to address this discrepant finding include use of single concentration analysis instead of saturation isotherms and an inadequate matching of factors such as age, gender, and postmortem interval.

In summary, five published postmortem studies have measured imipramine binding. Thus far, four of the five studies reported a decrease in imipramine binding and one study found an increase.

In addition to assessing postmortem presynaptic function of the 5-HT system in suicide, it is possible to measure postsynaptic 5-HT binding sites using ligands such as ^{3}H-spiroperidol, ^{3}H-ketanserin, or ^{125}I-LSD. Binding of 5-HT$_2$ in animals has been reported to be downregulated or reduced in response to chronic antidepressant treatment, and lesioning of 5-HT nuclei produces up-regulated or increased 5-HT$_2$ receptor binding (Brunello et al. 1982; Peroutka and Snyder 1980).

Table 3. Postmortem receptor studies of completed suicides: serotonergic receptor findings

Study	Findings
Impramine binding	
Stanley et al. (1982)	↓ ^{3}H-imipramine binding in cortex
Paul et al. (1984)	↓ ^{3}H-imipramine binding in hypothalamus
Perry et al. (1983)[a]	↑ ^{3}H-imipramine binding in cortex
Crow et al. (1984)	↓ ^{3}H-imipramine binding in cortex
Meyerson et al. (1982)	↕ ^{3}H-imipramine binding in cortex
5-HT$_2$ binding	
Stanley and Mann (1983)	↑ 5-HT binding in cortex
Mann et al. (1986)	↑ 5-HT binding in cortex
Meltzer et al. (1987)	↑ 5-HT binding in cortex
Owen et al. (1983)	Increased but not significantly
Cheetam et al. (1987)	↓ 5-HT binding in cortex

Note. 5-HT = serotonin.
[a]Depressed dying of natural causes.

Stanley and Mann (1983) measured 5-HT$_2$ binding in the frontal cortex of suicide victims compared with controls; both groups were matched for age, sex, postmortem interval, and suddenness of death (nonpharmacologic). The study found a significant increase in the number of 5-HT$_2$ binding sites in the frontal cortex of suicide victims, with no change in binding affinity.

Because many of the brains had also been used in the previous report on imipramine binding by Stanley et al. (1982), it was possible to assess the degree to which these measures of receptor function correlated. The number of binding sites (B_{max}) for 5-HT$_2$ and imipramine showed a trend for a negative correlation ($r = -.42$, $p > .10$). Such a relationship supports the suggestion that the increase in 5-HT$_2$ binding might reflect a compensatory increase in postsynaptic binding sites secondary to a reduction in presynaptic input. It may be that despite the compensatory postsynaptic changes, there is still an overall hypofunction of the serotonergic system. Thus reduced levels of 5-HIAA in the CSF of suicide attempters as well as reduced levels of

5-HT and 5-HIAA in the brains of suicide victims are consistent with a hypofunctioning serotonergic system.

Subsequent to the study done by Stanley and Mann (1983), there have been five additional reports of 5-HT$_2$ binding in suicides. Owen et al. (1983) reported a nonsignificant increase in 5-HT$_2$ binding in nonmedicated suicide victims. Crow et al. (1984) found no change in 5-HT$_2$ binding between suicides and controls. In a larger series of suicide victims and controls, Mann et al. (1986) found a significant increase in suicide victims of 5-HT$_2$. Meltzer et al. (1987) also reported a significant increase in 5-HT$_2$ binding in frontal cortex. A significant decrease in 5-HT$_2$ binding in the frontal cortex of depressed suicide victims was reported by Cheetam et al. (1987) (Table 3).

In addition to serotonergic binding sites, several groups have measured muscarinic and beta-adrenergic binding sites in the brains of suicide victims (Table 4). Three studies have examined muscarinic binding sites in the frontal cortices and other regions of the brains of suicide victims (Kaufman et al. 1984; Meyerson et al. 1982; Stanley 1984). The rationale for these studies was suggested by the choliner-

Table 4. Postmortem receptor studies of completed suicides: nonserotonergic receptor findings

Study	Findings
Muscarinic binding	
Stanley (1984)	No change in muscarinic cholinergic receptor binding in cortex
Kaufman et al. (1984)	No change in muscarinic cholinergic receptor binding
Meyerson et al. (1982)	↓ Muscarinic cholinergic receptor binding
Beta-adrenergic binding	
Zanko and Biegon (1983)	↑ Beta-receptor binding
Mann et al. (1986)	↑ Beta-receptor binding
Biegon (1987)	↑ Beta-receptor binding
Meyerson et al. (1982)	No change in beta-receptor binding
CRF binding	
Nemeroff et al. (1988)	↓ CRF binding sites in frontal cortex

Note. CRF = corticotropin-releasing factor.

gic-adrenergic imbalance theory postulated by Janowsky et al. (1972) and by the known high proportion of suicides that are diagnosed as suffering from an affective disorder.

In a study comparing a large group of suicide victims and nonsuicide controls, Stanley (1984) found no difference between the number of binding sites in the frontal cortex for the two groups. Similarly, no changes in binding affinity were observed between the two groups. This finding was replicated by Kaufman et al. (1984), who determined the binding of quinuclidinyl benzilate (QNB), a muscarinic antagonist, in three brain regions (including the frontal cortex) in suicide victims. They found no differences in binding parameters for either group in any of the brain regions studied. In contrast to the findings observed in the two previously described studies, Meyerson et al. (1982) reported a significant increase in QNB binding sites in a small group of suicide victims compared with a control group that was not matched for age, gender, and postmortem interval.

In an attempt to understand the functional status of central noradrenergic neurons in suicidal behavior, Mann et al. (1986) measured beta-adrenergic receptors in suicide victims. They noted a significant increase in specific beta-adrenergic binding in suicide victims compared with controls. It has been suggested that alterations in beta-adrenergic receptors might be linked to the therapeutic actions of antidepressant drugs (Sulser and Robinson 1978).

Zanko and Biegon (1983) reported an increased number of binding sites (B_{max}) with no change in K_d in a small series of six suicide victims and matched controls. Biegon (1987) reported on a new series of suicide cases with increased beta-receptor binding. In contrast with the above studies, Meyerson et al. (1982) reported no alteration in beta-receptor binding in suicide victims. Thus three of four studies measuring beta-adrenergic receptors have reported an increase in binding in suicide victims. It should be noted that antemortem use of antidepressants would not explain the receptor alterations observed in the three previous studies because data from animal studies indicate that chronic antidepressant treatment results in down-regulation of beta-adrenergic receptors (Sulser and Robinson 1978).

It is interesting to note that the combination of 5-HT_2 binding data together with the results obtained for beta-adrenergic binding may provide additional sensitivity and specificity in the identification of suicide victims. For example, in the study of Mann et al. (1986), victims were found to have increases in both 5-HT_2 and beta-adrenergic binding. Conversely, no suicide victims had low levels of both receptor types. These findings may have potential therapeutic and forensic applications.

In addition to those studies that have measured receptor sites for the biogenic amines in suicide victims, a recent study measured binding sites for corticotropin-releasing factor (CRF) (Nemeroff et al. 1988). In studies of depression, the levels of CRF in the CSF have been reported to be significantly elevated relative to normal controls (Nemeroff et al. 1984) and to those of schizophrenic patients (Banki et al. 1987). CRF binding sites in the frontal cortex of suicide victims were found to be lower than in nonsuicidal controls (Nemeroff et al. 1988). The findings of the above studies suggest that the increased levels of CRF observed in depression may subsequently result in a down-regulation of CRF receptors in suicide victims, many of whom would be diagnosed as depressed. However, a separate study that measured CSF levels of CRF in depressed patients who were either suicidal or nonsuicidal found no difference between the groups (Arato et al. 1986). Both groups of depressed patients, however, did have significantly higher levels of CRF compared to nondepressed controls. The results of that study suggest that CRF changes may be associated with a depressive disorder rather than suicidal behavior (Table 4).

5-HT and Suicide: Clinical Implications

The evidence that suicidal behavior is associated with abnormalities of the serotonergic system raises the question of how these important findings can be translated into clinically useful applications. One important implication has been alluded to: Suicide and attendant behaviors may be viewed as an independent disorder, the etiology and course of which are not invariably tied to the primary psychiatric disorder, such as depression or schizophrenia. Focusing on suicidal behavior alone has led to the observation of its association with altered serotonergic activity. This evidence, that suicide may be separated from other diagnostic entities on at least one biologic parameter, suggests that its course may be independently targeted in treatment. It also suggests that treatment of associated psychiatric diagnoses may not be sufficient to protect adequately against eventual suicide (Blumenthal and Kupfer 1986). The shift in emphasis toward such a view of suicide may facilitate our treatment and prevention of this behavior. In addition to affecting attitudes toward suicidal behavior, however, the data discussed in this chapter may also provide specific new tools for treating and predicting suicidal behavior.

The usefulness of antidepressant drugs and neuroleptic agents in the treatment of depression and psychosis has provided many of the current insights into what brain mechanisms may underlie these behavioral abnormalities. It was the empirical demonstration of the usefulness of antidepressants and neuroleptics that led to etiologic theories based on their known actions in the brain.

With the emerging evidence for a "serotonin-suicide connection," this process may be reversed. That is, observations about altered neurochemical processes in suicidal behavior may allow development of pharmacologic treatments for this behavior. Pharmacologic interventions in suicidal patients may be tailored to effect changes in the serotonergic system. Although there is little evidence as of yet that this will be an effective strategy in the reduction of suicidal behavior, the possibilities are compelling. The advent of a variety of medications that specifically target the serotonergic system makes this approach possible.

Paramount among the clinical problems associated with suicidal behavior is our poor ability to predict suicidal risk (Lettieri 1974; Pokorny 1983). Although a variety of factors that significantly correlate with suicide have been isolated (Platts 1984; Sainsbury 1973), the correlations are too weak to be of real clinical utility (Cohen 1986). Furthermore, they tend to be greatly overpredictive, falsely identifying too many people as suicide risks. Markers of abnormal serotonergic activity may help solve this dilemma. Although, as an isolated factor, serotonergic function is itself an inadequate predictor, in combination with other identifying (behavioral) factors the predictability of suicide may be sufficiently enhanced to become clinically meaningful (Blumenthal, this volume).

Treatment Implications: Targeting Suicidality

Apart from viewing suicide as a response to stress, treatment of the suicidal patient has traditionally focused on the psychiatric syndrome that dominates the clinical presentation. For example, suicidal patients with major depression are treated for their depressive syndrome. Although precautions are taken to protect the patient from expression of suicidal impulses, the primary therapeutic interventions are usually directed at treating depression. The implicit reasoning is that if the depression remits, the suicidal urges and the risk of suicidal behavior may also remit. The treatment of psychotic patients (with or without depression) is approached in a similar manner when suicidal behavior is present. Attention is directed at diminishing expressions of the psychosis. Antipsychotic agents may be used to treat the psychosis, while psychosocial interventions may target the presumed stressors in the patient's life.

Although this approach appears logical and recognizes the meaning that suicidal feelings have for the patient, it nevertheless treats suicidal impulses only as epiphenomena of the depression and psychosis. Yet the recent evidence that suicidality may be associated with a functional lesion of the serotonin system—a lesion that is at least partially independent of depression or any other specific psychiatric syndrome—suggests that suicidal behavior may be addressed independently of any one psychiatric diagnosis. Indeed, optimal therapeutic outcome may require that treatments targeted at suicidal behavior be considered separately from treatment of the underlying syndrome.

The association between suicidality and altered serotonergic function implies that medications with specific effects on the serotonergic system may alter the expression of suicidal behavior. If suicidality can be specifically treated, our ability to help suicidal patients would not be limited to the treatment of associated psychiatric disorders. In addition to the potential for saving lives, this capability could greatly expand the capacity to help certain patients. For example, a schizophrenic patient may be refractory to the antipsychotic effects of neuroleptics. Psychotic symptoms may greatly disrupt the life of such a patient. But if suicidal behavior in this patient could be independently treated, the patient may have an amelioration of the morbid risk of suicide, despite ongoing psychosis.

In another example, the risk for acting on suicidal impulses is a common feature among patients with borderline personality disorders. For this reason, as well as others, these patients are frequently difficult to treat. Often these patients require hospitalization for control of suicidal behavior. For these patients in particular, hospitalization for suicidal behavior can be disruptive to treatment and may require active interventions that are often inconsistent with long-term treatment objectives. Reduction of suicidal risk may allow such patients to continue treatment outside of the hospital with fewer disruptions to the therapeutic process. In general, the reduction of suicidal behavior among these patients can greatly reduce the stress and stress for their families and therapists during the protracted period of time often needed for the treatment of this disorder.

The neurochemical findings described in this chapter provide a rational basis for considering pharmacologic approaches to the problem of suicide. It is important to emphasize, however, that evidence for decreased turnover of 5-HT does not mean low 5-HT causes suicidal behavior. Several factors confound such a simple conclusion. First, the association between 5-HT as indicated by low levels of CSF 5-HIAA and suicide does not necessarily indicate a causal relationship. Suicidality and altered serotonergic function may both result from a common—and, as yet, undetermined—cause. Second, decreased turnover of 5-HT may represent the brain's attempt to compensate for a pathologic increase in serotonergic activity, or alternatively, may reflect a compensation for a lesion in another neurotransmitter system. Third, alterations in neurotransmitter concentration are not the only determinants of neurotransmitter activity. Changes in sensitivity of a variety of neurotransmitter receptors can alter the level of activity of the system despite a constant concentration of the neurotransmitter itself. Nevertheless, given the existing body of data, pharmacologic manipulation of the serotonergic system is the logical point at which to initiate treatment studies. Therefore, various approaches to altering the activity of the serotonergic system should be systematically evaluated.

This strategy has been tentatively explored already in a preliminary study (Meyendorff et al. 1986). Meyendorff et al. administered fenfluramine, a 5-HT-depleting agent, to eight suicidal patients. After 4 weeks of treatment, ratings of suicidal thinking and depression were significantly improved. Measures of central nervous system (CNS) serotonin (CSF 5-HIAA) were significantly diminished compared to baseline measures before treatment. Although a hopeful beginning, several factors necessitate caution in interpreting the results of this study. Small sample size, lack of a control group, and concurrent improvement in depression warrant caution in drawing a conclusion that serotonergic manipulation alone selectively modifies suicidality.

It is important to note that in this study, fenfluramine, a drug that *depletes* the brain of 5-HT, did not exacerbate suicidality. This suggests that lowering brain 5-HT does not cause suicidal behavior or ideation. Further support of this observation is derived from a study in which DeLisi et al. (1982) gave parachlorophenylalanine (PCPA) to seven schizophrenic patients. PCPA is an inhibitor of the first step in the conversion of tryptophan to 5-HT. Thus PCPA significantly reduces the amount of 5-HT available within the CNS. Despite this action of PCPA, there was no significant change in any symptom among the patients treated by DeLisi et al. (including no evidence of increased depression or suicidality). In 1966, Cremata and Koe reported the first use of PCPA in six healthy male volunteers. Neither depression nor suicidal ideation was reported as a side effect for any of the subjects, although substantial decreases in blood and urine 5-HIAA were documented. These observations support the notion that lowering CNS 5-HT does not encourage suicidal behavior, despite the finding of low 5-HIAA in suicidal patients.

For nearly two decades, investigators have considered the hypothesis that 5-HT is an important factor in the genesis of depression (Meltzer and Lowry 1987). This theory has generated a number of studies in which "specific" serotonergic antidepressants have been compared to nonspecific antidepressants. In general, these studies have examined the efficacy of these agents in patients who are grouped by evidence for low or high activity of either the serotonergic or adrenergic systems.

Although some individual studies have suggested that markers of neurotransmitter activity—such as CSF 5-HIAA or 3-methoxy-4-hydroxyphenyleneglycol (MHPG)—may predict responders to drugs whose activities are primarily serotonergic or adrenergic, as a group these investigations offer contradictory or poorly replicable findings. In addition, some of the so-called specific agents that have been used are not entirely specific. For example, chronic administration of the 5-HT reuptake blocker zimelidine will result in down-regulation of beta-adrenergic receptor binding sites (Ross et al. 1981).

These kinds of investigations may be now undertaken in regard to the effect of serotonergically active agents on the expression of suicidal behavior. Several questions particularly need to be answered. Do medications that have specific effects on the serotonergic system have "anti-suicidal" effects that are independent of their antidepressant effects? Do measures of the serotonergic system (such as CSF 5-HIAA) predict subgroups of patients whose suicidal behavior may be altered by such medications?

As discussed above, suicidality may have an organic etiology and clinical course that may differ from the associated psychiatric illness. Judging the efficacy of these drugs solely on the basis of their effect on depressive symptoms may obscure their specific effects on suicidal behavior. In addition, the emergence of drugs that are more specific for the serotonergic system (e.g., fluoxetine, citalopram) makes such research strategies more practical.

Strategies for Pharmacologic Manipulation of the Serotonergic System

Specific manipulation of the serotonergic system can be approached in a variety of ways (Table 5). Some of these approaches involve the sites of action for currently available antidepressants. However, the agents in common clinical use at this time are generally not specific to the serotonergic system.

5-HT Precursors. 5-HT is synthesized in a two-step enzymatically catalyzed conversion of tryptophan to 5-HT. Tryptophan is available in many foods in standard diets, particularly dairy and poultry products. It is also commonly marketed in tablet or capsule form in drug stores and "health food" stores. Promoted by vitamin "faddists" and nutritionally oriented therapists for years, it has been investigated for potential antidepressant and sedative properties (Cole et al. 1980). Tryptophan has been shown to increase 5-HT in the CNS (Gillman et al. 1981). Behavioral effects of tryptophan supplementation in laboratory animals have been documented (Valzelli

Table 5. Potential neuronal sites for modification of serotonergic function

5-HT precursors
  Tryptophan
  5-HTP + carbidopa

Inhibition of 5-HT reuptake into the presynaptic neuron
Inhibition of monoamine oxidase enzymes that catabolize monoamine   neurotransmitters
Release of neurotransmitter from presynaptic neurons
Presynaptic autoreceptors that modulate neurotransmitter release
Postsynaptic receptors

Note. 5-HT = serotonin; 5-HTP = 5-hydroxytryptophan.

1967). Despite some encouraging reports (Gelenberg et al. 1982), it has not proven to have reliable antidepressant effects in human subjects. This may be due, in part, to the variable entry of tryptophan across the blood-brain barrier (which partially depends on plasma concentrations of amino acids that compete for the same active transport mechanism).

This problem has prompted investigational use of 5-hydroxytryptophan (5-HTP), which results from the hydroxylation of tryptophan and is the intermediate stage between tryptophan and 5-HT. When given orally in combination with carbidopa, CNS concentrations of 5-HT are more reliably increased. Studies of the antidepressant properties of 5-HTP + carbidopa may be more promising (Bryerley et al. 1987). There have been no investigations yet of a potential specific effect on suicidal behavior.

Inhibition of 5-HT Reuptake Into the Presynaptic Neuron. Inhibition of reuptake into the presynaptic neuron is one pharmacologic effect of many standard tricyclic antidepressants (TCAs). Although many of the available TCAs inhibit the reuptake of 5-HT, most have effects on uptake of other neurotransmitters as well, particularly adrenergic monoamines. Even some (e.g., zimelidine) that have no direct effect on reuptake of other neurotransmitters affect beta-adrenergic receptors. These mixed effects make assessment of the clinical impact of changes in 5-HT hard to assess. More specific 5-HT reuptake blockers (e.g., clomipramine, fluoxetine) are now emerging. Clinical studies of their use in obsessive-compulsive disorder suggest that they have different clinical effects from the less specific reuptake inhibitors (Ananth et al. 1981).

Inhibition of Monoamine Oxidase (MAO) Enzymes That Catabolize Monoamine Neurotransmitters. This is the mode of action of the MAO inhibitor class of antidepressants. Similar to the standard TCAs, these drugs are nonspecific in their activity, affecting changes in several different monoamine neurotransmitters. As more selective MAO inhibitors become available, specific effects in the serotonergic system may become practical. There has been a report of a positive correlation between MAO-B and 5-HT turnover in the brain (Adolfsson et al. 1978).

Potentiation of Release of Neurotransmitter From Presynaptic Neurons. Fenfluramine has a twofold action on serotonin. It both blocks reuptake and potentiates 5-HT's release from the presynaptic neuron into the synaptic cleft. This has the immediate effect of increasing available 5-HT in the synaptic space. When administered chronically, however, there is a depletion of 5-HT.

Presynaptic Autoreceptors That Modulate Neurotransmitter Release. Neurotransmitter binds with autoreceptors on the surface of the presynaptic cell. Partly through this mechanism, release of neurotransmitter from the neuron is subject to feedback control. Antagonism or agonism of these autoreceptors provides another means of modulating the amount of extraneuronal 5-HT.

Postsynaptic Receptors. Interneuronal transmission is accomplished as neurotransmitter binds to postsynaptic receptors. Drugs that have direct agonistic or antagonistic effects on these receptors may have direct effects on postsynaptic neurons of the serotonergic system.

It is important to emphasize that each of these target sites of interneuronal transmission may have effects on the others. For example, TCAs that acutely inhibit neurotransmitter reuptake and MAO inhibitor agents that inhibit catabolism cause a "down-regulation" of postsynaptic (5-HT_2) receptors after chronic administration. This decrease in the number of postsynaptic receptor sites has been interpreted as a compensation for the increased availability of synaptic neurotransmitter. (This effect, which has a better temporal relationship with clinical antidepressant effects than do the acute effects of these medications, has been speculated to be responsible for the therapeutic effect of antidepressant drugs.)

Tests of Serotonergic Activity

In addition to its direct therapeutic implications, the association of 5-HT and suicide may enhance our clinical ability to predict which of our patients may be at greater risk for suicide. The capability for predicting suicide risk may have significant impact on treatment planning. Critical junctures in the management of potentially suicidal patients are complicated by our poor ability to predict suicide risk. The decision to hospitalize is often based on this concern. Although clinicians often tend to err on the side of conservative management (i.e., to admit the patient to the hospital when in doubt), many patients who do not exhibit warning signs of suicidal risk make precipitous suicide attempts. Similarly, decisions to discharge from the hospital are frequently based on similar concerns. Often patients might be treated in an office or clinic setting while living at home with family. However, when the morbid risk of suicide cannot be excluded, the patient must remain in the hospital. Effective and efficient use of the decision to admit or discharge from the hospital is limited by our ability to gauge suicide risk more accurately.

Measures of serotonergic function, in conjunction with other clinical and behavioral observations, may significantly increase our ability to predict the risk of suicidal behavior in an individual patient. As suggested above, this expanded ability to predict suicidal behavior may have significant impact on important junctures in clinical treatment, particularly decisions related to hospital admission and discharge.

Another potential use of assessing serotonergic function may be an enhancement of the clinician's capacity to tailor specific pharmacologic interventions on the basis of serotonergic profiles. Several attempts have been made to match patients with treatments on the basis of neurotransmitter activity. For example, some have characterized depressed patients by the urinary tract excretion of the epinephrine and norepinephrine metabolite MHPG. Others have compared patients on the basis of CSF MHPG and CSF 5-HIAA. As mentioned above, individual studies have suggested that such data may be used to select specific agents based on their relative activity in the serotonergic or adrenergic systems. Unfortunately, no systematic picture has emerged from these studies. However, as newer, more specific agents emerge, and as the suicidality is focused on rather than the global spectrum of depressive symptoms, this strategy may yet prove useful.

Variables that affect CSF concentrations of 5-HIAA have been well examined (Stanley and Winchel 1989). This technique has emerged as a useful measure of central serotonergic activity. CSF, however, can be obtained only by lumbar puncture. A lumbar puncture is not yet frequently performed, nor is it an easily accepted procedure in clinical psychiatry. Other methods of assessing the state of the serotonergic system have been explored. These are described below.

Neuroendocrine Challenge Tests. The secretion of various hormones can be influenced by 5-HT. This has prompted the use of neuroendocrine challenge tests as a functional measure of the activity of the serotonergic system. In these tests, agents that affect serotonergic activity are administered. Concentrations of various endocrine products are measured before and after administration of the provocative agent. Although baseline measures of these products, such as prolactin, growth hormone, and cortisol, may vary little among patients with altered serotonergic function, the response to challenge tests may provide markers of altered serotonergic activity. In this way, altered serotonergic activity in suicidal patients may be reflected in patterns of neuroendocrine response to challenge tests of this type. This too is currently being used to study patients with suicidal behavior (Meltzer et al. 1984), as well as other syndromes such as depression (Heninger et al. 1984), obsessive-compulsive disorder (Charney et al. 1988), and personality disorders (Coccaro et al. 1987). Provocative agents used in these studies include the 5-HT precursor tryptophan; fenfluramine, which is a 5-HT releasing agent as well as an indirect agonist; and direct agonists such as m-CPP and MK-212.

These challenge tests may prove of clinical utility in demonstrating which patients have alterations in serotonergic activity, and therefore may be at greater risk for suicidal behavior. A drawback of these challenge tests is that serotonergic influences are only one factor in the feedback control mechanisms that mediate production of these hormones. Although they may emerge as useful markers of suicidal risk, there are difficulties in extrapolating to specific neuroendocrine or serotonergic deficits.

Other neuroendocrine measures have been investigated in this regard. Several studies indicate high excretion of cortisol in suicidal patients (Bunney and Fawcett 1965; Ostroff et al. 1982; Prasad 1985). However, the validity of an association between suicidal behavior and high cortisol has been cast in doubt. Traskman et al. (1980) found no change in CSF cortisol in suicidal patients who were also depressed. Additionally, Banki et al. (1984) and Boorsbank et al. (1972) found no association between suicidal behavior and CSF cortisol.

It is generally accepted that the dexamethasone suppression test (DST) is abnormal in about 50% of patients with melancholic depression. Some studies indicate that abnormal DST results may provide a marker of suicidal tendencies (Agren 1983; Banki et al. 1984; Coryell and Schesser 1981; Targum et al. 1983). Because of the high rate of abnormal DST results among patients with major depression (Arana and Baldessarini 1987), it is unlikely that this factor alone will provide a highly specific predictor of suicidality among individuals with this disorder. As an additional item in a "profile" of risk factors, however, it may add to our ability to determine which patients are at significantly greater risk for suicidal behavior. Among patients with other diagnoses, however, an abormal DST—should it prove to be associated with suicidal behavior—may add more powerfully to a predictive profile because of the much lower percentage of patients who have abnormal DST results. Among individuals with schizophrenia, for example, the DST is reported to be abnormal in 13% on the average (Arana and Baldessarini 1987). If an abnormal DST result is predictive of suicide, the specificity of this measure for suicide will be much greater in diagnostic groups other than depression, which has an average of 44% abnormal DST results (range, 34% to 78%) (Arana and Baldessarini 1987). Further research is needed before the usefulness of the DST as a marker of suicidality can be determined.

CLINICAL USEFULNESS: CURRENT PROSPECTS

The association between altered 5-HT turnover and the risk for suicidal behavior provides a window through which we may begin to view the biologic determinants of suicide. It may be found, however, that clinical applications of these observations may precede our understanding of the pathophysiology of biochemical contributions to suicidal behavior. When combined with the study of behavioral and environmental correlates of increased suicide risk, studies of the serotonergic system may significantly enhance our ability to predict who may be at greater risk for suicidal behavior.

It should be noted that studies of biologic markers of suicidal behavior have been performed in patients who have ongoing suicidal ideation or who have made previous suicide attempts. To draw inferences about serotonergic turnover prior to the suicide attempt is tempting, but such inferences are not currently justified by the existing body of data.

Among the clinical observations made about suicidal patients, it is often said that the risk of suicide may increase in the first few days following initiation of antidepressant treatment. This apparent but undocumented risk has been speculatively tied to the increased energy and agitation that often occurs before the onset of improved mood. In these first days of exposure to the monoamine reuptake blockade common to many of these agents, increased 5-HT is available in the interneuronal synaptic space. Could increased suicidality be related to the presence of 5-HT in a "too sensitive" system? Is decreased 5-HIAA evidence of the body's attempt to "turn down" the system? Although no laboratory data exist to support such a conclusion, it is raised to underscore the limits on what conclusions can be drawn from what is already known.

The ability to predict an individual's risk for suicidal behavior on the basis of this biologic parameter alone is also severely limited. Several options exist, however, for increasing the predictive power of this tool. As other biologic correlates are investigated, such as neuroendocrine challenge tests, some may emerge that have predictive value regarding suicide. Such correlates, when combined with measures of the serotonergic system, may add significantly to predictive power.

Behavioral correlates of suicide may also be examined. As specific behavioral correlates of suicide are elucidated, they may contribute to the development of an at-risk "profile," the predictive power of which results from the accumulated sensitivity of both behavioral and biologic correlates (Blumenthal, this volume). Such behavioral correlates may be based on current behavior, but may also emerge from past history. In addition, behavioral features of certain character disorders (such as impulsive acts) may provide evidence of increased risk for suicidal behavior.

Specific biologic measures may not ultimately provide very sensitive "markers" for the prediction of suicidal behavior in large numbers of potential attempters. Despite this limitation, clinical utility may still be found for certain populations of patients. Data suggest that, at the lower ranges of CSF 5-HIAA concentration, the predictive power of this measure may be much enhanced (Stanley 1987). For these patients in particular, measures of serotonergic dysfunction may indeed provide a sensitive tool for predicting suicide risk. For other patients, the elucidation of other predictive factors in addition to 5-HIAA may be necessary to yield a helpful predictive tool. Identification of biologic factors associated with suicidal behavior holds promise for the development and application of pharmacologic treatments as part of suicide prevention.

REFERENCES

Adolfsson R, Gottfries CG, Oreland L, et al: Monoamine oxidase activity and serotonergic turnover in human brain. Prog Neuropsychopharmacol Biol Psychiatry 2:225–230, 1978

Agren H: Symptom patterns in unipolar and bipolar depression correlating with monoamine metabolites in the cerebrospinal fluid, II: suicide. Psychiatry Res 3:225–236, 1980

Agren H: Life at risk: markers of suicidality in depression. Psychiatr Dev 1:87–103, 1983

American Psychiatric Association: Diagnostic and Statistical Manual of Mental Disorders, 3rd Edition, Revised. Washington, DC, American Psychiatric Association, 1987

Ananth J, Pecknold JC, Van Densteen N, et al: Double blind comparative study of clomipramine and amitriptyline in obsessive neurosis. Progress in Neuro-Psychopharmacology 5:257–262, 1981

Arana GW, Baldessarini RJ: Clinical use of the dexamethasone suppression test in psychiatry, in Psychopharmacology: The Third Generation of Progress. Edited by Meltzer HY. New York, Raven, 1987, pp 609–616

Arato M, Banki CM, Nemeroff CB, et al: Hypothalamic-pituitary-adrenal axis and suicide, in Psychobiology of Suicidal Behavior. Edited by Mann JJ, Stanley M. New York, New York Academy of Sciences, 1986, pp 263–270

Asberg M, Thoren P, Traskman L, et al: Serotonin depression: a biochemical subgroup within the affective disorders? Science 191:478–480, 1976

Ashby P, Verrier M, Warsh JJ, et al: Spinal reflexes and the concentration of 5-HIAA, MHPG, and HVA in lumbar cerebrospinal fluid after spinal lesions in man. J Neurol Neurosurg Psychiatry 39:1191–1200, 1976

Banki CM: Factors influencing monoamine metabolites and tryptophan in patients with alcohol dependence. J Neural Transm 50:89–101, 1981

Banki CM, Arato M, Papp Z, et al: The effect of dexamethasone on cerebrospinal fluid monoamine metabolites and cortisol in psychiatric patients. Pharmacopsychiatria 16:77–81, 1983

Banki CM, Arato M, Papp Z, et al: Biochemical markers in suicidal patients: investigations with cerebrospinal fluid amine metabolites and neuroendocrine tests. J Affective Disord 6:341–350, 1984

Banki C, Arato M, Kilts C: Aminergic studies and cerebrospinal fluid cautions in suicide, in Psychobiology of Suicidal Behavior. Edited by Mann JJ, Stanley M. New York, New York Academy of Sciences, 1986, pp 221–230

Banki CM, Bissett G, Arato M, et al: CSF corticotropin-releasing factor-like immunoreactivity in depression and schizophrenia. Am J Psychiatry 144:873–877, 1987

Barraclough B, Bunch J, Nelson B, et al: A hundred cases of suicide: clinical aspects. Br J Psychiatry 125:355–374, 1974

Berrettini W, Nurenberger J, Narrow W, et al: Cerebrospinal fluid studies of bipolar patients with and without a history of suicide attempts, in Psychobiology of Suicidal Behavior. Edited by Mann JJ, Stanley M. New York, New York Academy of Sciences, 1986, pp 197–201

Beskow J, Gottfries CG, Roos BE, et al: Determination of monoamine and monoamine metabolites in the human brain: post mortem studies in a group of suicides and a control group. Acta Psychiatr Scand 53:7–20, 1976

Biegon A: Beta receptor changes in suicide victims. Grand rounds presentation, Rockefeller University, 1987

Blumenthal SI, Kupfer DJ: Generalizable treatment strategies for suicidal behavior, in Psychobiology of Suicidal Behavior. Edited by Mann JJ, Stanley M. New York, New York Academy of Sciences, 1986, pp 327–340

Boorsbank BW, Brammall MA, Cunningham AE, et al: Estimation of corticosteroids in human cerebral cortex after death by suicide, accident or disease. Psychol Med 2:56–65, 1972

Bourne HR, Bunney WE Jr, Colburn RW, et al: Noradrenaline, 5-hydroxytryptamine, and 5-hydroxindoleacetic acid in the hindbrains of suicidal patients. Lancet 2:805–808, 1968

Brown GL, Goodwin FK, Ballenger JC, et al: Aggression in humans correlates with cerebrospinal fluid amine metabolites. Psychiatry Res 1:131–139, 1979

Brown GL, Ebert MH, Goyer PF, et al: Aggression, suicide, and serotonin: relationships of CSF amine metabolites. Am J Psychiatry 139:741–746, 1982

Brunello N, Chuang EM, Costa E: Different synaptic location of mianserin and imipramine binding sites. Science 215:1112–1115, 1982

Bryerley WF, Judd LL, Reimherr FW, et al: 5-Hydroxytryptophan: a review of its antidepressant efficacy and adverse effects. J Clin Psychopharmacol 7:127–137, 1987

Bunney WE, Fawcett JA: Possibility of a biochemical test for suicidal potential. Arch Gen Psychiatry 13:232–239, 1965

Charney DS, Goodman WK, Price LH, et al: Serotonin function in obsessive-compulsive disorder: a comparison of the effects of tryptophan and M-chlorophenylpiperazine in patients and healthy subjects. Arch Gen Psychiatry 45:177–185, 1988

Cheetam SC, Cross JA, Crompton MR, et al: Serotonin and GABA function in depressed suicide victims. Abstract, International Conference on New Directions in Affective Disorders, Jerusalem, 1987

Coccaro EF, Siever LI, Klar H, et al: Serotonergic studies in DSM-III personality disorder: evidence for involvement in aggression and impulsivity. Abstract, American College of Neuropsychopharmacology, San Juan, Puerto Rico, 1987

Cochran E, Robins E, Grote S: Regional serotonin levels in brain: a comparison of depressive suicides and alcoholic suicides with controls. Biol Psychiatry 11:283–294, 1976

Cohen J: Statistical approaches to suicidal risk factor analysis, in Psychobiology of Suicidal Behavior. Edited by Mann JJ, Stanley M. New York, New York Academy of Sciences, 1986, pp 34–41

Cole JO, Hartmann E, Brigham P: Psychopharmacology update. McLean Hospital Journal 59:37–71, 1980

Coryell W, Schesser MA: Suicide and the dexamethasone suppression test in unipolar depression. Am J Psychiatry 138:1120–1121, 1981

Cremata VY, Koe BK: Clinical-pharmacological evaluation of P-parachlorophenylalanine: a new serotonin-depleting agent. Clin Pharmacol Ther 7:768–776, 1966

Crow TJ, Cross AJ, Cooper SJ, et al: Neurotransmitter receptors and monoamine metabolites in the brains of patients with Alzheimer-type dementia and depression and suicides. Neuropharmacology 23:1561–1569, 1984

Curzon G, Gumpert EI, Sharpe DM: Amine metabolites in the lumbar CSF of humans with restricted flow of CSF. Nature; New Biology 231:189, 1971

DeLisi LE, Freed WJ, Gillin C, et al: Parachlorophenylalanine trials in schizophrenic patients. Biol Psychiatry 17:471–477, 1982

Gelenberg AJ, Gibson JC, Wojcik JD: Neurotransmitter precursors for the treatment of depression. Psychopharmacol Bull 18:7–18, 1982

Gillman PK, Bartlett JR, Bridges PK, et al: Indolic substances in plasma, CSF and frontal cortex of human subjects infused with saline or tryptophan. J Neurochem 37:410–417, 1981

Goldney R: Loss of control in young women who have attempted suicide. J Nerv Ment Dis 170:198–201, 1982

Goodwin FK: Suicide, aggression and depression: a theoretical framework for future research, in Psychobiology of Suicidal Behavior. Edited by Mann JJ, Stanley M. New York, New York Academy of Sciences, 1986, pp 351–356

Heninger GR, Charney DS, Sternberg DE: Serotonergic function in depression: prolactin response to intravenous tryptophan in depressed patients and healthy subjects. Arch Gen Psychiatry 41:398–402, 1984

Jamison KR: Suicide and bipolar disorders, in Psychobiology of Suicidal Behavior. Edited by Mann JJ, Stanley M. New York, New York Academy of Sciences, 1986, pp 301–315

Janowsky DS, El-Yousef MK, Davis JM, et al: A cholinergic-adrenergic hypothesis of mania and depression. Lancet 2:632–635, 1972

Kaufman CA, Gillin JC, Hill B, et al: Muscarinic binding in suicides. Psychiatry Res 12:47–55, 1984

Korpi ER, Kleinman JE, Goodman SI, et al: Serotonin and 5-hydroxindoleacetic acid in brains of suicide victims: comparison in chronic schizophrenic patients with suicide as cause of death. Arch Gen Psychiatry 43:594–600, 1986

Langer SZ, Moret C, Raisman R, et al: High-affinity [³H] imipramine binding in rat hypothalamus: assocation with uptake of serotonin but not of norepinephrine. Science 210:1133–1135, 1980

Lettieri D: Suicidal death prediction scales, in The Prediction of Suicide. Edited by Beck A, Resnick H, Lettieri D. Bowie, MD, Charles Press, 1974, pp 163–192

Linnoila M, Virkkunen M, Scheinin M, et al: Low cerebrospinal fluid 5-hydroxyindoleacetic acid concentration differentiates impulsive from nonimpulsive violent behavior. Life Sci 33:2609–2614, 1983

Lloyd KG, Farley IJ, Deck JH, et al: Serotonin and 5-hydroxyindoleacetic acid in discrete areas of the brainstem of suicide victims and control patients. Adv Biochem Psychopharmacol 11:387–397, 1974

Mann JJ, Stanley M (eds): Psychobiology of Suicidal Behavior. New York, New York Academy of Science, 1986

Mann JJ, Stanley M, McBride PA, et al: Increased serotonin$_2$ and beta$_1$-adrenergic receptor binding in the frontal cortices of suicide victims. Arch Gen Psychiatry 43:954–959, 1986

McEntee WI, Mair RG: Memory impairment in Korsakoff's psychosis: a correlation with brain noradrenergic activity. Science 202:905–907, 1978

Meltzer HY, Lowry MT: The serotonin hypothesis of depression, in Psychopharmacology: The Third Generation of Progress. Edited by Meltzer HY. New York, Raven, 1987, pp 513–526

Meltzer HY, Perline R, Tricou BJ, et al: Effect of 5-hydroxytryptophan on serum cortisol levels in major affective disorders, II: relation to suicide, psychosis and depressive symptoms. Arch Gen Psychiatry 41:379–387, 1984

Meltzer HY, Nash JF, Ohmori T, et al: Neuroendocrine and biochemical studies in serotonin and dopamine in depression and suicide. Abstract, International Conference on New Directions in Affective Disorders, Jerusalem, 1987

Meyendorff E, Jain A, Traskman-Bendz L, et al: The effects of fenfluramine on suicidal behavior. Psychopharmacol Bull 22:155–159, 1986

Meyerson LR, Wennogle LP, Abel MS, et al: Human brain receptor alterations in suicide victims. Pharmacol Biochem Behav 17:159–163, 1982

Miles C: Conditions predisposing to suicide: a review. J Nerv Ment Dis 164:231–246, 1977

Monk M: Epidemiology, in A Handbook for the Study of Suicide. Edited by Perlin S. New York, Oxford University Press, 1975, pp 185–211

Montgomery SA, Montgomery D: Pharmacological prevention of suicidal behaviour. J Affective Disord 4:291–298, 1982

Muscettola G, Wehr T, Goodwin FK: Effect of diet on urinary MHPG excretion in depressed patients and normal control subjects. Am J Psychiatry 134:914–916, 1977

National Center for Health Statistics: Health, United States (DHHS Publ No PHS-85-1232). Washington, DC, U.S. Government Printing Office, 1984

Nemeroff CB, Widerlov E, Bissette G, et al: Elevated concentrations of CSF corticotropin-releasing factor-like immunoreactivity in depressed patients. Science 226:1342–1344, 1984

Nemeroff CB, Owens MJ, Bissett G, et al: Reduced corticotropin releasing factor (CRF) binding sites in the frontal cortex of suicides. Arch Gen Psychiatry 45:577–579, 1988

Ninan PT, Van Kammen DP, Scheinin M, et al: CSF 5-hydroxindoleacetic acid levels in suicidal schizophrenic patients. Am J Psychiatry 141:566–569, 1984

Ostroff RB, Giller E, Bonese K, et al: Neuroendocrine risk factors of suicidal behavior. Am J Psychiatry 139:1323–1325, 1982

Owen F, Cross AJ, Crow TJ, et al: Brain 5-HT$_2$ receptors and suicide. Lancet 2:1256, 1983

Palaniappan V, Ramachandran V, Somasundaram O: Suicidal ideation and biogenic amines in depression. Indian Journal of Psychiatry 25:286–292, 1983

Pare CMB, Yeung DP, Price K, et al: 5-Hydroxytryptamine, noradrenaline, and dopamine in brainstem, hypothalamus, and caudate nucleus of controls and of patients committing suicide by coal-gas poisoning. Lancet 2:133–135, 1969

Paul SM, Rehavi M, Skolnick P, et al: High affinity binding of antidepressants to a biogenic amine transport site in human brain and platelet: studies in depression, in Neurobiology of Mood Disorders. Edited by Post RM, Ballenger JC. Baltimore, Williams & Wilkins, 1984

Perez de los Cobos JZ, Lopez-Ibor Alino JJ, Saiz Ruiz J: Correlatos biologicos del suicidio y la agesividad en depresiones mayores (con melancolia): 5-HIAA en LCR, DST, y respuesta terapeutica a 5-HTp. Presented to the

First Congress of the Spanish Society for Biological Psychiatry, Barcelona, 1984

Perlin S, Schmitt S: Psychiatry, in A Handbook for the Study of Suicide. Edited by Perlin S. New York, Oxford University Press, 1975, pp 147–163

Peroutka SJ, Snyder SH: Regulation of serotonin ($5HT_2$) receptors labeled with [^{3}H] spiroperidol by chronic treatment with antidepressant amitriptyline. J Pharmacol Exp Ther 215:582–587, 1980

Perry EK, Marshall EF, Blessed G, et al: Decreased imipramine binding in the brains of patients with depressive illness. Br J Psychiatry 142: 188–192, 1983

Pickar D, Roy A, Breier A, et al: Suicide and aggression in schizophrenia: neurobiologic correlates, in Psychobiology of Suicidal Behavior. Edited by Mann JJ, Stanley M. New York, New York Academy of Sciences, 1986, pp 189–196

Platts S: Unemployment and suicidal behaviour: a review of the literature. Soc Sci Med 19:93–115, 1984

Pokorny AD: Prediction of suicide in psychiatric patients: report of a perspective study. Arch Gen Psychiatry 40:249–257, 1983

Post RM, Goodwin FK, Gordon EK, et al: Amine metabolites in human cerebrospinal fluid: effects of cord transection and spinal fluid block. Science 179:897–899, 1973

Prasad AJ: Neuroendocrine differences between violent and non-violent parasuicides. Neuropsychobiology 13:157–159, 1985

Raisman R, Sechter D, Briley MS, et al: High-affinity ^{3}H-imipramine binding in platelets from untreated and treated depressed patients compared to healthy volunteers. Psychopharmacology 75:368–371, 1981

Rehavi M, Skolnick P, Paul SM: Solubilization and partial purification of the high affinity [^{3}H] imipramine bindiing site from human platelets. FEBS Leh 150:514–518, 1982

Robins E: The Final Months. New York, Oxford University Press, 1981

Ross SB, Hall H, Renyi AL, et al: Effects of zimeldine on serotonergic and noradrenergic neurons after repeated administration in the rat. Psychopharmacology 72:219–225, 1981

Roy A: Suicide in chronic schizophrenia. Br J Psychiatry 141:171–177, 1982

Roy A, Ninan P, Mazonson A, et al: CSF monoamine metabolites in chronic schizophrenic patients who attempt suicide. Psychol Med 15:335–340, 1985

Roy-Byrne P, Post RM, Rubinow DR, et al: CSF 5-HIAA and personal and family history of suicide in affectively ill patients: a negative study. Psychiatry Res 10:263–274, 1983

Sainsbury P: Suicide: opinions and facts. Proceedings of the Royal Society of Medicine 66:579–587, 1973

Secunda SK, Cross CK, Koslow S, et al: Biochemistry and suicidal behavior in depressed patients. Biol Psychiatry 21:756–767, 1986

Shaw DM, Camps FE, Eccleston EG: 5-Hydroxytryptamine in the hind-brain of depressive suicides. Br J Psychiatry 113:1407–1411, 1967

Stanley M: Cholinergic receptor binding in the frontal cortex of suicide victims. Am J Psychiatry 141:1432–1436, 1984

Stanley M: Preliminary biochemical and behavioral findings in suicide attempers. Presentation, American College of Neuropsychopharmacology, San Juan, Puerto Rico, 1987

Stanley M, Mann JJ: Increased serotonin-2 binding sites in frontal cortex of suicide victims. Lancet 2:214–216, 1983

Stanley M, Mann JJ: Biological factors associated with suicide, in American Psychiatric Press Review of Psychiatry, Vol 7. Edited by Frances AJ, Hales RE. Washington, DC, American Psychiatric Press, 1988, pp 334–352

Stanley M, Winchel RM: Antemortem and post mortem measures of CNS serotonergic function: methodologic issues, in New Directions in Affective Disorders. Edited by Lerer B, Gershon S. New York, Springer-Verlag, 1989, pp 54–59

Stanley M, Virgilio J, Gershon S: Tritiated imipramine binding sites are decreased in the frontal cortex of suicides. Science 216:1337–1339, 1982

Stanley M, McIntyre I, Gershon S: Post mortem serotonin metabolism in suicide victims. Abstract, American College of Neuropsychopharmacology, San Juan, Puerto Rico, 1983

Stanley M, Traskman-Bendz L, Dorovini-Zis K: Correlations between aminergic metabolites simultaneously obtained from human CSF and brain. Life Sci 37:1279–1286, 1985

Sulser F, Robinson SE: Clinical implications of pharmacological differences among antipsychotic drugs, in Psychopharmacology: A Generation of Progress. Edited by Lipton MA, DiMascio A, Killam KF. New York, Raven, 1978, pp 943–952

Targum SD, Rosen L, Capodanno AE: The dexamethasone suppression test in suicidal patients with unipolar depression. Am J Psychiatry 140:877–879, 1983

Traskman L, Tybring G, Asberg M, et al: Cortisol in the CSF of depressed and suicidal patients. Arch Gen Psychiatry 37:761–767, 1980

Traskman L, Asberg M, Bertilsson K, et al: Monoamine metabolites in CSF and suicidal behavior. Arch Gen Psychiatry 38:631–636, 1981

Tsuang MT: Suicide in schizophrenics, manics, depressives, and surgical controls: a comparison with general population suicides. Arch Gen Psychiatry 35:153–155, 1978

Valzelli L: Drugs and aggressiveness. Advances in Pharmacology 5:79–108, 1967

Van Praag HM: Depression, suicide and the metabolism of serotonin in the brain. J Affective Disord 4:275–290, 1982

Van Praag HM: CSF 5-HIAA and suicide in non-depressed schizophrenics. Lancet 2:977–978, 1983

Virkkunen M, Nuutila A, Goodwin FK, et al: Cerebrospinal fluid monoamine metabolite levels in male arsonists. Arch Gen Psychiatry 44:241–247, 1987

Zanko MT, Biegon A: Increased β adrenergic receptor binding in human frontal cortex of suicide victims. Abstract, Annual Meeting of the Society of Neuroscience, Boston, 1983

Chapter 5

Genetic Factors in Suicide: Family, Twin, and Adoption Studies

Seymour S. Kety, M.D.

SUICIDE IS AN example of deviant behavior where both environmental and genetic factors may be important or necessary, and neither alone may be sufficient. The literature over many years has cited a large number of socioenvironmental factors that are associated with suicide (Dublin 1963), and several chapters in this volume deal with these influences in great detail. There are marked differences in the rates for suicide according to age, religion, the country in which the study is carried out, and the particular period in that country's history. For example, in the United States, there has been a striking increase in adolescent suicides in the past three decades. Such marked variations cannot be explained on the basis of genetic variance because the genes do not vary so widely from one country to another, nor do they vary within a country from one time to another. There are also personal factors associated with suicide: marital status, financial circumstances, unemployment, parental loss, and others that influence the risk. In addition, there are important psychiatric risk variables, especially a previous history or concurrent presence of depression or schizophrenia (Black and Winokur, this volume; Roy 1982; Tsuang 1978).

The plausibility that significant cultural influences and devastating personal experiences could cause suicide, at a time when single causes sufficed for explanations, diminished the motivation to seek other types of influence. The "nature versus nurture" question, now thought to be obsolete, appeared to be settled in favor of environmental factors.

EVIDENCE FROM TWIN STUDIES

Hypotheses suggesting the operation of genetic influences in suicide were infrequently proposed and inadequately examined. Although families with a high incidence of suicide were known and sometimes reported in the literature, this could be explained on the basis of cultural and psychological attributes shared by a family without invoking their genetic endowment. It was to be expected that genetic factors, if present in suicide, would be clearly demonstrated by studies on twins. It was therefore very significant that Kallmann and Anastasio (1947), who found high concordance rates for schizophrenia and manic-depressive illness in monozygotic twins, found no concordance at all for suicide, concluding that genetic factors did not operate significantly in that behavioral deviance.

However, 20 years later, a review of later studies revealed an 18% concordance rate for suicide in a total of 51 monozygotic twin pairs and no dizygotic twins concordant for suicide (Haberlandt 1967). Juel-Nielsen and Videbech (1970) found a significant number of concordant monozygotic twin pairs with suicide. In no series is the concordance rate as high as it is for depression or schizophrenia; this is probably because the risk of suicide itself in the population is quite low compared to that of schizophrenia or manic-depressive illness. Furthermore, an environmental stressor that may have been a necessary contributing factor to the suicide of one twin may not have been present in the experience of the other. It is also possible that suicide in one twin actually diminishes the possibility of suicide in the remaining twin through psychological mechanisms.

ADOPTION STUDIES

Because of the obvious ways in which suicidal risk and behavior in twins and in members of a family could be enhanced or attenuated by psychological interactions between them, studies of adopted individuals and their biologic and adoptive relatives with respect to attempted and completed suicide are of interest. Two such studies have been completed, both utilizing a national sample of individuals legally adopted in Denmark between 1925 and 1948. Because of the excellent adoption and population records maintained in that country (Kety et al. 1968), as the basis of one study it was possible to identify the biologic and adoptive parents, siblings, and half-siblings of a proband group consisting of 57 adoptees who had committed suicide (Schulsinger et al. 1979). For the second study, 71 adoptees who had suffered a depressive illness were selected (Wender et al. 1986). For each study, an equal number of matched control adoptees were selected, and searches were made of vital statistics and hospital records for evidence of attempted or completed suicide in their biologic or adoptive relatives.

The results of the study by Schulsinger et al. (1979) are presented in Table 1. In the biologic relatives of the adoptees who had committed suicide, there was a 4.5% incidence of suicide compared to an incidence of less than 1% in the biologic relatives of the controls. There were no suicides in the adoptive relatives of either group. The psychiatric register was searched for indications of depression or other mental illness in those relatives who had committed suicide. In approximately 50%, no such history was found. Although that does not exclude the possibility that a brief period of depression could have preceded the suicide, it was suggested that there is a type of suicide that is not necessarily associated with mental illness.

The prevalence of suicide in relatives of adoptees selected for depression and of their control adoptees from the study of Wender et al. (1986) is presented in Table 2. There were 19 suicides in the relatives as a whole, 15 of which were in the biologic parents, siblings, and half-siblings of the depressed adoptees. The highly significant concentration of suicide found in both studies occurred in people who were related only genetically to adoptees who had committed suicide or suffered from depression. They did not rear them, were not reared with them, and did not live in the same family environment. In almost all cases, the biologic relatives were unaware of the whereabouts of the adoptee or what had happened to him or her.

Table 1. Incidence of suicide in all identified relatives of 57 adoptees who committed suicide and 57 matched controls

Adoptees	Biologic relatives	Adoptive relatives
Suicide	12/269 (4.5%)	0/148 (0%)
Control	2/269 (0.7%)	0/150 (0%)
	$P < .01$[a]	

[a]Fisher's exact, one-tailed *t* test.
Source. From Schulsinger F, Kety SS, Rosenthal D, Wender PH: A family study of suicide, in Origin, Prevention and Treatment of Affective Disorders. Edited by Schou M, Stromgren E. New York, Academic, 1979. (Used with permission.)

Table 2. Incidence of suicide in the relatives of 71 adoptees who have suffered a depressive illness and 71 matched controls

Adoptees	Biologic relatives	Adoptive relatives
Depressed	15/387 (3.9%)	1/180 (0.6%)
Control	1/344 (0.3%)	2/169 (1.2%)
	$P < .01^a$	

^{a}Fisher's exact, one-tailed t test.
Source. Adapted from Wender PH, Kety SS, Rosenthal D, Schulsinger F, Ortmann J, Lunde I: Psychiatric disorders in the biological and adoptive families of adopted individuals with affective disorders. Arch Gen Psychiatry 43:923–929, 1986. (Used with permission.)

One would not, of course, conclude from such results that suicide is entirely a genetically determined pattern of behavior in the face of the vast literature, which supports the operation of a number of crucial environmental factors. It is more likely that of all individuals who are subjected to some stressful life process or event, those who commit suicide have a genetic predisposition to do so. That raises the question: What may that predisposition be?

NATURE OF THE GENETIC PREDISPOSITION

There is accumulating evidence from analyses of blood, cerebrospinal fluid, and postmortem brain samples—for metabolites of serotonin or measurement of its receptors—that suggests that some deficiency in serotonin activity somewhere within the brain may be associated with suicide.

Among these studies, an especially interesting one was carried out on a group of normal volunteers (Buchsbaum et al. 1976). Blood samples were analyzed for platelet monoamine oxidase, and a questionnaire about the individual's family and patterns of behavior was completed. The groups with the highest and lowest levels of monoamine oxidase were then compared with respect to their answers to the questionnaires. Among a number of findings, the most interesting one pertinent to this discussion is that those students with the lowest levels of this enzyme in their platelets had eight times the prevalence of suicide in their families compared to the students with high levels of the enzyme. Such results certainly suggest that serotonin metabolism may have some role in suicide, possibly in the expression of the genetic factors involved, since monoamine oxidase is an important enzyme in the further metabolism and inactivation of serotonin.

RELATION OF SUICIDE TO DEPRESSION AND IMPULSIVE BEHAVIOR

We can also ask: What is the behavioral trait that is genetically transmitted? Is it depression itself that sometimes leads directly to suicide? This, of course, would be an easy conclusion to draw since there is such a high incidence of suicide in depression and also of depression preceding suicide. Robins (1981), who studied 134 suicides exhaustively, found that a diagnosis of clinical depression could be made in the majority of such individuals. It has been pointed out (Carlson 1984), however, that whereas 62% of those over 60 years of age were diagnosed in that series with affective disorder, that was true for only 24% of those under 40 years. Instead, in the latter age group, 54% had histories that could be interpreted as showing violence or impulsivity.

If the incidence of suicide in the biologic relatives of depressed adoptees is broken down according to the type of affective disorder diagnosed in the adoptee (Table 3), it can be seen that whether the adoptees' diagnoses were affective reaction, neurotic depression, bipolar depression, or unipolar depression, there was a significant concentration of suicide in the biologic relatives of each group. It is also interesting that the very highest incidence of suicide was in the biologic relatives of the adoptees with a very transient syndrome, which in Denmark was called "affect reaction." This is usually initiated by a serious suicide attempt, followed by a depression of very brief duration with only rare recurrence. These individuals did not reappear in the psychiatric register. It was apparently an impulsive act

Table 3. Incidence of suicide in the biologic relatives of depressive and control adoptees

Diagnosis of adoptee	Biologic relatives	P^a
Affective reaction	5/66 (7.6%)	.0004
Neurotic depression	3/127 (2.4%)	.056
Bipolar depression	4/75 (5.3%)	.0036
Unipolar depression	3/139 (2.2%)	.067
No mental illness	1/360 (0.3%)	

[a]Fisher's exact, one-tailed *t* test compared with biologic relatives of control adoptees with no known history of mental illness.
Source. Adapted from Wender PH, Kety SS, Rosenthal D, Schulsinger F, Ortmann J, Lunde I: Psychiatric disorders in the biological and adoptive families of adopted individuals with affective disorders. Arch Gen Psychiatry 43:923–929, 1986. (Used with permission.)

almost always precipitated by some stressful life event. There was more than three times the prevalence of suicide in the biologic relatives of these adoptees than in those of the unipolar depressions, which would be the paradigm of severe chronic depressive illness.

Roy (1983) and Tsuang (1983) simultaneously and independently found significantly higher risk for suicidal behavior in the families of patients who committed suicide than in the relatives of those who did not. In a study on suicide and family loading for affective disorders, Egeland and Sussex (1985) reviewed all the suicides over a 100-year period in the Old Order Amish population. The vast majority (92%) of the 26 suicides were diagnosed with a major affective disorder and occurred in multigenerational families, with heavy loading for bipolar, unipolar, and other affective-spectrum disorders. The authors argued that the role of inheritance for suicide in these extended pedigrees provides presumptive evidence of genetic factors in both suicide and affective disorders. Thus there appears to be a genetic factor favoring suicide that may operate independently of, or additively with, depression or other major psychosis. It is an interesting possibility that the genetic predisposition to suicide may represent a tendency to impulsive behavior, of which suicide is a prime example. There have been a number of studies compatible with that suggestion. Brown et al. (1982) found diminished levels of 5-hydroxyindoleacetic acid in the cerebrospinal fluid of individuals who were not depressed but who were characterized by impulsive or sociopathic behavior. Lithium, which is often effective in the prophylaxis of manic-depressive disorder, has also been found to be effective in impulsive and aggressive behavior (Sheard et al. 1976). It would be difficult to find out in a controlled manner, but interesting to know, whether antidepressant drugs or precursors that act primarily to enhance the activity of serotonin in the brain are capable of suppressing suicidal tendencies specifically.

We cannot dismiss the possibility that the genetic factor in suicide is an inability to control impulsive behavior, while depression and other mental illness, as well as overwhelming environmental stress, serve as potentiating mechanisms that foster or trigger the impulsive behavior, directing it toward a suicidal outcome. In any case, suicide illustrates better than any of the mental illnesses that are more difficult to define and ascertain, the very crucial and important interactions between genetic factors and environmental influences.

References

Brown GL, Ebert MH, Goyer PF, et al: Aggression, suicide, and serotonin: relationship to CSF amine metabolism. Am J Psychiatry 139:741–746, 1982

Buchsbaum MS, Coursey RD, Murphy DL: The biochemical high-risk paradigm: behavioral and familial correlates of low platelet monoamine oxidase activity. Science 194:339–341, 1976

Carlson GA: More analysis of Eli Robins' suicide data. Am J Psychiatry 141:323, 1984

Dublin L (ed): Suicide: A Sociological and Statistical Study. New York, Ronald Press, 1963

Egeland JA, Sussex JN: Suicide and family loading for affective disorders. JAMA 254:915–918, 1985

Haberlandt W: Aportacion a la genetica del suicidio. Folio Clin Int 17:319–322, 1967

Juel-Nielson N, Videbech T: A twin study of suicide. Acta Genet Med Gemellol (Roma) 19:307–310, 1970

Kallmann F, Anastasio M: Twin studies on the psychopathology of suicide. J Nerv Ment Dis 105:40–55, 1947

Kety SS, Rosenthal D, Wender PH, et al: The types of prevalence of mental illness in the biological and adoptive families of adopted schizophrenics, in The Transmission of Schizophrenia. Edited by Rosenthal D, Kety SS. Oxford, Pergamon, 1968

Robins E (ed): The Final Months: A Study of the Lives of 134 Persons Who Committed Suicide. New York, Oxford University Press, 1981

Roy A: Risk factors for suicide in psychiatric patients. Arch Gen Psychiatry 39:1089–1095, 1982

Roy A: Family history of suicide. Arch Gen Psychiatry 40:971–974, 1983

Schulsinger F, Kety SS, Rosenthal D, et al: A family study of suicide, in Origin, Prevention, and Treatment of Affective Disorders. Edited by Schou M, Stromgren E. New York, Academic, 1979

Sheard M, Marini J, Bridges C, et al: The effect of lithium on impulsive aggressive behavior in man. Am J Psychiatry 133:1409–1413, 1976

Tsuang MT: Suicide in schizophrenics, manics, depressives, and surgical controls: a comparison with general population suicide mortality. Arch Gen Psychiatry 35:153–155, 1978

Tsuang MT: Risk of suicide in the relatives of schizophrenics, manics, depressives, and controls. J Clin Psychiatry 44:396–400, 1983

Wender PH, Kety SS, Rosenthal D, et al: Psychiatric disorders in the biological and adoptive families of adopted individuals with affective disorders. Arch Gen Psychiatry 43:923–929, 1986

Chapter 6

Suicide and Psychiatric Diagnosis

Donald W. Black, M.D.
George Winokur, M.D.

SUICIDE ACCOUNTS FOR more than 28,000 deaths in the United States annually, ranking eighth in frequency among causes of death (Weed 1985). Compared with other causes of death, suicide creates a disproportionate amount of turmoil for families and friends and arouses curiosity in the lay public. The popular news media are often filled with heartbreaking stories of inexplicable suicides. Most stories inevitably focus on unfortunate marital, social, occupational, or medical stresses the victim may have suffered, often while ignoring a history of mental illness. Research has shown, however, that the large majority of suicides have a major mental illness (Buda and Tsuang, this volume). Thus, while suicide may result from a complex matrix of biologic, social, and psychological factors, clinical variables, particularly psychiatric diagnosis, are now being viewed as increasingly important.

TYPES OF STUDIES ON SUICIDE

Suicide has been studied in many different ways. Most methods involve studies of general or clinical populations. An example of the former is the study of suicides reported to and identified by a coroner or medical examiner. Using a "psychological autopsy" method, survivors and other informants are contacted and interviewed to learn more about the victim. Hospital and clinic records may be gathered as well. The result of this inquiry is, in effect, an interview of the suicide by proxy, with the aim of learning about the suicide victim's mental condition at the time of the act. The second type of study draws on the clinical population. Persons treated at psychiatric hospitals or in mental health clinics are followed-up. Patterns of death among the deceased are studied. Causes of death, including suicide, may then be compared with matched controls or to the general population.

General Population Studies

Six studies that provide clinical information on suicides have been reported in the past 30 years: Robins et al. (1959), Dorpat and Ripley (1960), and Rich et al. (1986), all in the United States; Barraclough et al. (1974) in Great Britain; Beskow (1979) in Sweden; and Chynoweth et al. (1980) in Australia (Table 1). Despite differences in methodology, diagnostic criteria, location of study, and year of study, all yield similar information. First, all the studies found that about 90% of suicides suffer from a major psychiatric illness at the time of the suicide. Roughly half of the suicides were clinically depressed at the time of suicide. About one-third of the suicides occurred in chronic alcoholic patients. Schizophrenia, organic mental disorders, substance abuse, and anxiety disorders are less common contributors to suicide. Few suicides occurred in persons judged not mentally ill, suggesting that the "rational" suicide is uncommon. The study by Rich et al. (1986) departs from these conclusions somewhat in reporting drug use disorders in 45% and alcoholism in 54% of suicides, problems particularly severe in persons younger than 30 years of age. These disconcerting findings may reflect the growing problem with drug abuse in the United States, a problem that may be worse in southern California, where the study was conducted.

Studies of suicides in the general population reveal that typical suicides are male (about two-thirds), over 40 years of age, and divorced (Barraclough et al. 1974; Chynoweth et al. 1980). Psychiatric diagnosis tends to differ by age. Dorpat and Ripley (1960) found the most common diagnosis in suicides under 40 years to be schizophrenia; in suicides 40 to 60 years, alcoholism; and in suicides over 60 years, some type of depression. Rich et al. (1986) found suicides younger than 30 years to have more substance use disorders and antisocial personality, and suicides over 30 years to suffer more affective disorder. Taken together, the six studies powerfully demonstrate that major psychiatric illness is, for practical purposes, *necessary* for the suicide. As Murphy (1983) has cogently observed, however, other factors must come into play, for a psychiatric diagnosis itself is not *sufficient* to cause suicide.

Table 1. Psychiatric diagnosis in six studies of suicides in the general population.

	Robins et al. (1959) St. Louis (N = 134)	Dorpat and Ripley (1960) Seattle (N = 114)	Barraclough et al. (1974) England (N = 100)	Beskow (1979) Sweden (N = 271)	Chynoweth et al. (1980) Australia (N = 135)	Rich et al. (1986) San Diego (N = 283)
Depression alone	NS	NS	64	NS	27	NS
Any depression	47	30	80	28	55	44
Alcohol abuse/dependence alone	NS	NS	4	NS	10[b]	NS
Any alcohol abuse/dependence	25	31	15	31	29[b]	54
Drug abuse/dependence	1	NS	4	6	NS	45
Organic disorders	4	4	1	2	NS	4
Schizophrenia	2	12	3	3	4	3
Anxiety disorders	NS	NS	3	9[c]	NS	<1
Personality disorders	NS	9	NS	4	3	5
Other disorders	19	19	1	13	12	5
Not mentally ill[a]	0	7	3	12	5	
Depression with alcohol abuse	NS	NS	10	NS	18[b]	NS

Note. NS = not specified.
[a] Includes medically ill. [b] Alcoholism and drug dependence are combined. [c] Defined as "neurotic, other than affective."

Clinical Population Studies

Studies of hospital or clinic populations have yielded different information. These studies (Black et al. 1985a; Kraft and Babigian 1976; Martin et al. 1985; Pokorny 1964; Roy 1982a; Sletten et al. 1972) tend to show that most suicides in psychiatric populations, including both inpatients and outpatients, have an affective disorder, schizophrenia, or alcoholism. Schizophrenia tends to be responsible for more suicides in clinical settings than in the general population. This finding reflects the overrepresentation of schizophrenia that occurs in the clinical population. On the other hand, schizophrenia is unlikely to contribute in a major way to suicides in the general population because it is relatively uncommon.

Other differences between clinical and general population suicides have been found. Suicides in clinical samples tend to show a more equal sex distribution, although men still predominate (Black et al. 1985a; Martin et al. 1985; Roy 1982a). For example, in a study of 68 suicides occurring in a clinical population (Black et al. 1985a), 37 were men and 31 were women. Compared with the general population, men had a 15-fold increase in suicide, and women a 41-fold increase. Mental illness appears to be a great leveler for suicide in the psychiatric population between men and women. Suicides in clinical samples also tend to be young and have greater relative risk for suicide than the aged (Black et al. 1985a; Martin et al. 1985). In fact, as psychiatric patients age, observed rates get closer to expected rates of suicide when comparisons are made with the general population. For example, in one study (Black et al. 1985a), the observed rate of suicide in men younger than 30 years is 25 times the expected rate and in women younger than 30 years 47 times the expected rate. A systematic decrease in the suicide rates occurs as psychiatric patients age; after 69 years, neither men nor women with a psychiatric disorder are more likely to commit suicide than persons in the general population. Roy (1982a) found other differences as well: suicides were more likely unmarried, unemployed, living alone, and depressed (regardless of diagnosis). Additionally, risk for suicide is greatest close to the time of ascertainment. In a study of 5,412 hospitalized patients, 68 persons committed suicide during the follow-up after discharge; 38% of suicides occurred in the first 6 months, 57% within the first year, and 79% by 2 years follow-up (Black et al. 1985a).

DIFFERENCES BETWEEN SUICIDE COMPLETERS AND ATTEMPTERS

Although many investigators tend to regard suicide attempts and completed suicide as the same, they are largely discrete phenomena

(Avery and Winokur 1978; Tefft et al. 1977). Nonetheless, up to one-third of patients who commit suicide have a history of suicide attempts (Barraclough et al. 1974; Robins et al. 1959). An estimated 1% of suicide attempters will go on to complete suicide each year, up to an asymptote of 10% (Ettlinger 1975).

Differences between completed suicide and suicide attempts largely involve demographics and clinical characteristics. In the general population, men are about two times as likely as women to commit suicide; suicides can occur at any age over 14 years, and nearly all completers are mentally ill at the time of their suicide (Barraclough et al. 1974; Beskow 1979; Chynoweth et al. 1980; Robins et al. 1959). Suicide completers generally plan their act, choose an effective means, and carry it out in private or make provisions to avoid interruption (Robins 1981). They are serious about ending their lives. In contrast, suicide attempters are three times as likely female and usually younger than 35 years (Clendenin and Murphy 1971; Kreitman 1977). They often act impulsively, make provisions for rescue, and use ineffective or slowly effective means (Bancroft et al. 1976; Clendenin and Murphy 1971). The purpose is, along with surviving, to have an impact on others (Murphy and Wetzel 1982). The act is often carried out in the presence of others or after others have been notified.

Suicide attempters and suicide completers also differ diagnostically. Somewhat fewer suicide attempters than completers are psychiatrically ill. Whereas suicide victims are likely to suffer from depression, alcoholism, or both, attempters' diagnoses may include depression (often a secondary depression), alcohol or drug abuse, and also diagnoses that are uncommon among successful suicides, such as somatization disorder (Briquet's syndrome) and antisocial personality (Woodruff et al. 1972). Weissman et al. (1989) have found that suicide attempts are frequent in panic disorder. In their study, 20% of patients with panic disorder had made suicide attempts, a finding that cannot be explained by co-existing major depression or alcohol/drug abuse. Murphy and Wetzel (1982) estimated that personality disorders may be present in up to 40% of the population of suicide attempters. It has been suggested that between 5% and 20% of suicide attempters have no mental illness, unlike the 3% to 12% of suicides thought not to be ill (Dahlgren 1945; Murphy and Wetzel 1982).

Schmidt et al. (1954) proposed classifying suicide attempts as serious or not serious. Serious attempts result in medically or surgically serious conditions (e.g., a penetrating gunshot wound) or are judged serious on psychological grounds (e.g., a depressed person who had carefully planned a suicide and carried out the attempt in private). Most suicide attempts are neither medically nor psychologically serious. In their 8-month follow-up, Schmidt et al. (1954) reported that two suicides had occurred among 109 patients who had attempted suicide; both had made serious attempts and both had psychiatric disorders: manic-depressive illness and chronic alcoholism. They also found that depression and dementia were more frequent in the serious group than in the nonserious group. In contrast, antisocial personality and alcoholism were significantly more frequent diagnoses in the nonserious group.

Affective Disorders

Affective disorders comprise the largest single diagnostic group among patients who commit suicide. In fact, because affective disorder and suicide are linked, suicidal ideation and behavior is included as a diagnostic criterion for the diagnosis of major depression (American Psychiatric Association 1987). Suicide in affective disorder patients invariably occurs during an episode of clinical depression; therefore, patients who are not depressed are probably not at increased risk for suicide (Dorpat and Ripley 1960). Symptomatically, depressions in suicides do not differ from those of living depressed controls, although they may be more severe (Barraclough et al. 1974). A history of attempted suicide is up to eight times more common among successful suicides, however (Barraclough et al. 1974).

When one considers that 50% or more of suicides have an affective disorder, it becomes clear how important depression is as a contributor to suicide. Guze and Robins (1970) estimated that, based on available data, 15% of all persons with major affective disorders (including both unipolar and bipolar) will ultimately commit suicide. The annual rate of suicide in depressed patients ranges from 3.5 to 4.5 times higher than that of other diagnostic groups and 22 to 36 times higher than the general population rate (Pokorny 1964; Temoche et al. 1964).

Among samples of depressed patients who have committed suicide, relatively few risk factors emerge. Murphy and Robins (1967) were unable to find differences in marital status, amount of physical illness, number of life stresses, or interpersonal conflicts between depressed suicide completers and depressed living controls. The major difference between the groups was that twice as many victims as controls were living alone. Whether living alone predisposes to suicide or merely reflects on the consequence of being depressed is unclear. In a sample of depressed patients, Fawcett et al. (1987) found that hopelessness, loss of pleasure or interest, and mood cycling during the index episode correlated with subsequent suicide; diagnostic subtype, marital status, suicidal ideation at intake, past suicide attempts, and medical severity of attempts did not correlate with suicide. There is some evidence that a family history of suicide increases the risk for suicide in depressed patients (Egeland and Sussex 1985).

The first 2 or 3 years of follow-up appear to be the period of greatest risk for suicide; after that an asymptote is reached (Guze and Robins 1970; Miles 1977). In a 30- to 40-year follow-up, Tsuang (1978) found that increased risk for suicide was largely limited to the first decade following first admissions. In the Collaborative Depression Study (Fawcett et al. 1987), nearly one-third of suicides occurred within the first 6 months, and one-half within the first year after intake.

Many depressed patients who commit suicide communicate their intent to others. Barraclough et al. (1974) reported that 30% of depressed patients had given warning; Robins et al. (1959) found that 68% of 60 manic-depressive patients had communicated suicidal ideas, most frequently through a direct and specific statement of their intent to commit suicide. Moreover, they found that communications were diverse, repeated, and expressed to different persons.

Subtypes of Affective Disorder

It is not clear whether one subtype of depression is more likely to lead to suicide than another. Two long-term studies of hospitalized depressed patients (Angst et al. 1979; McGlashan 1984) showed that those with bipolar disorder have lower rates of suicide than those with unipolar disorder, although three other studies (Perris and D'Elia 1966; Tsuang 1978; Weeke and Vaeth 1986) failed to show any difference in suicides between unipolar and bipolar patients. On the other hand, two studies, one of a psychiatric practice population (Morrison 1982) and the other of an affective disorders clinic population (Dunner et al. 1976), showed bipolar patients at higher risk for suicide than unipolar patients. In the latter study, patients with bipolar II disorder had greater risk than patients with bipolar I. In a study of death rates in 1,593 patients with major affective disorders, similar rates of suicide were found in unipolar and bipolar depressed patients; however, when unipolar and bipolar patients were compared (both manic and depressed phases combined), bipolar patients had lower rates of suicide (Black et al. 1987). This finding was almost entirely due to the low risk of suicide in mania. The authors hypothesized that persons with bipolar disorder possibly spend less time at risk for suicide than persons with unipolar disorder because they have both manic and depressive episodes; therefore, in a short-term follow-up, patients with bipolar disorder appear to have lower risk for suicide. However, long-term follow-up studies, such as the Iowa 500 (Tsuang 1978), show that patients with primary unipolar depression and these with bipolar disorder are ultimately at similar risk for suicide (9.3% versus 11.1%, respectively).

Another unresolved question has been whether persons with primary depressive disorder have lower risk for suicide than persons with secondary depressive disorder. Martin et al. (1985) reported that, in a psychiatric clinic population, persons with secondary depressive disorder were at greater risk for suicide than those with primary depressive disorder. The authors postulated that, because persons with primary depressive disorder appear to respond better to antidepressant medication, their finding probably represents a benefit of the modern treatment era. On the other hand, one study (Black et al. 1987) found no difference in the suicide rates between those with primary and those with secondary depressive disorders. It is likely that if differences do exist, they are minor and unimportant.

Psychotic Affective Disorder

Psychosis apparently does not predispose to suicide in patients with diagnosed affective disorders. In a reanalysis of 134 suicides occurring in St. Louis in the 1950s, Robins (1986) noted that 16% of 63 affective patients were psychotic at the time of the suicide, and most were not manifestly "crazy" at the time of death. Black et al. (1988) followed 1,593 patients with major affective disorder (both unipolar and bipolar) and found that psychotic patients were not overrepresented among the suicides. Wolferdof et al. (1987) also failed to show any excess of suicide among psychotic depressed patients during a 3-year follow-up. It is possible that a difference in suicide outcome would emerge during a longer follow-up. However, in a 30- to 40-year follow-up of delusional depressed patients, Coryell and Tsuang (1982) found no significant difference in the suicide rate between those with psychotic and those with nonpsychotic primary unipolar depression (8.4% versus 10.0%, respectively).

These findings may not be true for hospitalized patients. Roose et al. (1983) found suicide 7.5 times more frequent among hospitalized psychotic than nonpsychotic depressed patients. Thus the dynamics of suicide may differ in the hospital from the dynamics outside the hospital.

ALCOHOLISM AND OTHER DRUG USE DISORDERS

Primary alcoholism is found in about one-third of suicides (Barraclough et al. 1974; Flavin et al., this volume; Robins et al. 1959).

Although chronic alcoholism may contribute to a quarter of suicides, alcohol itself, as measured in terms of blood alcohol, plays a role in many more suicides (Goodwin 1973). Indeed, intoxication may be associated with suicide in as many as 90% of alcoholic patients; only 40% of nonalcoholic patients have been reported as drinking at the time of suicide (Dorpat and Ripley 1960). It has been estimated that about 10% of chronic alcoholic patients will commit suicide (Miles 1977).

Alcoholic suicides differ in many ways from depressed suicides. Alcoholic patients often suffer chaotic personal lives filled with personal tragedy, probably resulting from their excessive drinking and its effect on their work, social relations, and physical health. Of importance, interpersonal loss within 6 weeks or less of their suicides has been found in up to one-third of alcoholic suicides (Murphy and Robins 1967). These losses are usually marital separation or divorce, or other disruptions such as breakup of nonmarital sexual relationships, estrangement from families, or recent bereavement. This finding was confirmed in a subsequent study where half of alcoholic suicide completers were found to have experienced a major interpersonal loss within a year of their death and 26% within 6 weeks or less (Murphy et al. 1979).

Miles (1977) observed that the incidence of suicide close to the time of original diagnosis is not as high in alcoholic patients as among depressed or schizophrenic patients; he concluded that suicide tends to be a long-term complication of alcoholism. Indeed, Robins et al. (1959) found duration from onset of alcoholism to suicide averaged 20 years. Dorpat and Ripley (1960) surmised that for alcoholic suicides "alcohol no longer served as an effective escape mechanism" (p. 354). They noted that, among these suicides, suicide occurred after years of progressive decline in their psychosocial adjustment, with 18% having recently lost jobs and 30% grieving over loss of a family member, usually through death or divorce. Goodwin (1973) specifically attributed suicide in alcoholic patients to the middle years; he explained that because alcoholic patients suffer an excess of death from causes other than suicide (e.g., accidents, cirrhosis), they are relatively unlikely to survive long enough to contribute many deaths by suicide in an aging population. Also, a sizable proportion of alcoholic patients recover spontaneously with treatment as they age, and recovered alcoholic patients are not replaced by new cases of the same age. Thus recoveries and early death can explain a declining contribution to suicide by aged alcoholic patients.

It is not known whether late-stage alcoholism is protective against suicide. Robins (quoted in Goodwin 1973) speculated that late-stage alcoholism might protect against suicide because later stages of alcoholism are associated with sufficient brain damage to "prevent the preparation necessary for successful suicidal behavior." Data are available to lend indirect support to this hypothesis. Excessive rates of suicide have been found among alcohol and other drug abusers (Black et al. 1985a), but not among a much older group of patients suffering alcoholic psychoses (i.e., hallucinosis, Korsakoff's psychosis, delirium tremens) (Black et al. 1985b).

Interestingly, depression is not a necessary accompaniment of suicide in alcoholic patients. In their study of 50 alcoholic suicides, Murphy et al. (1979) reported that one-fourth of those studied did not exhibit a depressive syndrome. Although the alcoholic patients may not have suffered from a major depressive illness, it is possible that they had depressive affect at the time, a finding that would be difficult to determine with certainty. Depressed alcoholic patients, however, were clinically similar to depressed suicides. Compared with living alcoholic patients, the alcoholic suicide victims were older, more likely divorced or widowed, and had histories of attempted suicide.

SCHIZOPHRENIA

Bleuler (1950) considered the suicidal drive to be "the most serious of schizophrenic symptoms" (p. 488). Nearly a century later, suicide remains of concern as a cause of early mortality in schizophrenic patients. Although between 2% and 12% of suicide victims have schizophrenia, approximately 10% of schizophrenic patients ultimately commit suicide (Miles 1977; Tsuang 1978). Some clinicians (Cohen et al. 1964; Lindelius and Kay 1973; Yarden 1974) have voiced concern that suicide among schizophrenic patients may be increasing since deinstitutionalization due to the increased stress from brief hospital stays and from living in the community (or on the streets) without adequate treatment. However, there is no evidence to support this assertion.

Research has identified a number of risk factors for suicide in schizophrenic patients, including male sex (Cohen et al. 1964; Roy 1982b; Breier and Astrachan 1984), age younger than 30 years (Breier and Astrachan 1984; Roy 1982b), white race (Breier and Astrachan 1984; Yarden 1974), unemployment (Roy 1982b), a chronic relapsing course (Farberow et al. 1966; Roy 1982b), prior depression (Cohen et al. 1964; Roy 1982b), past treatment for depression (Roy 1982b), depression during the last episode of illness (Roy 1982b), and a recent discharge (Roy 1982b). More than half of schizophrenic patients in some samples had made serious suicide attempts (Breier and Astrachan 1984; Cohen et al. 1964; Warnes 1968).

Almost 75% to 90% of victims are male, a preponderance that has led one investigator to question whether female schizophrenic patients are at any increased risk (Miles 1977). Most schizophrenic patients who kill themselves are young. In a recent study (Black and Winokur 1988), no suicides occurred among chronic schizophrenic patients after age 40. One conclusion from this study is that risk for suicide in a schizophrenic illness is age dependent and may be due to changes that occur in the character of schizophrenia over the years. These changes include a tendency toward less depression and more negative symptoms, such as asociality and amotivation (Pfohl and Winokur 1983), which may lessen the risk of suicide. Absolute age at time of suicide may be less meaningful than the number of years that have elapsed between onset of the illness and suicide. The majority of suicides occur early in the course of illness, particularly the first decade (Lindelius and Kay 1973). Virkkunen (1974) determined that most suicides occur, on average, after 6 or 7 years of illness. As women develop schizophrenia later than men (Loranger 1984), this difference in age of onset is reflected in age at suicide; women kill themselves an average of 6 years later than men (Black and Winokur 1988; Virkkunen 1974).

Schizophrenic patients with a high level of education appear to be at greater risk for suicide (Drake et al. 1984; Farberow et al. 1966; Sletten et al. 1972). This may be due to the "awareness of pathology" that may develop, including feelings of inadequacy and hopelessness, fear of disintegration, and a realization that many of their expectations will never be met (Drake et al. 1984; Warnes 1968). Unlike most psychiatric patients who commit suicide, schizophrenic patients apparently fail to communicate their suicidal intentions to the same degree; the suicide may be unexpected and inexplicable (Allebeck et al. 1987; Breier and Astrachan 1984). Schizophrenic patients are reported to use more highly lethal suicide methods (Breier and Astrachan 1984), although this has been disputed (Black 1988).

Several uncontrolled reports have suggested that paranoid schizophrenic patients are at higher risk for suicide than other subgroups (Achté et al. 1966; Levy and Southcombe 1953; Virkkunen 1974); Noreik (1975) observed that hebephrenic patients specifically have a lower rate than paranoid patients. Bolin et al. (1968) found no difference in suicide rates between these subtypes. Although there is no agreement on which subtype creates the greatest risk, Roy (1982b) found that schizophrenic patients who commit suicide are likely to have a chronic course with many exacerbations and remissions. Risk for suicide is highest early after hospital discharge, with as many as 50% occurring within the first 3 months (Roy 1982b). Although intense psychotic behavior has been implicated in many schizophrenic suicides, several well-controlled studies do not support a link between psychosis and suicide (Breier and Astrachan 1984; Roy 1982a). Thus it is unlikely that suicide is precipitated by psychosis in most cases.

Among suicides, a prior history of attempts has generally indicated a high risk for suicide. However, since twice as many schizophrenic patients attempt suicide as complete it, the predictive power of this variable is limited (Roy 1982b).

OTHER CLINICAL CONDITIONS

Organic mental disorders contribute about as often to suicide as schizophrenia in the general population, but much less in clinical samples (Black et al. 1985b; Martin et al. 1985). A number of specific neurologic diseases that cause mental impairment are reported to be associated with high suicide rates, including brain trauma (Achté et al. 1971), convulsive disorders (Barraclough 1987), Huntington's chorea (Chandler et al. 1960), Parkinson's disease (Mindham 1970), and multiple sclerosis (Müller 1949). The absolute number of suicides associated with these conditions is small, either because the rate is only moderately increased or because the conditions themselves are uncommon.

Other clinical conditions have also been linked to suicide. In a heterogeneous sample of "severe neurotics," Sims and Prior (1978) reported an excess of suicides. Subsequent investigators have broken this category down. Coryell et al. (1982) found significant rates of suicide among 113 patients with panic disorder followed for 35 years but in other studies (Coryell 1981, 1983) failed to find excess suicides in either Briquet's syndrome (somatization disorder) or obsessive-compulsive disorder. Long-term follow-up studies of patients with obsessive-compulsive disorder confirm that suicide occurs infrequently. As Goodwin et al. (1969) observed, this appeared true "despite the frequency with which suicide may figure in obsessional thinking" (p. 185). A superimposed depressive syndrome is probably a necessary accompaniment of suicide in persons with these conditions.

Personality disorder has also emerged as the major diagnosis in many suicide victims in general population samples (Beskow 1979; Dorpat and Ripley 1960; Rich et al. 1986). Personality disorder has also demonstrated excess suicides in clinical samples (Black et al. 1985a; Martin et al. 1985; Pokorny 1964). Aside from antisocial personality (and perhaps borderline personality disorder), personality disorders have not been studied sufficiently to establish them as valid psychiatric disorders and so the contribution of a primary personality disorder to suicide statistics is unclear. Nonetheless, many researchers

(McCulloch et al. 1967; Ovenstone and Kreitman 1974; Seager and Flood 1965) have detected personality disorder in up to one-third to one-half of persons who had committed suicide. These persons tend to be young, to come from broken homes, and to have had a chaotic life-style in which violence and substance abuse were common.

Of specific personality disorders that have been studied, border-line personality has been associated with a suicide rate ranging from 4% to 10% in three studies (Akiskal et al. 1985; Paris et al. 1987; Pope et al. 1983), and antisocial personality has been associated with a 5% suicide rate (Maddocks 1970; Miles 1977). On the other hand, suicide attempts in antisocial personality disorder are common, often repetitive, usually nonserious, and may be precipitated by difficulties in important relationships (Garvey and Spoden 1980).

Drug use disorders also contribute to suicide in the general population (Barraclough et al. 1974; Beskow 1979; Rich et al. 1986; Robins et al. 1959) and in clinical populations (Black et al. 1985d; Martin et al. 1985; Roy 1982a; Sletten et al. 1972). These disorders may be responsible for a growing percentage of suicides, particularly among the young (Rich et al. 1986). Miles (1977) suggested that drug use may be the single most important factor behind the increase in suicides among youth in the United States.

Other disorders have also been linked to excessive suicides, including depressive neurosis (Black et al. 1985c; Kraft and Babigian 1976; Miles 1977), acute schizophrenia (Black et al. 1985c), schizoaffective disorders (Berg et al. 1983; Tsuang et al. 1979), adjustment disorders (Black et al. 1985c), and conversion reactions (Stefansson et al. 1976). These conditions have not been sufficiently studied to establish them as valid psychiatric disorders so that, as with personality disorder, their contribution to suicide statistics is unclear.

DISORDERS OF CHILDREN AND ADOLESCENTS

Suicide is uncommon in childhood and early adolescence. However, among 15- to 24-year-olds, death by suicide is the third most frequent cause of death, ranking behind death by accidents and homicide. The rate among boys is higher than for girls, due in part to boys using more violent methods than girls (e.g., shooting or hanging). This appears to be changing; more girls are now using violent means of committing suicide (Shaffer 1974; Shafii et al. 1985). Further, national statistics have shown that although suicide rates are relatively stable in older age groups, rates among young white males are increasing.

Little is known about causes of suicide in childhood and adolescence. This topic is covered in greater detail in Brent and Kolko's chapter in this volume. Using a psychological autopsy method,

Shaffer (1974) studied 30 completed suicides in children under the age of 15. Although diagnoses were not assigned, affective symptoms had occurred in 13% of the suicide victims, antisocial symptoms alone in 17%, and mixed antisocial and affective symptoms in 57%. Shafii et al. (1985) studied 20 children and adolescents who committed suicide. They also found a high incidence of antisocial symptoms (70%), frequent use of nonprescribed drugs or alcohol (70%), and "inhibited personality" (65%). In a subsequent report, which included an additional case, they reported that 95% of the suicide victims had a serious mental disorder (Shafii et al. 1988). The presence of two or more mental disorders occurred in 81%; 76% had a mood disturbance (major depression or dysthymia), 62% had a diagnosis of substance abuse, and 29% had a diagnosis of a personality disorder. Rich et al. (1986) did not specifically study children or adolescents, but compared 133 suicides occurring in persons under 30 years of age with 150 suicides in persons aged 30 years and older; 30 victims were aged 15 to 24. There were few diagnostic differences between the groups, except for significantly higher rates of substance use disorders and antisocial personality in the younger group and more affective disorders in the older group.

Among the limited conclusions that can be drawn from these studies are that children and young adults who commit suicide are likely to be seriously mentally ill, but other factors may play more of a role than in adult suicides. For example, in the younger group, imitation may play more of a role (Gould, this volume; Phillips and Carstensen 1986), and suicide is likely to be associated with drug abuse or personality disturbance. Unfortunately, none of these associations are strong enough for reliable detection of the few youths at risk for suicide.

Kuperman et al. (1988) followed up a clinical sample of formerly hospitalized children and adolescents. They found significant risk of suicide among patients with schizophrenic or organic mental disorders. In contrast to follow-up studies of adult inpatients, they were unable to associate suicide with a primary affective disorder, substance abuse, or neurosis. They concluded that schizophrenia and organic mental disorders carry substantial risk for suicide among younger patients in a clinical setting.

IMPLICATIONS FOR CLINICIANS

Because suicide is a relatively rare event, it is not always possible to identify in advance those who will commit suicide. Thus predicting suicide demands the skills of a clairvoyant—skills that psychiatrists do not typically possess. However, assessing clinical risk is an important aspect of the clinician's evaluation of the patient (Murphy 1983). Research has identified clinical, historical, and social information that helps alert clinicians to heightened risk for suicide in a given patient (Blumenthal, this volume). Psychiatric diagnosis is perhaps the most important signal to alert the physician to suicidal behavior over the life cycle. Most patients who commit suicide suffer major psychiatric illness, most commonly depression or alcoholism.

REFERENCES

Achté K, Stenbäck A, Teräväinen H: On suicides committed during treatment in psychiatric hospitals. Acta Psychiatr Scand 42:272–284, 1966

Achté KA, Lonnqvist J, Hillborm E: Suicides following war brain injuries. Acta Psychiatr Scand 225:7–94, 1971

Akiskal HS, Chen SE, Davis GC: Borderline: an adjective in search of a noun. J Clin Psychiatry 546:41–48, 1985

Allebeck P, Varla A, Kristjansson E, et al: Risk factors for suicide among patients with schizophrenia. Acta Psychiatr Scand 76:414–419, 1987

American Psychiatric Association: Diagnostic and Statistical Manual of Mental Disorders, 3rd Edition, Revised. Washington, DC, American Psychiatric Association, 1987

Angst J, Felder W, Frey R: The course of unipolar and bipolar affective disorders, in Origin, Prevention, and Treatment of Affective Disorder. Edited by Schou M, Strömgren E. London, Academic, 1979, pp 215–226

Avery D, Winokur G: Suicide, attempted suicide, and relapse rates in depression: occurrence after ECT and antidepressant therapy. Arch Gen Psychiatry 35:749–753, 1978

Bancroft JHJ,Skrimshire AM, Simkin S: The reasons people give for taking overdoses. Br J Psychiatry 128:538–548, 1976

Barraclough BM: Suicide rate of epilepsy. Acta Psychiatr Scand 76:339–345, 1987

Barraclough B, Bunch J, Nelson B, et al: A hundred cases of suicide: clinical aspects. Br J Psychiatry 125:355–373, 1974

Berg E, Lindelius R, Petterson V, et al: Schizoaffective psychoses: a long-term follow-up. Acta Psychiatr Scand 67:389–398, 1983

Beskow J: Suicide and mental disorder in Swedish men. Acta Psychiatr Scand (Suppl) 277:1–138, 1979

Black DW: Mortality in schizophrenia: the Iowa record linkage study. Psychosomatics 29:55–60, 1988

Black DW, Winokur G: Age, mortality, and chronic schizophrenia. Schizophrenia Research 1:267–272, 1988

Black DW, Warrack G, Winokur G: The Iowa record linkage study, I: suicide and accidental death among psychiatric patients. Arch Gen Psychiatry 42:71–75, 1985a

Black DW, Warrack G, Winokur G: The Iowa record linkage study, II: excess mortality among patients with organic mental disorders. Arch Gen Psychiatry 42:78–81, 1985b

Black DW, Warrack G, Winokur G: The Iowa record linkage study, III: excess mortality in patients with "functional" disorders. Arch Gen Psychiatry 42:82–88, 1985c

Black DW, Winokur G, Warrack G: Suicide in schizophrenia: the Iowa record-linkage study. J Clin Psychiatry 46 (sec 2):14–17, 1985d

Black DW,Winokur G, Nasrallah A: Suicide in subtypes of major affective disorder: comparison with general population suicide mortality. Arch Gen Psychiatry 44:878–880, 1987

Black DW, Winokur G, Nasrallah A: Effect of psychosis on suicide risk in 1593 patients with unipolar and bipolar affective disorders. Am J Psychiatry 145:849–852, 1988

Bleuler E: Dementia Praecox, or the Group of Schizophrenias. New York, International Universities Press, 1950

Bolin RK, Wright RE, Wilkinson MN, et al: Survey of suicide among patients on home leave from a mental hospital. Psychiatr Q 42:81–89, 1968

Breier A, Astrachan BM: Characterization of schizophrenic patients who commit suicide. Am J Psychiatry 141:206–209, 1984

Chandler J, Reed T, DeJong R: Huntington's chorea in Michigan, III: clinical observations. Neurology 10:148–153, 1960

Chynoweth R, Tonge JI, Armstrong J: Suicide in Brisbane: a retrospective psychosocial study. Aust N Z J Psychiatry 14:37–45, 1980

Clendenin WW, Murphy GE: Wrist cutting: new epidemiological findings. Arch Gen Psychiatry 25:465–469, 1971

Cohen S, Leonard CV, Farberow NL, et al: Tranquilizers and suicide in the schizophrenic patient. Arch Gen Psychiatry 11:312–321, 1964

Coryell W: Diagnosis specific mortality: primary unipolar depression and Briquet's syndrome (somatization disorder). Arch Gen Psychiatry 38:939–942, 1981

Coryell W: Mortality after 30 or 40 years: panic disorder compared with other psychiatric illnesses, in Psychiatry Update: The American Psychiatric Association Annual Review, Vol 3. Edited by Grinspoon L. Washington, DC, American Psychiatric Press, 1984, pp 460–467

Coryell W, Tsuang MT: Primary unipolar depression and the prognostic importance of delusions. Arch Gen Psychiatry 39:1181–1184, 1982

Coryell W, Noyes R, Clancy J: Excess mortality in panic disorder. Arch Gen Psychiatry 39:701–703, 1982

Dahlgren KG (ed): On Suicide and Attempted Suicide: A Psychiatrical and Statistical Investigation. Lund, Sweden P, Lindstedts University-Bokhandel, 1945

Dorpat L, Ripley HS: A study of suicide in the Seattle area. Compr Psychiatry 1:349–359, 1960

Drake RE, Gates C, Cotton PG: A suicide among schizophrenics: who is at risk? J Nerv Ment Dis 172:613–617, 1984

Dunner DL, Gershon ES, Goodwin FK: Heritable factors in the severity of affective illness. Biol Psychiatry 11:31–42, 1976

Egeland JA, Sussex JN: Suicide and family loading for affective disorders. JAMA 254:915–918, 1985

Ettlinger R: Evaluation of suicide prevention after attempted suicide. Acta Psychiatr Scand (Suppl) 260:1–135, 1975

Farberow NL, Shneidman ES, Neuringer C: Case history and hospitalization factors in suicides of neuropsychiatric hospital patients. J Nerv Ment Dis 142:32–44, 1966

Fawcett J, Scheftner W, Clark D, et al: Clinical predictors of suicide in patients with major affective disorders: a controlled prospective study. Am J Psychiatry 144:35–40, 1987

Garvey MJ, Spoden F: Suicide attempts in antisocial personality disorder. Compr Psychiatry 21:146–149, 1980

Goodwin DW: Alcohol, suicide and homicide. Quarterly Journal of Studies on Alcohol 34:144–164, 1973

Goodwin DW, Guze SB, Robins E: Follow-up studies in obsessional neurosis. Arch Gen Psychiatry 20:182–187, 1969

Guze, SB, Robins E: Suicide and primary affective disorders. Br J Psychiatry 117:437–438, 1970

Kraft DP, Babigian HM: Suicide by persons with and without psychiatric contacts. Arch Gen Psychiatry 33:209–215, 1976

Kreitman N (ed): Parasuicide. New York, John Wiley, 1977

Kuperman S, Black DW, Burns TL: Excess suicide among formerly hospitalized child psychiatry patients. J Clin Psychiatry 49:88–93, 1988

Levy S, Southcombe RH: Suicide in a state hospital for the mentally ill. J Nerv Ment Dis 117:504–514, 1953

Lindelius R, Kay DWK: Some changes in the pattern of mortality in schizophrenia in Sweden. Acta Psychiatr Scand 49:315–323, 1973

Loranger AW: Sex difference in age at onset of schizophrenia. Arch Gen Psychiatry 41:157–161, 1984

Maddocks PD: A five year follow-up of untreated psychopaths. Br J Psychiatry 116:511–515, 1970

Martin RL, Cloninger CR, Guze SB, et al: Mortality at a follow-up of 500 psychiatric outpatients, II: cause-specific mortality. Arch Gen Psychiatry 42:58–66, 1985

McCulloch J, Phillip AE, Carstairs GM: The ecology of suicidal behavior. Br J Psychiatry 113:313–319, 1967

McGlashan TH: Chestnut Lodge follow-up study, II: long term outcome of schizophrenia and the affective disorders. Arch Gen Psychiatry 41:586–601, 1984

Miles CP: Conditions predisposing to suicide: a review. J Nerv Ment Dis 164:231–246, 1977

Mindham RH: Psychiatric symptoms in parkinsonism. J Neurol Neurosurg Psychiatry 33:188–191, 1970

Morrison JR: Suicide in a psychiatric practice population. J Clin Psychiatry 43:348–352, 1982

Müller R: Studies on disseminated sclerosis with special reference to symptomatology, course, and prognosis. Acta Med Scand (Suppl) 133:1–214, 1949

Murphy GE: Problems in studying suicide. Psychiatr Dev 1:339–350, 1983

Murphy GE, Robins E: Social factors in suicide. JAMA 199:303–308, 1967

Murphy GE, Wetzel RD: Family history of suicidal behavior among suicide attempters. J Nerv Ment Dis 170:86–90, 1982

Murphy GE, Armstrong JW, Hermele SL, et al: Suicide and alcoholism: interpersonal loss confirmed as a predictor. Arch Gen Psychiatry 36:65–69, 1979

Noreik K: Attempted suicide and suicide in functional psychoses. Acta Psychiatr Scand 52:81–106, 1975

Ovenstone IMR, Kreitman N: Two syndromes of suicide. Br J Psychiatry 124:336–345, 1974

Paris J, Brown R, Nowlis D: Long-term follow-up of borderline patients in a general hospital. Compr Psychiatr 28:530–535, 1987

Perris C, D'Elia G: A study of bipolar (manic-depressive) and unipolar recurrent depressive psychoses X. Mortality, suicide, and life cycles. Acta Psychiatr Scand (Suppl) 42:172–183, 1966

Pfohl B, Winokur G: The micropsychopathology of hebephrenic/catatonic schizophrenia. J Nerv Ment Dis 171:296–300, 1983

Phillips DP, Carstensen LL: Clustering of teenage suicides after television news stories about suicide. N Engl J Med 15:685–689, 1986

Pokorny AD: Suicide rates in various psychiatric disorders. J Nerv Ment Dis 139:499–506, 1964

Pope HG, Jonas JM, Hudson JI, et al: The validity of DSM-III borderline personality disorder. Arch Gen Psychiatry 40:23–30, 1983

Rich CL, Young D, Fowler RC: San Diego suicide study, I: young vs. old subjects. Arch Gen Psychiatry 43:577–582, 1986

Robins E (ed): The Final Months: A Study of the Lives of 134 Persons Who Committed Suicide. New York, Oxford University Press, 1981

Robins E: Psychosis and suicide. Biol Psychiatry 21:665–672, 1986

Robins E, Murphy GE, Wilkinson JR, et al: Some clinical considerations in the prevention of suicide based on a study of 134 successful suicides. Am J Public Health 49:888–899, 1959

Roose SP, Glassman AH, Walsh BT, et al: Depression, delusions, and suicide. Am J Psychiatry 140:1159–1162, 1983

Roy A: Risk factors for suicide in psychiatric patients. Arch Gen Psychiatry 39:1089–1095, 1982a

Roy A: Suicide in chronic schizophrenia. Br J Psychiatry 141:171–177, 1982b

Schmidt EH, O'Neal P, Robins E: Evaluation of suicide attempts as a guide to therapy: clinical and follow-up study of 109 patients. JAMA 155:549–557, 1954

Seager CP, Flood RA: Suicide in Bristol. Br J Psychiatry 111:919–932, 1965

Shaffer D: Suicide in childhood and early adolescence. J Child Psychol Psychiatry 15:275–291, 1974

Shafii M, Carrigan S, Whittinghill JR: Psychological autopsy of completed suicide in children and adolescents. Am J Psychiatry 142:1061–1064, 1985

Shafii M, Steltz-Lenarsky J, Derrick AM, et al: Comorbidity of mental disorders and the post-mortem diagnoses of completed suicide in children and adolescents. J Affective Disord 15:227–233, 1988

Sims A, Prior P: The pattern of mortality in severe neuroses. Br J Psychiatry 133:249–305, 1978

Sletten IW, Brown ML, Evenson RC, et al: Suicide in mental hospital patients. Diseases of the Nervous System 33:328–334, 1972

Stefansson JG, Messina JA, Meyerowitz S: Hysterical neurosis, conversion type: clinical and epidemiologic considerations. Acta Psychiatr Scand 53:119–138, 1976

Tefft BM, Pederson AM, Babigian HM: Patterns of death among suicide attempters, a psychiatric population, and a general population. Arch Gen Psychiatry 34:1155–1161, 1977

Temoche A, Pugh TF, MacMahon B: Suicide rates among the current and former mental institution patients. J Nerv Ment Dis 138:124–130, 1964

Tsuang MT: Suicide in schizophrenics, manics, depressives, and surgical controls. Arch Gen Psychiatry 35:153–155, 1978

Tsuang MT, Dempsey FM, Fleming JA: Can ECT prevent premature death and suicide in schizoaffective patients? J Affective Disord 1:167–171, 1979

Virkkunen M: Suicides in schizophrenia and paranoid psychoses. Acta Psychiatr Scand 250:1–305, 1974

Warnes H: Suicide in schizophrenics. Diseases of the Nervous System (Suppl) 29:35–40, 1968

Weed JA: Suicide in the U.S., 1958–1982, in Mental Health, United States. Washington, DC, National Institute of Mental Health, 1985, pp 135–169

Weeke A, Vaeth M: Excess mortality of bipolar and unipolar manic-depressive patients. J Affective Disord 11:227–234, 1986

Weissman MM, Klerman GL, Markowitz JS, et al: Suicidal ideation and suicide attempts in panic disorder and attacks. N Engl J Med 321:1209–1214, 1989

Wolferdorf M, Keller F, Steiner B, et al: Delusional depression and suicide. Acta Psychiatr Scand 76:359–363, 1987

Woodruff RA, Clayton PJ, Guze SB: Suicide attempts and psychiatric diagnosis. Diseases of the Nervous System 33:617–621, 1972

Yarden PE: Observations on suicide in chronic schizophrenics. Compr Psychiatry 15:325–333, 1974

Chapter 7

Personality and Suicide

Scott J. Goldsmith, M.D.
Minna Fyer, M.D.
Allen Frances, M.D.

THERE ARE APPROXIMATELY 29,000 completed suicides each year in the United States, and 8 to 10 times that many attempts (Adam 1985). Throughout the life cycle, psychiatric illness puts a person at greatly increased risk for suicide (see Black and Winokur, Chapter 6; Brent and Kolko, Chapter 11; Osgood and Thielman, Chapter 13, this volume). Robins et al. (1959) found that 93% of those in the general population who died by suicide were suffering from a psychiatric disorder at the time of death. Martin et al. (1985) found in a follow-up study of 500 psychiatric outpatients that suicide rates were nearly 15 times that expected by comparison with matched controls. Although overall suicide rates have remained relatively constant, rates in younger groups have risen dramatically in the last two decades, with suicide being the third leading cause of death in people between the ages of 15 and 34 (Black et al. 1985). It is of interest to note that this is precisely the age group most likely to present with florid symptoms of personality disorder.

Most studies of suicide in psychiatric populations have focused on Axis I disorders and have shown an increased risk of suicide in patients with primary affective disorder (Guze and Robins 1970; Pokorny 1964; Roy 1983; Weissman 1974), schizophrenia (Kraft and Babigian 1976; Miles 1977; Roy 1982), and substance abuse (James 1967; Noble et al. 1972; Vaillant 1966). These issues are addressed comprehensively in other chapters in this book.

A much smaller body of work has examined suicide in relation to Axis II personality disorder diagnoses and other personality variables. The relationships between suicidal behavior and personality are not as well established as those between suicide and Axis I illness, but a number of fascinating and convergent leads have emerged. Results of some investigators (Black et al. 1985; Martin et al. 1985) suggest that patients with personality disorders account for a significant proportion of completed suicides among psychiatric patients. When compared with those who have completed suicide, an even larger percentage of those who have attempted suicide appears to suffer from personality disorders. Moreover, evidence suggests that the presence of a concurrent personality disorder may increase the risk of suicide in patients with certain Axis I disorders (Alessi et al. 1984; Crumley 1979; Friedman et al. 1982, 1983). Finally, there are two personality disorders that are by far the ones most frequently associated with both suicide attempts and successful suicides.

In this chapter we will begin with a definition of personality disorder and discuss issues of evaluation that pertain to the assessment of suicide risk. Next, methodological problems in the research will be identified, and the available data relating suicidal behavior with personality will be summarized. We will conclude with a discussion of the clinical implications of these findings.

PERSONALITY DISORDERS

According to DSM-III-R (American Psychiatric Association 1987), personality disorders are patterns of inflexible and maladaptive personality traits that result in significant impairment in social and occupational functioning and/or subjective distress. By definition, these are not time-limited syndromes, the beginning and end of which can be clearly demarcated during isolated periods of adult life. Rather, they are chronic behavior patterns with an early and insidious onset that become evident by late adolescence or early adulthood. The presence of a personality disorder tends to create and exacerbate stress by provoking aversive reactions in others; by leading to a failure to make optimal social, occupational, or other life decisions; and by creating situations that are problematic, pathogenic, and fulfilling of a person's worst fantasies.

The diagnosis of personality disorders has been receiving increasing attention (Vaillant and Perry 1985; Widiger and Frances 1987). Prior to DSM-III (American Psychiatric Association 1980), these diagnoses were often overlooked in the presence of other conspicuous or prominent clinical syndromes, including suicidality (Coyne 1976;

Frances and Widiger 1986). The inclusion of a separate axis and the development of relatively explicit criteria for the diagnosis of personalty disorders in DSM-III was instrumental in the development of increased clinical and research interest. The multiaxial evaluation offered by DSM-III and DSM-III-R recognizes the contribution and interrelationship of long-term trait factors in the development of psychiatric symptoms and disorders. The diagnosis of a personality disorder on Axis II is particularly important because it may alter the presentation, course, and treatment of an Axis I clinical syndrome and may be a contributing factor for suicidality (Gunderson and Siever 1985; Millon 1981; Pfohl et al. 1986).

In DSM-III-R, personality disorders are grouped into three clusters: 1) the odd or eccentric (schizotypal, schizoid, and paranoid); 2) the anxious or fearful (avoidant, dependent, obsessive-compulsive, and passive aggressive), and 3) the one cluster that has been shown to be associated with suicidal behavior—the dramatic, emotional, or erratic (histrionic, narcissistic, antisocial, and borderline). Although this grouping has only limited empirical support (Kass et al. 1983; Millon 1981), it does serve a heuristic purpose. Space limitations do not allow for a detailed review of the personality disorders themselves. However, a description of their theoretical background, empirical support, and criteria sets can be obtained elsewhere (Frances and Widiger, in press). It is worth keeping in mind, however, that the assessment of these disorders involves the assessment of chronic and pervasive traits rather than states or situations.

There are a number of ways to conceptualize the possible causal relationships between personality disorders and suicidality (Frances et al. 1986):

1. *Suicidal behavior may be an inherent component of certain personality disorders in the same way that suicidal behavior is included in the definition of major depressive disorder.* In keeping with this, DSM-III included suicidal behavior as a criterion for two personality disorders: borderline and histrionic, although DSM-III-R has eliminated this from the latter personality disorder in an attempt to delineate these two more clearly. Obviously, whenever suicidal behavior forms part of the definition of a disorder, this may produce an artifactual co-variance between that disorder and suicide that should be confirmed independently of the definitional association.
2. *Personality disorder may directly predispose to suicidal behavior or to a particularly lethal form of suicide attempt.*
3. *Personality disorders may predispose to Axis I disorders (e.g., depression), which then independently increase the risk of suicide.*

4. *Personality disorders might influence the expression of an Axis I disorder.* Most patients with major depression do not commit suicide. The presence of a personality disorder may help to determine whether a given depressed individual is likely to attempt or succeed at suicide.
5. *Personality traits, rather than personality disorders, may better predict suicidal behavior.* Since suicide is not diagnostically specific for Axis I disorders, it is perhaps unrealistic to expect any pure correlation with Axis II disorders. Combinations of personality traits that cut across traditional diagnostic categories might better predict suicidal behavior. For example, the trait of impulsivity might make it particularly likely for an individual to commit suicide, especially if depressed, manic, schizophrenic, or abusing substances.
6. *Axis I conditions that are associated with suicide may predispose to increased prevalence of Axis II disorders, which may or may not then independently contribute to increased risk of suicide.*
7. *Any association between suicide and personality disorder may be no more than coincidental.*

It is not possible, given our current level of understanding of the relationship of personality disorders to Axis I syndromes and to suicide, to choose from among these alternatives. It is useful to keep in mind that many different causal relationships may be possible.

Methodological Issues

There are a number of methodological issues that make research into the relationship of personality disorder and suicide difficult to conduct and interpret. Most basic are the definitional and assessment problems. Only recently have reliable methods of measuring personality been available, and the validity of these methods must still be established. Moreover, it is also difficult to define and classify the broad spectrum of suicidal behaviors, which may range from fleeting ideation to completed suicide. The available literature suggests that completers and attempters represent two separate but overlapping populations (Robins et al. 1957; Stengel 1969) and that attempters do not greatly resemble completers in demographic, diagnostic, psychological, or personality variables (Adam 1985; Kreitman 1981; Pallis and Birtchnell 1977; Stengel 1969).

Studies have also suffered from the effects of what are often of necessity retrospective designs. In the case of completed suicides, postmortem psychological autopsies consist of reviews of available records and interviews with those who knew the victim. In attempted suicides, assessments are often brief and must be conducted under emergency conditions, which make the diagnosis of personality disorder a problematic endeavor. People are often secretive about their unsuccessful suicide attempts so that only those patients who come to the attention of mental health professionals are available for possible consideration.

Because suicide is a relatively rare event, prospective study will always pose great difficulties and is not performed very often. There are extremely few studies of suicidal behavior in an identified personality population, and these have been conducted in an open and informal manner using samples with retrospective personality disorder diagnoses. Despite these obstacles, attempts to analyze the relationship between personality and suicidality have yielded compelling and converging data worth noting and applying to clinical practice.

PERSONALITY DISORDERS AND SUICIDE

There is good evidence suggesting that two of the personality disorders, borderline personality disorder (BPD) and antisocial personality disorder (ASPD), predict both suicide attempts and completions. Although this point will be addressed later in this chapter and will be discussed in greater detail in other chapters of this volume, it is worth keeping in mind that often the relationship between personality and suicide is mediated through the comorbidity of personality disorder with substance abuse and affective disorder.

Borderline Personality Disorder

BPD is characterized by a pattern of intense and chaotic relationships, affective instability, fluctuating and extreme attitudes regarding other people, impulsivity, direct and indirect self-destructive behavior, and lack of a clear or certain sense of identity, life plan, or values. Table 1 presents the criteria for DSM-III-R diagnosis.

The DSM-III-R criteria make the diagnosis of BPD explicit and reliable, but there is a persistent controversy whether it is best conceived as a "subaffective" or a personality disorder (Akiskal et al. 1985; Gunderson and Siever 1985) or whether it represents some overlap between the two. Certainly, BPD identifies a very heterogeneous group of patients and overlaps with just about every other personality disorder and many Axis I conditions as well (Fyer et al. 1988).

Worth noting is the overlap between aspects of borderline behavior and histrionic personality behavior. While suicidal gestures were considered part of this overlap in DSM-III, this was deleted as an aspect of histrionic personality disorder in DSM-III-R to clarify BPD diagnosis further.

Table 1. DSM-III-R criteria for borderline personality disorder

---

A pervasive pattern of instability of mood, interpersonal relationships, and self-image, beginning by early adulthood and present in a variety of contexts, as indicated by at least *five* of the following:
  (1) a pattern of unstable and intense interpersonal relationships characterized by alternating between extremes of overidealization and devaluation
  (2) impulsiveness in at least two areas that are potentially self-damaging, e.g., spending, sex, substance abuse, shoplifting, reckless driving, binge eating (Do not include suicidal or self-mutilating behavior covered in [5].)
  (3) affective instability: marked shifts from baseline mood to depression, irritability, or anxiety, usually lasting a few hours and only rarely more than a few days
  (4) inappropriate, intense anger or lack of control of anger, e.g., frequent displays of temper, constant anger, recurrent physical fights
  (5) recurrent suicidal threats, gestures, or behavior, or self-mutilating behavior
  (6) marked and persistent identity disturbance manifested by uncertainty about at least two of the following: self-image, sexual orientation, long-term goals or career choice, type of friends desired, preferred values
  (7) chronic feelings of emptiness or boredom
  (8) frantic efforts to avoid real or imagined abandonment (Do not include suicidal or self-mutilating behavior covered in [5].)

Source. Reprinted from American Psychiatric Association 1987, with permission.

Although BPD patients engage in a great deal of self-destructive behavior, it has been presumed that these actions are not likely to be lethal (Gunderson and Elliot 1985; Gunderson and Singer 1975; Perry and Klerman 1978; Spitzer et al. 1979). There have, in fact, been surprisingly few studies of completed suicide in BPD patients to support these assumptions. Available data, however, indicate that BPD carries a significant comorbidity with suicidality, almost comparable to that of affective disorder and schizophrenia. Akiskal et al. (1985) found a 4% rate of complete suicide in a 6- to 36-month follow-up of BPD patients. In a 4- to 7-year follow-up, Pope et al. (1983) found a rate of 7.4%. In a 15-year follow-up, Stone (1986) found a 9.5% rate of completed suicide. The average age at death for these patients was 27 years (Stone 1986). In other 15-year follow-up studies, Paris et al. (1988) found an 8.5% rate of suicide and McGlashan (1986) found a 3% rate. The low rate in the McGlashan study is probably an artifact related to the referral patterns of the hospital in which it was conducted. Chestnut Lodge tended to receive patients who had failed at many other treatments in other hospitals, a "screening" process that probably filtered out the more suicidal BPD patients by selecting for patients who had been chronically in supervised settings.

Several studies suggest that the combination of BPD and affective disorder is particularly lethal. Among 76 adolescent inpatients, Friedman et al. (1982) found that patients who met criteria for both BPD and major affective disorder made more frequent and more lethal attempts. Conversely, a study of 53 depressed inpatients (Friedman et al. 1983) found that the 36 who also met criteria for BPD made more serious and numerous suicide attempts. Among 180 BPD patients, Fyer et al. (1988) found a difference in suicidal behavior between those with and those without concurrent affective disorder. For that sample, 19% had no history of suicide, 32% had made only gestures, and 49% had made serious attempts. However, significantly more of those with affective disorder made serious attempts (56%) than those without an affective diagnosis (37%), and fewer of the affective BPD patients had no history of suicide. Of note again is that a large percentage of these patients are also substance abusers, which may play an additional role in increased suicidality.

The clinical implications of these data in evaluating both the suicidal patient for personality disorder and in evaluating the BPD patient for suicidality will be considered later in this chapter.

Antisocial Personality Disorder

ASPD was among the first described and is among the most researched of the personality disorders. In 1801, a character type defined by a pattern of immoral behavior that was without impairment in reasoning was delineated by Pinel, and later termed "moral insanity" by U'Prichard (1835). Checkly (1941) provided the most influential formulation, emphasizing the psychological traits of guiltlessness, egocentricity, incapacity for love, superficial charm, lack of remorse or shame, lack of insight, and failure to learn from past experience. ASPD was the first personality disorder to be formally recognized within psychiatry and was included in all versions of the DSM.

The criteria for DSM-III diagnosis of ASPD were based in large part on the systematic research of Robins (1985), which demonstrated a temporal stability in the antisocial behavior pattern. However, this work has been criticized for underemphasizing some of the traits suggested by Checkly (1941). As currently defined, ASPD is a pattern of socially irresponsible, exploitative, and guiltless behavior, evident in the tendency to fail to conform to the law, to fail to sustain consistent employment, to exploit and manipulate others for personal gain, to deceive, and to fail to develop stable relationships. The DSM-III-R criteria for ASPD are presented in Table 2.

A controversy in the DSM-III-R diagnostic classification of ASPD is whether there is too much emphasis on delinquent-criminal behavior (Frances 1980; Hare 1983). Many people with "psychopathic" personalities do not follow a criminal career and can be exploitative, deceptive, and irresponsible in socially acceptable professions. DSM-III-R criteria may overemphasize criminality and underemphasize

Table 2. DSM-III-R criteria for antisocial personality disorder

A. Current age at least 18.
B. Evidence of conduct disorder with onset before age 15, as indicated by a history of *three* or more of the following:
   (1) was often truant
   (2) ran away from home overnight at least twice while living in parental or parental surrogate home (or once without returning)
   (3) often initiated physical fights
   (4) used a weapon in more than one fight
   (5) forced someone into sexual activity with him or her
   (6) was physically cruel to animals
   (7) was physically cruel to other people
   (8) deliberately destroyed others' property (other than by fire-setting)
   (9) deliberately engaged in fire-setting
   (10) often lied (other than to avoid physical or sexual abuse)
   (11) has stolen without confrontation of a victim on more than one occasion (including forgery)
   (12) has stolen with confrontation of a victim (e.g., mugging, purse-snatching, extortion, armed robbery)
C. A pattern of irresponsible and antisocial behavior since the age of 15, as indicated by at least *four* of the following:
   (1) is unable to sustain consistent work behavior, as indicated by any of the following (including similar behavior in academic settings if the person is a student):
     (*a*) significant unemployment for six months or more within five years when expected to work and work was available
     (*b*) repeated absences from work unexplained by illness in self or family
     (*c*) abandonment of several jobs without realistic plans for others
   (2) fails to conform to social norms with respect to lawful behavior, as indicated by repeatedly performing antisocial acts that are grounds for arrest (whether arrested or not), e.g., destroying property, harassing others, stealing, pursuing an illegal occupation
   (3) is irritable and aggressive, as indicated by repeated physical fights or assaults (not required by one's job or to defend someone or oneself), including spouse- or child-beating
   (4) repeatedly fails to honor financial obligations, as indicated by defaulting on debts or failing to provide child support or support for other dependents on a regular basis
   (5) fails to plan ahead, or is impulsive, as indicated by one or both of the following:
     (*a*) traveling from place to place without a prearranged job or clear goal for the period of travel or clear idea about when the travel will terminate
     (*b*) lack of a fixed address for a month or more
   (6) has no regard for the truth, as indicated by repeated lying, use of aliases, or "conning" others for personal profit or pleasure
   (7) is reckless regarding his or her own or others' personal safety, as indicated by driving while intoxicated, or recurrent speeding
   (8) if a parent or guardian, lacks ability to function as a responsible parent, as indicated by one or more of the following:
     (*a*) malnutrition of child
     (*b*) child's illness resulting from lack of minimal hygiene
     (*c*) failure to obtain medical care for a seriously ill child
     (*d*) child's dependence on neighbors or nonresident relatives for food or shelter
     (*e*) failure to arrange for a caretaker for young child when parent is away from home
     (*f*) repeated squandering, on personal items, of money required for household necessities

Table 2.   DSM-III-R criteria for antisocial personality disorder, *continued*

(9) has never sustained a totally monogamous relationship for more than one year
(10) lacks remorse (feels justified in having hurt, mistreated, or stolen from another)
D. Occurrence of antisocial behavior not exclusively during the course of
   schizophrenia or manic episodes.

Source. Reprinted from American Psychiatric Association 1987, with permission.

problems with bonding, learning from past experience, impulsivity, aggressivity, and lack of guilt.

Of note as well is that there is some evidence of a biologic predisposition to ASPD, be it genetic (Brantley and Sutker 1984) or, more specifically, based in low cortical arousal and reduced inhibitory anxiety (Fowles 1984; Gorenstein and Newman 1980), which in turn contribute to an impulsive, sensation-seeking life-style with a failure to respond to aversive consequences. Like BPD, ASPD also appears to be associated with alcohol abuse, resulting in a mutually interactive effect. Alcoholism may either result from or contribute to the development of an antisocial life-style. Alcoholic patients with ASPD are particularly prone to violent crimes.

Most clinicians associate ASPD with externally directed violence. The fact that ASPD is also a potent predictor of suicide is much less well known. Reports of the suicide rate among patients with ASPD vary considerably, and most investigators have not used the DSM-III criteria for study purposes. Miles (1977) estimated that 5% of ASPD patients eventually die by suicide. Maddocks (1970) further found that while 5% successfully suicided, 46% made suicide attempts. Robins (1966) found a lower rate, with only 11% of ASPD patients attempting suicide, and a completed suicide rate that was not different from normal controls. From a different vantage point, Woodruff et al. (1972) studied a series of 500 psychiatric patients and found that 23% of 71 suicide attempters met ASPD criteria and constituted the entire ASPD population in the sample of 500.

It has also been observed that ASPD and criminality may be predictors of *recurrent* suicide attempts, and that suicide attempts are often made in the setting of interpersonal difficulties. In one study (Garvey and Spoden 1980), 72% of 29 ASPD individuals made a total of 63 suicide attempts, yet only 3 were serious and none used violent methods. Of note was that half of the ASPD attempters indicated that their most recent attempt was preceded by a crisis in a significant relationship. Robins (1966) found that only 1 of 16 ASPD patients had made a serious suicide attempt compared with 80% of controls with affective disorder. ASPD patients were also younger than affective controls, and findings also showed that 85% of ASPD patients consumed alcohol just prior to suicide attempts. Attempts were often precipitated by anger and frustration in love or marital relationships. Batchelor (1954) studied 42 suicide attempters with "psychopathic states" and found that the majority of attempts were precipitated by difficulties in relationships, that almost half had made previous attempts, and that most used nonviolent means. However, at least one-third of attempts were felt to be serious.

Given these data, it may be reasonable to assume that although the lifetime risk of successful suicide in ASPD individuals is appreciable, many attempts made by them are intended to manipulate those around them.

The relationship between substance abuse, ASPD, and suicidality cannot be overemphasized. One study of 155 polydrug abusers with suicidal behavior found 29% to receive a diagnosis of ASPD, and these patients made more serious attempts (Ward and Schuckit 1980). In a sample of 533 opiate addicts (Rounsaville et al. 1982), there was a 17% lifetime prevalence of suicide attempts, with 60% of attempters meeting DSM-III criteria for ASPD. Yet in this study, 87% of attempters also had a diagnosis of depression and 32% had alcoholism.

In summary, suicide attempts in ASPD appear to be common, repetitive, usually not serious, and are often precipitated by difficulties in important relationships. These data must be integrated with the caution that the combination of ASPD and other disorders may have a significantly different pattern and outcome of suicidality. The 5% rate of successfully completed suicide in ASPD may represent primarily those individuals who also have concurrent affective disorder, substance abuse, and/or other personality disorders that increase risk for successful suicide.

Personality Traits and Suicide

Rather than assessing for the presence of a categorical personality disorder (e.g., an Axis II diagnosis) in suicidal individuals, or for the rate of suicide in those with personality disorder, the psychological literature has more often measured specific personality dimensions or traits in suicide attempters and/or completers. Attempters have more disturbed personality profiles; they are also more likely to be women, to be under 24 years of age, to be receiving "neurotic" or personality disorder diagnoses, and to commit public, impulsive, suicidal acts using less lethal means (Clayton 1985). Suicide completers are more likely to be men, to be older, to have an Axis I diagnosis (particularly depression or alcoholism), to make private and violent attempts, and to use lethal means.

There has been increasing interest in the relationship between suicide and aggression. This interest may have originally stemmed from the psychodynamic formulations of depression and suicide as forms of "hostility turned toward the self" (Abraham 1927; Freud 1916). Data have shown that suicidal individuals have significantly greater aggression or hostility (Cantor 1976; Conte and Plutchik 1974; Murthy 1969; Vinoda 1966), impulsivity (Cantor 1976), social withdrawal or interpersonal difficulty (Farberow and Devries 1967; Rushing 1969; Nelson et al. 1977; Topol and Reznikoff 1982), low self-esteem (Kamano and Crawford 1966; Wetzel 1975; Neuringer 1974a, 1974b; Wilson et al. 1971), dependency (Birtchnell 1981; Braaten and Darling 1962; Paykel and Dienelt 1971; Pallis and Birtchnell 1977), hopelessness (Cantor 1976; Crook et al. 1975; Paykel and Dienelt 1971), external locus of control, rigid cognitive style, and poor problem solving (Birtchnell 1981).

Although many studies have attempted to use the Minnesota Multiphasic Personality Inventory (MMPI) (Hathaway and McKinley 1951) to differentiate between suicidal and nonsuicidal patients, the results have been inconclusive (Pallis and Birtchnell 1977). Likewise, studies of hysterical personality traits and suicide (Gunderson and Kolb 1978; Keltikangas-Jarvinen 1978; Spitzer et al. 1979; Weissman et al. 1973) are inconsistent. Studies using the Eysenck Personality Inventory (1968) have found consistently high neuroticism, psychoticism, and introversion scores in suicidal subjects (Colson 1972; Irfani 1978; Mehryar et al. 1977; Pallis and Jenkins 1977).

A particularly interesting recent finding is the correlation between the personality dimension of aggressive impulsivity in suicidal and violent individuals and the biologic finding of low central nervous system serotonin turnover (Brown et al. 1979, 1982). This association seems to hold up in impulsive personality disorder patients even in the absence of an Axis I diagnosis of affective disorder. Serotonin dysfunction in these patients appears to represent more of a trait than a state condition. It has been postulated that some central problem in serotonergic metabolism may contribute to the individual's traits of impulsivity and aggressiveness. When these personality traits coexist in a patient suffering from a clinical depression, the threshold to suicidal behavior may be lowered; this represents a particularly lethal combination of factors.

YOUTH SUICIDE: PART OF A CONTINUUM

How does this discussion pertain to youth suicide, which has become a special and growing problem for the clinician? A central question that arises is whether or not personality can be accurately assessed in youth. According to DSM-III-R, most personality disorders are difficult to diagnose until age 18, and youthful manifestations of ASPD are considered under the rubric of conduct disorder. In children and teenagers, it is especially problematic to sort out the influences of Axis I conditions from personality, and social and situational difficulties from both of these. In addition, developmental changes can often be mistaken for personality traits, making many teenagers seemingly eligible for diagnoses ranging from narcissistic personality disorder to BPD to ASPD, for which they will no longer qualify once they grow out of that stage or leave a stressful situation.

However, two studies of personality in youth suicide provide data that suggest that there is considerable overlap in personality predictors between youths and adults. Bergstrand and Otto (1962) found that a series of 500 cases of young suicide attempters were most often termed infantile and hysterical. Shaffer (1974) found that the most common personality descriptions among adolescent suicide attempters were paranoid, impulsive, self-critical, and uncommunicative; of these, 75% showed antisocial and/or affective symptoms.

It is somewhat problematic to compare these studies with studies of adults given different classification symptoms; however, despite these difficulties, there are data to suggest that problems with aggression manifest themselves in early life and that many children and teenagers with conduct disorder, itself a high risk factor for suicide, go on to develop adult ASPD (Frances and Blumenthal 1986). Likewise, suicidality in BPD and ASPD patients is often worse early in the course of these disorders, furthering the association of these two personality disorders with youth suicide. Finally, there is evidence for a cohort effect demonstrating the increasing incidence of conduct disorder among younger populations. This effect parallels and may in part account for a similar cohort effect in the rates of youth suicide. Thus the personality areas that have the greatest predictive value for adult suicide appear to have precursors in youth that are stable throughout the life cycle (Blumenthal and Kupfer 1988; Frances and Blumenthal 1986).

Of note also is that the perfectionist, self-critical posture of many adolescents may amplify suicidality in this age group, as apparently minor stresses to an adult may precipitate a crisis in the adolescent.

Personality and Suicide: Clinical Guidelines

It is clear that personality disorders may play an important role in the prediction of suicide and that certain personality disorders increase lifetime suicide risk. The clinician should view this from two vantage points. In assessing the suicidal patient, it is important to determine whether the patient meets criteria for BPD or ASPD. This will help to guide one's interventions both in assessing risk and in planning an approach to the suicidal patient. The target of acute treatment is generally not the personality disorder, but rather to reduce the acute risk of suicide.

Given that both BPD and ASPD improve on long-term follow-up and that the major morbidity of both is suicide within the third decade, management of suicide attempts often becomes an integral part of the treatment of these Axis II disorders. In this section, the assessment of personality in the suicidal patient will be addressed, followed by a consideration of the different interventions that may be dictated by this assessment.

Assessment Issues

Often an assessment of the suicidal patient is undertaken in a crisis setting, necessitating that management decisions be made swiftly. While it is not the purpose of this discussion to outline a comprehensive approach to the suicidal patient, it should be underscored that even in the most hectic settings (e.g., an emergency room), some personality assessment of the suicidal patient is essential. This should be undertaken even if a suicide attempt has been made and the patient is to be admitted to the hospital. Even the preliminary diagnosis of a personality disorder may influence the risk assessment and approach to treatment of a suicide attempt in a particular patient. Further, the comorbidity between affective disorders, substance abuse, and personality disorder is sufficiently high as to suggest the value of some evaluation of the latter in suicide assessment. Personality assessment will serve as one among many predictors in the assessment of suicidality, along with a consideration of other factors—including Axis I illness, previous suicide attempts, concomitant substance abuse, severity of intention and plan, family history, and many others that have been covered elsewhere in this volume.

Since BPD and ASPD are most closely correlated with suicidal behavior, it is essential to assess a patient for at least these two disorders. In situations where time is limited, this can be done by conducting a careful clinical interview, with consideration of DSM-III-R criteria for these disorders. Fortunately, of all the personality disorders, BPD and ASPD have the most extensive research literature and the highest diagnostic reliability. A preliminary diagnosis based on DSM-III-R criteria has a good likelihood of being reasonably accurate and meaningful, particularly if the clinician systematically asks about the items in the criteria set and assures that the behaviors are long standing.

In the situations that call for a more thorough Axis II evaluation, a variety of measures can be used (for review, see Widiger and Frances 1987), ranging from self-report scales of personality traits such as the MMPI to more comprehensive interview formats such as the Personality Disorder Examination (PDE) (Loranger et al. 1985). In addition, there are specific instruments designed to assess both the broad spectrum of personality disorders, as well as BPD and ASPD in particular (Jacobsberg et al. 1989).

Often, however, a patient will either be unwilling (e.g., uncooperative) or unable (e.g., being treated medically for a suicide attempt) to be assessed using even a brief interview. In these situations, available family members or significant others should be consulted to complete both the suicide and personality evaluation. Many of the instruments for personality assessment (e.g., the PDE) have been designed with alternative versions for significant others to fill out.

Management Issues

The Borderline Personality Disorder Patient

There is no one accepted treatment for suicidality in BPD patients, just as there is no one accepted treatment for BPD itself. In part, this may be due to the heterogeneity of BPD patients. Further, since there is clear comorbidity between BPD and many Axis I disorders, the assessment of suicidality may differ at various stages of the patient's clinical course and life cycle. In these ways, Axis I and Axis II illnesses each confound the ability to assess the other.

In assessing the BPD patient for suicidality, there are a number of reasons why it is vital to take a careful history of previous treatments. First, suicidality in BPD patients often occurs in the context of, and sometimes is a complication of, an ongoing treatment. Hence, it is essential to check with a patient's treating therapist to determine the specific meaning of the suicidality/suicide attempt and the consequences of such for the treatment. Further, a history of past suicide attempts and their subsequent treatment is essential. For instance, many BPD patients use suicidality as a means of gaining a hospital admission. While this may at times be appropriate for the patient, it is important to assess this before a decision for admission is made. It is generally advisable to admit BPD patients to the hospital when they exhibit great resistance to hospitalization and to avoid hospitalizations whenever possible when the patient appears to be using the suicidal behavior to manipulate the environment. Of course, the decision not to hospitalize has risks and must be carefully considered and compared with alternatives that make sense to both the patient and the clinician. Often this will involve a crisis intervention format involving the mobilization of significant others.

One of the most salient questions in making such decisions is the extent to which a hospitalization might be counterproductive. Sometimes hospitalizations will foster more impulsive behavior and make recovery a dangerous and seemingly impossible task for the patient and clinician. Brief hospitalizations of BPD patients can be a useful adjunct to outpatient treatment. Patients are admitted explicitly for a brief stay to protect from suicidal impulses. A frequent target of inpatient treatment in these patients is the management of the substance abuse often associated with BPD. Suicidality in BPD patients should be viewed as a symptom to be worked with, as the management of suicidality is often an integral part of the treatment plan. The clinician should also keep in mind that these patients, especially when suicidal, often engender countertransferential anger in the treating therapist or evaluator (Maltsberger and Buie 1974). The evaluator who does not keep this in mind runs the risk of conveying the covert and dangerous message that it would be desirable for the patient to in fact kill him- or herself.

In addition to the issues discussed concerning the management of acute suicidality in the BPD patient, there are many reported approaches for the treatment of chronic suicidality in BPD patients. Many of these approaches may also prove useful in the management of acute suicidality in these patients. For example, pharmacotherapy of this disorder, when administered skillfully and targeted to particular symptoms, often proves very helpful in reducing impulsivity and accompanying self-destructive behavior. Low-dose neuroleptics may be particularly helpful for those BPD patients who are prone to cognitive slippage or psychotic-like disorganization in the context of interpersonal stress. Antidepressants may be useful in treating the depression that often accompanies BPD, although there are some reports of behavioral disinhibition and the potential for more impulsive behavior while on antidepressants (Soloff et al. 1987). Monoamine oxidase inhibitors appear at times to be especially useful, although again the potential for acting out by not adhering to the tyramine-free diet should be considered. Additionally, lithium may be helpful for the cyclothymic BPD patient, and carbamazepine may be differentially useful for those with violent outbursts.

As in all suicidal patients, medications should be prescribed according to the clinician's assessment of risk of overdose. The patient should receive only small amounts of the medication at a time. Where possible, particularly for young people, medication should be supervised by an entrusted relative. Side effects should be monitored carefully as well; these patients will often be very sensitive to side effects. Adequate trials of medication are often hampered by a patient's noncompliance secondary to side effects. Also, it is important to realize that any successful trial of medication must take place in the context of an ongoing treatment relationships. Personality disorders are chronic so that any assessment of success will primarily focus on the amelioration of accompanying Axis I syndromes and target behaviors.

Various psychotherapeutic approaches to BPD have also been proven effective and may curtail chronic suicidality. Linehan (1981) described a behavioral-cognitive approach to these patients in which self-destructive thoughts and behaviors are identified and worked with to provide the patient with new methods for dealing with them. Insight-oriented or supportive psychotherapy can also be helpful, but should be undertaken as a long-term process, with the expectation that the course may be very difficult. Kernberg (1984), Masterson (1976), and Adler and Buie (1979) describe different psychodynamic approaches to these patients.

The Antisocial Personality Disorder Patient

ASPD has been recognized as an extremely difficult and refractory personality disorder to treat. Often the ASPD patient may experience a greater satisfaction outwitting the therapist than in demonstrating effective positive changes. The target of treatment must be the accompanying suicidal behavior, affective disorder, and substance abuse, *not* the underlying personality disorder.

There are reports that both lithium and propranolol are useful for violent episodes in ASPD patients, but these have been largely uncontrolled studies undertaken in prison and hospital settings. Suicidality in ASPD individuals often arises in the setting of substance abuse, depression, or anxiety and is exacerbated by confinement, social failure, and abuse. In these situations, treatment will be more successful if the clinician avoids the temptation to treat the Axis II illness and focuses instead on the depression and inordinate losses so common in these patients.

Although a correctional facility may often be the only means of controlling some ASPD patients, hospitalization may be necessary in situations where suicidality is an issue. In these situations, the clinician faces two difficult questions. First, to what extent is the ASPD patient feigning suicidality? Often the ASPD patient will seek admission to a psychiatric hospital for secondary gain to avoid confrontations with enemies or with legal authorities. Second, unless admitted to a specialized treatment setting, such as a substance abuse program or a ward designed to treat similar patients, the ASPD patient is often a very destructive influence on other patients. The ASPD patient can become a "wolf among the sheep" of innocent staff and defenseless psychiatric patients. Hence in some circumstances, suicidality might be better addressed in a treatment program within a correctional environment or through outpatient crisis intervention.

As in the treatment of BPD patients, therapists must be careful to monitor their own responses to these patients. Reactions of therapists may range from disgust and moral condemnation to fantasies that one can change the course of the ASPD patient's life by developing an alliance that has never been possible before. In either case, when these patients present as suicidal, it is also common for the clinician to vent frustration by giving an implicit or even explicit message that suicide may be a desirable option.

SUMMARY

Personality and personality disorders are chronic patterns of thought, behavior, and interpersonal interaction that tend to improve with age, however slowly, through the life cycle. We have addressed the interplay between personality and suicidality both in the clinical and research arenas of psychiatric practice. While questions regarding the relationship between personality and suicide are conceptually difficult, and have hence been infrequently addressed, it seems clear that personality traits, particularly aggression and impulsivity, and personality disorders, particularly BPD and ASPD, are essential to assess in the thorough evaluation of the suicidal patient.

Specifically, it is important to identify BPD and ASPD because these often dictate different treatment approaches to suicidality. Conversely, suicidality in these two populations poses a challenge, as attempts to treat Axis II disorders often involve the management of chronic suicidality.

Many questions remain as to the extent to which suicidal thought and behavior are related to personality, and in turn to other behaviors (most particularly substance abuse). Studies designed to elucidate this relationship further will be of considerable clinical importance and interest.

REFERENCES

Abraham K: Notes on the psychoanalytic investigation and treatment of manic-depressive insanity and allied conditions, in Selected Papers. Edited by Jones E. London, Hogarth Press, 1927, pp 137–156

Adam KS, Attempted Suicide. Psychiatr Clin North Am 8:183–201, 1985

Adler G, Buie DH: The psychotherapeutic approach to aloneness in the borderline patient, in Advances in Psychotherapy of the Borderline Patient. Edited by LeBoit J, Capponi A. New York, Jason Aronson, 1979, pp 433–448

Akiskal HS, Chen SE, Davis GC, et al: Borderline: an adjective in search of a noun. J Clin Psychiatry 46:41–48, 1985

Alessi, NE, McManus M, Brickman A, et al: Suicidal behavior among serious juvenile offenders. Am J Psychiatry 141:286–287, 1984

American Psychiatric Association: Diagnostic and Statistical Manual of Mental Disorders, 3rd Edition. Washington, DC, American Psychiatric Association, 1980

American Psychiatric Association: Diagnostic and Statistical Manual of Mental Disorders, 3rd Edition, Revised. Washington, DC, American Psychiatric Association, 1987

Batchelor IRC: Psychopathic states and attempted suicide. Br Med J 1:1342–1347, 1954

Bergstrand OG, Otto U: Suicidal attempts in adolescence childhood. Acta Paedopsychiatr 31:397–411, 1962

Birtchnell J: Some familial and clinical characteristics of female suicidal psychiatric patients. Br J Psychiatry 138:381–390, 1981

Black DW, Warrack G, Winokur G: The Iowa Record Linkage Study, I: suicides and accidental deaths among psychiatric patients. Arch Gen Psychiatry 42:71–75, 1985

Blumenthal SJ, Kupfer DJ: Overview of early detection and treatment strategies for suicidal behavior in young people. Journal of Youth and Adolescence 17:1–23, 1988

Braaten LJ, Darling CD: Suicidal tendencies among college students. Psychiatr Q 36:665–692, 1962

Brantley P, Sutker P: Antisocial behavior disorders, in Comprehensive Handbook of Psychopathology. Edited by Adams H, Sutker P. New York, Plenum, 1984, pp 439–478

Brown GL, Goodwin FK, Ballenger JC, et al: Aggression in human correlates with cerebrospinal fluid amine metabolites. Psychiatry Res 1:131–139, 1979

Brown GL, Ebert MH, Goyer PF, et al: Aggression, suicide, and serotonin: relationships to CSF amine metabolites. Am J Psychiatry 139:741–746, 1982

Cantor PC: Personality characteristics found among youthful female suicide attempters. J Abnorm Psychol 85:324–329, 1976

Checkly H (ed): The Mask of Sanity. St. Louis, MO, CV Mosby, 1941

Clayton PJ: Suicide. Psychiatr Clin North Am 8:203–214, 1985

Colson CE: Neuroticism, extraversion and repression-sensitization in suicidal college students. British Journal of Social and Clinical Psychology 11:88–89, 1972

Conte HR, Plutchik R: Personality and background characteristics of suicidal mental patients. J Psychiatr Res 10:181–188, 1974

Coyne J: Toward an interactional description of depression. Psychiatry 39:28–40, 1976

Crook T, Raskin A, Davis D: Factors associated with attempted suicide among hospitalized depressed patients. Psychol Med 5:381–388,1975

Crumley FE: Adolescent suicide attempts. JAMA 241:2404–2407, 1979

Eysenck SBG, Eysenck HJ: The measurement of psychoticism: a study of factor stability and reliability. British Journal of Social and Clinical Psychology 7:286–294, 1968

Farberow, NL, Devries AG: An item differentiation analysis of MMPIs of suicidal neuropsychiatric hospital patients. Psychol Rep 20:607–617, 1967

Fowles D: Biological variables in psychopathology, in Comprehensive Handbook of Psychopathology. Edited by Adams H, Sutke P. New York, Plenum, 1984, pp 77–110

Frances A: The DSM-III personality disorders section: a commentary. Am J Psychiatry 137:1050–1054, 1980

Frances A, Blumenthal SJ: Personality disorders and characteristics in youth suicide. Paper presented at the National Conference on Risk Factors for Youth Suicide, Bethesda, MD, May 8–9, 1986

Frances A, Widiger T: The classification of personality disorders: an overview of problems and solutions, in Psychiatry Update: American Psychiatric Association Annual Review, Vol 5. Edited by Frances AJ, Hales RE. Washington, DC, American Psychiatric Press, 1986, pp 240–257

Frances A, Widiger T: Personality disorders, in Treatment of Mental Disorders. Edited by Griest J, Jefferson J, Spitzer R. New York, Oxford University Press (in press)

Frances A, Fyer MR, Clarkin J: Personality and Suicide. Ann NY Acad Sci 487:281–293, 1986

Freud S: Mourning and melancholia, in Collected Papers, Vol 4. Edited by Jones E. London, Hogarth Press, 1916, pp 15–27

Friedman RC, Clarkin JF, Corn R, et al: DSM-III and affective pathology in hospitalized adolescents. J Nerv Ment Dis 170:511–521, 1982

Friedman RC, Aronoff MS, Clarkin JF, et al: History of suicidal behavior in depressed borderline inpatients. Am J Psychiatry 140:1023–1026, 1983

Fyer MR, Frances AJ, Sullivan T, et al: Comorbidity of borderline personality disorder. Arch Gen Psychiatry 45:348–352, 1988

Garvey MJ, Spoden F: Suicide attempts in antisocial personality disorder. Compr Psychiatry 21:146–149, 1980

Gorenstein E, Newman J: Disinhibitory psychopathology: a new perspective and a model for research. Psychol Rev 87:301–315, 1980

Gunderson JG, Elliot G: The interface between borderline personality disorder and affective disorder. Am J Psychiatry 142:277–288, 1985

Gunderson JF, Kolb JE: Discriminating features of borderline patients. Am J Psychiatry 135:792–796, 1978

Gunderson J, Siever L: Relatedness of schizotypal to schizophrenic disorders: editor's introduction. Schizophr Bull 11:532–537, 1985

Gunderson JF, Singer MT: Defining borderline patients: an overview. Am J Psychiatry 132:1–10, 1975

Guze SN, Robins E: Suicide and primary affective disorders. Br J Psychiatry 117:437–438, 1970

Hare R: Diagnosis of antisocial personality disorder in two prison populations. Am J Psychiatry 140:887–890, 1983

Hathaway SR, McKinley JC: Minnesota Multiphasic Personality Inventory: Manual for Administration and Scoring. Minneapolis, MN, University of Minnesota Press, 1951

Irfani S: Personality correlates of suicidal tendency among Iranian and Turkish students. J Psychol 99:151–153, 1978

Jacobsberg L, Goldsmith S, Frances A: Assessment of DSM-III personality disorders, in Measuring Mental Illness: Psychometric Assessment for Clinicians. Edited by Wetzler S. Washington, DC, American Psychiatric Press, 1989, pp 139–159

James I: Suicide and mortality amongst heroin addicts in Britain. Br J Addict 62:391–398, 1967

Kamano DK, Crawford CS: Self-evaluations of suicidal mental hospital patients. J Clin Psychol 22:278–279, 1966

Kass F, Spitzer R, Williams J: An empirical study of the issue of sex bias in the diagnosis criteria of DSM-III Axis II personality disorders. Am Psychol 38:799–801, 1983

Keltikangas-Jarvinen L: Personality of violent offenders and suicidal individuals. Psychiat Fennica 57–63, 1978

Kernberg O: Severe Personality Disorders: Psychotherapeutic Strategies. New Haven, Yale University Press, 1984

Kraft D, Babigian H: Suicide by persons with and without psychiatric contacts. Arch Gen Psychiatry 33:209–215, 1976

Kreitman N: The epidemiology of suicide and parasuicide. Crisis 2:1–13, 1981

Linehan MM: A social-behavioral analysis of suicide and parasuicide: implications for clinical assessment and treatment, in Depression: Behavioral and Directive Intervention Strategies. Edited by Clarkin JF, Glazer HI. New York, Garland Publishing, 1981, pp 229–294

Loranger AW, Susman VL, Oldham JM, et al: Personality Disorder Examination (PDE): A Structured Interview for DSM-III-R Personality Disorders. White Plains, NY, The New York Hospital-Cornell Medical Center, Westchester Division, 1985

Maddocks PD: A five year follow-up of untreated psychopaths. Br J Psychiatry 116:511–515,1970

Maltsberger JT, Buie DH: Countertransference hate in the treatment of suicidal patients. Arch Gen Psychiatry 30:625–633, 1974

Martin RL, Cloninger CB, Guze SB, et al: Mortality in a follow up of 500 psychiatric outpatients, II: cause-specific mortality. Arch Gen Psychiatry 42:58–66, 1985

Masterson JF: Psychotherapy of the Borderline Adult: A Developmental Approach. New York, Brunner/Mazel, 1976

McGlashan TH: The Chestnut Lodge follow up study, III: long term outcome of borderline personalities. Arch Gen Psychiatry 43:20–30, 1986

Mehryar AH, Hekmat H, Khajavi F: Some personality correlates of contemplated suicide. Psychol Rep 40:1291–1294, 1977

Miles CP: Conditions predisposing to suicide: a review. J Nerv Ment Dis 164:231–246, 1977

Millon T (ed): Disorders of Personality: DSM III, Axis II. New York, John Wiley, 1981

Murthy VN: Personality and the nature of suicidal attempts. Br J Psychiatry 115:791–795, 1969

Nelson VL, Nielsen EC, Checketts KT: Interpersonal attitudes of suicidal individuals. Psychol Rep 40:983–989, 1977

Neuringer C: Attitude toward self in suicidal individuals. Suicide Life Threat Behav 4:96–106, 1974a

Neuringer C: Self- and other appraisals by suicidal, psychosomatic and normal hospitalized patients. J Consult Clin Psychol 42:306, 1974b

Noble P, Hart T, Nation R: Correlates and outcome of illicit drug use by adolescent girls. Br J Psychiatry 120:497–504, 1972

Pallis DJ, Birtchnell J: Seriousness of suicide attempt in relation to personality. Br J Psychiatry 130:253–259, 1977

Pallis DJ, Jenkins JS: Extraversion, neuroticism, and intent in attempted suicides. Psychol Rep 41:19–22, 1977

Paris J, Brown R, Nowlis D: Long term follow up of borderline patients in a general hospital. Compr Psychiatry 29:147–150, 1988

Paykel ES, Dienelt M: Suicide attempts following acute depression. J Nerv Ment Dis 153:234–243, 1971

Perry JC, Klerman GL: The borderline patient: a comparative analysis of four sets of diagnostic criteria. Arch Gen Psychiatry 35:141–150, 1978

Pfohl B, Corywell W, Zimmerman M, et al: DSM-III personality disorders: diagnostic overlap and internal consistency of individual DSM-III criteria. Compr Psychiatry 27:21–34, 1986

Pinel P: Abhandlung uber Geisteverirrungen oder Manie. Wien, Carl Schaumburg, 1801

Pokorny AD: Suicide rates in various psychiatric disorders. J Nerv Ment Dis 139:499–506, 1964

Pope HG Jr, Jonas JM, Hudson JI, et al: The validity of DSM-III borderline personality disorder: a phenomenologic, family history, treatment response, and long-term follow-up study. Arch Gen Psychiatry 40:23–30, 1983

Robins L: Epidemiology of antisocial personality disorder, in Psychiatry, Vol 3. Edited by Michels R, Cavenar J. Philadelphia, JB Lippincott, 1985, pp 1–14

Robins LN (ed): Deviant Children Grown Up. Baltimore, Williams & Wilkins, 1966

Robins E, Schmidt EH, O'Neal P: Some interrelations of social factors and clinical diagnosis in attempted suicide: a study of 109 patients. Am J Psychiatry 114:221–231, 1957

Robins E, Gassner S, Kayes J, et al: The communication of suicidal intent: a study of 134 consecutive cases of successful (completed) suicide. Am J Psychiatry 115:724–733, 1959

Ross MW, Clayer JR, Campbell RL: Parental rearing patterns and suicidal thoughts. Acta Psychiatr Scand 67:429–433, 1983

Rounsaville BJ, Weissman MM, Kleber H, et al: Heterogeneity of psychiatric diagnosis in treated opiate addicts. Arch Gen Psychiatry 39:161–166, 1982

Roy A: Suicide in chronic schizophrenia. Br J Psychiatry 141:171–177, 1982

Roy A: Suicide in depressives. Compr Psychiatry 24:487–491, 1983

Rushing WA: Deviance, interpersonal relations and suicide. Human Relations 22:61–76, 1969

Shaffer D: Suicide in childhood and early adolescence. J Child Psychol Psychiatry 15:275–291, 1974

Soloff PH, George A, Nathan RS, et al: Behavioral dyscontrol in borderline patients treated with amitriptyline. Psychopharmacol Bull 1:177–181, 1987

Spitzer RL, Endicott J, Gibbon M: Crossing the border into borderline personality and borderline schizophrenia: the development of criteria. Arch Gen Psychiatry 36:17–24, 1979

Stengel E (ed): Suicide and Attempted Suicide. Baltimore, Penguin, 1969

Stone MH: Exploratory psychotherapy in schizophrenia-spectrum patients: a reevaluation in the light of long-term follow-up of schizophrenia and borderline patients. Bull Menninger Clin 50:287–306, 1986

Topol P, Reznikoff M: Perceived peer and family relationships, hopelessness and locus of control as factors in adolescent suicide attempts. Suicide Life Threat Behav 12:141–150, 1982

U'Prichard JC: A Treatise on Insanity. London, Sherwood, Gilbert, & Piper, 1835

Vaillant G: Twelve year follow up of New York narcotic addicts, I: the relation of treatment to outcome. Am J Psychiatry 122:727–737, 1966

Vaillant G, Perry J: Personality disorders, in Comprehensive Textbook of Psychiatry, Vol 1, 4th Edition. Edited by Kaplan H, Sadock B. Baltimore, Williams & Wilkins, 1985, pp 958–981

Vinoda KS: Personality characteristics of attempted suicide. Br J Psychiatry 112:1143–1150, 1966

Ward NG, Schuckit MA: Factors associated with suicidal behavior in polydrug abusers. J Clin Psychiatry 41:379–385, 1980

Weissman MM: The epidemiology of suicide attempts, 1960 to 71. Arch Gen Psychiatry 30:737–746, 1974

Weissman MM, Fox K, Klerman GL: Hostility and depression associated with suicide attempts. Am J Psychiatry 130:450–455, 1973

Wetzel RD: Self-concept and suicide intent. Psychol Rep 36:279–282, 1975

Widiger T, Frances A: Interviews and inventories for the measurement of personality disorders. Clin Psychol Rev 7:49–75, 1987

Wilson LT, Braucht GN, Miskimins RW, et al: The severe suicide attempter and self-concept. J Clin Psychol 27:307–309, 1971

Woodruff RA Jr, Clayton PJ, Guze SB: Suicide attempts and psychiatric diagnosis. Diseases of the Nervous System 33:617–621, 1972

Chapter 8

Substance Abuse and Suicidal Behavior

Daniel K. Flavin, M.D.
John E. Franklin, Jr., M.D.
Richard J. Frances, M.D.

JOHN BERRYMAN WAS a 20th-century American poet who won the 1965 Pulitzer Prize in Letters/American Poetry for his work *The Dream Songs* (Berryman 1969). John Berryman was also an alcoholic who committed suicide in 1972 by jumping from a bridge onto a bank of the Mississippi River. His father had died by committing suicide. A gifted artist heavily influenced by Yeats and Auden, John Berryman was known for his experimentation within traditional poetic forms; much of his work reflected the complex interplay of tensions associated with his alcohol use. As Gilmore (1987) noted: "Even within a single poem, Berryman could be both honest and evasive about his drinking, both blind and perceptive" (p. 121). Berryman's later work provides a poignant look into the tenuous nature of his sobriety and recovery. In his poem "Of Suicide" (Berryman 1970), he wrote (third, fourth, and sixth stanzas deleted):

> Reflexions [sic] on suicide, & on my father, possess me.
> I drink too much. My wife threatens separation.
> She won't "nurse" me. She feels "inadequate".
> We don't mix together.

> It's an hour later in the East.
> I could call up Mother in Washington, D.C.
> But could she help me?
> And all this postal adulation & reproach?

. . . .

I don't entirely resign. I may teach the Third Gospel
this afternoon. I haven't made up my mind.
It seems to be sometimes that others have easier jobs
& do them worse.

. . . .

Rembrandt was sober. There we differ. Sober.
Terrors came on him. To us too they come.
Of suicide I continually think.
Apparently he didn't. I'll teach Luke.

In a study of premature mortality in 27 prominent American
authors known for their excess drinking, at least 3 were found to have
died by their own hand: Berryman, Hart Crane, and Ernest Heming-
way (Davis 1986). This study emphasized not only the tragic personal
toll on the lives of these individuals and their families, but also the
social cost of alcohol abuse and dependence.

Suicide accounts for 25,000 to 30,000 deaths in the United States
annually (Clayton 1985) and is the eighth leading cause of death in the
United States. The use of alcohol and/or other psychoactive substances places an individual at higher risk for suicide and other forms
of self-destructive behavior whether or not a diagnosis of psychoactive substance abuse or dependence is present. Alcohol use has been
associated with up to one-half of all suicides; it is also of interest that
the use of intoxicants in violence-prone individuals represents the
single most important factor in homicide (Langevin et al. 1982; Rushing 1968). An analysis of nearly 3,400 violence-related deaths in Erie
County, New York, during the period of 1973 to 1983 in which victims'
blood alcohol concentrations were measured found suicide to be the
cause of death in 21%. One-third of these had been drinking immediately prior to their death and nearly one-quarter were legally intoxicated (Abel and Zeidenberg 1985). As Vaillant (1983) has pointed out
however, the use of alcohol does not necessarily indicate the presence
of a clinically defined problem with abuse or dependence.

The incidence of alcohol dependence in suicide victims ranges
from 15% to 26.9%, with an average across studies of 21.1%. Among
causes of death in alcoholics, the percentage thought to have died by
suicide ranges from 2% to 56%, with a mean of 17.6% (Roy and
Linnoila 1986). Thus the use of alcohol or other drugs may be a risk
factor for self-destructive behavior even in the absence of a clinically
defined abuse or dependence problem; clearly, the suicide rate is
substantially raised among individuals who are alcohol dependent.

Annually, approximately 100,000 deaths in the United States are
alcohol-related (Ravenholt 1984). Given the forensic difficulties inher-

ent in the classification of suicide, it is difficult to estimate the number of additional fatalities that may be related to self-destructive behavior associated with vehicular accidents (in which blood alcohol concentrations are not measured), drownings, fires, falls, boating or aviation accidents, or serious medical illness with or without concurrent organic mental changes.

Menninger (1938) conceived of alcoholism and other addictions as a protracted form of suicide; he noted that the self-destructive behavior was "accomplished in spite of and . . . by means of the very device used by the sufferer in relieving his pain." Such a formulation ignores the paradox of the circumscribed nature of risk-taking in addicts not typically characterized by other stigmata of major mental illness (Galanter and Castaneda 1985). Indeed, the majority of individuals addicted to alcohol or other drugs do not suffer from a coexistent major psychiatric disorder. A more sophisticated understanding of the etiologic relationship of psychoactive substance use and suicide is predicated on the establishment of a multifaceted model of psychoactive substance use and dependence from a biopsychosocial perspective, its etiology, the clarification and standardization of nosology and research methodology, more sensitive methods of detecting suicidal behavior, more accurate forensic classification, and an understanding of the interplay between other known risk factors such as gender, age, recent loss, psychiatric illness, organic mental disorders, family history, physical illness, and other drug use.

In this chapter, the available literature on psychoactive substance use and various forms of self-destructive behavior will be reviewed. Emphasis will be given to alcohol use, abuse, and dependence for two reasons: 1) the far greater magnitude of alcohol use and alcohol-related problems vis-à-vis other drug-related problems and 2) the greater emphasis in the literature thus far with regard to alcohol use as it interfaces with suicidal behavior. Specific reference will be given to the relationship between alcohol and other drug use and major psychiatric disorders, the emergence of research into biologic markers, the needs of special populations, and the importance of social support systems. We conclude with an examination of diagnostic and management issues faced by clinicians of all disciplines who work in this area.

PSYCHOACTIVE SUBSTANCE USE AND SUICIDE

Alcohol Use, Abuse, and Dependence

As early as 1911, Bleuler (1911/1951) speculated on the role of "alcoholic melancholia" in suicide. Since that time, the psychiatric literature has demonstrated a close association between alcohol use, abuse, and dependence and self-destructive behavior. Galanter and Castaneda (1985) noted that two factors account for this relationship: 1) the high suicide rate among chronic alcoholics, and 2) alcohol intoxication at the time of the suicide attempt or completion. Several retrospective studies have concluded that alcoholism is second only to the affective disorders in psychiatric diagnoses associated with suicide in adults (Barraclough et al. 1974; Robins et al. 1954). More men than women commit suicide in both alcoholic and nonalcoholic populations; whites commit suicide more frequently than blacks (Goodwin 1983).

In general, the prevalence of attempted suicide, estimated to be from 600 to 800 per 100,000, is significantly greater than completions (O'Brien 1977). Of those who are successful at taking their own life, 30% to 40% have previously attempted it (Ottosson 1979). Weissman (1974) noted that drug overdoses, frequently accompanied by alcohol use, account for 70% to 90% of all unsuccessful attempts. Alcohol abuse has been reported to be more frequent among those who attempt suicide than completers (Goodwin 1983). Those alcoholics who commit suicide, according to Teft et al. (1974), frequently choose violent deaths by the use of firearms, hanging, or drowning and usually suffer from affective disorders. Miles (1977) estimated the suicide rate for alcoholics to be 270 per 100,000 per year, and there are between 6,200 and 13,000 alcoholic suicides each year.

Determining the frequency of suicide among alcoholics is a complex task; epidemiologic studies come from different countries and employ different follow-up methods and varying follow-up times. Study series are frequently drawn from different types of institutions and often vary in the criteria used to diagnose alcoholism. The result is that the comparative analysis of such studies is difficult if not impossible; only the most global conclusions can be reached, and statistical results vary widely. Keeping this caveat in mind is helpful in examining how data are gathered about how often alcoholics or other drug-dependent individuals commit suicide. This is done in basically two ways: 1) by examining follow-up studies in alcoholics reporting mortality and causes of death, and 2) by examining studies on suicide in the general population to find out the number of alcoholics among the victims.

Roy and Linnoila (1986) noted that, as of their writing, a total of 21 follow-up studies appeared in the international literature reporting on 27,956 alcoholics. The percentage of alcoholics reported to have died by their own hand ranged from 2% to 56%, with a mean of 17.7%. Five general population studies from four countries reported on 748 suicide victims; 158 (21.1%) were thought to be alcoholic. Twelve studies reported sex distribution; 87.4% of the victims were men. Five studies recording age noted a mean of 46.8 years in suicide victims. Risk factors associated with an increased likelihood of suicide included single, divorced, or widowed marital status; race; and previous suicide attempt (36.5% of 104 alcoholic suicides in which these data were recorded). The postdischarge period was also noted to be a time of increased risk for suicide. Goodwin (1973) commented previously that the greater number of alcoholic suicides in the middle-age years may be secondary to two factors: 1) decreased longevity from a number of associated health or other causes, and 2) lower recovery rates among alcoholics.

Other investigators have attempted to examine those clinical factors that may be predictive of suicidal behavior. In a study of 262 patients admitted to a Veterans Administration Hospital alcoholism rehabilitation center, Black et al. (1986) examined those factors distinguishing alcoholics with a history of suicide attempts from nonattempters. They concluded that the best predictors of suicidal behavior included: 1) the amount of alcohol consumed within a 24-hour period, 2) a previous history of alcoholism treatment, 3) a previous history of other drug use, and 4) a high Hamilton Rating Score for Depression (Hamilton 1960) on admission. In a study of 913 primary alcoholics entering an alcoholism treatment program, Schuckit (1986) noted that 17% had attempted suicide. Compared to other primary alcoholics, those with histories of suicide attempts were more likely to have had early life difficulties with police, school, and parents; were more likely to have reported more misuse of drugs; and were much more likely to have an alcoholic or depressed close relative. Among a series of 50 completed alcoholic suicides, 92% were found to have had a history of communicating in some manner their self-destructive thoughts before taking their lives (Murphy et al. 1979).

The presence of interpersonal conflict and loss of a close interpersonal relationship have emerged as significant clinical indicators of increased suicidal risk. Robins et al. (1954) retrospectively studied a series of 134 consecutive suicides, 31 of whom met criteria for the diagnosis of alcoholism. The authors found that approximately one-half had experienced the loss of a close relationship within a year before their death, in contrast to fewer than 20% of those with a depressive illness who committed suicide (Murphy and Robins 1967). Approximately one-third of the alcoholics had experienced this loss within 6 weeks of their death. As Murphy (1986) noted, the loss of autonomy or loss of control of the relationship as well as shame played a significant role in some of the suicides. In addition, most of the alcoholics had experienced some significant medical or psychosocial problem within the year before their death. Nearly three-quarters of the victims in Murphy's study were depressed; this was not found to be related to the presence of interpersonal loss.

Beck et al. (1982) studied 76 male and 29 female outpatient alcoholics using the Scale for Suicidal Ideation, the Beck Hopelessness Scale, and the Beck Depression Inventory (Beck et al. 1961, 1974, 1979). They concluded that hopelessness was the critical link in the relationship between depression and suicidal ideation.

The incidence of major affective disorders in alcoholic individuals who attempt or commit suicide has not been extensively addressed in the literature. In a review of four studies examining this question, Roy and Linnoila (1986) observed that 63 of 111 (56.8%) alcoholic suicides were assessed as having an associated depressive syndrome. Whitters et al. (1985) found that the majority of suicide attempters in a study of alcoholic inpatients had a lifetime diagnosis of major depression. Significantly more of those attempters had reported vegetative signs and symptoms of major depression. Berglund (1984) reported that among alcoholics who committed suicide (compared with those who had not taken their lives) a significant number were rated at the time of their first admission as having slight depression, irritability, dysphoria, aggressiveness, and lability of affect.

Alcoholics are most likely clinically depressed at the time of suicide. Silver et al. (1971) found a positive relationship between the depth of depressed mood and suicidal intent in alcoholics. Nakamura et al. (1983) described a subset of alcoholics whose depression has as a central feature the recognition of helplessness in the face of an addictive disease.

Determining whether or not a coexistent affective disorder is primary or secondary may have predictive value. Martin et al. (1985) noted that alcoholics with a secondary affective disorder may carry a greater overall mortality than those with a coexistent primary affective disorder. Schuckit and Winokur (1972) suggested that female alcoholics in the latter group may carry a better overall prognosis. The length of alcohol use may explain in part this relationship. Cadoret and Winokur (1974) found that 62% of males who had secondary depression had alcoholic histories of greater than 10 years. Hamm et al.'s (1979) study noted that clinical depressions are not common in young healthy male alcoholics not seeking treatment. Schuckit (1983) suggested that the effect of alcohol on mood in suicidal alcoholics with depression is often complicated by concomitant drug use.

Mayfield and Montgomery (1972) delineated two types of suicidal attempts in alcoholics: the "abreaction" attempt and the suicide attempt occurring within the depressive syndrome of chronic intoxication. The abreaction attempt is an abrupt suicidal attempt while intoxicated. These attempts usually are impulsive and occur more in the context of interpersonal conflict; an analogy may be drawn to so-called crimes of passion seen in homicide, where intensive stimuli may produce a dissociated state resulting in violence. In their study of 34 suicide attempts, Mayfield and Montgomery noted that 26 were intoxicated at the time of the attempt. Attempts that occur in the context of a major affective disorder are, in general, more pernicious and typically occur after several weeks of escalating motor retardation and withdrawal. Alcohol can potentiate other methods of suicide and may also complicate the "safe" execution of an otherwise ambivalent suicidal gesture.

While acknowledging the significant contribution of alcohol to trauma, cirrhosis, and violent death, Vaillant (1983) pointed out that caution should be used in interpreting statistics. As previously noted, he commented that there are important differences between intoxication and alcoholism per se, differentiating between an alcohol-associated phenomenon and the same occurring in an alcoholic. He also argued the following perspective: while it is true that among young alcoholics the death rates from suicide, accidents, and cirrhosis are roughly 10 times the expected (compared to a rate of twice that expected for heart disease), the total excess mortality from heart disease over the life span may exceed that from cirrhosis or suicide in alcoholics (Vaillant 1983, p. 162).

Perhaps far more pernicious is the presence of indirect or covert suicidal ideation or intent. Patients with serious medical complications related to their alcohol use, or who suffer serious neuropsychological sequelae of their use, should be carefully evaluated for the presence of suicidal ideation. An analogy can be drawn with the smoker who cannot stop smoking despite advancing restrictive airway disease. Such may be a manifestation of denial or of covert suicidal intent or may be related to significant organic impairment associated with substance use.

Additionally, alcohol use can complicate the course of other major medical illnesses and contribute to risk-taking behavior of many, and sometimes bizarre, varieties. For example, within a 1-year time period on an inpatient alcoholism treatment program, three cases of alcohol-dependent homosexual men were diagnosed who had an associated secondary depression related to chronic alcohol ingestion and who were actively seeking to contract acquired immune deficiency syndrome (AIDS) as a means of committing suicide (Flavin et al. 1986). Depressive mood and suicidal ideation were directly proportional to their alcohol intake; the use of alcohol was associated with markedly impaired judgment during which they engaged in high-risk sexual activity. Interestingly, two of the three acknowledged passive homicidal ideation during these episodes, realizing they could function as both repository and dispenser of human immunodeficiency virus (HIV). Asch (1980) described this phenomenon in terms of the hidden executioner, a projection of murderous impulses onto another, as though to seek out an executioner. The interplay of underlying psychopathology, alcohol use, and other factors such as interpersonal loss, unemployment, physical debilitation, societal prejudice, and lack of social support structures may all combine to increase the likelihood of self-destructive and possible other-destructive behaviors in high-risk individuals.

It is difficult to estimate the incidence of hidden suicides in accidents of all varieties, and to what extent alcohol or other drug use may play a role. Selzer et al. (1967) noted that psychopathology plays a specific role in accidents occurring in some alcoholics, related to the likelihood of expressing evidence of underlying illness while intoxicated. Tabachnink et al. (1966) found that 50% of accident victims had used alcohol before their accident and that at least half of these were individuals described as impulsive in nature. Tsuang et al. (1985) noted similar patterns of low frustration tolerance on the Minnesota Multiphasic Personality Inventory (MMPI) (Hathaway and McKinley 1951) in comparing alcoholics and accident victims. What is unclear, however, is what contribution alcohol per se made to the noted pathology or pathologic behavior. Tsuang et al. (1985) also noted several studies comparing coroner reports that indicated that 50% of accidents and suicides are alcohol related. Combs-Orme et al. (1983) found that one-third of fatally injured adult pedestrians had positive blood alcohol levels.

Other Drug Use and Self-Destructive Behavior

Suicide and suicide attempts accompany the use of drugs other than alcohol. Suicide risk among drug abusers is estimated to be at least 12 times that of the general population (Frances et al. 1986). Interestingly, among this population, male and female patients presented differing self-destructive portraits. For example, drug-abusing males were less likely to use firearms in suicide attempts and were more likely to attempt suicide by overdose than their female counterparts. Anecdotally, an increased frequency of suicide attempts has been observed in patients seen during phase I of cocaine withdrawal (Gawin and Kleber 1986).

Individuals who attempt suicide by the nonprescribed use of drugs of any class, such as by overdose, should be evaluated for the presence of an alcohol and/or other drug abuse problem. In 1983, the Drug Abuse Warning Network (a system monitoring the nonmedical use of drugs through 76 coroners' offices and 760 emergency rooms across the country) reported 2,975 deaths from drug abuse and

108,585 drug abuse incidents (National Institute on Drug Abuse 1984). Of the incidents, 39% were classified as attempted suicide; of the deaths reported, 37% were classified as suicide. Of those persons whose deaths were classified as suicide by drug overdose, 53% were female; two-thirds of those attempting suicide were female. Alcohol was involved in 21% of suicides and 20% of attempts. Caution must be exercised in any attempt to extrapolate these data to the population as a whole, but such data provide additional information about drug-related suicide attempts.

In a study of 155 polydrug abusers, Ward and Schuckit (1980) noted that drug use patterns associated with serious suicidal activity included a preference for depressant drugs, a history of withdrawal from barbiturates, and a lower frequency of phencyclidine use. Diagnostic factors associated with an increase in suicidal behavior included a history of depression in the subject's mother and a diagnosis of antisocial personality in the subjects themselves. Weissman et al. (1979) at the University of Pennsylvania attempted to isolate variables differentiating drug abusers attempting suicide from nonabusers who made an attempt. Although they found that drug abuse status was not a significant contributor to the severity of suicidal intent, they noted that hopelessness among drug abusers accounted for a significant proportion of the variations of intent and represents an important target for therapeutic intervention.

Much of the literature devoted to substance abuse and dependence and self-destructive behavior has concentrated on those addicted to opiates. Estimates of the incidence of suicide among heroin addicts range from 82 to 350 per 100,000, depending on the study population (Keeler et al. 1979). Suicide rates are markedly increased and range from 7% to 25% (Miles 1977). Vaillant (1966), for example, reported a rate of 7% in 100 opiate addicts, the majority of whom were jailed; in a much larger cohort considered to be at greater risk, rates of between 23% and 25% were reported by Bewley et al. (1968) and James (1967). Vaillant (1966) noted that suicide among addicts generally occurred at an earlier age than in alcoholics, with all in his study dying before age 40. Emery et al. (1981) found that suicidal intent correlated more with hopelessness than depressed mood in their population of 191 heroin addicts.

Murphy et al. (1983) studied the lifetime prevalence rates of suicide attempts in a sample of 533 treated opiate addicts and evaluated the clinical characteristics of those who reported having made a suicide attempt. In this sample, 17.3% reported having made at least one suicide attempt, a rate more than four times higher than that found in the community surveyed. Those who had attempted suicide reported more drug overdoses and had a clinical profile characterized by fewer resources and liabilities. Specifically, the authors noted a childhood history of more severe familial disruption; a higher rate of depression and alcoholism in the family; a history of heavier concomitant alcohol, sedative, and amphetamine abuse; an increased frequency of coexistent psychiatric disorders; and poorer psychosocial functioning. A study of 278 patients enrolled in a methadone maintenance program suggested similar risk factors as being operative in both control and methadone-maintained patients (Moore et al. 1979).

Within the adolescent population, the suicide rate in the United States has tripled over the past 30 years (Brent and Kolko, Chapter 11, this volume; Pfeffer 1985). Despite the magnitude of the problem, it has also begun to generate systematic research study. Tonkin (1987) reviewed the literature on risk-taking behavior in adolescents. The use of alcohol and drugs in this age group is closely related to the presence of suicidal behavior and psychopathology (McKenry et al. 1983). In the San Diego suicide study, Fowler et al. (1986) noted that 53% of 133 consecutive youth suicides had a principal psychiatric diagnosis of substance abuse; 24% had an additional principal diagnosis of atypical depression, atypical psychosis, or adjustment disorder with depression. The relationship of the substance abuse problem to the additional Axis I diagnosis was usually obscure; it tended to be chronic, with the use of multiple substances being the norm. Alcohol, marijuana, and cocaine were the most frequently used substances. In a study of 20 children and adolescents who committed suicide, Shafii et al. (1985) found that 70% suffered from drug or alcohol abuse problems. A similar association has been noted by others (e.g., Rydelius 1984).

PSYCHOACTIVE SUBSTANCE USE AND MOOD DISORDERS

The Role of Alcohol

Depression is a major risk factor for suicide (Black and Winokur, Chapter 6 this volume). Studies suggest that 60% to 80% of adults who end their lives by suicide suffer from an affective disorder (Barraclough et al. 1974; Dorpat and Ripley 1960; Robins et al. 1954). Depression is a common symptom in both alcoholics and users of psychoactive drugs. Understanding the relationship between the affective disorders, other psychopathology, and psychoactive substance use is crucial given the contributions of each to self-destructive behavior. In this section we will review the literature on the association between psychoactive substance use and mood disorders.

Individuals presenting for substance abuse treatment commonly complain of depressed mood, sleep and appetite disturbance, decreased energy, decreased libido and diminished sexual potency, as well as feelings of helplessness, loss of control, and hopelessness. A number of studies have documented the frequency of depressed mood in association with substance abuse, particularly with the use of alcohol (Mirin and Weiss 1986). In this case, the affective disorder may be primary (occurring in the absence of a preexisting psychiatric disorder) or secondary to the toxic effects of the drug. In most cases of depression occurring in alcoholics, symptoms improve within several weeks of abstinence. It has been noted, however, that in approximately 5% of males and 25% to 50% of female alcoholics, the depression may persist in the absence of alcohol (Zimberg 1982). Determining whether the affective disorder is primary or secondary may be a difficult task; making an accurate diagnosis depends on the chronological sequence of drug use and onset of depressive symptomatology, a careful evaluation of the depressive episode, and a careful family history. Andreasen and Winokur (1979) commented that depressive symptoms are usually more severe if the disorder is primary. In a study of alcoholics with and without secondary depression, Weissman et al. (1977) found similar demographic characteristics, antisocial problems, and family histories of affective disorder.

Although efforts to standardize and clarify nosology with regard to alcohol-related problems and depression have represented a much-needed advance, serious methodological problems exist in the literature, limiting the conclusions that can be drawn from many studies. For example, depending on the instruments used, methods of measuring depression in alcoholics have produced estimates ranging from 3% to 98% (Keeler et al. 1979; Petty and Nasrallah 1981; Pottenger et al. 1978). Weissman and Myers (1980) noted inconsistent associations between alcoholism and depression, resulting from variable methods of assessing depressive illness. Hesselbrock et al. (1983) found depression in the same group of alcoholics 62% of the time using the MMPI, 54% of the time using the Beck Depression Inventory (Beck et al. 1961), and 27% of the time utilizing DSM-III (American Psychiatric Association 1980) criteria. Others have suggested that depression may be overrepresented in treatment populations studied because individuals who seek treatment may be more likely to be depressed (O'Sullivan 1984).

It is known that while low doses of alcohol may have stimulant activity in the central nervous system (CNS), higher doses, either in prolonged or chronic use, are associated with depressive activity (Mirin and Weiss 1986). Within alcoholic populations, several studies have demonstrated the latter finding. McNamee et al. (1968), for example, demonstrated that subjects dependent on alcohol experienced an increase rather than a decrease in symptoms of anxiety associated with a depressive disorder during intoxication. Tamerin and Mendelson (1969) noted that prolonged drinking in an experimental situation produced progressively depressed mood. They concluded that the anxiety-reduction model was inadequate in delineating motivation for alcohol use in this population. Other evidence suggests that the use of alcohol in alcoholics may be more palliative than euphoric (Mayfield and Allen 1967). Caution is necessary in extrapolating data from carefully controlled in vitro studies to natural environments with different cues and stimuli.

Various experts have suggested that a postcessation evaluation period of up to 6 months may be necessary since a protracted alcohol withdrawal phenomenon can mimic a primary major affective disorder. The majority of authors are in agreement that most depressive symptoms associated with alcohol use are secondary to the depressant effects of the drug. Nakamura et al. (1983) found that, at the end of 4 weeks of treatment, only 4 of 62 patients with depression initially experienced residual symptoms. Hatsukami and Picheur (1982) noted that the rates of depressive symptoms in subjects abstinent up to 1, 6, and 12 months after discharge were no higher than in the general population.

Other evidence seems to be at odds with these observations. Pottenger et al. (1978) studied 61 outpatients and found that 57% were depressed, with symptoms persisting over a 1-year follow-up period. Another study of 72 alcoholics with an average of 64 months of sobriety concluded that 15% of patients had serious depressive symptoms that began after a mean of 35 months of sobriety (Behar et al. 1984). Possible explanations for the discrepancies noted here include selection bias and predisposition for depressive diathesis.

Until recently, the literature examining the relationship between preadolescent and adolescent alcohol use was sparse. Famularo et al. (1985) reported on 10 cases of preadolescent alcohol abuse and dependence. The authors noted an impressive prevalence of affective disorder among the patients and their families, as well as the presence of additional DSM-III diagnoses on Axis I or Axis II.

Other Drug Use

The literature examining the relationship between drugs other than alcohol and affective disorders until recently has been sparse and primarily anecdotal in nature. Recent investigations, however, promise to expand our knowledge in this area.

Mirin and Weiss (1986) reported on data from an ongoing study of affective disorder in patients admitted to the Drug Dependence Treatment Unit at McLean Hospital. Specifically, they examined the epidemiologic, laboratory, and clinical presentations of affective disorders in individuals abusing stimulants, depressants, and the opiates. Of individuals using CNS depressants seeking treatment, approximately one-half received a DSM-III Axis I diagnosis in addition to substance abuse disorder; 18% were diagnosed as having a concurrent major or atypical depression and 6% as having a bipolar or cyclothymic illness. The majority of the remaining patients were diagnosed as having a generalized anxiety or panic disorder (Mirin et al. 1984a, 1984b). Weiss and Rosenberg (1985) had noted earlier that 22.6% of their study population of 84 alcoholics met DSM-III criteria for anxiety or panic disorder, usually antedating the onset of problematic drinking. Of interest is the observation by the authors of the McLean study that the incidence of Axis I pathology was quite low among abusers of methaqualone.

Among stimulant abusers, the prevalence of affective disorders is less apparent. In two studies, Mirin et al. (1984a, 1984b) reported on data gathered from 36 stimulant abusers, over 80% of whom preferred cocaine as their primary drug of choice. Nearly one-third of these patients received a current diagnosis of unipolar depression, with bipolar disorder diagnosed in an additional 22%. Of particular note was the higher rate of affective disorder in this group (vis-à-vis the general population and other drug groups) and in their same-sex first-degree relatives (Weissman et al. 1982). Despite attempts to subtype cocaine abusers, relatively few controlled studies of the effects of stimulants on patients with underlying affective disorders have been done.

Affective illness may follow stimulant withdrawal (Schildkraut et al. 1971). While in most cases this is transient, in some individuals the withdrawal process may unmask an underlying primary affective disorder, which the patient may have been attempting to self-medicate. Laboratory studies suggest that the postwithdrawal depression is accompanied by alterations in catecholamine homeostasis similar to that seen in some types of uncomplicated depressive disorders (Mirin and Weiss 1986).

Signs and symptoms of major depression can complicate the diagnosis of opiate intoxication or withdrawal. Whereas the psychoanalytic literature viewed opiate use as a form of self-medication (Wurmser 1974), this view has been challenged by more recent studies. Rounsaville et al. (1979), for example, in a study of opiate addicts entering a multimodality treatment program, found that 17% met Research Diagnostic Criteria (RDC) (Spitzer et al. 1978) for current major depression, while the incidence of bipolar illness equaled that of the general population. In a subsequent study, the same authors noted that the combined lifetime occurrence of affective disorder in a group of 533 opiate addicts was 73.4%; the majority experienced their initial depressive episode after the onset of opiate abuse (Rounsaville et al. 1982). Dackis and Gold (1984) linked depressive symptoms in detoxified opiate addicts to chronic opiate withdrawal at the level of the CNS opiate receptor. The withdrawal process may also serve to unmask an underlying affective disorder. The topic of psychopathology in opiate addicts is comprehensively reviewed elsewhere (Kosten and Rounsaville 1986).

PSYCHOACTIVE SUBSTANCE ABUSE AND OTHER PSYCHIATRIC DISORDERS

In addition to the major affective disorders, a review of the differential diagnosis of substance-induced organic mental disorders includes personality disorders (especially borderline and antisocial varieties), delirium- or nondrug-induced organic mental disorders, schizophrenia, temporal lobe epilepsy, panic disorders, generalized anxiety disorder, and attention-deficit disorder (residual type). In the pediatric population, mental retardation, specific developmental disorders, conduct disorder, oppositional disorder, and attention-deficit disorder are additional diagnostic considerations. Alcohol and other drug abuse must be considered in the process of diagnostic decision making when any of the above diagnoses are considered to avoid making a delayed or inappropriate diagnosis. The appropriate diagnosis and treatment of psychiatric disorders is a cornerstone in the prevention of suicide (Blumenthal, Chapter 26, this volume).

Alcoholics with coexistent Axis I or Axis II diagnoses are being recognized more frequently. One study demonstrated, through the use of a structured interview, evidence for coexistent psychiatric problems in 50% of a sample of 71 female alcoholics (Halikas et al. 1983). In this population, affective disorder was most common, followed by anxiety disorder (10%) and psychotic symptoms prior to treatment (6%). In the Hesselbrock et al. (1985) alcoholism-treatment patient sample, depression was the most frequently diagnosed entity; nearly twice as many women as men experienced symptoms of an anxiety disorder, including phobias and panic disorder. Bedi and Halikas (1985) found a lifetime rate of affective disorder of 43% in alcoholic females and 29% in alcoholic males.

Antisocial personality disorder has been diagnosed in up to 25% of alcoholics and in 6% of suicides (Cadoret et al. 1984; Martin et al. 1985; Miles 1977). Schuckit (1985) found that the best outcome results for a sample of 577 Veterans Administration hospital patients were in primary alcoholic patients and the worst in those with antisocial personality disorders. The latter group tended to be younger, less well educated, and more likely to have reported secondary affective episodes, suicide attempts, psychiatric hospitalizations, and coexistent abuse of other drugs. Nace et al. (1983) found that 12% of alcoholic patients were diagnosed as having a borderline personality disorder. These patients were significantly younger and more likely to have had a history of suicide attempts in addition to being more sensitive to affective stimuli. Masterson (1972) gave many case examples of the use of a variety of substances by borderline adolescents in attempts to discharge anger, overcome boredom, or ward off painful affects. Loranger and Tulis (1985) pointed out the high rate of alcoholism found in the families of 83 women with a DSM-III diagnosis of borderline personality compared to bipolar or schizophrenic patients.

Research in the area of personality characteristics of alcoholics has been summarized by Nerviano and Gross (1983), Bartsch and Hoffman (1985), and Cloninger (1987). The latter author's work is unique in his attempt to bridge clinically observable personality characteristics with specific subtypes of alcoholism and specific neurotransmitter systems. Such promising work may have a direct impact on treatment research in the future.

A variety of substances—including marijuana, the hallucinogens, and amphetamines—may produce psychotic symptoms. An increased frequency of substance abuse has been noted in patients with schizophrenia (Alterman 1985; Alterman et al. 1982; Roy 1986b). In their review of 72 drug abusers with psychotic symptoms, Tsuang et al. (1982), noted that drug abusers with psychoses of longer duration were more likely to have schizoid or paranoid premorbid personalities, poor insight, and disorganized thought processes.

Hartocollis (1982) studied the personality characteristics of adolescent problem drinkers. Those studied tended to act out and to ignore social customs and mores. Further, a review of the hospital records of 100 adolescents between the ages of 13 and 18 showed that when a dual diagnosis was made, conduct disorder was the secondary diagnosis in nearly one-half of the cases. This raises the question of specific subtypes of conduct disorders associated with the later development of alcoholism and other substance abuse problems (Morrison and Smith 1987). Both conduct disorder and alcohol abuse are major risk factors for youth suicide. Their co-occurrence is a particularly lethal combination (Blumenthal and Kupfer 1988).

Biologic Markers

Research examining the presence of various biologic markers in suicide, aggressive behavior, and the use of alcohol and other drugs can be divided into several categories: genetic studies, cerebrospinal fluid (CSF) studies, postmortem studies in alcoholic suicides, neuroendocrine research, studies of glucose metabolism, and platelet monoamine oxidase research. These studies have been reviewed elsewhere (Fowler et al. 1986; Garvey et al. 1983; Roy and Linnoila 1986; Stanley et al. 1986).

In animal studies, alterations in central indoleamine and catecholamine turnover have been noted to be caused by alcohol. Serotonin may play a role in the regulation of aggressive (and possibly suicidal) behavior. In a study of 68 depressed patients, Asberg et al. (1976) found that significantly more of the patients with decreased levels of 5-hydroxyindoleacetic acid (5-HIAA) had attempted suicide by a violent method. Conflicting reports since this initial study have been published, however.

Takahashi and Yamama (1974) proposed that an alteration of brain serotonin metabolism may be a factor associated with abstinence and depressive symptoms as well as suicidal ideation in alcoholics. Several researchers have commented on an inverse correlation between length of abstinence and 5-HIAA levels in the CSF. Ballenger et al. (1979) suggested that alcoholics may have preexisting low levels of serotonin centrally, raised in a transient fashion by alcohol consumption, only to lead to further depletion of serotonin in the CNS. Genetic strains of rats preferring alcohol to water have lower brain serotonin levels (Ballenger et al. 1979). Postmortem studies also suggest that there may be a subgroup of alcoholics who exhibit suicidal behavior with a decrease in serotonin turnover (Roy and Linnoila 1986). Branchey et al. (1984) reported decreased tryptophan ratios in a subgroup of alcoholics at risk for depression, suicide, and aggressive behavior.

Neuroendocrine studies have recently emphasized the blunted response of thyroid-stimulating hormone (TSH) in response to thyroid-releasing hormone. This has been noted in up to 40% of depressed patients and has been observed in alcoholic patients as well (Roy and Linnoila 1986). Linkowski et al. (1983) concluded that patients with a history of violent suicide attempts had a blunted TSH response when compared with depressed patients. Such studies need to be replicated among alcoholics who have made suicide attempts.

Other research has examined glucose metabolism and platelet monoamine oxidase activity. Virkkunen (1982) examined glucose metabolism and insulin secretion among violent and impulsive offenders, concluding that alterations in mean peak insulin levels were affected in those with an early history of onset of alcohol abuse. Initial enthusiasm about the significance of low platelet monoamine oxidase activity in alcoholics and in their blood relatives has waned more recently given the fact that blood platelet activity may not reflect CNS catecholamine metabolism and the nonspecific nature of a decreased platelet monoamine oxidase level (Roy and Linnoila 1986). Crawley et al. (1985) reviewed the literature on animal models of self-destructive behavior and suicide. Implications of the use of these biologic markers in treatment and prevention awaits further research.

The association of peptic ulcer disease and suicide in alcoholics has sparked interest in the last several years. Berglund (1984) found peptic ulcers to be predictive of suicide in 21% of alcoholics versus 7% in controls. Overall, 10% of patients who committed suicide in this study had a history of peptic ulcer disease. In a more recent study, the same author noted that suicide occurred in 17% of a study population with peptic ulcer disease versus 6% in those without (Berglund 1986). Knop and Fischer (1981) studied 1,000 patients with a history of Billroth II resection; 13% of these patients committed suicide, and alcoholism was found in 50% of these patients (developing after surgery in the majority). The significance of these interesting findings needs further investigation.

SOCIAL SUPPORT NETWORKS AND CLINICAL MANAGEMENT

As noted earlier, suicide often follows either real or perceived rejection, loss, or humiliation in both alcoholic and nonalcoholic populations. Both interpersonal loss and a sense of hopelessness seem to be emerging as perhaps the most significant factors to be evaluated in any potentially suicidal person. In addition to previously referenced work by Murphy (1986), other authors have noted the importance of these risk factors (Adam, Chapter 3; Blumenthal, Chapter 26, this volume; Fawcett et al. 1969). Beck et al. (1982) concluded that hopelessness is a better indicator of suicidal risk in outpatient alcoholics than is the level of depression or the number of past attempts. In a prospective study of 88 alcoholics, Berglund (1984) found that alcoholics who later attempted suicide had a higher percentage of dysphoric symptoms and were more brittle and sensitive to others. Steer et al. (1982) found intrapunitive self attitudes as a factor in depression experienced by some alcoholics. In a study of 69 surviving suicidal patients with alcoholism, Bascue and Epstein (1980) noted that past attempters continued to view themselves as a suicidal risk.

Evaluation of an individual's social support network is crucial in assessing risk and appropriate treatment. Alcoholics or other drug users may often alienate natural support systems; a careful assessment of family and social support structure dynamics may dictate that rapid stabilization of these networks is necessary. Support systems can include family, significant others, Alcoholics Anonymous, schools, workplace, professional and/or community organizations.

Early identification is the key concept in intervention to prevent suicide or other forms of self-destructive behavior.

The clinician working with alcoholics and other drug users or abusers is often faced with difficult diagnostic and management decisions involving the patient and the patient's social support network. For example, managing the suicidal intoxicated individual requires immediate intervention to protect the individual from self-harm. This may require involuntary hospitalization, after consideration of risk factors and clinical parameters, including prior attempts, recent history of loss (be it real or perceived), a sense of hopelessness, the presence of coexistent Axis I or Axis II psychopathology, the nature of social support structures and interpersonal relationships, the presence of other drug use, the subjective perception of intent on the part of the patient, frequency of intoxication, level of insight, gender, age, the presence of physical illness, and neuropsychiatric impairment. Close cooperation between community services personnel and local care givers is necessary both in the immediate and long-term care of those individuals who may continue to be at risk for self-destructive behavior on a chronic basis. The appropriate management of the so-called dually diagnosed patient requires astute diagnostic acumen, quality multidisciplinary care, and the skillful application of treatment options.

The inappropriate use of alcohol and other drugs affects the entire family and social support structure. When overt self-destructive behavior complicates the clinical picture, the needs of families become even more intense. The concept of codependency, stressing the role of family and significant others in the addiction process and their needs, underscores the necessity of treating family members as well as the identified patient. Family members may themselves have alcohol- or other drug-related problems and emotional disturbances or may be children of alcoholics. Alterations of homeostatic equilibrium within the family system as one family member recovers often may be met with resistance or emerging psychopathology in other family members. Al-Anon and related groups are a mainstay of treatment for family members; Children of Alcoholics groups may also be of major importance in treatment planning for some family members.

Treatment plans must be tailored to suit individual needs. For example, a treatment approach emphasizing confrontation may have negative effects on the severely depressed alcoholic contemplating suicide, but may be indicated in approaching some patients without significant coexistent psychopathology. Patients who in the past were considered inappropriate candidates for psychotherapy may in some cases benefit from such a modality. For example, Woody et al. (1983) emphasized that suicide is not uncommon among individuals with antisocial personality disorder and depression and/or substance abuse; these individuals may significantly benefit from psychotherapy. Some patients may require the judicious use of medications in addition to Alcoholics Anonymous and other elements of treatment. This may include the use of psychotropics for coexistent primary psychiatric disorders. The potential benefits of disulfiram in this population must be weighed against potential risks, such as exacerbation of mood disturbances or complicating psychotic illnesses. Appropriate matching of patients with treatment modalities is necessary, as is solid clinical research in this area. Given our current level of sophistication, the therapist in conjunction with the patient must decide on which approach or combination of approaches is best.

The presence or absence of neuropsychological deficits is especially important in assessing risk and in planning management of the self-destructive substance-using patient. The literature in this area has been reviewed by a number of authors (National Institute on Alcohol Abuse and Alcoholism 1987). An individual who is organically impaired either as a direct result of substance abuse or from coexistent physical illness may be at a higher risk for self-destructive behavior. Chabon and Robins (1986) demonstrated that cognitive distortions among drug abusers in recovery who are depressed and suicidal may respond to cognitive therapy.

Special note needs to be made of the needs of traditionally underserved groups, such as women, the elderly, minorities, the socially disenfranchised, and physicians. Increased rates of suicide are associated with problem drinking among the elderly, especially in those with primary affective disorders (Schuckit and Miller 1976). Schuckit and Paster (1978) noted that alcoholics over age 65 reported significantly more suicide attempts. In addition, they are more susceptible to falls, other trauma, self-neglect, confusion, and social isolation.

More men than women are found among alcoholic suicides; this is thought to reflect on the fact that suicide is found more among men than women as is alcoholism. Barraclough et al. (1974) concluded that the sex of an alcoholic does not predispose to suicide. Other authors disagree. Knop and Fischer (1981) and Nicholls et al. (1974) noted a doubled rate of suicide among male alcoholics. Differences between male and female alcoholics include family history of affective disorder, drinking behavior, and gender-related effects of alcohol (Roy and Linnoila 1986). Perhaps because of the emphasis or greater visibility of alcohol-related problems in men, the needs of chemically dependent women have been, until recently, ignored to a large extent.

The needs of racial and ethnic minorities have recently received more attention in the literature; for example, the problem of alcohol abuse and dependence among Native Americans is significant. According to the Indian Health Service, recent studies have noted that 5 of the 10 leading causes of death among Native Americans are alcohol related (National Institute on Alcohol Abuse and Alcoholism 1987). These include accidents, cirrhosis, alcohol dependence, suicide, and homicide. Accidents account for one-fifth of all deaths among American Indians; 75% of these are alcohol related. Suicide accounts for approximately 2% of all deaths, a rate twice that of the national average. The Indian Health Service estimates that 80% of these are alcohol related (National Institute on Alcohol Abuse and Alcoholism 1987). Westermeyer (1974) provided the caveat, however, that historically some tribes have had higher rates of suicide and that only recently has there been an association with alcohol use. Homicide accounts for 2% of all Indian deaths; in more than 90% of these either the victim or the assailant had consumed alcohol (Andre 1979).

Among physicians, the disorders most commonly associated with suicide are alcoholism, other drug abuse, and depression (Holmes and Rich, Chapter 22, this volume; Murray 1983; Roy 1985). Interviews of the survivors of 249 physicians whose suicides were reported in the *Journal of the American Medical Association* between 1965 and 1967 revealed that alcohol or drug abuse was a significant factor in 40% (Blachly et al. 1968). A significant relationship was also found in a study done by the Oregon Board of Medical Examiners (Cranshaw et al. 1980). Physicians' spouses are also at increased risk for suicide. This has been related to the high rates of substance abuse in this group (Sakinofsky 1980).

Indirect or covert suicidal ideation poses a particular challenge to the clinician working in this field. Since the patient may not be aware of self-destructive impulses, the clinician's sensitivity and creativity can help elicit suicidal intent and bring it to the patient's attention in a meaningful fashion. The following case illustrates this point.

Clinical Case Summary

A 37-year-old unemployed bisexual married man without formal psychiatric history presented to the alcoholism treatment service with a 7-year history of alcohol dependence characterized by increased tolerance, mild withdrawal symptoms on cessation of use, blackouts, and loss of control with significant psychosocial sequelae. For 2 to 3 years prior to admission, he complained of lability of mood and more recently noted more pervasive features suggestive of a major depression. He acknowledged several failed attempts to take his own life; his suicidal ideation remained and seemed to escalate as his alcohol consumption increased. One year prior to admission, he began having high-risk sexual encounters in an attempt to become infected with HIV associated with AIDS. Alcohol allowed him an opportunity to distance himself from his actions. High-risk contacts were circumscribed within the context of intoxication, coupled with remorse while sober. He acknowledged the presence of sexual identity conflict, subjectively perceived as ego-dystonic, but was unable to acknowledge his covert self-destructive activity until after 3 weeks in treatment.

Such a clinical scenario illustrates the fact that suicide is a multifaceted phenomenon that interfaces, at times intimately, with entities with which it is not readily identified, requiring a creative vigilance on the part of the clinician and an appreciation of the role of alcohol and substance abuse in the genesis of psychopathology and associated suicidal ideation. In the case above, a multidisciplinary approach to treatment, including Alcoholics Anonymous, individual supportive psychotherapy, and family referral to Al-Anon, met with improved mood and successful termination of all substance use and high-risk activity for over 1 year. At the time AIDS-related complex was diagnosed, he returned to alcohol use and complained of overt suicidal ideation, necessitating intensification of his outpatient treatment. The management of suicidal ideation, especially in the context of a prolonged physical illness, requires a long-term commitment on the part of the treating therapist or program.

Conclusion

The appropriate management of substance-abusing patients requires a multidisciplinary team approach to assess risk, to evaluate environmental factors, and to develop and administer a comprehensive treatment plan. Consideration of prior attempts, frequency of intoxication, the presence and severity of coexisting psychiatric disorders, other drug use, level of patient insight, recent loss, the degree of hopelessness, and the quality of social support systems are mandated in the complete assessment of any patient at risk for self-harm. Early identification, appropriate interventions, and flexibility in the selection of treatment options define optimal clinical care for this group. Consideration must be given to the needs of populations who have been traditionally underserved in our society, as well as to family members and significant others.

References

Abel EL, Zeidenberg P: Age, alcohol and violent death: a postmortem study. J Stud Alcohol 46:228–231, 1985

Alterman AI (ed): Substance Abuse and Psychopathology. New York, Plenum, 1985

Alterman AI, Erdlen DL, LaPorte DJ, et al: Effects of illicit drug use in an inpatient psychiatric population. Addict Behav 7:231–242, 1982

American Psychiatric Association: Diagnostic and Statistical Manual of Mental Disorders, 3rd Edition. Washington, DC, American Psychiatric Association, 1980

Andre JM: The epidemiology of alcoholism among American Indians and Alaska Natives. Albuquerque, NM, Indian Health Service, 1979

Andreasen NC, Winokur G: Secondary depression: familial, clinical, and research perspectives. Am J Psychiatry 136:62–66, 1979

Asberg M, Traskman L, Thoren P: 5-HIAA in the cerebrospinal fluid: a biochemical suicide predictor? Arch Gen Psychiatry 33:1193–1197, 1976

Asch SS: Suicide and the hidden executioner. International Review of Psychoanalysis 7:51–60, 1980

Ballenger J, Goodwin F, Major L, et al: Alcohol and central serotonin metabolism in man. Arch Gen Psychiatry 36:224–227, 1979

Barraclough B, Bunch J, Nelson B, et al: A hundred cases of suicide: clinical aspects. Br J Psychiatry 125:355–373, 1974

Bartsch TW, Hoffman JJ: A cluster analysis of a million clinical multiaxial inventory (MCMI) profiles: more about a taxonomy of alcoholic subtypes. J Clin Psychol 41:707–713, 1985

Bascue LO, Epstein L: Suicide attitudes and experiences of hospitalized alcoholics. Psychol Rep 47:1233–1234, 1980

Beck AT, Ward CH, Mendelson M: An inventory for measuring depression. Arch Gen Psychiatry 4:461–471, 1961

Beck AT, Weissman A, Lester D, et al: The measurement of pessimism: the Hopelessness Scale. J Consult Clin Psychol 42:861–865, 1974

Beck AT, Kovaks M, Weissman A: Assessment of suicidal intention: the Scale for Suicidal Ideation. J Consult Clin Psychol 47:343–382, 1979

Beck AT, Steer RA, McElroy MG: Relationships of hopelessness, depression and previous suicide attempts to suicidal ideation in alcoholics. J Stud Alcohol 43:1042–1046, 1982

Bedi A, Halikas JA: Alcoholism and affective disorder. Alcoholism 9:133–134, 1985

Behar D, Winokur G, Berg CJ: Depression in the abstinent alcoholic. Am J Psychiatry 141:1105–1107, 1984

Berglund M: Suicide in alcoholism, a prospective study of 88 suicides, I: the multidimensional diagnosis at first admission. Arch Gen Psychiatry 41:888–891, 1984

Berglund M: Suicide in male alcoholics with peptic ulcers. Alcoholism 10:631–634, 1986

Berryman J: The Dream Songs. New York, Farrar, Straus, and Giroux, 1969

Berryman J: Of Suicide, in Love and Fame. Edited by Berryman J. New York, Farrar, Straus, and Giroux, 1970

Bewley TH, Ben-Arie O, James IP: Morbidity and mortality from heroin dependence, I: survey of heroin addicts known to home offices. Br Med J 1:725–726, 1968

Blachly P, Disher W, Roduner G: Suicide by physicians. Bulletin of Suicide 1:1–18, 1968

Black DW, Yates W, Petty F, et al: Suicidal behavior in alcoholic males. Compr Psychiatry 27:227–233, 1986

Bleuler E (ed): Textbook of Psychiatry. Translated by Brill A. New York, Dover, 1911/1951

Blumenthal SJ, Kupfer DJ: Overview of early detection and treatment strategies for suicidal behavior in young people. Journal of Youth and Adolescence 17:1–23, 1988

Branchey L, Branchey M, Shaw S, et al: Depression, suicide, and aggression in alcoholics and their relationship to plasma amino acids. Psychiatry Res 12:219–226, 1984

Cadoret R, Winokur G: Depression in alcoholism. Ann NY Acad Sci 233:34–39, 1974

Cadoret R, Troughton E, Widmer R: Clinical differences between antisocial and primary alcoholics. Compr Psychiatry 25:1–8, 1984

Chabon B, Robins CJ: Cognitive distortions among depressed and suicidal drug abusers. Int J Addict 21:1313–1329, 1986

Clayton P: Suicide. Psychiatr Clin North Am 8:203–214, 1985

Cloninger CR: A systematic method for clinical description and classification of personality variants: a proposal. Arch Gen Psychiatry 44:573–588, 1987

Combs-Orme T, Taylor JR, Scott EB, et al: Violent deaths among alcoholics, a descriptive study. J Stud Alcohol 44:938–949, 1983

Cranshaw R, Bruce J, Eracker P, et al: An epidemic of suicide among physicians on probation. JAMA 243:1915–1917, 1980

Crawley JN, Sutton ME, Pickar D: Animal models of self-destructive behavior and suicide. Psychiatry Clin North Am 8:299–310, 1985

Dackis CA, Gold MS: Depression in opiate addicts, in Substance Abuse and Psychopathology. Edited by Mirin SM. Washington, DC, American Psychiatric Press, 1984, pp 19–40

Davis WM: Premature mortality among prominent American authors noted for alcohol abuse. Drug Alcohol Depend 18:133–138, 1986

Dorpat TL, Ripley HS: A study of suicide in the Seattle area. Compr Psychiatry 1:349–359, 1960

Emery GD, Steer RA, Beck AT: Depression, hopelessness, and suicidal intent among heroin addicts. Int J Addict 16:425–429, 1981

Famularo R, Stone K, Popper C: Preadolescent alcohol abuse and dependence. Am J Psychiatry 142:1187–1189, 1985

Fawcett J, Leff M, Bunney WE Jr: Suicide: clues from interpersonal communication. Arch Gen Psychiatry 21:129–137, 1969

Flavin DK, Franklin JE, Frances RJ: The acquired immune deficiency syndrome and suicidal behavior in alcohol-dependent homosexual men. Am J Psychiatry 143:1440–1442, 1986

Fowler RC, Rich CL, Young D: San Diego suicide study, II: substance abuse in young cases. Arch Gen Psychiatry 43:962–965, 1986

Frances R, Franklin J, Flavin D: Suicide and alcoholism. Ann NY Acad Sci 487:316–326, 1986

Galanter M, Castaneda R: Self-destructive behavior in the substance abuser. Psychiatr Clin North Am 8:251–261, 1985

Garvey MJ, Tuason VB, Hoffman N, et al: Suicide attempters, nonattempters, and neurotransmitters. Compr Psychiatry 24:332–336, 1983

Gawin FH, Kleber HD: Abstinence symptomatology and psychiatric diagnosis in cocaine abusers. Arch Gen Psychiatry 43:107–113, 1986

Gilmore TB: John Berryman and drinking: from jest to sober earnest, in Alcoholism and Drinking in Twentieth Century Literature. Edited by Gilmore TB. Chapel Hill, NC, University of North Carolina Press, 1987, pp 119–144

Goodwin D: Alcohol in suicide and homicide. Quarterly Journal of Studies on Alcohol 34:144–156, 1973

Goodwin DW: Alcoholism and suicide: associated factors, in The Encyclopedic Handbook of Alcoholism. Edited by Pattison E, Kaufman E. New York, Gardner Press, 1983

Halikas JA, Herzog MA, Mirassou MM, et al: Psychiatric diagnoses among female alcoholics, in Currents in Alcoholism, Vol 8. Edited by Galanter M. New York, Grune & Stratton, 1983

Hamilton M: A rating scale for depression. J Neurol Neurosurg Psychiatry 23:56–62, 1960

Hamm J, Major LF, Brown G: The quantitative measurement of depression and anxiety in male alcoholics. Am J Psychiatry 136:580–582, 1979

Hartocollis PC: Personality characteristics in adolescent problem drinkers. J Am Acad Child Adolesc Psychiatry 21:348–353, 1982

Hathaway SR, McKinley JC: Minnesota Multiphasic Personality Inventory: Manuel for Administration and Scoring. Minneapolis, MN, University of Minnesota Press, 1951

Hatsukami D, Picheur RW: Post treatment depression in an alcohol and drug abuse population. Am J Psychiatry 139:1563–1566, 1982

Hesselbrock MN, Hesselbrock VM, Tennen H, et al: Methodological considerations in the assessment of depression in alcoholics. J Consult Clin Psychol 51:399–405, 1983

Hesselbrock MN, Meyer RE, Keener JJ: Psychopathology in hospitalized alcoholics. Arch Gen Psychiatry 42:1050–1065, 1985

James IP: Suicide and mortality amongst heroin addicts in Britain. Br J Addict 62:391–398, 1967

Keeler M, Martin H, Taylor C: Are all recently detoxified alcoholics depressed? Am J Psychiatry 136:586–588, 1979

Knop J, Fischer A: Duodenal ulcer, suicide, psychopathology and alcoholism. Acta Psychiatr Scand 63:346–355, 1981

Kosten TR, Rounsaville BJ: Psychopathology in opioid addicts. Psychiatr Clin North Am 9:515–532, 1986

Langevin R, Paitich D, Orchard B, et al: The role of alcohol, drugs, suicide attempts and situational strains in homicide committed by offenders seen for psychiatric assessment: a controlled study. Acta Psychiatr Scand 66:229–242, 1982

Linkowski P, van Wettere J, Kerkhofs M, et al: Thyrotrophin response to thyreostimulun in affectively ill women: relationship to suicidal behaviour. Br J Psychiatry 143:401–405, 1983

Loranger AW, Tulis EH: Family history of alcoholism in borderline personality disorders. Arch Gen Psychiatry 42:153–157, 1985

Martin RL, Cloninger R, Guze SB, et al: Mortality in a follow-up of 500 psychiatric outpatients, I: total mortality. Arch Gen Psychiatry 43:47–54, 1985

Masterson JF (ed): Treatment of the Borderline Adolescent. New York, Wiley Interscience, 1972

Mayfield D, Allen D: Alcohol and affect: a psychopharmacological study. Am J Psychiatry 11:1346–1351, 1967

Mayfield DG, Montgomery D: Alcoholism, alcohol intoxication, and suicide attempts. Arch Gen Psychiatry 27:349–353, 1972

McKenry PC, Tischler CL, Kelley C: The role of drugs in adolescent suicide attempts. Suicide Life Threat Behav 13:166–175, 1983

McNamee HB, Mello N, Mendelson JH: Experimental analysis of drinking patterns of alcoholics: concurrent psychiatric observations. Am J Psychiatry 124:1063–1069, 1968

Menninger K (ed): Man Against Himself. New York, Harcourt Brace, 1938

Miles CP: Conditions predisposing to suicide: a review. J Nerv Ment Dis 164:231–246, 1977

Mirin SM, Weiss RD: Affective illness in substance abusers. Psychiatr Clin North Am 9:503–514, 1986

Mirin SM, Weiss RD, Sollogub A, et al: Affective illness in substance abusers, in Substance Abuse and Psychopathology. Edited by Mirin SM. Washington, DC, American Psychiatric Press, 1984a, pp 57–77

Mirin SM, Weiss RD, Sollogub A, et al: Psychopathology in the families of drug abusers, in Substance Abuse and Psychopathology. Edited by Mirin SM. Washington, DC, American Psychiatric Press, 1984b, pp 79–106

Moore JT, Judd LL, Zung WW, et al: Opiate addiction and suicidal behaviors. Am J Psychiatry 136:1187–1189, 1979

Morrison MA, Smith QT: Psychiatric issues of adolescent chemical dependence. Pediatr Clin North Am 34:461–480, 1987

Murphy GE, Suicide in alcoholism, in Suicide. Edited by Roy A. Baltimore, Williams & Wilkins, 1986, pp 89–96

Murphy GE, Robins E: Social factors in suicide. JAMA 199:303–308, 1967

Murphy GE, Armstrong JW, Hermele SL, et al: Suicide and alcoholism, interpersonal loss confirmed as a predictor. Arch Gen Psychiatry 36:65–69, 1979

Murphy SL, Rounsaville BJ, Eyre S, et al: Suicide attempts in treated opiate addicts. Compr Psychiatry 24:79–89, 1983

Murray R: The mentally ill doctor: causes and consequences. Practitioner 227:65–75, 1983

Nace EP, Saxon JJ Jr, Shore N: A comparison of borderline and nonborderline alcoholic patients. Arch Gen Psychiatry 40:54–56, 1983

Nakamura MM, Overall JE, Hollister LE, et al: Factors affecting outcome of depressive symptoms in alcoholics. Alcoholism 7:188–193, 1983

National Institute on Alcohol Abuse and Alcoholism: Sixth Special Report to the Congress: Alcohol and Health (DHHS Publ No ADM-87-1519). Washington, DC, U.S. Government Printing Office, 1987

National Institute on Drug Abuse: Drug Abuse Warning Network: Annual Data, 1983 (DHEW Publ No ADM-84-13537). Rockville, MD, 1984

Nerviano V, Gross H: Personality types of alcoholics on objective inventories. J Stud Alcohol 44:837–851, 1983

Nicholls P, Edwards G, Kyle E: Alcoholics admitted to four hospitals, in England, II: general and cause-specific mortality. Quarterly Journal of Studies on Alcohol 35:841–855, 1974

O'Brien JP: Increase in suicide attempt by drug ingestion: the Boston experience, 1964–1974. Arch Gen Psychiatry 34:1165–1169, 1977

O'Sullivan K: Depression and its treatment in alcoholics: a review. Can J Psychiatry 29:379–384, 1984

Ottosson JO: The suicidal patient. Can the psychiatrist prevent his suicide?, in Origin and Treatment of Affective Disorders. Edited by Schon M, Stromgren E. New York, Academic, 1979

Petty F, Nasrallah HA: Secondary depression in alcoholism: implications for future research. Compr Psychiatry 22:587–595, 1981

Pfeffer CR: Self-destructive behavior in children and adolescents. Psychiatr Clin North Am 8:215–226, 1985

Pottenger M, McKernon J, Patrie LE, et al: The frequency and persistence of depressive symptoms in the alcohol abuser. J Nerv Ment Dis 166:562–570, 1978

Ravenholt RT: Addiction mortality in the United States, 1981: tobacco, alcohol and other substances. Pop Dev Rev 101:697–724, 1984

Robins E, Murphy G, Wilkinson R, et al: Some clinical considerations in the prevention of suicide based on a study of 134 successful suicides. Am J Public Health 49:888–899, 1954

Rounsaville BJ, Weissman MM, Rosenberger PH, et al: Detecting depressive disorders in drug abusers: a comparison of screening instruments. J Affective Disord 1:255–267, 1979

Rounsaville BJ, Weissman MM, Kleber H, et al: Heterogeneity of psychiatric diagnosis in treated opiate addicts. Arch Gen Psychiatry 39:161–168, 1982

Roy A: Suicide in doctors. Psychiatr Clin North Am 8:377–387, 1985

Roy A: Genetics of suicide. Ann NY Acad Sci 487:97–105, 1986a

Roy A: Suicide in Schizophrenics, in Suicide. Edited by Roy A. Baltimore, Williams & Wilkins, 1986b, pp. 97–112

Roy A, Linnoila M: Alcoholism and Suicide. Suicide Life Treat Behav 16:244–273, 1986

Rushing WA: Individual behavior and suicide, in Suicide. Edited by Gibbs JP. New York, Harper & Row, 1968

Rydelius PA: Deaths among child and adolescent psychiatric patients. Acta Psychiatr Scand 70:119–126, 1984

Sakinofsky I: Suicide in doctors and wives of doctors. Canadian Family Physician 26:837–844, 1980

Schildkraut JJ, Watson R, Draskoczy PR: Amphetamine withdrawal: depression and M.H.P.G. excretion. Lancet 2:485–486, 1971

Schuckit M: Alcoholic patients with secondary depression. Am J Psychiatry 140:711–714, 1983

Schuckit MA: The clinical implications of primary diagnostic groups among alcoholics. Arch Gen Psychiatry 42:1043–1049, 1985

Schuckit M: Primary men alcoholics with histories of suicide attempts. J Stud Alcohol 47:78–81, 1976

Schuckit MA, Miller PL: Alcoholism in elderly men: a survey of a general medical ward. Ann NY Acad Sci 273:558–571, 1976

Schuckit MA, Paster PA: The elderly as a unique population. Alcoholism 2:31–38, 1978

Schuckit MA, Winokur G: A short-term follow-up on women alcoholics. Diseases of the Nervous System 33:672–678, 1972

Selzer ML, Payne CE, Westervelt FH, et al: Automobile accidents as an expression of psychopathology in an alcoholic population. Quarterly Journal of Studies on Alcohol 28:505–516, 1967

Shafii M, Carringan S, Whittinghill J, et al: Psychological autopsy of completed suicide in children and adolescents. Am J Psychiatry 142:1061–1064, 1985

Silver MA, Bohnert M, Beck AT, et al: Relation of depression of attempted suicide and seriousness of intent. Arch Gen Psychiatry 25:573–576, 1971

Spitzer RL, Endicott J, Robins E: Research Diagnostic Criteria: rationale and reliability. Arch Gen Psychiatry 35:773–782, 1978

Stanley M, Stanley B, Traskman-Bendz L, et al: Neurochemical findings in suicide completers and suicide attempters. Suicide Life Threat Behav 16:286–300, 1986

Steer RA, McElroy MG, Beck AT: Structure of depression in alcoholic men: a partial replication. Psychol Rep 50:723–728, 1982

Tabachnick N, Litman RE, Osman M, et al: Comparative psychiatric study of accidental and suicidal death. Arch Gen Psychiatry 14:60–68, 1966

Takahashi S, Yamama H: CSF monoamine metabolism in alcoholism: a comparative study with depression. Folin Psych Neuro Japan 28:347–354, 1974

Tamerin JS, Mendelson JH: The psychodynamics of chronic inebriation: observations of alcoholics during the process of drinking in an experimental group setting. Am J Psychiatry 125:886–899, 1969

Teft BM, Penderson AM, Babigian HM: Patterns of death among suicide attempters: a psychiatric population and a general population. Arch Gen Psychiatry 34:1155–1161, 1974

Tonkin RS: Adolescent risk-taking behavior. J Adolesc Health Care 8:213–220, 1987

Tsuang MT, Simpson JC, Kronfol Z: Subtypes of drug abuse with psychosis: demographic characteristics, clinical features, and family history. Arch Gen Psychiatry 39:141–147, 1982

Tsuang TM, Boor M, Fleming JA: Psychiatric aspects of traffic accidents. Am J Psychiatry 142:538–546, 1985

Vaillant GE: A twelve-year follow-up of New York narcotic addicts, I: the relation of treatment to outcome. Am J Psychiatry 122:231–246, 1966

Vaillant GE (ed): The Natural History of Alcoholism. Cambridge, Harvard University Press, 1983

Virkkunen M: Reactive hypoglycemic tendency among habitually violent offenders: a further study by means of the glucose tolerance test. Neuropsychobiology 8:35–40, 1982

Ward NG, Schuckit M: Factors associated with suicidal behavior in polydrug abusers. J Clin Psychiatry 41:379–385, 1980

Weiss KJ, Rosenberg DJ: Prevalence of anxiety disorder among alcoholics. J Clin Psychiatry 46:3–5, 1985

Weissman AN, Beck AT, Kovacs M: Drug abuse, hopelessness and suicidal behavior. Int J Addict 14:451–464, 1979

Weissman M: The epidemiology of suicide attempts, 1960 to 1971. Arch Gen Psychiatry 30:737–746, 1974

Weissman MM, Myers JK: Clinical depression in alcoholism. Am J Psychiatry 137:372–373, 1980

Weissman MM, Pottenger M, Kleber H, et al: Symptom patterns in primary and secondary depression, a comparison of primary depressives with depressed opiate addicts, alcoholics and schizophrenics. Arch Gen Psychiatry 34:854–862, 1977

Weissman MM, Kidd KK, Prusoff BA: Variability in rates of affective disorders in relatives of depressed and normal probands. Arch Gen Psychiatry 39:1397–1403, 1982

Westermeyer J: The drunken Indian: myths and realities. Psychiatric Annals 4:29–36, 1974

Whitters A, Cadoret R, Widmer R: Factors associated with suicide attempts in alcohol abusers. J Affective Disord 9:19–23, 1985

Woody GE, Luborsky L, McLellan AT, et al: Psychotherapy for opiate addicts. Arch Gen Psychiatry 40:639–645, 1983

Wurmser L: Psychoanalytic considerations of the etiology of compulsive drug use. J Am Psychoanal Assoc 22:820–843, 1974

Zimberg S: The Clinical Management of Alcoholism. New York, Brunner/ Mazel, 1982, pp 43–44

Chapter 9

Medical Illness and Suicide

Thomas B. Mackenzie, M.D.
Michael K. Popkin, M.D.

IT IS A CLINICAL maxim that medical illness is a risk factor for suicide. In other words, the presence of a disturbance in physical health is believed to result in a higher rate of suicide. To the extent that suicide represents a confluence of factors that diminish a person's will to live, it seems indisputable that a medical illness with pain, disfigurement, restricted function, and/or fear of dependence would increase the risk of suicide. As intuitive as this concept may seem, designing studies that forge a link between suicide and medical illness while controlling for other variables has been difficult. Efforts to establish such a link are divisible into those that consider medical illness as a generic entity and those that restrict study to a specific disease or condition (e.g., cancer, hypertension, head trauma).

SUICIDE AND GENERIC MEDICAL ILLNESS

Attempts to study generic medical illness as a risk factor for suicide have generally sought to show that the frequency of physical illness among suicides is greater than the frequency in a control group. Demographic, psychiatric, and medical data from consecutive suicides in a particular locale are analyzed, and the percentage of suicides with a physical illness determined. The most important requirement of these studies is the inclusion of a satisfactory control population. The control group must be matched for other risk factors associated with suicide (e.g., age, sex, marital status, psychopathology, substance abuse).

Table 1 presents the results of 11 studies in which the frequency of medical illness in a series of suicides was studied in the United States, Great Britain, Sweden, and South Africa. A mean of 43% of suicides across studies (range, 20% to 70%) were judged to be suffering from medical illness at the time of death. None of the studies had a well-matched control group. Data from the 1974 U.S. National Health Survey (Wilder 1977) estimated that 14% of the population (excluding those living in institutions) experienced some degree of activity limitation due to chronic disease or impairment other than a mental disorder. Although the mean of the 11 studies is three times this figure, the difference cannot be considered conclusive in the absence of a matched control group.

Five of the studies summarized in Table 1 attempted to grade the importance of medical illness in the suicide. In a mean of 25% of suicides, a medical illness was deemed important. Notably, data from three studies concluded that no more than 5% of suicides occurred in the context of terminal illness (Robins et al. 1959; Sainsbury 1956; Seager and Flood 1965). In other words, the relationship between suicide and medical illness was not limited to persons who were told or correctly discerned that death was imminent. These figures indicate that so-called rational suicides, expressing a considered decision to forego the pain and dependence of dying, account for no more than 5% of suicides. This is consistent with the observation of Brown et al. (1986) that thoughts of suicide among terminally ill patients occurred only in those who were depressed.

In a vast majority of the suicides in the presence of medical illness, a psychiatric disorder was judged to be present. The series of Dorpat et al. (1968) and Robins et al. (1959) suggest that at least 70% of such patients were suffering from depression or alcoholism. Dorpat et al. (1968) concluded that all suicides in their sample had a psychiatric illness.

The available literature sheds little light on the precise role or mechanism by which generic medical illness affected the onset or progression of psychopathology or the occurrence of suicide itself. Information on whether the medical illness predated the depression or vice versa is absent. What percentage of the depressions would have been diagnosed as organic mood disorders is also obscure. Sainsbury (1956) and Robins et al. (1959) reported that 4% of the suicides had cognitive dysfunction, raising the possibility that these patients were hallucinatory, deluded, or grossly impaired with respect to memory, judgment, or impulse control. Cavan (1928) specu-

Table 1. Relationship of medical illness to suicide

Study	Location	Period of study	Number of suicides	Physical illness present (%)	Physical illness important (%)	Physical illness teminal (%)
Cavan (1928)	Chicago	1923	391	23	16	NA
Sainsbury (1956)	London	1936–1938	390	NA	29	NA
Tuckman and Lavell (1958)	Philadelphia	1951–1955	319	43	NA	NA
Stewart (1957)	England	1952–1957	65	68	NA	NA
Registrar General (Foreign Letters 1957)	England	1955	5043	28[a]	NA	NA
Robins et al. (1959)	St. Louis	1956–1957	134	46	21	4
Seager and Flood (1965)	England	1957–1961	325	20	11	4
Rorsman et al. (1982)	Sweden	1957–1972	28	57	NA	NA
Barraclouch et al. (1974)	England	1966–1968	100	NA	NA	6
Dorpat et al. (1968)	Seattle	1968	80	70	51	NA
Gangat et al. (1987)	South Africa	1982–1984	47	50	NA	NA

Note. NA = not available.
[a]Associated with surgical operations, childbirth, and chronic pain or illness.

lated that medical illness led to suicide when an individual's capacity to endure severe pain was surpassed. She found that 3% of the suicides in her series were the result of pain. Since 10 of 11 of these victims were male, she concluded that pain was a more significant risk factor in males.

Gangat et al. (1987) found that 65% of persons who committed suicide in the presence of medical illness were taking a prescribed medication with the potential for precipitating depression. Their data suggest that the potency of medical illness as a risk factor may in some cases be attributable to the use of medications that precipitate depression.

Dorpat et al. (1968) and Sainsbury (1956) found that the prevalence of medical illness was higher in male than female suicide, suggesting that illness may be a more significant risk factor in males. However, Robins et al. (1959) reported a greater prevalence of medical illness in females than males, and Seager and Flood (1965) found no difference between men and women, leaving the issue unresolved.

Robins et al. (1959) found that cardiovascular and gastrointestinal diseases were the most prevalent in their series. Seager and Flood (1965) reported that three-quarters of the illnesses present at the time of suicide were chronic. This suggests a physical illness usually exerts its effect in a lingering rather than abrupt fashion.

As a result of his study, Sainsbury (1956) reported that suicide attempts related to medical illness were more likely to be lethal; thus the ratio of attempted to completed suicide was low.

Variation Across the Life Cycle

Dorpat et al. (1968) noted that the percentage of suicides with a significant medical condition increased with age (13.3% under 39 years old versus 69.7% over 60). This finding suggests that the risk of suicide associated with medical illness may vary across the life cycle. Klerman (1987) seems to support this pattern when he cites medical illness as a risk factor for adults 30 years and over, but not for adolescents and youth under the age of 30 years. It is tempting to speculate that adolescents and young adults would somehow be more resistant to the risk imposed by medical illness or that the elderly, with fewer resources to cope with medical illness, might be more vulnerable. However, such a conclusion needs to be tempered by the recognition that the prevalence of medical illness increases with age, and the concurrence of medical illness and suicide among the elderly could reflect that factor alone. On the other hand, one might speculate that adolescents, preoccupied with issues of identity and emancipation, would have difficulty adjusting to the demands imposed by chronic medical illness. This might take the form of careless or defiant administration of self-care as well as disguised suicide. Stearns (1959) noted this pattern in young diabetics. However, firm epidemiologic evidence supporting this pattern is lacking.

SUICIDE AND SPECIFIC MEDICAL ILLNESS

Researchers have also examined the relationship between specific medical illnesses and the risk of suicide. This approach offers an opportunity to elucidate the mechanisms that might link a specific pathophysiology with suicide.

Acquired Immune Deficiency Syndrome (AIDS)

Studying New York City residents, Marzuk et al. (1988) determined that the relative risk of suicide in men with AIDS aged 20 to 59 years was 36 times that of men aged 20 to 59 years without the diagnosis. All suicides had occurred within 9 months of diagnosis, and none of the victims at autopsy appeared to have an advanced form of the disease. Three of the suicides, or 25%, occurred on an inpatient medical ward, all three by jumping from a window. In 5 of 12 cases, the patient had seen a psychiatrist within the preceding 96 hours. A recent psychiatric tabloid (Pierce 1987) reported seven suicides over a 2 1/2-month period in Miami among people who tested positive for the human immuno-deficiency virus (HIV). The article pointed out that none of the seven had received posttest counseling. AIDS-related suicides are likely to be attributed to the psychosocial turmoil attendant to learning that one has a highly lethal disease. However, recent evidence suggests that the HIV may affect central nervous system function early in the course of the illness and, in so doing, predispose seropositive individuals to catastrophic reactions by compromising memory, mood, or impulse control (Grant et al. 1987). Thus clinical evaluation must attend to cognitive function as well as psychosocial distress. As seropositive individuals develop AIDS, the contemporary stigmata attached to this diagnosis may drive some to suicide. With disease progression, virtually 100% of patients will develop brain changes consistent with subacute encephalitis (Gabuzda and Hirsch 1987). This may be marked by cognitive deficits, memory loss, depression, personality changes, or psychosis. Any of these symptoms might increase the risk of suicide.

In addition to being a potential risk factor for suicide, contraction of AIDS may be a means of suicide. Four cases have been described wherein alcoholic, homosexual males consciously sought infection with HIV as a means of committing suicide (Flavin et al 1986; Frances et al. 1985). In at least two of the cases there was a deliberate attempt to spread the disease to others as well (Flavin et al. 1986).

Cancer

Campbell (1966) checked suicides from 1959 to 1962 against the Connecticut Tumor Registry and concluded that male cancer patients of all ages had a greater risk of suicide than the general population. An increased risk was not found for female patients.

Among cancer patients in Finland, Louhivuori and Hakama (1979) found that the number of suicides was higher in both men and women. The excessive risk was confined to the first 5 years of follow-up and was greater for those patients with nonlocalized disease. Among patients with localized disease, digestive organ cancer showed the highest risk of suicide. Patients who received chemotherapy or no treatment had a higher risk of suicide than patients treated with surgery and/or radiation, even when extent of disease was taken into account.

Fox et al. (1982) studied the suicide rate in 144,530 persons with cancer identified in Connecticut from 1940 through 1969. Male, but not female, cancer patients were at increased risk of suicide. The risk of suicide in men was the greatest soon after diagnosis.

Whitlock (1978) observed 21 neoplasms among 273 suicides (7.7%) and only 3 (1.1%) neoplasms among a matched group of accident victims. This difference was significant even when benign neoplasms (4 in the suicide group, 1 in the accident victims) were excluded. The author pointed out that a premorbid diagnosis of cancer had not been made in 7 of the malignant cases. Although the victims may have been aware of their diagnosis, it is also possible that the tumors exerted a paraneoplastic effect and thereby altered mental function.

Using a case-control methodology involving 22,000 New York residents, Marshall et al. (1983) found more cancer patients among those who suicided than among those who died in a motor vehicle accident or from myocardial infarction. The effect was observed in both males and females, but was greater in males. No effect of disease stage or lag between diagnosis and death was observed.

Farberow et al. (1963) reported that patients with cancer were overrepresented among suicides in Veterans Administration (VA) general medical and surgical hospitals. Of the 32 cancer suicides identified, 29 were judged to have been in critical medical condition at the time of suicide. Bolund (1987) also found that a high percentage (67%) of cancer suicides were in an advanced or terminal phase.

Collectively, these studies indicate that the incidence of suicide in males with cancer is increased in the period following diagnosis and extending for as long as 5 years. The data for women are suggestive, but not conclusive. There is some evidence that the patients who underwent chemotherapy were at highest risk, suggesting that chemotherapy either induces an organic mental disorder (including organic mood disorders) conducive to suicide or that the use of chemotherapy is correlated with a poor prognosis and an attendant sense of hopelessness. Data from Louhivuori and Hakama (1979), Bolund (1987), and Farberow et al. (1963) indicating that the risk of suicide in cancer patients is directly related to the severity of disease favor the latter explanation. Louhivuori and Hakama (1979) suggested that gastrointestinal cancers confer the greatest relative risk of suicide.

In 17 (28%) of 80 completed suicides, Dorpat et al. (1968) noted the presence of a severe and morbid fear of cancer. Since only 6 patients actually had a malignancy, it appears that 65% with such a fear had no evidence of the condition. Brown and Pisetsky (1960) also emphasized the importance of a fear of cancer in patients who commit suicide. Since somatic concerns, such as cancerphobia, are often a symptom of depression, it seems likely that the patients in these studies suffered from a depressive illness manifested principally by fear of cancer.

Diabetes Mellitus

Entmacher et al. (1985) of the Joslin Clinic reported on the causes of death among a large series of the clinic's diabetic patients for three periods. For the interval 1950–1959, 0.3% of 9,925 deaths were identified as suicide. For the period 1960–1968, the figure was 0.3% of 7,160 deaths and for 1969–1979 the percentage was 0.5% of 4,290 deaths. In the last of these intervals, diabetic ketoacidosis (DKA) accounted for 1.2% of deaths, hypoglycemia 0.4%, accidents 1.7%, "other causes" 2.4%, and "diabetes and unknown" 0.5%.

Tunbridge (1981) examined factors contributing to the deaths of 448 diabetics under the age of 50, who died in England, Wales, or Northern Ireland in 1979. DKA caused 16% and hypoglycemia 4% of the deaths. No deaths in the series were conclusively identified as suicides; however, an overdose of drugs was central to DKA in one case. In addition, Tunbridge reported that patients' neglect of their diabetes was contributory in 27% of deaths and that personality factors and domestic difficulties, which may have delayed seeking medical attention, were relevant in 25% of cases. Of the 17 hypoglycemic deaths, most of the patients had either "personality problems or psychiatric disorders"; 6 had made previous suicide attempts.

In 1982, Teutsch et al. (1984) studied 35 deaths of diabetic patients who were using continuous subcutaneous insulin-infusion pumps. Only 1 death, that of a 26-year-old white male, was attributed to suicide.

In each of the above studies, the rate of suicide appears quite modest. This is surprising, given factors such as increased rates of cognitive dysfunction (Perlmuter et al. 1984; Ryan et al. 1985) and mood disorder (Popkin et al 1988) in diabetes. However, one must consider issues of underreporting on death certificates and also the contention that discontinuation of therapy is one of the two commonest causes of severe DKA (Beigelman 1971). Cohen et al. (1960) found that such omissions accounted for 25% of all DKA episodes. Similarly, deaths from hypoglycemia may represent the consequence of intentional insulin overdose. Stearns (1959) described such self-destructive behaviors in young diabetics.

Epilepsy

In their review of suicide and epilepsy, Matthew and Barabas (1981) concluded that the suicide rate among epileptic patients was higher than in the general population. Consolidating mortality statistics from several studies of epileptic populations, the authors calculated that 5.0% of deaths in epileptic patients were suicides. This figure was contrasted with an overall suicide rate of 1.4% for the United States population. However, such a comparison is misleading. The percentage of total deaths accounted for by suicide is influenced by the number of deaths from other causes and varies significantly with age. The 5.0% rate in epileptic patients must be compared with the rate in an age-matched control group. For instance, in the United States, the percentage of suicides among deaths in whites aged 25 to 29 years is 15.4% (National Center for Health Statistics 1982), a rate three times the rate cited for epilepsy.

Blumer and Benson (1982) drew attention to the view held by European clinicians that the incidence of suicide may be heightened following improvement of chronic temporal lobe epilepsy. These authors advanced two explanations for this phenomenon: 1) that the suicide is related to suddenly having to live without a recognized handicap, or 2) that a suicidal depression emerges in the absence of recurrent convulsions.

Head Injury

Achte et al. (1971) described a 25-year follow-up of 6,498 Finnish veterans who had received a head injury during World War II. Nine percent had suicided, yielding an average yearly incidence of 66 per 100,000, roughly twice that of the Finnish population. The rate per 100,000 approached 400 in those who had shown psychotic symptoms following the injury. Suicide was not associated with a specific site of injury, but did correlate positively with severity. Dementia and a change in character after a head injury were ominous signs, enhancing the suicide rate. Nearly 60% of the suicides had threatened self-harm and 25% had made previous attempts. Alcohol abuse was overrepresented in those who committed suicide.

Huntington's Chorea

In his original description of Huntington's chorea, George Huntington (1872) identified a tendency toward suicide as characteristic of the disease. Chandler et al. (1960) reported that suicide was an important cause of death in noninstitutionalized patients with Huntington's, accounting for 7.8% of deaths in males and 6.4% of deaths in females. The mean age at death in Chandler et al.'s patients was 53 years old. These percentages of death by suicide are considerably higher than the 1.3% (National Center for Health Statistics 1982) observed for persons aged 55 to 64 years old living in the United States. Dewhurst et al. (1970) speculated that a substantial fraction of suicides may occur in the prodromal stage of the illness.

The mechanisms by which Huntington's confers an increased risk of suicide is most probably through the production of an organic mental disorder with a prominent affective disturbance (McHugh and Folstein 1975).

Hypertension

Stewart (1960) reported that 27% of suicide victims who came to autopsy had hypertension with cardiac hypertrophy. He found that in a majority of cases the hypertension had developed recently and had been rapidly progressive. He predicted that the observed rate of hypertension would exceed that in the general population but provided no comparison figures. No mention was made of how many individuals were taking amine-depleting agents at the time of their suicide. In a retrospective chart review, Levitan (1983) found that hypertensive patients had a significantly higher rate of attempted suicide or suicidal ideation than a group of patients with cholelithiasis matched for a 20-year age range. None of the patients who developed suicidal ideation following the discovery of hypertension had been treated with amine-depleting agents, such as reserpine.

Multiple Sclerosis

Miles (1977) reported that multiple sclerosis may be associated with an increased suicide rate, citing two studies to support this possibility. Muller (1949) reviewed the course of 810 persons found to have multiple sclerosis between the years of 1920 to 1945. Of 190 patients who had died, 5 had committed suicide, yielding a death rate from suicide of 2.6%. In a 6-year follow-up of 295 patients with multiple sclerosis, Kahana et al. (1971) found that 17% of all deaths were suicides, nearly three times the 6.6% rate for whites 40 to 44 years of age (National Center for Health Statistics 1982).

Peptic Ulcer

In a three-decade follow-up of 1,000 patients who had undergone a Billroth II procedure for treatment of peptic ulcer, Knop and Fischer (1981) reported a nearly fourfold increase in the relative risk of suicide for both men and women. The suicides had a significantly increased frequency of psychiatric hospitalization compared with the survivors and those who had died of natural causes. One-third of the suicides had a diagnosis of alcoholism, as opposed to 8.7% of the entire study population.

Viskum (1975) followed up all patients admitted to the hospital over a 14-year period in whom X-ray examination of the stomach and duodenum had revealed evidence of peptic ulcer disease or whose upper gastrointestinal symptoms could not be otherwise explained. Men, but not women, had a greater than expected number of deaths from suicide. The suicide rate was not related to surgical treatment. Compared to the general population, the study population had an excess of nonpsychotic mental disorders. No data on the substance use history of those who committed suicide were presented.

Berglund (1986) carried out a 12- to 25-year follow-up of male alcoholics in Sweden. The relative risk of suicide in the entire group was 10 times that of the general population. However, the suicide rate among those with peptic ulcer disease with and without gastric surgery was 30 times that of the general population. In other words, peptic ulcer disease in men conferred a risk of suicide in this population beyond that associated with alcoholism alone. Since alcoholic men with and without ulcer disease showed similar mortality rates (excluding suicide) and social prognosis among survivors, Berglund concluded that peptic ulcer disease was not simply a marker for severity of alcohol abuse.

The incidence of suicide in males with peptic ulcer disease with and without gastric surgery is increased. The data for women are inconclusive. Alcoholism is overrepresented in the patient group with peptic ulcer who commit suicide. However, it appears that the risk conferred by peptic ulcer disease is independent of the risk associated with alcoholism.

Premenstrual Syndrome

There is no firm epidemiologic evidence linking the premenstrual syndrome (PMS), called late luteal phase dysphoric disorder in DSM-III-R (American Psychiatric Association 1987) if emotional symptoms are prominent, with an increased risk of suicide. To the extent that PMS has been linked to the occurrence of major depression, a secondary effect reflecting the association of depression and suicide can be assumed (Mackenzie et al. 1986; Schuckit et al. 1975; Wetzel et al. 1975). However, this effect has not been quantitated. Most research has examined the role of menstrual cycle phase in the timing of suicidal behavior. The effect is not a change in overall risk but a fluctuation in risk. Using uterine tissue to determine cycle phase, Mackinnon and Mackinnon (1956) found that suicides clustered in the middle luteal phase. Other studies reviewed by Wetzel and McClure (1972) have reported an increased frequency of suicide during the menstrual phase of the cycle.

Pulmonary Disease

Retrospective accounts of suicide on medical-surgical hospital wards have identified dyspnea as a risk factor for suicide (Farberow et al. 1966; Glickman 1980; Salmon et al. 1982). Surprisingly, however, most studies of consecutive suicides in community settings have not discerned a higher than expected rate of pulmonary disease. Sawyer et al. (1983) reported on three attempted suicides and one completion among 43 patients with chronic obstructive pulmonary disease (COPD) who had enlisted in a nocturnal oxygen rehabilitation study. The authors hypothesized that when the hope engendered by a new treatment faded, the patients became discouraged and hopeless, leading to suicidal behavior in four instances. In contrast, Levitan (1983) compared patients with COPD and those with cholelithiasis and found that the rate of suicidal thinking was equal. In that study, asthma had a significantly greater association with suicidal thinking than COPD. Lewiston and Rubinstein (1987) proposed that a depression-suicide factor was partially responsible for a 200% increase in the annual number of asthma deaths in children between 1977 and 1983. The article did not present specific suicide rates.

The available data do not provide epidemiologic support for a relationship between pulmonary disease and suicide. However, the experience of clinicians points strongly to dyspnea, whether a consequence of COPD or asthma, as a symptom that can enhance the risk of suicide.

Rheumatoid Arthritis

Dorpat et al. (1968) found an increased prevalence of rheumatoid arthritis (15%) in their series of consecutive suicides when contrasted with the prevalence in their nonmatched control population (2% to 3%). The authors felt that this reflected years of pain and progressive disability as well as increasing isolation from other people. Whether any of the patients with rheumatoid arthritis were taking steroids or other immunosuppressive agents was not specified. Pokorny (1960) noted that 6 of 44 suicides among patients in a VA hospital had bone or joint disease, not otherwise specified, compared to 2 of 44 ex-patients who served as controls. No specific relationship between joint disease and suicide was postulated.

Spinal Cord Injury

Wilcox and Stauffer (1972) followed up 420 patients who had been hospitalized with spinal cord injury. Four years after hospitalization, 14% of the patients had died. Of these, 18% had committed suicide. For the United States population as a whole, 1.4% of all deaths were suicides (National Center for Health Statistics 1982). Ducharme and Freed (1980) reviewed 158 deaths after initial hospitalization among spinal cord injured patients registered with the National Spinal Cord Injury Data Research Center. Nine percent of the deaths were suicides, 80% occurring during the first 3 follow-up years. This is probably a conservative percentage, since in more than 38% of all the deaths, insufficient information was available to judge the precise cause. The authors, like Wilcox and Stauffer (1972), pointed out that the possibilities for indirect suicide created by spinal cord injury are considerable. They also commented on the clinical observation that there is an inverse relationship between suicide and severity of injury.

Assessing the risk of suicide associated with spinal cord injuries per se is complicated by the reality that persons who sustain injuries are drawn from an impulsive, self-destructive population that might be expected to have a high suicide rate independent of spinal cord injury. However, the data indicate that once injured, the spinal cord patient is at increased risk of suicide. Crude calculations based on the data of Wilcox and Stauffer (1972) suggest that the incidence of suicide per 100,000 (not counting indirect suicide) in the spinal cord injured may be as high as 600 per year, 60 times the overall rate for the general population (National Center for Health Statistics 1982). Thus it seems likely that the incidence of suicide is increased in spinal cord injured patients. Importantly, less severe injury may confer just as much or more risk than severe injury.

SUICIDE IN MEDICAL-SURGICAL HOSPITALS

A number of researchers have studied suicide occurring in medical-surgical hospitals. Although this approach does not quantify the risk of suicide in medical illness, it elucidates the phenomenology of suicide in the medically ill, allowing construction of a high-risk profile. This in turn increases the chance that the suicidal patient will be identified and effective measures taken.

Pollack (1957) reviewed the clinical records of 11 men who committed suicide from 1948 to 1953 in a VA hospital. Ten of the 11 died as a result of a fall. Signs of delirium were evident in 7 of 11 patients. Significantly, 6 of the patients had respiratory problems, suggesting that discomfort in breathing might have been an intolerable burden. One of the patients had a malignancy, 1 was judged to have been critically ill, and 3 had a history of alcohol abuse. Although 9 had a significant neuropsychiatric history, suicide attempts had not been a prominent feature of their prior behavior. Only one patient had been admitted following a suicide attempt, suggesting that persons admitted for medical treatment of a suicide attempt were underrepresented among those who killed themselves in the hospital. This may not reflect a reduction in risk immediately after a suicide attempt as much as it signifies prompt implementation of psychiatric care. Unambiguous signs of severe emotional disturbance appeared at least 24 hours before the suicide in 10 of 11 patients, with 7 of these 10 showing frankly psychotic behavior. The psychotic behavior was attributed to an organic mental disorder in 7 patients.

Friedman and Cancellieri (1958) reviewed Fordham Hospital records from 1954 to 1957. In that period, three males attempted suicide by jumping, two successfully. None of them had shown signs of organic impairment or depression, and none had been admitted because of a suicide attempt. The authors reported that of 272 persons admitted following an ingestion of poison, none of the 250 who survived made a subsequent attempt in the hospital.

Brown and Pisetsky (1960) studied the records of 16 patients who committed suicide on the medical-surgical wards of the Bronx VA Hospital in the period 1947 through 1958. All victims were chronically ill: 5 had a malignancy and 6 had central nervous system syndromes. Severe, chronic, or terminal illness with pain, dyspnea, and disfigurement was common. The fraction of patients with a past neuropsychiatric history was not specified. Apparently none had been admitted for treatment of a suicide attempt. The authors did not comment on the relationship of the suicides to psychiatric diagnosis and judged that most of the suicides were rational. They predicted that since advancing medical technology leaves old age and chronic disease in its wake, the rate of suicide in medical-surgical hospitals would increase. In 1979, the same authors (Pisetsky and Brown 1979) reported that there had actually been a relative decline in suicide in the hospital where their original study had been done. They attributed the decline to greater alertness to the mental state of the patient and effective efforts to deal with problems on the part of medical staffs.

Farberow et al. (1963) examined 32 suicides in VA general medical-surgical hospitals during the years 1955 through 1960 in patients who had cancer. Unlike Pollack's (1957) study, the condition of 91% was rated critical at the time of their suicide. The percentage of men under 45 years old in the suicide group was greater than that of the overall VA cancer population. Hemapoietic cancers contributed disproportionately to suicide in the younger suicide group (under 45 years old), whereas cancer of the larynx and pharynx (i.e., the neck region) contributed disproportionately to suicide in the older group. The investigators compared the suicide group with a group matched for diagnosis, severity, age, race, and religion, although not for hospital. The suicide patients showed a pattern of overinvolvement in treatment, with a need to control it and, in many cases, with complaining and demanding behavior. Compared to controls, the suicides were noted to have more tension in their family life; indications of unusual emotional disturbances appeared in 20 suicides and only 10 controls. The suicide patients demonstrated significantly less tolerance for pain. Twenty-eight percent had threatened suicide and 2 had made a previous attempt. This contrasts with Pollack (1957) and Brown and Pisetsky (1960), who found talk of suicide to be uncommon. Seventeen suicides and 14 controls had notations of depression in their records.The authors did not find a relationship between suicide and confusion. They even speculated that confusion might have acted to preclude suicide attempts: 8 of the suicides as opposed to 15 of the controls were judged to have been confused.

Farberow et al. (1966) studied suicide in VA patients with cardiorespiratory illness. Compared to a matched control group, the 45 patients who committed suicide were more emotionally disturbed; more hostile, depressed, and anxious over their illness; more often seen as dependent and complaining; more alert and aware; and more troubled by insomnia. The suicides were judged to have poorer interpersonal relationships with the staff and tended to see the hospital as indifferent toward them. The hospital staff saw these patients as difficult problems and reacted to them with less support than was offered to the controls. Alcoholism was not overrepresented in the suicide group. The amount of difficulty breathing experienced by the two groups was not significantly different. A personality pattern, which the authors labeled dependent-dissatisfied, emerged among the suicides. This personality was associated with disturbed interpersonal relations both in and outside the hospital. Most (56%) of the patients committed suicide by jumping; cutting and hanging occurred next most often. The authors did not indicate how many of the suicides had a past neuropsychatric history, had been admitted for treatment of suicide attempts, or had an organic mental disorder secondary to respiratory failure. The mechanism by which respiratory insufficiency may contribute to a suicidal outcome has been discussed by Salmon et al. (1982).

Shneidman et al. (1970) described 12 suicides among patients on general medical-surgical wards in Los Angeles County during the period 1963–1964. Despite the fact that this study included all hospitals in the area (not just VA hospitals), 11 were men. The median stay in the hospital from admission to suicide was only 3 days. Ten patients leaped to their deaths. Four were judged to have been confused and 7 depressed. Two suicides were related to alcohol. None of the patients had been hospitalized because of a suicide attempt. Past neuropsychiatric history was not specified. The authors noted that suicide in the hospital was a rare event, but pointed out that in the period of the study there were more than 150 suicides within 2 months of discharge from a medical-surgical hospital.

In a report of suicides submitted to the VA Central Research Unit, Farberow et al. (1971) concluded that the suicide rate per 100,000 for patients treated in general medical-surgical hospitals was 6 per year. They noted that this figure was impressively low, especially considering the physical pain and emotional distress caused by physical illness.

Glickman (1980) described 22 patients who committed suicide while being treated on the nonpsychiatric services of Kings County Hospital Center in New York between 1963 and 1978; 73% were male. Nineteen of the 22 killed themselves by jumping out a window. Five were originally admitted following a suicide attempt. In reviewing the suicide population, the author concluded that almost all had one of the following characteristics: 1) dyspnea, 2) organic brain syndrome, 3) alcoholism, 4) poor medical prognosis, or 5) admission for treatment of previous suicide attempt. Only two had a malignancy. According to the author, patients with delirium tremens on an open ward were at highest risk for suicide. In contrast to the view that confusion may confer protection, most of them attempted suicide within the first 24 hours of their delirium.

When Reich and Kelly (1976) reviewed records at the Peter Bent Brigham Hospital in Boston between 1967 and 1973, they identified 17 attempts, but no completions. Thirteen of the 17 were females and the predominant methods were self-cutting and ingestions. The one-story construction of the hospital precluded jumping, the most common method at multistoried hospitals. The authors related the attempts to imminent discharge or change in social support rather than to changes in physical condition, depression, or cognitive impairment.

Demographic and clinical analysis of persons who commit suicide while in a general medical-surgical hospital suggests several things. The overall suicide rate appears to be low. The overwhelming majority of suicides are male. Lethal falls are the most common means of death. Most of the patients who commit suicide are chronically and severely ill. Few have been admitted for treatment of a suicide attempt. Notes or explanations are rarely left. Many of the suicides appear in the context of organicity or alcoholism. The perpetrators are often demanding and dissatisfied. A rapid depressive and/or psychotic decompensation may precede the suicide. Cancer and dyspnea are overrepresented.

SUICIDE AND MEDICAL PROCEDURES

The incidence of suicide in relationship to certain medical procedures has received attention. For example, Fawcett (1972) predicted that urologic surgery might precipitate severe depression in men and, thereby, substantially increase the risk of suicide. Abram et al. (1971) reported an increased rate of suicide in patients on renal dialysis. The risk may be particularly high in young persons who suffer graft failure after renal transplantation and are forced to resume dialysis (Washer et al. 1983). However, the magnitude of the relative risk, while undoubtedly significant, has been difficult to ascertain precisely (Levy 1979). As DiBiance (1979) pointed out, this is at least partially because a definition of suicidal behavior is a point of disagreement among researchers in the field. For some clinicians, death related to nonadherence to a medical regimen is considered suicide; for others, lethal noncompliance must be accompanied by symptoms of depression to be judged suicide.

ASSESSMENT OF SUICIDE RISK IN THE PATIENT WITH MEDICAL ILLNESS

Risk Factors

Prevention of suicide requires knowledge of the characteristics that can increase its risk. The literature dealing with suicide in patients with medical illness indicates that the following may signal an increased risk of suicide: advancing age; male gender; a painful, terminal illness; dyspnea; depression; psychosis; organic mental disorder; alcoholism; demanding, complaining behavior; poor interpersonal relations; access to lethal means; AIDS; cancer; peptic ulcer; spinal cord injury; head injury; Huntington's chorea; inadequate sedation; weak physician-patient bond; and failure to monitor the patient's emotional state.

Clinical Interview

Identification of high-risk cases on an actuarial basis must be combined with a thorough clinical interview (Hendren, Chapter 10, this volume). The presence of a significant medical illness expands the scope of the standard interview. Of initial concern is whether the patient acknowledges having an illness. If a patient maintains that there is no illness or that it is trivial, this degree of denial should not be accepted without additional inquiry. The object of persistence is not to breach the denial but to examine the patient's thought processes as well as indicate a willingness to discuss the extent and seriousness of the illness. Patients may have been conditioned to deny illness through experiences with family, friends, or medical personnel. Exploration of denial can also be accomplished by introducing hypothetical questions about how the patient would respond to future illness. The degree to which denial should be challenged depends on the implications it carries. If it is seriously disrupting care, firm dissent may be necessary. If the denial assists the patient to manage anxiety in an adaptive fashion, such as optimism that one will recover from a myocardial infarction, no challenge is indicated.

If the patient recognizes the presence of an illness, the patient's view of its seriousness and its potential impact on living patterns should be established. It is important to determine how the patient perceives the future: will the illness remain the same, get better or worse? If better, has the patient any doubts? If worse, over what time course does the subject expect the change to occur? What is the most troubling aspect of the change? Does the patient believe that this outcome is inevitable or does the patient maintain some hope? Patients often fear pain and dyspnea, but just as frequently they fear loss of autonomy and becoming a burden. Ascertaining how much "strength" a patient has left will help gauge how the patient expects to respond to changes. An alternative approach is to ask how much more the patient can tolerate. Inquiry about whether doctors have been able to help allows exploration of whether the patient trusts the physician to treat pain vigorously and provide accurate information. If the patient believes he or she is seriously ill, it may be important to understand the patient's concept of death. A concept that emphasizes escape and peace may be more conducive to suicide than one involving punishment or stigmatization for suicide. A thorough assessment of the patient's social and religious resources should be made. It should be established whether the patient is looking forward to goals or landmarks. Their absence is a worrisome situation. A detailed account of ideas about, of plans for, or attempts at suicide should be sought. Careful attention must be paid to incompletely treated medical symptoms such as pain, dyspnea, insomnia, and nausea and to whether the patient believes that any of the drugs being taken are causing disconcerting side effects. As in any psychiatric interview, a detailed assessment of affect and cognition should take place. The latter is of special significance. Subtle cognitive deficits are difficult to detect retrospectively and are hence almost certainly underestimated in case and epidemiologic studies of suicide. Minor disturbances in gathering, processing, and acting on relevant data could certainly contribute to the emergence of suicidal intent.

A corroborative history should be sought routinely but is especially important if the patient minimizes or denies the medical illness and its implications. Even if collateral sources are unfamiliar with the patient's thinking, they may be able to describe changes in energy, sleep, motivation, appetite, libido, and so on, which permit a longitudinal construction of the patient's course.

Diagnostic Issues

An overwhelming majority of persons with medical illness who commit suicide are suffering from depression and/or alcoholism. Thus evidence relevant to these diagnoses must be sought with diligence. How to classify depression associated with medical illness has been a long-standing matter of debate (Popkin et al. 1987). One dimension of the debate focuses on when to use the category organic mood disorder. Ultimately, this hinges on the uncertain matter of when central nervous system dysfunction satisfactorily accounts for a depressed mood. One can take the position that any evidence of dysfunction (e.g., abnormal electroencephalogram, widened cortical sulci, enlarged ventricles, increased protein in the cerebrospinal fluid, abnormal neuropsychological performance, focal or lateralizing neurologic examination, elevated thyroid-stimulating hormone) is sufficient to make a diagnosis of organic mood disorder. A more conservative approach is to insist on a distinct chronological relationship between depressive symptoms and neurologic dysfunction, the identification of a syndrome well established in the literature to cause depression, or the resolution of the mood disturbance with treatment of the medical illness. The latter approach allows a more rigorous subtyping of organic mood disorder and potential refinement of drug treatment in these types. As Popkin et al. (1985) have pointed out, tricyclic antidepressants do not appear to have the same efficacy in the depressed medically ill as they do in groups with major depression. This may be due to a less than optimal match between the central nervous system mechanism involved in a specific case and the type of antidepressant regimen prescribed.

It should be emphasized that somatic treatment of depression is not contingent on whether the etiology is considered reactive or endogenous. While it is possible that depressive syndromes that emerge following loss of health, autonomy, financial security, and so on are less responsive to antidepressants, this is by no means a sufficient certainty to deprive patients of what may be life-saving or life-enhancing treatment. Even if one's remaining life span is measured in weeks, the difference between spending that time adapting to the personal tasks at hand (e.g., writing a will, communicating affection and thanks) or being plagued by dysphoria or sleeplessness is significant.

The use of alcohol or other drugs to manage pain, insomnia, or dysphoria must always be considered when assessing a patient with medical illness. These substances may exacerbate depression and compound cognitive dysfunction as well as serving as a means for suicide.

Rational Suicide

Evaluation of persons with serious medical illness inevitably raises the problem of rational suicide. Siegel (1986) outlined the defining characteristics of rational suicide as: 1) the individual possesses a realistic assessment of the situation; 2) the mental processes leading to a decision to commit suicide are unimpaired by psychological illness or severe emotional distress; and 3) the motivational basis of the decision would be understandable to the majority of uninvolved observers from the community or social group. The moral and ethical dimensions of this question have been admirably reviewed by Engelhardt

(1986). For clinical purposes it is most important to realize that studies of suicide indicate that terminal medical illness is rarely a sufficient explanation and that a vast majority of suicides show psychopathology that would enhance the risk of suicide. Thus the conditions set forth by Siegel are rarely met.

Nevertheless, rational suicides do appear to occur, and they present the clinician with vexing problems, especially when the mode of self-harm is discontinuation of an established medical treatment, continuation of which would offer survival. It is a well-established judicial principle that a patient may refuse any medical treatment, even if the alternative is death, provided that the individual's ability to reason is not disturbed. This places a burden on the clinician to determine whether the refusal is a rational and considered decision, not unduly influenced by disturbances in mood or cognition, which to some degree are nearly inevitable in severe physical illness. This judgment is made even more difficult if the individual in question has a history of impulsive, dramatic, or self-destructive behavior. Discussion of the patient's decision with family and friends may be necessary, even if this is forbidden by the individual. If the contribution of psychopathology to the patient's decision cannot be satisfactorily gauged, the clinician may elect to seek the advice of a hospital ethics committee.

MANAGEMENT AND TREATMENT

Medical-Surgical Units

Management of the suicidal patient in a medical-surgical hospital usually requires the assistance of a psychiatric consultant and is well set forth by Missel (1978) in his discussion of suicide risk in rehabilitation settings and by Slaby (1987) in his analysis of the emergency treatment of the depressed patient with physical illness. It is crucial that the patient in the hospital be protected from upper-story windows without shatterproof glass or safety screens, open stairwells, and laundry chutes. Suicidal patients may behave impulsively and for that reason should be constantly supervised by staff or sitters when on medical-surgical units (Goldberg 1987). Anxious, depressed, or confused patients should be given adequate doses of psychotropic medication. Overhead bars, cords, scissors, razors, and other sharp implements should be removed. Personal supplies of potentially harmful substances should be confiscated. An effort to increase the patients' sense of mastery over their circumstances has been cited as useful by Dubovsky (1978). Concerns about the patient's safety should be directly discussed with the patient and, in most cases, the patient's family. Opportunities, such as the care conference described by Cohen and Merlino (1983), for staff to discuss their reactions to caring for the suicidal patient may help generate a consistent approach to the patient. If a patient's medical problems can be managed on a psychiatry service (and this varies from site to site), strong consideration should be given to transferring a suicidal patient to such a service.

Treatment Approaches

Somatic treatment should be aimed at 1) identifying agents that may be causing dysphoria, insomnia, nausea, or agitation; 2) adjusting medical regimens to reduce pain, insomnia, nausea, diarrhea, and constipation; and 3) initiating treatment for depression, anxiety, or psychosis.

When prescribing tricyclic antidepressants, the clinician must consider that the elderly may require a lower dosage, that the physically ill may have little cognitive reserve and hence be especially susceptible to delirium, that the patient may be receiving other anticholinergic agents, and that there may be medical conditions that limit the use of specific antidepressants. Although the tricyclic antidepressants may exacerbate epilepsy, worsen pulmonary functions by drying mucous membranes, or compromise cardiac conduction, careful use of these agents remains a reasonable first-line treatment. The most serious contraindication is the presence of cardiac conduction defects. Use in these instances should follow consultation with a cardiologist. Careful monitoring is necessary since even judicious use of these agents may produce delirium, urinary retention, severe obstipation, postural hypotension with ataxia, and cardiac arrhythmias. If, as occurs in at least half of cases (Popkin et al. 1985), tricyclics are not effective, alternative agents such as stimulants, monoamine oxidase inhibitors, or lithium deserve consideration, depending on the patient's specific medical condition.

A National Institute of Mental Health Consensus Conference (1985) on electroconvulsive therapy (ECT) concluded that increased intracranial pressure was an absolute contraindication and space-occupying lesions in the brain, a recent myocardial infarction, and large aneurysms were relative contraindications to the use of ECT. The report also indicated that the efficacy of ECT in patients with major depression that is nonendogenous or nonmelancholic was not well studied. Weiner (1982), however, found no evidence that the presence of medical illness diminished the therapeutic efficacy of ECT. ECT may become the treatment of choice in the depressed medically ill if drug trials are contraindicated, poorly tolerated, or ineffective, or if therapeutic response within a week is critical.

Psychotherapy should be supportive and nonjudgmental. Feelings of guilt and shame in those afflicted with medical illnesses are quite common. Such reactions are supported by societal tenets that, perhaps self-servingly, view medical illness as exclusively an outcome of profligate behavior. Cognitive-behavioral strategies may help certain patients to recognize maladaptive percepts regarding their illness. The therapist's response to talk of suicide must recognize that suicidal thoughts have diverse meanings: a quantification of distress, a method of arousing support, or a declaration of intent. Identifying which of these meanings predominates will assist in offering a satisfactory mix of empathy, concern, and protection.

Outpatient Management

Outpatient management of a potentially suicidal patient with a significant medical illness requires close collaboration among persons rendering treatment. This begins with ascertaining the name and professional identity of every person involved in all aspects of management. Physicians must take care not to duplicate prescriptions, especially for analgesics or hypnotics, written by colleagues. This is best accomplished by agreeing on which drugs each physician will prescribe in advance. Since changes in medication regimen or medical status may herald significant shifts in mental state and risk of suicide, such information must be promptly available to all caretakers. Psychotropic medications should be dispensed in limited quantities without automatic refills. Firearms in the home should be disarmed or relinquished. Fashioning a contract wherein the patient agrees to call for help if he or she becomes self-destructive is a common, if unproven, management practice. It generally assumes the existence of a crisis line that is staffed 24 hours a day. Who might answer such calls and what they will know about the clinical situation should be made clear to the patient in advance.

CONCLUSION

Medical illness appears to enhance the relative risk of death by suicide. This effect is more notable in men and in the elderly. Jumping from heights is the most common method in patients hospitalized on medical-surgical units. Chronic, incurable, and painful conditions seem to be associated with the greatest risk. AIDS, cancer, peptic ulcer, spinal cord injury, Huntington's chorea, head injury, and renal dialysis are specifically associated with increased rates of death by suicide. The relationship of suicide to multiple sclerosis, premenstrual syndrome, pulmonary disease, rheumatoid arthritis, epilepsy, diabetes mellitus, and hypertension is less clear and requires clarification.

The mechanism by which medical illness increases the relative risk of suicide appears to depend on the illness. In most cases, the victim has shown evidence of a mental disorder, most often depression. Alcoholism is also common, especially in those with peptic ulcer. In other cases, central nervous system impairment, either structural or metabolic, seems to be the operative mechanism. The neuropsychological dysfunction may be global, as in delirium, or limited to thought and/or affect, as is often the case in Huntington's chorea. The occurrence of rational suicide in relation to medical illness appears to be unusual.

It is possible that the suicide rate is increased in some diseases because of associated treatment. For example, the use of reserpine in a group of hypertensive patients may precipitate depression with suicidal intent. Careful scrutiny of treatment modalities is indicated in any disease positively related to suicide.

Little research on the psychiatric histories of persons who commit suicide in relationship to medical illness has been conducted. The literature describes some suicides as having a positive neuropsychiatric history, often alcoholism, but these studies are a minority. Some patients who suicide are noted to be demanding and difficult when confronted with medical illness. Apparently, few have made prior suicide attempts. How many have had full-blown depressive episodes well in advance of their medical illness or have a positive family history of suicide or affective disorder is unknown.

A clinical knowledge of the conditions and circumstances that increase the risk of suicide in the medically ill is a firm foundation for attempts to prevent suicide in this group.

REFERENCES

Abram HS, Moore GL, Westervelt FB: Suicidal behavior in chronic dialysis patients. Am J Psychiatry 127:1199–1204, 1971

Achte KA, Loongvist J, Hillbom E: Suicides following war brain-injuries. Acta Psychiatr Scand (Suppl) 225:7–94, 1971

American Psychiatric Association: Diagnostic and Statistical Manual of Mental Disorders, 3rd Edition, Revised. Washington, DC, American Psychiatric Association, 1987

Barraclough B, Bunch J, Nelson B, et al: A hundred cases of suicide: clinical aspects. Br J Psychiatry 125:355–373, 1974

Beigelman PM: Severe diabetic ketoacidosis (diabetic coma). Diabetes 20:490–500, 1971

Berglund M: Suicide in male alcoholics with peptic ulcers. Alcoholism (NY) 10:631–634, 1986

Blumer D, Benson DF: Psychiatric manifestations of epilepsy, in Psychiatric Aspects of Neurological Disease, Vol 2. Edited by Benson DF, Blumer D. New York, Grune & Stratton, 1982

Bolund C: Suicide and cancer, II: medical and care factors in suicides by cancer patients in Sweden, 1973–1976. Journal of Psychosocial Oncology 48:33–38, 1987

Brown JH, Henteleff P, Barakat S, et al: Is it normal for terminally ill patients to desire death? Am J Psychiatry 143:208–211, 1986

Brown W, Pisetsky JE: Suicidal behavior in a general hospital. Am J Med 29:307–315, 1960

Campbell PC: Suicide among cancer patients. Connecticut Health Bulletin 80:207–212, 1966

Cavan RS (ed): Suicide. Chicago, University of Chicago Press, 1928

Chandler JH, Reed TE, DeJong RN: Huntington's chorea in Michigan. Neurology 10:148–153, 1960

Cohen AS, Vance VK, Runyan JW Jr, et al: Diabetic acidosis: an evaluation of the cause, course and therapy of 73 cases. Ann Intern Med 52:55–86, 1960

Cohen MA, Merlino JP: The suicidal patient on the surgical ward: a multi-disciplinary case conference. Gen Hosp Psychiatry 5:65–71, 1983

Dewhurst K, Oliver JE, McKnight AL: Socio-psychiatric consequences of Huntington's disease. Br J Psychiatry 116:255–258, 1970

DiBiance JT: The hemodialysis patient, in Suicide: Theory and Clinical Aspects. Edited by Hankoff LD, Einsidler B. Littleton, MA, PSG Publishing, 1979

Dorpat TL, Anderson WF, Ripley HS: The relationship of physical illness to suicide, in Suicidal Behaviors: Diagnosis and Management. Edited by Resnik HLP. Boston, Little, Brown, 1968

Dubovsky SL: Averting suicide in terminally ill patients. Psychosomatics 19:113–115, 1978

Ducharme SH, Freed MM: The role of self-destruction in spinal cord injury mortality. Science Digest, Winter 1980, pp 29–38

Engelhardt HT: Suicide and the cancer patient. CA 36:105–109, 1986

Entmacher PS, Krall LP, Kranczer SN: Diabetes mortality from vital statistics, in Joslin's Diabetes Mellitus, 12th Edition. Edited by Marble A, Krall LP, Bradley RF. Philadelphia, Lea & Febiger, 1985

Farberow NL, Shneidman ES, Leonard CV: Medical Bulletin 9: Suicide among general medical and surgical hospital patients with malignant neoplasms. Washington, DC, Department of Medicine and Surgery, Veterans Administration, February 1963, pp 1–11

Farberow NL, McKelligott JW, Cohen S, et al: Suicide among patients with cardiorespiratory illnesses. JAMA 195:422–428, 1966

Farberow NL, Ganzler S, Cutter F, et al: An eight-year survey of hospital suicides. Suicide Life Threat Behav 1:184–202, 1971

Fawcett J: Suicidal depression and physical illness. JAMA 219:1303–1306, 1972

Flavin DK, Franklin JE, Frances RJ: The acquired immune deficiency syndrome (AIDS) and suicidal behavior in alcohol-dependent homosexual men. Am J Psychiatry 143:1440–1442, 1986

Foreign Letters: United Kingdom. JAMA 163:1176, 1957

Fox BH, Stanek EJ, Boyd SD, et al: Suicide rates among cancer patients in Connecticut. J Chronic Dis 35:89–100, 1982

Frances RJ, Wikstrom T, Alcena V: Contracting AIDS as a means of committing suicide. Am J Psychiatry 142:656, 1985

Friedman JH, Cancellieri R: Suicidal risk in a municipal general hospital. Diseases of the Nervous System 19:556–560, 1958

Gabuzda DH, Hirsch MS: Neurological manifestations of infection with human immunodeficiency virus: clinical features and pathogenesis. Ann Intern Med 107:383–391, 1987

Gangat AE, Naidoo LR, Simpson MA: Iatrogenesis and suicide in South African Indians. S Afr Med J 71:171–173, 1987

Glickman LS (ed): Psychiatric Consultation in the General Hospital. New York, Marcel Dekker, 1980

Goldberg RJ: Use of constant observation with potentially suicidal patients in general hospitals. Hosp Community Psychiatry 38:303–305, 1987

Grant I, Atkinson JH, Hesselink JR, et al: Evidence for early central nervous system involvement in the acquired immunodeficiency syndrome (AIDS) and other human immunodeficiency virus (HIV) infections. Ann Intern Med 107:828–836, 1987

Huntington G: On chorea. Medical and Surgical Reports. 26:317–321, 1872

Kahana E, Leibowitz U, Alter M: Cerebral multiple sclerosis. Neurology 21:1179–1185, 1971

Klerman GL: Clinical epidemiology of suicide. J Clin Psychiatry [Suppl] 48:33–38, 1987

Knop J, Fischer A: Duodenal ulcer, suicide, psychopathology and alcoholism. Acta Psychiatr Scand 63:346–355, 1981

Levitan H: Suicidal trends in patients with asthma and hypertension: a case study. Psychother Psychosom 39:165–170, 1983

Levy NB: Psychological problems of the patient on hemodialysis and their treatment. Psychother Psychosom 31:260–266, 1979

Lewiston NJ, Rubinstein S: The young Damocles: the adolescent at high risk for serious or fatal status asthmaticus. Clin Rev Allergy 5:273–284, 1987

Louhivuori KA, Hakama M: Risk of suicide among cancer patients. Am J Epidemiol 109:59–65, 1979

Mackenzie TB, Wilcox K, Baron H: Lifetime prevalence of psychiatric disorders in women with perimenstrual difficulties. J Affective Disord 10:15–19, 1986

Mackinnon PCB, Mackinnon IL: Hazards of the menstrual cycle. Br Med J 1:555, 1956

Marshall JR, Burnett W, Brasure J: On precipitating factors: cancer as a cause of suicide. Suicide Life Threat Behav 13:15–27, 1983

Marzuk PM, Tierney H, Tardiff K, et al: Increased risk of suicide in persons with AIDS. JAMA 259:1333–1337, 1988

Matthews WS, Barabas G: Suicide and epilepsy: a review of the literature. Psychosomatics 22:515–524, 1981

McHugh PR, Folstein MF: Psychiatric syndromes of Huntington's chorea: a clinical and phenomenologic study, in Psychiatric Aspects of Neurologic Disease. Edited by Benson DG, Blumer D. New York, Grune & Stratton, 1975

Miles CP: Conditions predisposing to suicide: a review. J Nerv Ment Dis 164:231–246, 1977

Missel JL: Suicide risk in the medical rehabilitation setting. Arch Phys Med Rehabil 59:371–376, 1978

Muller R: Studies on disseminated sclerosis with special reference to symptomatology, course and prognosis. Acta Med Scand [Suppl] 222:1–214, 1949

National Center for Health Statistics: Vital Statistics of the United States 1978, Vol II: Mortality Part A. Hyattsville, MD, U.S. Department of Health and Human Services, 1982

National Institute of Mental Health Consensus Conference: Electronconvulsive therapy. JAMA 254:2103–2108, 1985

Perlmuter LC, Hakami MK, Hodgson-Harrington C, et al: Decreased cognitive function in aging non-insulin-dependent diabetic patients. Am J Med 77:1043–1048, 1984

Pierce C: Underscore urgency of HIV counseling. Clinical Psychiatry News 15:1, 29, 1987

Pisetsky JE, Brown W: The general hospital patient, in Suicide: Theory and Clinical Aspects. Edited by Hankoff LD, Einsidler B. Littleton, MA, PSG Publishing, 1979

Pokorny AD: Characteristics of forty-four patients who subsequently committed suicide. Arch Gen Psychiatry 2:314–323, 1960

Pollack S: Suicide in a general hospital, in Clues to Suicide. Edited by Shneidman ES, Farberow NL. New York, McGraw-Hill, 1957

Popkin MK, Callies AL, Mackenzie TB: The outcome of antidepressant use in the medically ill. Arch Gen Psychiatry 42:1160–1163, 1985

Popkin MK, Callies AL, Colon EA: A framework for the study of medical depression. Psychosomatics 28:27–33, 1987

Popkin MK, Callies AL, Lentz RD, et al: Prevalence of major depression, simple phobia and other psychiatric disorders in patients with long-standing type I diabetes mellitus. Arch Gen Psychiatry 45:64–68, 1988

Reich P, Kelly MJ: Suicide attempts by hospitalized medical and surgical patients. N Engl J Med 294:298–301, 1976

Robins E, Murphy GE, Wilkinson RH, et al: Some clinical considerations in the prevention of suicide based on a study of 134 successful suicides. Am J Public Health 49:888–899, 1959

Rorsman B, Hagnell O, Lanke J: Violent death and mental disorders in the Lundby study: accidents and suicides in a total population during a 25-year period. Neuropsychobiology 8:233–240, 1982

Ryan C, Vega A, Drash A: Cognitive deficits in adolescents who developed diabetes early in life. Pediatrics 75:921–927, 1985

Sainsbury P (ed): Suicide in London. New York, Basic Books, 1956

Salmon JA, Hajek PT, Rachut E, et al: Mortality conference: suicide of an "appropriately" depressed medical inpatient. Gen Hosp Psychiatry 4:307–313, 1982

Sawyer JD, Adams KM, Conway WL, et al: Suicide in cases of chronic obstructive pulmonary disease. Journal of Psychiatric Treatment and Evaluation 5:281–283, 1983

Schuckit MA, Daley V, Herrman G, et al: Premenstrual symptoms and depression in a university population. Diseases of the Nervous System 36:516–517, 1975

Seager CP, Flood RA: Suicide in Bristol. Br J Psychiatry 111:919–932, 1965

Shneidman ES, Farberow NL, Litman RE (eds): The Psychology of Suicide. New York, Science House, 1970

Siegel K: Psychosocial aspects of rational suicide. Am J Psychother 40:405–418, 1986

Slaby AE: The emergency treatment of the depressed patient with physical illness. Int J Psychiatry Med 17:71–83, 1987

Stearns S: Self-destructive behavior in young patients with diabetes mellitus. Diabetes 8:379–382, 1959

Stewart I: Organic disease and suicide. Lancet 1:1355, 1957

Stewart I: Suicide: the influence of organic disease. Lancet 2:919–920, 1960

Teutsch SM, Herman WH, Dwyer DM, et al: Mortality among diabetic patients using continuous subcutaneous insulin-infusion pumps. N Engl J Med 310:361–368, 1984

Tuckman J, Lavell M: Study of suicide in Philadelphia. Public Health Rep 73:547–553, 1958

Tunbridge WM: Factors contributing to deaths of diabetics under fifty years of age. Lancet 2:569–572, 1981

Viskum K: Ulcer, attempted suicide and suicide. Acta Psychiatr Scand 51:221–227, 1975

Washer GF, Schroter GP, Starzl TE, et al: Causes of death after kidney transplantation. JAMA 250:49–54, 1983

Weiner RD: The role of ECT in the treatment of depression in the elderly. J Am Geriatr Soc 30:710–712, 1982

Wetzel RD, McClure JN: Suicide and the menstrual cycle: a review. Compr Psychiatry 12:369–374, 1972

Wetzel RD, Reich T, McClure JN, et al: Premenstrual affective syndrome and affective disorder. Br J Psychiatry 127:219–221, 1975

Whitlock FA: Suicide, cancer, and depression. Br J Psychiatry 132:269–274, 1978

Wilcox NE, Stauffer ES: Follow-up of 423 consecutive patients admitted to the Spinal Cord Center, Rancho Los Amigos Hospital, 1 January to 31 December 1967. Paraplegia 10:115–122, 1972

Wilder CS: Limitation of activity due to chronic conditions, United States, 1974, Vital and Health Statistics: Series 10, data from the National Health Survey: No 111 (DHEW Publ No HRA-77- 1537). Rockville, MD, June 1977

Strategies for Assessment and Management of Suicidal Patients Over the Life Cycle

Assessment and Interviewing Strategies for Suicidal Patients Over the Life Cycle

Robert L. Hendren, D.O.

ONE OF THE clinician's most important skills in assessing suicidal behavior is the ability to interview patients effectively. Research has indicated that a clinician's manner of communicating with a patient significantly affects the adequacy of the clinical interview, the accuracy of detection of psychological disturbance, the patient's understanding and compliance with the clinician's advice, and the patient's satisfaction (Sanson-Fisher and Maguire 1980). The purposes of the interview are to establish an interaction between the clinician and the patient, to gather necessary data, and to develop a treatment relationship that will enable the patient to accept the clinician's help.

In this chapter, interviewing principles for suicidal behavior are discussed using a developmental approach. Each age group across the entire life cycle has specific risk factors that must be evaluated. A clinician's interviewing style should be modified to the developmental level of the patient to be effective in gathering critical information. Examples of age-specific techniques for use with children, adolescents, adults, and the elderly are provided. Assessment of risk factors and coping abilities of individuals at each developmental level are outlined, and specific guidelines for behavior assessment and effective communication are presented.

Techniques of Communication

The initial presentation of the person with suicidal thoughts varies, and interview styles should be adapted accordingly to establish rapport and gather accurate information. During this first interview, the primary goal is to identify relevant problems systematically while maintaining an empathic working relationship with the patient. This is most likely to occur if the interviewer 1) allows the patient to tell his or her own story while maintaining structure in the interview, 2) employs language appropriate to the patient's age and background, 3) uses tact in framing questions that relate to sensitive matters, 4) moves effectively from one area of questioning to another, 5) allows the patient to express feelings, and 6) conveys an understanding and empathy for the patient's feelings. At the end of the interview, the clinician should provide closure in a way that the patient feels understood and has an understanding of what the next steps will be in the treatment plan. This is most likely to occur if the interviewer informs the patient of the proposed interventions and asks for the patient's response to these recommendations. If it seems likely that the patient will refuse the suggested interventions and the patient is of danger to him- or herself, then additional clinical support should be enlisted before presenting the patient with this information in the final portion of the interview.

The effective interviewer must also be aware of process communications during the interview. Process refers to what happens during the interview that elucidates the patient's and interviewer's emotional reactions to questioning and to the subjects being discussed. Process is particularly evidenced by the sensitivity and sensibility that evolve "beneath the surface" and "between the lines" of the actual verbal exchange. Process communications are often revealed in body language, symbolic reference to past events, avoidance of certain topics, and the interviewer's own emotional reactions. Awareness of these often subtle clues to the patient's feelings is essential to an effective interviewing relationship with the potentially suicidal patient.

Development of open and productive communication with the patient can be guided by specific techniques of asking questions. Interviewing strategies that fit the interviewer's style and comfort should be developed. Specific techniques of communicating are listed in Table 1.

For a person in a high-risk category, such as medical illness, open-ended questions can lead to more direct questions about suicide. Examples include: How are things going? How are your spirits

Table 1. Techniques of communicating

FACILITATION is verbal or nonverbal communication that *encourages the patient to elaborate* on something that he or she said. The patient's last word may be repeated, a questioning look given, or a question asked; for example, "Can you say more about that?"

OPEN-ENDED QUESTIONS are requests stated in general terms for *nonspecific information*; for example, "Tell me more about your sad feelings."

DIRECT QUESTIONS are those that ask the patient for *specific information;* for example, "Do you have a plan for taking your own life?"

SUPPORT comprises both verbal and nonverbal expressions that indicate the interviewer's *interest* and *concern* and *willingness to help* the patient. (Support should not be offered before the patient has expressed his or her feelings.) An example of a supportive statement is "Even though things seem hopeless right now, there are ways that we can help you feel better soon."

EMPATHY is communication that expresses *understanding of and sympathy for the patient's feelings* and the patient's need to express those feelings. (As with support, empathy offered before the patient has told the clinician of his or her feelings is not as effective as it is when offered after.) An example is "I would guess you must have felt very hurt when your girlfriend broke up with you."

REFLECTION is a response from the physician that *repeats, mirrors,* or *echoes* a portion of what the patient has just said; for example, "You said your depression began after your mother died?"

SILENCE is a nonverbal communication that may express a range of responses from total disinterest to active concern. Ideally, silence on the part of the interviewer *leads to very useful information* in that it gives the patient a chance to explore and express deeper, less obvious concerns.

CLARIFICATION is a response that asks the patient for further information and explanation. An example is "How bad have your depressed feelings been?"

CONFRONTATION is a technique that brings the patient face-to-face with or calls attention to some aspect of his or her behavior, appearance, or manner including inconsistencies and contradictions in what the patient has said. An example of a confrontational statement is, "You've told me that you plan to kill yourself, but you say I shouldn't worry about you."

SUMMATION *reviews the information* that has been given by the patient; for example, "Let me see if I have this right—you have been more depressed since your friend committed suicide and have considered taking your own life as well."

INTERPRETATION is a *formulation* by the interviewer of data, events, or thoughts into terms that make the patient aware of their interrelationship. (Interpretations should be used cautiously, especially until the interviewer knows the patient and has established reasonably good rapport.) An example is, "I wonder if your mother's suicide when she was your age is part of what's leading to your suicidal feelings now?"

Source. Adapted from Hendren (1987).

holding up? Do you feel depressed, down in the dumps, or sad? How bad does it get? Are you spending more time alone than usual? Have you gotten so low that you wished you were dead or thought of taking your life? How would you do it? If you were to kill yourself, how do you think it would affect your family? Have you written a note? Is there anything that will help you keep from harming yourself? Have you ever tried to hurt yourself before, even in small ways like taking a few pills?

The clinician should remember that many patients deny suicidal ideation when first asked, and, therefore, the topic should be reassessed at various points during the interview, particularly after rapport has been established. It is the rare severely depressed patient who has not had some fleeting thoughts of suicide. Therefore, total denial of suicidal ideation should be a red flag to the interviewer (Shea 1988).

When the presenting complaint is suicidal thoughts or behavior, questions should be more direct from the beginning. This communicates to the patient that you take these thoughts seriously and want to understand them. For example: Do you have a plan to take your life? Do you feel hopeless about the future? Do you think you are a burden to your loved ones and that you would be better off dead? Have you attempted suicide before? Do you know anyone who has attempted suicide?

A determination of social supports and stressors should also be made. This can often be accomplished by interviewing collateral informants. With regard to stressful life events, the clinician should evaluate such potential stressors as job loss, family disruption, recent losses, or humiliating life experiences. An evaluation of social supports should include an assessment of significant interpersonal relationships; a lack of family, friends, or a confidant; whether the person lives alone; and societal supports such as community or religious affiliations. A hostile interpersonal environment significantly increases suicide risk.

An assessment of the patient's defense mechanisms is useful for determination of the accuracy of information received from the patient and the patient's coping ability. Defenses such as denial, projection, splitting, and acting out are more pathologic and indicate a greater risk and a reduced ability to cope with stress. Healthier defenses such as sublimation, rationalization, humor, and altruism are usually indicative of less risk and greater coping ability (Vaillant et al. 1986). The more rational the suicide appears to the patient, the more concerned the interviewer should become. This is especially the case when patients imagine that their death will serve a humanistic purpose (e.g., "It's the only way I can help my wife") (Shea 1988).

INTERVIEWING PRINCIPLES FOR SUICIDAL ASSESSMENT

In most psychiatric settings, it is important to gather a complete history from the patient and the family to establish a diagnosis and to make treatment recommendations. However, when the clinician is evaluating suicidal behavior, expediency is often crucial, and the assessment process may need to be abbreviated. The clinician's knowledge of specific risk factors for the patient under evaluation becomes extremely important in guiding the interview and assessing suicidal potential. Although as much of the information as possible should come from the patient, family members and friends often must be asked to corroborate, refute, or add information. The interview also should include a mental status examination and an assessment of social support systems.

Risk factors that a clinician should keep in mind to expedite the interviewing process include the presence of psychiatric illnesses, particularly depression, alcoholism, and schizophrenia (Black and Winokur, Chapter 6, this volume). Certain personality factors, such as hostility and hopelessness, have been shown to distinguish depressed individuals who are suicidal from those who are not (Hendin 1986). Delusional depressed patients were found to be five times more likely to kill themselves than depressed patients who were not delusional (Roose et al. 1983). The suicide rate has been found to be 10 times greater among alcoholics than among nonalcoholics (Hendin 1986), and one retrospective study of suicide found a history of alcoholism in approximately 25% of all cases (Robins 1981).

In a follow-up study, Motto et al. (1985) identified 15 variables as significant predictors of suicidal outcome. Included were older age, certain higher level and lower level occupations, and increased financial resources coupled with threatened financial loss. Other variables were emotional disorders in the family, bisexual or homosexual orientation, previous psychiatric hospital admissions, and special recent stresses. Mental status findings that were predictive included ideas of persecution or reference, suicidal impulse, suicidal intent, increased sleep, and weight gain or loss. A negative reaction to the patient by the interviewer was also found to be predictive of suicide.

Other high-risk categories include certain professionals (especially physicians who are in poor physical health), persons who have undergone medical care within the past 6 months, and, of course, persons who have previously attempted suicide (Hendin 1986). Social isolation, the inability to accept help, a high risk–low rescue suicidal plan, low self-worth, and the wish to be reunited with a lost loved one are also associated with increased risk (Bhatia et al. 1986; Jacobs 1983). Certain variables result in greater risk in different age groups. These will be discussed later in this chapter.

Estimation of a patient's ability to cope is another essential component of the initial interview. While psychiatric illnesses involve higher suicidal risk, some suicide attempts occur in persons who are not psychiatrically ill. An estimation of the current stresses and losses, along with a history of how the person has coped with previous crises, is crucial to the evaluation of suicidal risk in every potentially suicidal patient regardless of the number of risk factors present.

During the interview, the clinician should also evaluate the extent of the lethality. This can range from fleeting thoughts of suicide to concrete plans with an accessible method. The clinician should determine how frequently and for how long the patient experiences thoughts of suicide, the concreteness of the suicide plan, and whether actions have been taken to carry out the plan. While patients may reveal bits of information about these elements, it is the responsibility of the clinician to pursue these questions tenaciously and persistently to assess accurately the lethality of the patient's suicidal crisis.

Another important aspect of the successful interview is the evaluation of the clinician's own feelings about the patient. Accurate and appropriate empathy is extremely valuable in establishing rapport and gathering information. When clinicians find they are losing empathy for their patients, it is important to consider the cause. They should ask themselves questions such as: What are my own beliefs about suicide? Do I feel that people who kill themselves are weak? Do I feel that suicide is a sin? Can I imagine killing myself? Have I known a friend, colleague, or family member who committed suicide? How do these feelings affect the way I approach this patient? (Shea 1988). The clinician should be aware that certain hostile patients can elicit angry feelings in the clinician as can patients who repeatedly attempt suicide. Hopeless patients can elicit feelings of hopelessness in those around them. Emotions commonly generated in clinicians evaluating and treating suicidal patients include hate, restlessness, fear, pity, and indifference (Maltsberger and Buie 1974). Additionally, uncovering serious suicidal ideation and plans from a patient may mean additional and taxing work for the clinician. The patient's family may be extremely demanding. When the patient or family resists treatment, the clinician may become involved in involuntary commitment proceedings. In other words, when the clinician does a thorough job in evaluating the patient, there may be a price to pay. These countertransference issues may emerge in such omissions as waiting until the end of the interview to inquire about suicidal thoughts, not inquiring at all, rushing through the assessment, framing questions in ways that will not elicit the needed information, and failure to establish a therapeutic rapport (Shea 1988).

There is a reduced occurrence of counterproductive interactions when the clinician is aware of his or her own feelings. When a clinician's feelings go beyond those that might normally be elicited by the patient's actions, introspective assessment of countertransference feelings is important. When the clinician becomes too angry, frustrated, anxious, or indifferent to deal effectively with a suicidal patient, consultation should be obtained.

A DEVELOPMENTAL APPROACH TO INTERVIEWING

Determination of the patient's developmental level should guide the clinician's interviewing approach (Table 2). The introduction to the patient, the questioning technique, and the analysis of subtle behavioral or historical clues will vary depending on whether the patient is a child, an adolescent, or an adult. Additionally, the interview should be directed toward determination of age-specific risk factors, discussed below. Family relationships are also important in a patient evaluation based on development.

Childhood

The diagnostic interview with a child requires modifications based on the child's use and understanding of language. Play and fantasy are often helpful in establishing initial rapport so that the child can speak comfortably. In young children, much of the interview might consist of metaphorical play, story telling, and projective free drawing. Children may deny suicidal thoughts when asked directly. This may be a result of immature language development, shyness, or psychological disturbance. Play observation and a history of the child's play are often helpful in revealing information not available in the verbal interview.

Four characteristics of play associated with suicidal risk have been described by Pfeffer (1986). Themes of loss and retrieval (e.g., jumping, hiding, and throwing) represent the child's conflicts with separation and autonomy. The repetition of dangerous and reckless behaviors can be seen in children who use their bodies as play objects. Suicidal children may often misuse toys and playthings in such ways as hitting and breaking. Finally, life-endangering acting out of omnipotent fantasies is yet another warning sign of suicidal risk in children. Although some of these play characteristics may be present in nonsuicidal children, or in suicidal children who are improving, the persistence and extent of these characteristics along with the assessment of other risk factors should help identify suicidal risk in younger children.

Table 2. Developmentally appropriate questions in suicidal assessment

	Child	Adolescent	Adult	Elderly
Family functioning	Do your mommy and daddy have bad fights?	How do you get along with your parents?	How have you been feeling about your spouse/children?	How often do you see or talk to your children?
Family history	Has anyone in your family ever died?	Do you know of anyone who has committed suicide?	Has anyone in your family ever been suicidal or severely depressed?	Has anyone in your family ever threatened to end their life?
Past attempts	Have you ever wanted to or tried to stop living?	Have you ever made a plan to kill yourself?	Have you ever thought you and everyone else would be better off if you were dead?	Have you ever gotten so down that you tried to take your own life?
Suicidal intent	What do you think will happen to you if you die?	Can you promise me that you won't hurt yourself at least until you meet with me again?	Do you have any hope that things will get better?	Would you hope to be reunited with your loved ones if you were to take your life?

Depressed	Do you feel sad a lot of the time?	Have you been more irritable and isolated recently?	Do you have trouble sleeping at night, loss of appetite, loss of concentration, and interests?	Have you been "down in the dumps" a lot?
Associated risk factors	Have you ever hurt yourself or someone else on purpose?	Do you or your friends use alcohol or recreational drugs?	How many alcoholic beverages do you drink in a day? week?	Has drinking alcohol ever interfered with your life? Would your family agree?
Social supports	Do your parents have any close friends or family who live nearby?	Do you have any close friends that you tell about these feelings?	How are things going for you at work?	What do you do for fun?
Coping ability	Is there anyone who really cares about you?	Is anything going well in your life?	What do you think will help you through this?	How have you dealt with tough times in the past?
Other	Has anything new or different happened to you or your family recently?	Do you know where to find a gun or rifle?	Have you ever been treated for a psychiatric disorder?	How is your health?

Children who are developmentally mature enough to use language should be evaluated in a verbal mode with language appropriate to their developmental level. The use of language helps the child identify and label disturbing feelings and develop new ways of dealing with conflicts. In addition, the clinician can often help parents understand the child's feelings when the conflicts can be expressed more directly with language.

Certain characteristics of the child and the child's family are associated with greater suicidal risk. Children with certain psychiatric disorders—such as depression, conduct disorder, specific developmental disorders, and adjustment disorder—are vulnerable to suicidal behavior. The severity of the depression in children has been found to be positively associated with the severity of suicidal tendencies (Carlson and Cantwell 1982). The extent of preoccupation with death, recent aggression, and previously stressful experiences (e.g., loss) have also been found to be significantly related to suicidal behavior in children (Pfeffer et al. 1986). The clinician may find certain psychometric inventories useful in evaluating suicide risk in children (see Appendix 1).

Suicidal children often report feeling sad, hopeless, and worthless (Pfeffer 1986). Children's feelings about the meaning of their death and their experiences with the death of relatives, friends, and pets are important to assess. If the child has actually attempted suicide, the child's reasons for this are also important to determine. For instance, was the act meant to hurt or frighten someone else? Did the child really expect to die? Does the child understand the finality of death? Answers to these questions aid in the determination of suicidal potential in the future.

While family assessment is valuable in all potentially suicidal individuals, for the suicidal child it is essential. Parents can provide important information about the child's general functioning, home and school environment, and recent stresses and losses that the child may not be able to describe fully. In addition, family turmoil, parental depression, and suicidal behavior in other family members are important risk factors for childhood suicidal behavior (Mattsson et al. 1969).

Much of the success of the clinician's intervention with a suicidal child depends on the relationship established with the child and the family during the interview. Children usually respond to a kind, nurturing person who understands their method of communication. Engaging the child and the family in a meaningful interview helps to ensure that treatment recommendations will be followed. If clinician-patient engagement does not occur, hospitalization becomes a necessity while the clinician continues trying to establish a working relationship with the child and the parents. Much of this relationship depends on the clinician's ability to use effective, age-appropriate means of communication.

Adolescence

Suicidal thoughts and behavior among adolescents have become more common in recent years (Brent and Kolko, Chapter 11, this volume). In a survey of 380 high school students in New York, 60% reported they had thought of killing themselves and almost 9% reported that they had made at least one attempt to kill themselves (Friedman et al. 1987). Fewer than half the attempters reached the attention of mental health professionals. A psychological autopsy of 20 children and adolescents aged 12 to 19 years who had committed suicide revealed that 85% of the victims had expressed suicidal ideation to others (Shafii et al. 1985). The detection of suicidal intent in adolescents depends in large part on the ability of the clinician to gather important information from the adolescent.

When approaching the suicidal screening of an adolescent, the evaluator should first be well informed about the risk factors for adolescent suicide. This enables the interviewer to ask the pertinent questions necessary to make an adequate assessment in a brief amount of time. Questions should be asked directly and simply. Most adolescents respond well to clearly stated questions and are likely to turn off an interviewer who tries to gather information with indirect and open-ended questions. It is important to take the adolescent's communication seriously. Hollow statements such as "You are so young and have your whole life ahead of you" or "Lots of adolescents feel suicidal but grow out of it" are likely to distance the adolescent.

Characteristics often associated with adolescent suicide include a history of suicidal threats and attempts, drug or alcohol abuse, depression, antisocial behavior, and inhibited personality (Shafii et al. 1985). The inhibited adolescent who does not share problems; is quiet, lonely, sensitive, and introverted; and has few close friends is at high risk. If these factors are also present with antisocial behavior, the adolescent is at even greater risk. School problems, recent stresses and losses, and angry outbursts are other characteristics frequently found in suicidal teenagers (Gispert et al. 1985). Recent direct or indirect exposure to suicide must also be considered as a risk factor (Gould and Shaffer 1986).

Some suicidal adolescents may present with a typical depression, exhibiting sadness, tearfulness, sleep and appetite disturbance, and feelings of hopelessness. However, the presentation of many other young people is characterized by anger, antisocial behavior, and denial of depression. Depression may emerge as a significant factor in these adolescents when questioned directly about recent stresses and losses. Suicidal thoughts may then be expressed.

It is essential to obtain a history of family functioning from the adolescent and the adolescent's family. Family disruption is frequently associated with suicidal feelings in the adolescent. Many attempts are precipitated by family fights. Suicidal behavior in parents, relatives, and friends and a parental history of emotional problems, absence, and abusiveness are found to be significant factors in completed suicides (Shafii et al. 1985). Thirty percent of adolescent runaways have attempted suicide and an additional 28% have suicidal ideation (Shaffer and Caton 1983). Although family problems may not initially be apparent, careful questioning often reveals marital discord, poor communication, parental depression, and acute or chronic stress in the family.

High functioning and gifted adolescents are often overlooked as potential suicide attempters because of their high intelligence and performance (Delisle 1986). The expectations and subsequent pressure placed on gifted adolescents by society, their families, and themselves are often great. The perception of failure in this population may be far different than among average students. Anxieties about their future may seem an unnecessary worry to those around them, but should be taken seriously by the evaluator. It is important to consider the meaning of failures, losses, and stresses in relationship to the adolescent's overview of the world when evaluating all teenagers. It is especially important when assessing suicidal potential in gifted adolescents since they may superficially appear to be coping well when compared to other teenagers.

The essential components of the interview to assess suicidal potential in an adolescent consist of a history of suicide attempts, family functioning, school performance, depression, psychiatric disturbance, drug and alcohol use, and stressful life events, including recent humiliating life events (Blumenthal and Kupfer 1988). Comparing this information with the risk factors previously described will help make a clinical prediction of risk. Further determinations to help guide the nature and extent of the intervention include the patient's 1) ability to promise abstention from suicidal behavior, 2) ability to give compliments to oneself and others, 3) capacity to identify and express feelings, and 4) capacity to plan ahead for suicidal situations (Rotheram 1987). The response to these questions will help in the determination of the adolescent's coping ability. Using this information, the clinician is then able to make an appropriate intervention to protect the adolescent from self-destruction while receiving treatment.

Adulthood

While adolescents who attempt suicide often express their anger overtly, suicidal adults are more likely to have a constriction of affective expression, with indirect hostility often directed toward themselves. Particular subgroups of the population are at greater risk than others. Former psychiatric inpatients are more likely than controls to commit suicide within 2 years of discharge (Winokur and Black 1987). This is especially so for those with a diagnosis of unipolar depression or alcoholism. Persons exhibiting signs of psychosis or dementia are also at high risk. As in other age groups, the most serious risk factor is a previous attempt. Suicide in close friends and family members also increases risk, especially around anniversaries of their death. The risk of suicide is also greater in adult white males, in persons over age 45, and in persons who have a detailed, highly lethal suicidal plan (Smith and Bope 1986). Medical illness increases the risk of suicide in adults (Mackenzie and Popkin, Chapter 9, this volume), especially if it leads to immobility, severe pain, loss of dignity, impaired judgment, or disfigurement. In a review of studies from the United States and Great Britain, Mackenzie and Popkin (1987) found physical illness to be present in 20% to 70% of suicides and to be an important risk factor in 11% to 51% of these cases. A number of studies indicate that the suicide rate is increased in patients with cancer, head injury, and peptic ulcer. Huntington's chorea, multiple sclerosis, and spinal cord injury are also associated with increased suicidal risk. Alcoholism, neurologic dysfunction, and severe or incapacitating medical conditions appear to link physical illness and suicide. Hospitalized patients at greatest risk of suicide include "accident victims" and patients who are belligerent, complaining, demanding, and dissatisfied with their medical care (McAlpine 1987).

In highly specialized subgroups of the adult population, suicide may have specific characteristics. For example, studies indicate that suicides among women physicians occur two to three times more often than in the general population (Holmes and Rich, Chapter 22, this volume). Psychiatrists are reported to have twice the frequency of other physicians (Simon 1986). Those male and female physicians at greatest risk show other signs of impairment, such as drug and alcohol abuse and depression prior to their attempt. High-risk periods occur when the physician is establishing a new practice after completion of residency and when the physician nears retirement.

In assessing suicidal potential in adults, it is important to ask directly about the patient's own opinion of his or her suicidal risk and to obtain a history of previous suicide attempts. The presence of social supports, a family history of suicide, symptoms of depression, recent losses, and use of alcohol and other drugs require direct inquiry (Blumenthal 1988; Jamison 1987). The clinician should evaluate the mental status of the patient and should specifically note whether there is evidence of hallucinations or delusions or other psychiatric impairment. The patient's sense of hopelessness should also be carefully evaluated as it has been shown to be the best long-term predictor of eventual suicide (Beck 1987).

The clinician should attempt to construct a clear understanding of the patient's suicidal thoughts to assess suicidal risk. Such a profile would include information about how often the patient has felt suicidal, how long episodes last, what is helpful in alleviating suicidal feelings, and the methods of suicide that have been considered. It is often helpful to ask patients to describe the fantasy of the suicide. This description should include how they would prepare for it and the patient's views regarding what would happen after the suicide. Very concrete plans, a wish to be reunited with a deceased loved one, putting one's affairs in order, and a feeling that "things would be better for everyone if I were dead" are ominous signs.

Older Age

The highest suicide rates are found in people over the age of 50. While this group makes up 26% of the United States population, it accounts for approximately 39% of the total deaths by suicide (Hendin 1986). Among this group, the highest rate occurs in white males.

Loneliness, isolation, and feelings of hopelessness and helplessness are the characteristics most frequently found in presuicidal elderly people (Achte and Karha 1985; Osgood and Thielman, Chapter 13, this volume). Often there is ambivalence in the wish to live or die. Loss, separation, and abandonment are themes common in the thinking of all suicidal people and are especially so in the elderly. Older people suffer many losses as friends and family die and as their bodily functions deteriorate. They are also closer to death because of their position in the life cycle. All of these risk factors, important at other developmental levels, become an everyday part of the life of the elderly. The ability to deal with these issues depends on the meaning and personal significance they have to each individual. Because previous coping ability is often predictive of current coping ability, a clinician should also attempt to assess how the elderly person adjusted to stress and loss at previous developmental levels. In this regard, it is also important to assess the strength of social supports currently available to the older person.

Depression is an important symptom of suicidal behavior in the elderly. Depressive disorders in older people often manifest themselves in somatic symptoms, such as tiredness, fatigue, lack of energy, agitation, fretfulness, and early morning insomnia (Achte and Karha 1985). Excessive complaints about bodily function are another clue to underlying depression. Confusion and memory loss may also be present. Poor health, loss of personal dignity, retirement from work and decreased income, and relocation to a new and possibly less comfortable environment are other contributors to depression in the elderly that may lead to suicidal behavior.

An older person is often reluctant to talk directly about suicidal feelings. Direct questions about suicide asked early in the interview are likely to be unanswered or answered in the negative. The interviewer should convey a sincere interest in the person and be patient and empathic as the older person tells of his or her life, losses, family, and concerns about bodily functions. Gentle questions about losses, depression, and, finally, suicidal thoughts are most apt to get accurate responses. Direct questions about risk factors such as substance abuse, depressive symptoms, and previous suicide attempts are best asked later in the interview, when rapport and trust have been established. Knowledge of the life of the individual makes possible an understanding of the subjective meanings of the life situations or crises being encountered, which, in turn, gives meaning to the suicidal behavior. At this point, too, interventions are more likely to be accepted.

SUMMARY

The assessment of suicidal potential with people of all ages is done most effectively by an empathic and knowledgeable interviewer. Knowledge of age-specific risk factors should guide the interviewer in gathering necessary information effectively. Coping ability, support systems, substance abuse, psychiatric illness including depression, and access to a lethal method are important factors to assess in all age groups. Clinicians use their craft to weigh these risk factors, historical information, and assessment of intervention resources to make judgments about relative risk and treatment strategies. Additionally, during the process of the interview, the clinician has helped the patient to share painful feelings that have often been shouldered alone. Using a life-cycle perspective, the interview with a child requires modifications based on the child's use and understanding of language. With younger children, much of the interview might consist of fantasy and play. Themes of loss, danger, and destruction are seen frequently in the play of suicidal children. In assessing suicidal potential in an adolescent, the interviewer should be direct and open. Previous suicide attempts, drug and alcohol abuse, depression, antisocial behavior, and an inhibited personality are associated with increased suicidal risk in teenagers. Suicidal adults are less likely than adolescents to express anger overtly and may direct hostility toward themselves. Former psychiatric inpatients and individuals with affective disorder, alcoholism, or certain medical illnesses are at high risk for suicide. Direct questions about the adults' opinion of their own suicidal risk is often a helpful predictor of risk. Individuals over 50 years of age have the highest suicide rates of any age group. Loneliness, isolation, loss, and hopelessness are frequently found in presuicidal elderly people. Excessive complaints about bodily function, tiredness, confusion, and agitation are clues to underlying depression in older individuals. The interviewer should gently and patiently establish rapport with the elderly person before asking direct questions about suicide.

The diagnostic interview is a critical element of suicide prevention. The clinician's ability to adapt his or her interviewing style to the patient's position in the life cycle leads to an accurate assessment of suicidal potential. A thorough diagnostic evaluation permits the clinician to construct interventions that will protect the patient from self-destruction while receiving appropriate treatment. Additionally, the clinician's sensitive and thorough questioning conveys to the patient that someone cares and, in this way, begins to form an important lifeline to a source of lifesaving support and treatment.

REFERENCES

Achte K, Karha E: Some psychodynamic aspects of the presuicidal syndrome with special reference to older persons. Crisis 7:24–32, 1985

Beck AT: Reported in Clinical Psychiatry News 15:17, 1987

Bhatia SC, Khan MH, Sharma A: Suicide risk: evaluation and management. Am Fam Physician 34:167–174, 1986

Blumenthal SJ: A guide to risk factors, assessment and treatment of the suicidal patient. Med Clin North Am 72:937–971, 1988

Blumenthal SJ, Kupfer DJ: Overview of early detection and treatment strategies for suicidal behavior in young people. Journal of Youth and Adolescence 17:1–23, 1988

Carlson GA, Cantwell DP: Suicidal behavior and depression in children and adolescents. Journal of the American Academy of Child Psychiatry 21:361–368, 1982

Delisle JR: Death with honors: suicide among gifted adolescents. Journal of Counseling and Development 64:558–560, 1986

Friedman JMH, Asnis GM, Boeck M, et al: Prevalence of specific suicidal behaviors in a high school sample. Am J Psychiatry 144:1203–1206, 1987

Gispert M, Wheeler K, Marsh L, et al: Suicidal adolescents: factors in evaluation. Adolescence 20:753–762, 1985

Gould MS, Shaffer D: The impact of suicide in television movies: evidence of imitation. N Engl J Med 325:690–694, 1986

Hendin H: Suicide: a review of new directions in research. Hosp Community Psychiatry 37:148–154, 1986

Hendren RL: Communication and interviewing, in Behavioral Science: A National Medical Series Book for NBME Study and Review. Edited by Wiener JM. Media, PA, Harwal Publishing, 1987, pp 197–209

Jacobs D: Evaluation and care of suicidal behavior in emergency settings. International Journal of Psychiatry 12:295–310, 1983

Jamison KR: Psychotherapeutic issues and suicide prevention in the treatment of bipolar disorders, in Psychiatry Update: American Psychiatric Association Annual Review, Vol 6. Washington, DC, American Psychiatric Press, 1987, pp 108–124

Mackenzie TB, Popkin MD: Suicide in the medical patient. International Journal of Psychiatry 17:3–22, 1987

Maltsberger JT, Buie DH: Countertransference hate in the treatment of suicidal patients. Arch Gen Psychiatry 30:625–633, 1974

Mattsson A, Seese LR, Hawkins JW: Suicidal behavior as a child psychiatric emergency. Arch Gen Psychiatry 20:100–109, 1969

McAlpine DE: Suicide: recognition and management. Mayo Clin Proc 62:778–781, 1987

Motto JA, Heilbron DC, Juster RP: Development of a clinical instrument to estimate suicide risk. Am J Psychiatry 142:680–686, 1985

Pfeffer CR: The Suicidal Child. New York, Guilford Press, 1986, pp 173–203

Pfeffer CR, Plutchik R, Mizruchi MS, et al: Suicidal behavior in child psychiatric inpatients and outpatients and in nonpatients. Am J Psychiatry 143:733–738, 1986

Robins E: The Final Months: A Study of the Lives of 134 Persons Who Committed Suicide. New York, Oxford University, 1981

Roose SP, Glassman AH, Walsh BT, et al: Depression, delusions, and suicide. Am J Psychiatry 140:1159–1162, 1983

Rotheram MJ: Evaluation of imminent danger for suicide among youth. Am J Orthopsychiatry 57:102–110, 1987

Sanson-Fisher R, Maguire P: Should skills in communicating with patients be taught in medical schools? Lancet 2:523–526, 1980

Shaffer D, Caton C: Runaway and Homeless Youth in New York City: A Report to the Ittleson Foundation, New York, 1983 (unpublished report)

Shafii M, Carrigan S, Whittinghill JR, et al: Psychological autopsy of completed suicide in children and adolescents. Am J Psychiatry 142:1061–1064, 1985

Shea SC: Psychiatric Interviewing: The Art of Understanding. Philadelphia, WB Saunders, 1988, pp 409–441

Simon W: Suicide among physicians: prevention and postvention. Crisis 7:1–13, 1986

Smith CW, Bope ET: The suicidal patient: the primary care physician's role in evaluation and treatment. Postgrad Med 79:195–202, 1986

Vaillant GE, Bond M, Vaillant CO: An empirically validated hierarchy of defense mechanisms. Arch Gen Psychiatry 43:786–794, 1986

Winokur G, Black DW: Psychiatric and medical diagnoses as risk factors for mortality in psychiatric patients: a case-control study. Am J Psychiatry 144:208–211, 1987

Chapter 11

The Assessment and Treatment of Children and Adolescents at Risk for Suicide

David A. Brent, M.D.
David J. Kolko, Ph.D.

SUICIDE IS NOW the second-leading cause of death among adolescents (Centers for Disease Control 1985; Shaffer and Fisher 1981). Suicidal behavior has also become increasingly common among youth (Hawton et al. 1981; Kosky 1987; O'Brien 1977; Weissman 1974; Wexler et al. 1978), and the assessment of suicidality among young people is the most common emergency encountered by child and adolescent psychiatrists (Mattsson et al. 1969; Shafii et al. 1979). Furthermore, a high proportion of child and adolescent psychiatric patients show evidence of serious suicidal ideation or behavior (Brent et al. 1986; Carlson and Cantwell 1982; Pfeffer 1982; Pfeffer et al. 1979, 1980; Ryan et al. 1987). Therefore, the assessment and diminution of suicidal potential among youthful psychiatric patients should be a task of the highest priority for the practicing child psychiatrist and health care professional.

In this chapter, we will review the descriptive epidemiology and associated risk factors for youthful suicide, suicidal behavior, and suicidal ideation. A discussion of the assessment of suicidal potential in youthful psychiatric patients, as well as a delineation of the contribution of psychosocial stressors, specific psychiatric syndromes, in-

---

This chapter is dedicated to the memory of Joaquim Puig-Antich, M.D. (1944–1989).

tercurrent medical illness, personality and cognitive style, and family and environmental factors to suicidal risk, will follow. In the second half of this chapter, the application of current knowledge about risk factors for suicide in psychiatric patients to the prevention of suicidality through empirically based psychiatric treatment of patients at high risk for suicide is discussed. In the last section of this chapter, the indications for psychiatric inpatient treatment are delineated. Finally, both somatic and psychosocial treatments are examined with respect to their potential effectiveness in diminishing the risk for subsequent suicide and suicidal behavior in psychiatric patients.

EPIDEMIOLOGY AND RISK FACTORS FOR YOUTHFUL SUICIDE

As noted above, suicide is the second-leading cause of death among adolescents 15 to 19 years old. Moreover, the rate of suicide in this age group has tripled in the past three decades from 2.6 to 8.5 per 100,000 (Centers for Disease Control 1985; Shaffer and Fisher 1981). Although some of this increase may be attributable to coroners' increasing willingness to render a verdict of suicide in an adolescent in recent years, there is no question that there has been a true increase in the youth suicide rate (Brent et al. 1987a; Kosky 1987; Sims 1974).

The reasons for this increase are unclear. Several investigators have hypothesized that a cohort effect has rendered the postwar generation of youth more vulnerable to depression and, consequently, suicide (Hellon and Solomon 1980; Klerman et al. 1985; Murphy and Wetzel 1980; Shaffer and Fisher 1981). The increase in the youthful suicide rate has also been linked to a parallel increase in the abuse of alcohol (Brent et al. 1987a) and greater availability of firearms (Brent et al. 1987a). Publicity about suicide has also been hypothesized to have fueled the increased rate among youth (Gould et al. 1987b; Shaffer and Fisher 1981), as have the increased divorce rate, increased mobility, and a decrease in religious affiliation (McAnarney 1979). Finally, the suicide rate among adolescents has been correlated with the proportion of adolescents in the total population. It has been suggested that the competition for scarce resources that is associated with larger birth cohorts has contributed to the increased rate of suicide observed among youth born after World War II (Holinger and Offer 1982). Table 1 presents the risk factors for suicide.

Age

Suicide is extremely rare among prepubertal children; among adolescents, the rate increases with increasing age (Shaffer and Fisher 1981). Most epidemiologic studies have not documented an increase in the suicide rate among 10- to 14-year-olds; this increase is confined to

Table 1. Risk factors for suicide

	Versus controls	Versus suicidal patients
Demographic		
Sex	Male	Male
Age	Older	Older
Ethnic group	White	−
	Native American	−
Psychiatric		
Any disorder	+	o
Affective disorder	+	o
Affective disorder with comorbidity	+	+
Bipolar disorder	+	+
Psychosis	+	+
Substance abuse	+	o
Conduct problems	+	?
Personality disorder	+	?
Past suicidal threats or behavior	+	o
Past psychiatric treatment	+	−
High suicidal intent/lethality	?	+
Family/environmental		
Family history of psychiatric disorder:		
Any disorder	+	o
Suicide	+	+
Suicidal behavior	+	o
Affective disorder	+	o
Other environmental		
Parental absence	+	o
Parental abuse	+	?
Numerous life stressors	+	?
Availability of firearms	?	+
Exposure to suicide	+	o
Medical		
Epilepsy	+	?
Perinatal stress	+	?

Note. + = risk factor more common in completed suicide. − = risk factor less common in completed suicide. o = no association. ? = association not yet investigated.
Source. Brent and Kolko 1990. Reprinted with permission from WB Saunders.

older adolescents and young adults (Brent et al. 1987a; Shaffer and Fisher 1981).

The relatively low rate of suicide among prepubertal children and younger adolescents deserves special consideration. While prepubertal children and younger adolescents frequently experience serious suicidal thoughts and impulses (Brent et al. 1986; Carlson and Cantwell 1982; Pfeffer 1982; Pfeffer et al. 1979, 1980; Ryan et al. 1987), this age group may be protected against suicide by their cognitive immaturity (Shaffer and Fisher 1981). As a result, they may be unable to plan and execute a lethal suicide act. Conversely, a greater-than-expected proportion of young adolescent suicide completers have been shown to have IQs above 130 (Shaffer 1974). Therefore, it is possible that intellectual precocity may override the putatively protective effects of cognitive immaturity. Other factors that may protect this age group against suicide include greater familial support and the relatively low incidence of depression in this age group (Shaffer and Fisher 1981).

Sex

The rate among males is much higher than among young females (Centers for Disease Control 1985; Shaffer and Fisher 1981). This may be related to males' propensity to resort to violent, irreversible methods of suicide, whereas female suicide attempters often engage in less lethal methods. Interestingly, in Asian countries such as Singapore and India, the rates among adolescents are comparable between males and females (Chia 1979; Kua and Tsoi 1985; Sathyavathi 1975).

Ethnicity

The suicide rate is higher among whites as compared to blacks (Earls et al., Chapter 21, this volume). It is among white males in whom the greatest increase in the suicide rate has been observed over the past three decades (Brent et al. 1987a; Murphy and Wetzel 1980). The gap between white and black suicide rates is greatest in the Southeastern United States and least in the urban North and Midwest (Shaffer and Fisher 1981). This geographic difference has been attributed to greater cultural assimilation by Northern blacks, with attendant loss of traditional forms of social support (Shaffer and Fisher 1981). Young Native Americans also show a very high rate of suicide, which varies greatly by tribe, with higher rates observed among youth in those tribes that have undergone more cultural assimilation and have associated high rates of alcoholism, delinquency, and family disorganization (Berlin 1987). A similar pattern has been observed among Micronesian adolescent and young adult males, who show an extraordinarily high suicide rate (Rubenstein 1983). The portion of the Micronesian archipelago with the highest suicide rates are those islands that are neither Westernized nor traditional, but are currently undergoing a cultural transition (Rubenstein 1983).

Marital Status

Although the rate of suicide is lower among married than among single adults, marriage appears to confer an increased risk for suicide in adolescence, particularly for females (Kreitman and Schreiber 1979). Unwed, pregnant young women are at increased risk (Blumenthal 1988).

Method

In the United States, firearms are the most common method of suicide among youth for both sexes. Other common methods of suicide in the United States, in descending frequency, include hanging, carbon monoxide poisoning, jumping, and overdose (Centers for Disease Control 1985; Shaffer and Fisher 1981). Suicides by firearms among youth have increased faster than suicide by other methods (Boyd 1983; Boyd and Moscicki 1986; Brent et al. 1987a) and appear to be a particularly common method of suicide when the victim was intoxicated (Brent et al. 1987a). There is evidence that the suicide rate by firearms is correlated with the production, sales, and ownership of guns (Kellerman and Reay 1986; Markush and Bartolucci 1984) and inversely correlated with the restrictiveness of gun control laws (Lester 1983; Lester and Murrell 1980). Moreover, in one study, after controlling for demographic and diagnostic variables, adolescent suicide victims were 2.5 times more likely to have a gun available to them in their homes than were hospitalized suicidal adolescents (Brent et al. 1988b). The British and Australian experience suggests that the availability of other methods of suicide (domestic gas and sedatives, respectively) can favorably influence the suicide rate (Goldney and Katsikitis 1983; Kreitman 1976).

Profile of Youthful Suicide Completers

There have been relatively few investigations into the characteristics of youth who commit suicide (Brent et al. 1988b; Shaffer 1974; Shaffer et al. 1985; Shafii 1986b; Shafii et al. 1985). In addition to these investigations are a few follow-up studies of youthful psychiatric patients (Otto 1972; Welner et al. 1979). Therefore, our picture of adolescent suicide at this point in time is incomplete.

Precipitants

In a study of the characteristics of 31 young adolescents who committed suicide in England and Wales, Shaffer (1974) noted that disciplinary crises, interpersonal loss, and interpersonal conflict were common precipitants for suicide. Other studies have indicated that interpersonal conflict and increased number of stressors seem to play a contributory role (Brent et al. 1988b; Shafii 1986b). One of the key elements in precipitants for adolescent suicide is that of humiliation (Blumenthal and Kupfer 1988).

Circumstances of the Suicide

There is evidence that youthful suicide victims are frequently intoxicated with alcohol (Brent et al. 1987a, 1988b; Friedman 1985). Despite the disinhibiting effects of alcohol, it appears that many adolescent suicides show evidence of high suicidal intent, as manifested by planning, leaving a note, choice of an irreversible method, and timing the suicide attempt so as to avoid discovery and rescue (Brent et al. 1988b; Shaffer 1974).

Psychiatric Variables

There is convergent evidence that the majority of adolescent suicide victims have at least one major psychiatric disorder at the time of death (Brent et al. 1988b; Shafii 1986b; Shafii et al. 1985). Both affective and antisocial symptomatology appear to play a role in adolescent suicide, often concurrently (Brent et al. 1988b; Blumenthal and Kupfer 1988; Shaffer 1974; Shafii 1986b; Shafii et al. 1985). In fact, in the studies where psychiatric diagnoses were rendered through use of the psychological autopsy approach, between 63% and 76% of suicide victims had an affective disorder (Brent et al. 1988b; Shafii 1986b), with one study indicating that more than one-fifth of suicide victims had a diagnosis of bipolar disorder (Brent et al. 1988b). Substance abuse was diagnosed in more than one-third of youthful suicide victims, both alone, and in combination with affective disorder (Brent et al. 1988b; Rich et al. 1986; Shafii 1986b; Shafii et al. 1985). Previous suicidality was noted in a substantial proportion (44% to 85%) of these victims (Brent et al. 1988b; Shaffer 1974; Shafii et al. 1985). Finally, while many of these victims had had at least one mental health contact (30% to 45%), few were actively engaged in treatment at the time of death (Brent et al. 1988b; Shaffer 1974; Shafii et al. 1985).

Social Functioning

The social adaptation and personality characteristics of youthful suicide victims have not been carefully assessed. However, a substantial minority appear to show academic and behavioral problems in school, antisocial behavior resulting in legal difficulties, and personality problems such as inhibition, perfectionism, and explosiveness (Shaffer 1974; Shafii et al. 1985).

Family History

The families of suicide completers appear to have very high rates of psychiatric disorder, particularly unipolar and bipolar disorders, antisocial personality disorder, and attempted and completed suicide (Brent et al. 1988b; Shaffer 1974; Shafii et al. 1985). The family history of suicide and suicidal behavior may confer a genetic risk to offspring and may also serve as a model for imitation (Blumenthal and Kupfer 1988; Shaffer 1974).

Family Environment

Shaffer (1974) noted a high prevalence of marital breakdown among the parents of young suicide victims. This relationship appears to be nonspecifically related to an increased risk for a variety of psychiatric disorders and may be a consequence of the parental tendency to psychiatric disorder as well. Suicide victims have been noted to experience more parental absence and abuse than controls (Shafii et al. 1985).

Exposure to Suicide

In addition to the familial aggregation of suicide, there is additional evidence that exposure to suicide may predispose to suicide as well as suicidal behavior among youth. There are reports of outbreaks of adolescent suicide and suicidal behavior far in excess of the expected frequency in several communities (e.g., suicide clusters) (Coleman 1987; Gould et al. 1987b; Robbins and Conroy 1983; Ward and Fox 1977). Adolescent completers are much more likely to have been exposed to a suicide than demographically matched friends, and the rate of suicide is increased in the close friends of suicide victims on follow-up (Shafii 1986a, 1986b; Shafii et al. 1985). Finally, there is evidence that media publicity about suicide is followed by an increase in suicide, regardless of whether such publicity is propagated by newspaper (Phillips 1974; Shepherd and Barraclough 1978), television news reports (Phillips and Carstensen 1986), or fictional television docudramas (Gould and Shaffer 1986). This increase appears to be confined to younger populations (Gould and Shaffer 1986; Phillips and Carstensen 1986; Shepherd and Barraclough 1978), appears to be proportional to the amount and type of publicity (i.e., more sensationalized) (Phillips 1974; Phillips and Carsensen 1986; Shepherd and Barraclough 1978), and may vary by locale (Gould et al. 1987a; Phillips and Paight 1987).

Medical Illness

The only medical illness that has been conclusively linked to suicide in the adolescent age group is that of epilepsy (Matthews and Barabas 1981; Silanpaa 1973). The use of phenobarbital as an anticonvulsant appears to increase the risk for depression and suicidal ideation among epileptic children (Brent et al. 1987b). Since depression and suicidal ideation are frequent precursors of suicide among youth, it is possible that phenobarbital may contribute to the high risk for suicide that has been described among young epileptic patients. In addition to the association between epilepsy and suicide, an increased risk of suicide has been noticed in adolescents who have previously experienced perinatal distress (Salk et al. 1985).

There have been no controlled investigations into the prevalence of physical illness in youthful suicide victims. Sathyavathi (1975) found that 29% of a series of 45 young suicide victims in India had some kind of physical illness; other studies have found much lower prevalences (Chia 1979; Shaffer 1974). Chronic physical illness appears to be a much more important contributory factor to suicide in older adults (Rich et al. 1986). However, as acquired immune deficiency syndrome (AIDS) becomes more prevalent in the adolescent population, this disorder may contribute to the suicide rate, as it has in older adults (Blumenthal 1988; Marzuk et al. 1988).

EPIDEMIOLOGY AND RISK FACTORS FOR SUICIDAL BEHAVIOR

Suicide attempters and completers are two distinct but overlapping populations. The two groups are distinct insofar as attempters tend to be primarily female, and only a minority (.1% to 10%) of youthful attempters go on to complete suicide (Blumenthal and Kupfer 1988; Goldacre and Hawton 1985; Otto 1972). However, the two groups overlap insofar as a large proportion of completers have made previous attempts, both groups show high rates of psychiatric disturbance, and the risk for suicide is elevated 100- to 1,000-fold in suicide attempters when compared to the population (Brent et al. 1988b; Goldacre and Hawton 1985; Otto 1972; Shaffer 1974; Shafii 1986b; Shafii et al. 1985). Table 2 presents the risk factors for suicidal behavior.

Descriptive Epidemiology

The rate of suicidal behavior among adolescents and young adults has shown a dramatic increase over the three decades following World War II (Hawton and Goldacre 1982; Hawton et al. 1981; Kosky 1987;

O'Brien 1977; Weissman 1974; Wexler et al. 1978). A study in the Oxford area of Great Britain indicates that the rates of attempted suicide increased from 97 to 131 per 100,000 among 12- to 15-year-olds from 1979, with similar increases in the rates of attempted suicide observed among 16- to 20-year-olds (277 to 341 per 100,000) (Hawton and Goldacre 1982). In Great Britain, intentional overdose is now the leading reason for admission to a hospital, accounting for 4.7% of all hospital admissions (Hawton and Goldacre 1982). The absolute prevalence of suicidal behavior is likely to be much higher than reflected in these figures, given that only as few as 12% of adolescent suicide attempters ever come to medical attention (Smith and Crawford 1986). Epidemiologic studies in public high schools, medical clinics, and community samples indicate that the prevalence of such behavior may be even more common than previously thought. The 12-month and lifetime prevalences of suicidal behavior are 4% and 8% to 9%, respectively, when high school students and pediatric clinic attendees were surveyed by self-report questionnaires (Harkavy-Friedman et al. 1987; Robins 1989; Smith and Crawford 1986). On the other hand, one community psychiatric epidemiologic survey reported a lifetime prevalence of suicide attempts of 3.5% as determined by psychiatric interviews (Velez and Cohen 1988).

Sex

Although females make suicide attempts much more frequently than males, some investigators report that the gap has narrowed in recent years (O'Brien 1977). The reported ratio of female to male attempters ranges from 3:1 to 9:1 (Garfinkel et al. 1982; Harkavy-Friedman et al. 1987; Hawton et al. 1982b, 1982c; Otto 1972; Smith and Crawford 1986). The reasons for the female preponderance of attempters are unknown, but may relate to females' preference for less lethal methods of suicidal behavior, their greater comfort with engaging in covert and overt help-seeking behavior, and their higher rate of affective disorder, of which suicidal behavior is frequently a symptom (Hawton et al. 1982c; Shaffer and Fisher 1981).

Age

Suicidal behavior is rare among prepubertal children, although suicidal thoughts are commonly found in psychiatrically referred patients in this age group (Brent et al. 1986; Carlson and Cantwell 1982; Pfeffer 1982; Pfeffer et al. 1979, 1980, 1984; Ryan et al. 1987). Within the adolescent age group, suicidal behavior becomes more frequent with increasing age (Carlson and Cantwell 1982; Hawton and Goldacre 1982: Robins 1989).

Table 2. Risk factors for suicidal behavior

	Versus controls	Versus nonsuicidal psychiatric patients	Repeated attempted	High intent/ high lethality
Demographic				
Sex	Female	Female	o	Male
Age	Older	Older	?	Older
Socioeconomic status	Lower	?	?	?
Psychiatric				
Any disorder	+	o	o	o
Chronic, severe disorder	+	+	+	+
Affective disorder	+	+	o	+
Substance abuse	+	+	o	o
Conduct disorder	?	+	o	?
Psychosis	+	?	?	?
Personality disorder	+	+	+	?
Past suicidal threats or behavior	+	+	+	?
Past psychiatric treatment	+	?	—	?
Psychological				
Hostility	+	+	+	?
Hopelessness	+	+	+	+
Poor social skills	+	+	+	?
Poor school performance	+	?	+	—
Impulsivity	+	+	+	?
Cognitive distortion/poor coping strategies		+	?	?

Family/environmental				
Family history of psychiatric disorder:				
Any psychiatric disorder	+	o	?	o
Suicide/suicidal behavior	+	+	?	+
Affective disorder	+	+	?	?
Alcohol/drug abuse	+	o	?	o
Other environmental				
Physical/sexual abuse	+	+	+	?
Discord	+	+	?	?
Parental absence/loss	+	o	+	?
Exposure to suicide behavior	+	?	?	?
Total life stressors	+	+	?	?
Medical				
Epilepsy (perhaps in concert with use of phenobarbital)	+	?	+	+

Note. + = risk factor associated with category. − = risk factor less common in completed suicide. o = no association. ? = association not yet investigated.

Source. Brent and Kolko 1990. Reprinted with permission from WB Saunders.

Race and Socioeconomic Status

Few epidemiologic studies have surveyed areas with large minority populations. However, in studies based on emergency rooms, suicidal behavior may be more prevalent among poor and minority youth (Garfinkel et al. 1982; Kosky 1983; Mattsson et al. 1969; McIntire and Angle 1970). One community survey found no association between socioeconomic status and suicide attempts (Velez and Cohen 1988).

Motivation

Suicide attempters show variable intent. In one consecutive series of adolescent attempters seen in a pediatric emergency room, only one-third wanted to die (Brent 1987). Often the motivation for the attempt is not to die, but rather a desire to influence significant others to gain attention, to communicate love or anger, or simply to escape a noxious situation (Hawton et al. 1982c). Most frequently, suicide attempts by adolescents are impulsive and result in little threat to life (Brent 1987; Hawton et al. 1982b, 1982c).

Precipitants

The precipitants for suicidal behavior among children and adolescents are similar to those for adolescent suicide. Frequently, interpersonal conflicts, either with a parent or a romantic attachment, are prominent (Brent et al. 1988b; Hawton et al. 1982a). Interpersonal loss, physical and sexual abuse, family discord, an unwanted pregnancy, and parental psychiatric illness have also been related to suicidal behavior among children and adolescents (Blumenthal and Kupfer 1988; Cohen-Sandler et al. 1982a, 1982b; Deykin et al. 1985; Garfinkel et al. 1982; Hawton et al. 1982a, 1982b, 1982c; Hibbard et al. 1988; Kosky et al. 1986; Pfeffer 1986; Taylor and Stansfeld 1984a; Tishler et al. 1981; Topol and Reznikoff 1982).

Method and Lethality

By far, the most common method of suicide attempts is that of intentional overdose (Brent 1987; Garfinkel et al. 1982). Wrist-slashing is the second most common method in most North American series (Brent 1987; Brent et al. 1988b; Garfinkel et al. 1982). There is some evidence that those suicide attempts that resemble completions in lethality (e.g., high degree of planning; use of lethal method such as hanging, carbon monoxide, jumping) resemble completers in diagnosis and family history and, in fact, are more at risk to finally complete suicide (Brent 1987; Garfinkel et al. 1982; Otto 1972). However, lethality and intent are only modesty correlated, unless the attempter has adequate knowledge of the lethality potential of the method chosen (Brent 1987; Beck et al. 1975a).

Intent

Suicidal intent, or the extent to which the attempter wished to die, is an extremely useful construct in the assessment of suicidal risk. High intent is characterized by premeditated attempts in which the attempter tries to minimize the possibility of rescue (e.g., timed so that discovery is unlikely, occurs in an isolated place) (Beck et al. 1974). High suicidal intent has been found to discriminate between youthful attempters and completers (Brent et al. 1988b) and to predict reattempts in adolescent self-poisoners (Hawton et al. 1982b).

Psychiatric Disorders

Although most studies of suicidal behavior in adolescents have focused on referred samples, there is evidence from samples drawn from emergency rooms, pediatric clinics, and community samples that depressive symptomatology, substance abuse, and conduct disorder are most closely related to suicidal behavior (Garfinkel and Garner 1982; Goldberg 1981; Pfeffer et al. 1984; Robins 1989; Smith and Crawford 1986; Velez and Cohen 1988). These results are convergent with those that have relied on either medically or psychiatrically referred samples (Brent 1987; Brent et al. 1986, 1988b; Carlson and Cantwell 1982; Crumley 1979; Pfeffer 1982; Pfeffer et al. 1979, 1980; Robbins and Alessi 1985).

Personality Characteristics

Studies of personality disorder among adolescent suicide attempters have been few, in part due to confusion with regard to the existence and assessment of personality disorder among adolescents. However, investigations have demonstrated that suicide attempters frequently have discordant and impaired interpersonal relationships with family and peers (Hawton et al. 1982a, 1982b, 1982c). Several studies have demonstrated a relationship between borderline personality disorder and suicidal behavior among adolescents in clinical samples, particularly if the personality disorder is comorbid with affective disorder (Crumley 1979; Gibbs 1981; McManus et al. 1984). Prepubertal suicidal children have also been reported to be more likely than nonsuicidal psychiatric controls to have a diagnosis of borderline personality disorder (Pfeffer 1982).

In addition to dimensional classifications of personality disorder among adolescent suicide attempters, there have been efforts to identify certain personality and cognitive traits that may predispose children and adolescents to suicidal behavior. Among these traits are hopelessness, impulsivity, external locus of control, poor affective modulation, cognitive rigidity, and poor social skills (Blumenthal and Kupfer 1988).

Hopelessness

Hopelessness has long been considered one of the key cognitive variables in the assessment and treatment of suicidal adults (Beck et al. 1975b, 1985). There is now accumulating evidence that this is the case among children and adolescents as well. Suicidal children and adolescents are more hopeless than nonsuicidal psychiatric controls, both in referred and in nonreferred samples (Asarnow et al. 1987; Brent et al. 1986; Kazdin et al. 1983; Pfeffer et al. 1979; Robins 1989; Smith and Crawford 1986; Topol and Reznikoff 1982). Moreover, hopelessness appears to be correlated with the severity of depression and suicidal ideation and to be predictive of recurrent suicidal behavior in adolescent suicide attempters (Brent et al. 1986; Hawton et al. 1982b; Pfeffer et al. 1979; Smith and Crawford 1986). Furthermore, hopelessness appears to differentiate those psychiatrically disturbed children and adolescents who have nonspecific thoughts about suicide from those who formulate a concrete suicidal plan or actually attempt suicide (Brent et al. 1986; Smith and Crawford 1986). Based on the work of Beck et al. (1974), it is likely that amelioration of hopelessness can significantly reduce the suicidal potential in patients at risk for suicide.

Impulsivity

The majority of suicide attempts among children and adolescents are unplanned (Brent 1987; Hawton et al. 1982b) and may reflect an underlying impulsive problem-solving style. Pfeffer et al. (1988) demonstrated that, in a community sample, those youth who have a tendency toward explosive, aggressive outbursts are at greatest risk for repetition or escalation of their suicidal behavior. In addition, the lethality of the behavior of impulsive, nonhopeless suicide attempters is much more likely to be a function of the dangerousness of the available method, rather than such "intrinsic" variables as intent, affective disorder, and family history of affective disorder (Brent 1987; Williams et al. 1977). Therefore, in addition to trying to reduce impulsivity among these youngsters, it is particularly critical to urge family members to secure, or preferably to remove, all potentially dangerous methods of suicide (e.g., firearms, drugs) from the home environment (Blumenthal and Kupfer 1988).

Cognitive Distortion and External Locus of Control

Suicidal children, when compared to chronically ill or normal children, tend to be repulsed by life and attracted to death (Orbach et al. 1983, 1984) and also tend to be more rigid in their approach to tasks and to generate fewer alternatives for problem solving (Orbach et al. 1987). For the suicidal children only, there was a relationship between cognitive rigidity and attractiveness of death (Orbach et al. 1987). Additionally, the use of cognitive mediational strategies to enhance personal coping has been less frequently found among inpatient children who were suicidal than among depressed controls (Asarnow et al. 1987). Negative self-attributions and other negative cognitive biases have been found more frequently among youthful suicide attempters than among psychiatric or normal controls (Asarnow et al. 1987; Rotheram and Trautman, unpublished manuscript, 1986; Trautman et al. 1984). External locus of control, which may be viewed as a correlate of both hopelessness and impulsivity, has also been found to be more frequent among adolescent attempters than among either psychiatric or normal nonsuicidal controls (Topol and Reznikoff 1982).

Poor Social Skills

As noted above, youthful suicide attempters appear to have more peer relationship problems than normal or nonsuicidal psychiatrically disturbed youth (Hawton et al. 1982a, 1982b, 1982c; Linehan et al. 1986; Rotheram and Trautman, unpublished manuscript, 1986; Stanley and Barter 1970) and are more likely to receive a diagnosis of a personality disorder (Crumley 1979; McManus et al. 1984). Indeed, the most common precipitant for suicidal behavior among adolescents appears to be interpersonal discord either with a peer or a family member (Brent et al. 1988b; Hawton et al. 1982a). Moreover, the interpersonal motivations of adolescent suicide attempters indicate implicitly these individuals' lack of skill in direct communication and negotiation with family members and peers (Hawton et al. 1982c). In fact, it has been demonstrated that self-poisoners show more deficits in interpersonal problem solving than psychiatric or normal controls (McLeavey et al. 1987).

Family History of Psychiatric Disorder

There is evidence that suicide attempters, like completers, have a high rate of affective disorder, alcohol and drug abuse, and suicide and suicidal behavior among their family members (Brent et al. 1988; Garfinkel et al. 1982; Pfeffer 1982; Pfeffer et al. 1979, 1980, 1983, 1984; Tishler and McKenry 1982; Tishler et al. 1981). Moreover, such family members are likely to be depressed and suicidal at the time of the child's presentation for treatment (Pfeffer et al. 1979, 1980, 1984; Tishler and McKenry 1982; Tishler et al. 1981). Additionally, the parents of depressed adolescent suicide attempters may have an earlier age of onset of psychiatric disorder than the parents of depressed, nonsuicidal psychiatric controls (Friedman et al. 1984).

Family Environment

In addition to a frank family history of psychiatric disorder, there is substantial evidence that familial discord and disruption serve as a key antecedent to suicidal behavior (Brent et al. 1988b; Hawton et al. 1982a; Hirschfeld and Blumenthal 1986; Robins 1989; Smith and Crawford 1986; Trautman and Shaffer 1984). Both Hawton et al. (1982a) and Taylor and Stansfeld (1984a) found that a disrupted relationship with parents was a common precipitant of suicide attempts among adolescent self-poisoners. Suicidal children and adolescents rate their family environments as less cohesive and more conflicted than do psychiatric controls (Asarnow et al. 1987; Topol and Reznikoff 1982). Furthermore, the relationship between suicidal youth and their parents is characterized by greater hostility and enmity (Kosky 1983; Kosky et al. 1986; Miller et al. 1982; Smith and Crawford 1986; Taylor and Stansfeld 1984a), overt conflict, excessive negative consequences, and limited mutual problem solving than are the parent-child relationships of nonsuicidal psychiatric and normal controls (Williams and Lyons 1976). In fact, attempters have had a greater exposure to family violence than psychiatric controls (Kosky 1983; Kosky et al. 1986; Myer et al. 1985; Tishler et al. 1981) and have more often been the victims of sexual or physical abuse than normal or psychiatric controls (Cohen-Sandler et al. 1982a, 1982b; Deykin et al. 1985; Green 1978; Hibbard et al. 1988; Kosky 1983; Myers et al. 1986; Roberts and Hawton 1980; Smith and Crawford 1986). The relationship between suicidality and abuse appears to be particularly strong in preschool and young school-age children (Rosenthal et al. 1986). Adolescents who have run away from home and are living on their own are also noted to be at higher risk for suicidal behavior (Robins 1989).

Not only are current discord and frank abuse risk factors for suicidal behavior, but the early life experiences of adolescents are also likely to predispose to suicidal behavior. For example, attempters are more likely than psychiatric or medical controls to have experienced the loss or separation from a parent (Garfinkel et al. 1982; Kosky 1983), particularly when the loss occurred before 12 years of age (Stanley and Barter 1970).

Other Environmental Influences

Exposure to suicide may also increase the risk for suicidal behavior. The airing of television docudramas about suicide was followed by an increase not only of suicide but of suicidal behavior as well, at least in the New York metropolitan area (Gould and Shaffer 1986). High-school students who are suicide attempters, when compared to non-attempters, are more likely to have known someone who has completed suicide or attempted suicide, both within and outside of their family (Harkavy-Friedman et al. 1987; Smith and Crawford 1986). In addition to the increased risk of intrafamilial assault, suicide attempters are also more likely to have experienced extrafamilial physical or sexual assault than nonattempters (Robins 1989; Smith and Crawford 1986).

Medical Illness

Children with epilepsy appear to be at higher risk, not only for suicide but for suicidal behavior as well. In one consecutive series of children and adolescents seen at a pediatric emergency room for suicide attempts, epileptic children were overrepresented by a factor of almost 16 (Brent 1986). There is evidence that this predisposition to suicidal behavior may be attributable in part to the use of phenobarbital as an anticonvulsant (Brent 1986; Brent et al. 1987b). There have been no other specific medical illnesses among children or adolescents with a documented increase in suicidal behavior, although there have been anecdotal reports of juvenile diabetic patients overdosing on their own insulin (Kaminer and Robbins 1988). However, a higher proportion of adolescent suicide attempters has been noted to have visited a general practitioner within the month previous to their attempt, and as many as one-third of this British series of 50 attempters were noted to have chronic (although unspecified) physical conditions (Hawton et al. 1982a).

Risk for Reattempts Among Youthful Suicide Attempters

There is a substantial risk among adolescent suicide attempters for reattempts. In follow-up studies ranging from 1 year to almost 3 years, the reattempt rate was between 6% and 15% per year (Chocquet et al. 1980; Cohen-Sandler et al. 1982a; Goldacre and Hawton 1985; Hawton et al. 1982b; McIntire et al. 1977; Stanley and Barter

1970). Predictors of reattempts include previous attempts, high suicidal intent, depression, substance abuse, personality disorder, hostility and aggression, hopelessness, noncompliance with treatment, social isolation, poor school performance, family discord, abuse and/or neglect, and parental psychiatric illness (Chocquet et al. 1980; Cohen-Sandler et al. 1982a; Gispert et al. 1987; Hawton et al. 1982b; McIntire et al. 1977; Stanley and Barter 1970). In one particularly large series, the risk for repetition was greatest within 3 months of the initial attempt (Goldacre and Hawton 1985).

Comparison of Attempters and Completers

There have been few studies that have compared adolescent completers and attempters. In one comparison of suicide completers and psychiatrically hospitalized suicidal adolescents (the majority of whom were attempters, the remainder had ideation with a plan or had made a suicidal threat), the characteristics of the two groups were remarkably similar with respect to high rates of affective disorder, family history of affective disorder and suicidality, and previous suicidal behavior (Brent et al. 1988b). On the other hand, after adjusting for demographic differences between the groups, several differences emerged. The completers were more likely to have shown high suicidal intent, to have never received psychiatric evaluation, to have had a gun available to them in their home, to have had a diagnosis of bipolar disorder, and to have affective disorder occurring with nonaffective comorbidity (i.e., affective disorder occurring with nonaffective disorder diagnoses such as conduct disorder, substance abuse, and attention deficit disorder) (Brent et al. 1988b). These variables are convergent with other prospective studies (see below) and therefore are likely to be risk factors for suicide among adolescent suicide attempters.

Risk for Suicide Among Adolescent Psychiatric Patients and Suicide Attempters

There have been few prospective studies of adolescent psychiatric patients and/or suicide attempters. Welner et al. (1979) reported a 7.7% fatality rate due to suicide in an 8- to 10-year follow-up of 77 former adolescent psychiatric inpatients (some of whom were initially suicidal). The risk was exceedingly high for bipolar and schizophrenic adolescents, a finding substantiated by others (Perris 1966). In follow-up studies of adolescent suicide attempters, the risk for suicide is substantially elevated above those of normal controls. Goldacre and Hawton (1985) found that 0.7% of male and 0.1% of female self-poisoners committed suicide over a 2.8-year follow-up. In a 10- to 15-year follow-up of adolescent suicide attempters, Otto (1972) found that 2.9% of females and 10% of males had died by suicide. The period of greatest risk for suicide in this study was within the first 2 years after the attempt. The characteristics of those who were most likely to have completed suicide were as follows: male sex, no apparent precipitant, high intent, "active" method (e.g., jumping), and bipolar or "psychotic" (probably schizophrenic) disorder. These results are in large part convergent with the comparison of adolescent suicide completers and attempters cited above (Brent et al. 1988b).

SUICIDAL IDEATION

Suicidal ideation is even more common than suicidal behavior. Community-based studies indicate that between 6.7% to 12% of children and adolescents have some form of serious suicidal ideation (Pfeffer et al. 1984; Velez and Cohen 1988). Suicidal ideation and behavior are about three to four times more common among psychiatric patients (Brent et al. 1986; Pfeffer et al. 1979; Ryan et al. 1987). Among psychiatric patients, suicidal ideation is most closely associated with depression, although it is associated with almost every type of psychiatric disorder (Brent et al. 1986). Suicidal ideation can be conceptualized as a spectrum from nonspecific (e.g., "Life is not worth living"), specific ("I wish I was dead"), ideation with an intent ("I'm going to kill myself"), to ideation with a plan ("I'm going to kill myself with pills"). Both hopelessness and the severity of depressive symptomatology are correlated with the severity of suicidal ideation (Brent et al. 1986; Carlson and Cantwell 1982; Pfeffer et al. 1979; Smith and Crawford 1986). Some investigators have found that those children and adolescents who engage in suicidal ideation are quite different from those who actually engage in suicidal behavior (Carlson and Cantwell 1982), with the ideators showing more depression and the attempters manifesting more conduct and impulse control disorders (Carlson and Cantwell 1982). On the other hand, others have found that suicidal ideation and attempts are a continuum and that in fact those children and adolescents with serious ideation are clinically indistinguishable from those who actually make suicide attempts (Brent et al. 1986; Pfeffer et al. 1979). The sampling frame may greatly influence these results, although community-based studies have tended to support the continuum viewpoint (Smith and Crawford 1986). Therefore, it follows that those with serious suicidal ideation, either with intent or a plan, should be considered to be at high potential to act on their suicidal thoughts (Table 3).

Table 3. Interviewing for suicidal ideation

Have you ever thought that life was not worth living?

Have you ever wished you were dead?

Have you ever thought about trying to hurt yourself?

Do you want to hurt yourself?

Have you thought of a way to hurt yourself?

Have you ever hurt yourself?

Source. Brent and Kolko 1990. Reprinted with permission from WB Saunders.

ASSESSMENT OF SUICIDAL POTENTIAL AND THE DECISION TO HOSPITALIZE

Risk Factors for Suicidal Behavior and Suicide

The assessment of the risk for suicidal behavior and suicide is in essence an assessment of the domains outlined above (see also Blumenthal, Chapter 26, this volume). It is clear from the text that the risk factors for suicidal behavior and for suicide are quite convergent with regard to major psychopathology, medical condition of epilepsy, and family history of suicide and psychiatric disorder. However, case-control and prospective studies indicate that the presence of certain factors renders suicide attempters particularly vulnerable to suicide: male sex, high intent/high lethality attempt, diagnoses of bipolar disorder, affective disorder with nonaffective comorbidity, psychoses, lack of compliance with psychiatric treatment, and availability of firearms in the home.

Psychiatric Inpatient Hospitalization

The assessment of the immediate and short-term potential of the patient for self-harm is the most important task of the psychiatrist evaluating a potentially suicidal adolescent. Psychiatric hospitalization is indicated for patients who, unless monitored in a structured and protective environment, are judged to be in imminent danger of suicide or suicidal behavior. Patients who are preoccupied with death, who show evidence of a suicidal plan and have intent to carry it out, and who have made suicide attempts of high intent or of extremely high lethality are best treated on an inpatient unit (Table 4). Further-

Table 4. Indications for psychiatric inpatient hospitalization

---

Characteristics of suicidality
  Inability to maintain a no-suicide contract
  Active suicidal ideation (with plan and intent)
  High intent or lethality suicide attempt

Psychiatric disorder
  Psychosis
  Severe depression
  Substance abuse
  Bipolar illness
  Serious aggression
  Previous attempts
  Previous noncompliance or failure with outpatient treatment

Family problems
  Abuse
  Severe parental psychiatric illness
  Family unable to monitor or protect patient or unwilling

Source.   Brent and Kolko 1990. Reprinted with permission from WB Saunders.

more, those patients whose psychiatric illnesses preclude outpatient treatment, such as those with active substance abuse, psychosis, and unstable (i.e., rapidly cycling or mixed state) bipolar disorder, are best initially stabilized in an inpatient facility. Other relative indications for hospitalization include a chaotic family that is unlikely to be able to sustain outpatient treatment and a history of previous attempts with failure to follow through with outpatient treatment.

One helpful clinical tool in the decision to hospitalize the patient rests on the clinician's judgment of the patient's ability to keep a "no-suicide" contract (Drye et al. 1973; Strayhorn 1982). This contract is an agreement between the patient, family, and therapist that the patient will not attempt suicide and that if the patient does feel suicidal, he or she will notify a significant other, as well as the therapist. It is helpful to go beyond a simple assertion on the part of the patient and test his or her resolve by asking what the patient would do if the precipitant (e.g., family discord) for the initial suicidal episode should recur (Rotheram 1987). The no-suicide contract is not foolproof, but it is a measure of the therapeutic alliance and should be viewed within the context of other clinical risk factors. If the patient and family can agree to the contract, and if there are no clinical contraindications (e.g., psychosis, active substance abuse, unstable bipolar disorder), then treatment can proceed on an outpatient basis.

Psychiatric hospitalization may be opposed by the patient, and if a no-suicide contract cannot be obtained and/or the patient has a dangerous constellation of risk factors, then an involuntary commitment should be sought. One exception to this manner of procedure is when both the patient and the family are adamantly opposed to hospitalization. In this case, the clinician must weigh the need of the patient for immediate protection against the possibility that commitment may alienate both the patient and family against subsequent psychiatric care. Unless the patient is an immediate suicidal risk, the clinician may be better off trying to arrange for close outpatient monitoring of the patient through a strong alliance with the family.

Hospitalization is at best a temporary respite from suicidality. The risk of suicide and suicidal behavior is greatest in the time immediately after discharge from the hospital, according to studies on adolescents and adults (Otto 1972; Pokorny 1960; Roy 1982). Therefore, linkages between inpatient and outpatient programs are essential, as is a clear discharge follow-up plan, so that treatment and monitoring of suicidal risk can continue uninterrupted after discharge from the hospital.

TREATMENT OF PATIENTS AT RISK FOR SUICIDE AND SUICIDAL BEHAVIOR

Psychiatric treatment of patients at high risk for suicide represents an opportunity to translate our knowledge, albeit incomplete, about risk factors for suicide into clinical practice (Blumenthal 1988). Psychiatric treatment of patients at high risk for suicide should focus on the amelioration of those risk factors that are most likely, if untreated, to result in a fatal outcome. In addition to focusing on treatment that targets these particular risk factors, we will first review some general principles in the management of youthful patients at high risk for suicide. These principles include the maintenance of the no-suicide contract, the availability of 24-hour clinical backup, steps to take to heighten compliance with treatment, the importance of involving the family, and the removal of lethal agents from the environment (Bluementhal and Kupfer 1988; Hawton and Catalan 1987; Pfeffer 1986).

No-Suicide Contract

We described above the importance of the no-suicide contract in the initial assessment of suicidal potential. However, the assessment of suicidality and the patient's current repertoire for coping with suicidal thoughts should be part of every session with a patient thought to be at high risk for suicide. This can be done without calling undue attention to suicide, particularly if a cognitive model of therapy is utilized. In cognitive therapy, assessment of a range of depressogenic and negative cognitions and the manner in which the patient copes with stressful situations is central to this mode of psychiatric intervention (Bedrosian and Epstein 1984).

Availability of 24-Hour Clinical Back-Up

The clinician also has responsibilities as a result of the no-suicide contract. Paramount among these is the agreement that the therapist or a designated substitute should be available to respond to the patient day or night. It is a rare psychiatrist who is truly available 24 hours a day, so the patient and his or her family should be given the number of a hospital with 24-hour emergency psychiatric coverage in addition to that of the treating professional.

Steps to Increase Compliance With Treatment

Suicidal patients are particularly noncompliant with treatment recommendations. Only about half of adolescent and young adults keep the first outpatient appointment, and only one-third complete as many as three outpatient sessions (Hawton et al. 1982a; Paykel et al. 1974; Taylor and Stansfeld 1984b; Trautman et al. 1984). This noncompliance is of particular concern given evidence that noncompliant suicidal patients are more likely to have more severe psychopathology, to have higher suicidal intent, to have more disturbed parents (Taylor and Stansfeld 1984b; Trautman et al. 1987), and to reattempt and to commit suicide as well (Greer and Bagley 1971; Kennedy 1972; Motto 1976; Welu 1977).

Therefore, certain steps that have been found to increase compliance in a variety of outpatient psychiatric settings should be taken (Table 5) (Baekeland and Lundwall 1975). First, there should be therapist consistency. Ideally the patient should be treated by the same person who performs the initial evaluation, or, at least, the patient should be introduced to the person who will provide treatment at the time of the initial assessment. Second, the patient should receive a definite appointment at the time of intake. Third, patients may need to be called to remind them of their appointment the day before. Fourth, patients should be scheduled in a timely fashion (i.e., within a week of intake). Fifth, no-shows should be pursued aggressively by phone and letter. Sixth, the type of treatment desired by the patient and family should be elicited, and an explicit contract made around what type of treatment will be provided. Seventh, significant others (e.g., family, professionals, friends) should be involved as necessary in the treatment. The last issue of family involvement deserves additional comment.

Table 5. Steps to maintain compliance with outpatient treatment

1. Continuity between evaluation and treatment

2. Patient given a definite appointment for follow-up at the time of intake

3. Patient called to be reminded of the appointment

4. Patient scheduled in a timely fashion

5. No-shows pursued by phone calls and letters

6. Explicit contracting between patient, family, and therapist about the type of treatment that is desired and what can be provided

7. Involvement of family members and other significant adults (e.g., teachers, physicians)

Source. Brent and Kolko 1990. Reprinted with permission from WB Saunders.

The Family's Role in Treatment

Involvement of the family is quite important in the treatment of suicidal youth. Apart from the fact that parents frequently provide payment and transportation, their inclusion in the treatment is vital to the initiation and ultimate success of any psychiatric intervention. There is evidence from studies of adult patients with affective disorders that family psychoeducation about the identified patient's illness and counseling about how best to interact with the patient increase compliance not only with clinic appointments but with use of medication, and the overall success rate of the treatment (Frank and Kupfer 1986; Frank et al. 1985; Haas et al. 1986; Miklowitz et al. 1986). Therefore, family psychoeducation about suicide psychiatric illness (e.g., affective disorder), and the type of treatments to be utilized will help to cement an alliance with the family and to increase compliance with the treatment regimen (Blumenthal and Kupfer 1986). Conversely, a negative parental attitude toward treatment is associated with noncompliance (Taylor and Stansfeld 1984b). Therefore, it is critical to consolidate the alliance between the clinician and the parents, and there should be proscribed times for feedback to the family about the progress of their child, with an opportunity for the parents to ask questions of the treating clinician.

There are other reasons why family involvement is particularly critical in the treatment of suicidal youth. Family conflict is one of the most frequent precipitants for suicide and suicidal behavior (Brent et al. 1988b; Cohen-Sandler et al. 1982a, 1982b; Hawton et al. 1982a; Kosky 1983; Kosky et al. 1986; Pfeffer 1986; Taylor and Stansfeld 1984a). Therefore, at the outset of treatment, it is important to try to arrange a "truce" around the most emotionally loaded issues of family conflict, through the use of techniques such as behavioral contracting (Patterson 1975).

Sometimes, the patient's and/or parent's irritability secondary to affective illness is highly contributory to the degree of familial discord (Weissman et al. 1973). In this case, behavioral contracting alone may not relieve the tension, but psychoeducation about the effects of living with a family member with a psychiatric illness may buy some time while the psychiatrist provides treatment (e.g., antidepressant treatment) for the ill family member. This underscores the importance of psychiatrically assessing the parents of the suicidal patient, since it is likely that at least one of them has serious psychiatric illness and/or suicidality of their own (Brent et al. 1988b; Pfeffer et al. 1979, 1980, 1984; Tishler and McKenry, 1982; Tishler et al. 1981). Moreover, there is evidence that parental psychopathology is associated with nonattendance in child psychiatric outpatients in general (Gould et al. 1985) and child and adolescent suicide attempters in specific (Taylor and Stansfeld 1984b; Trautman et al. 1987). The proper identification and treatment of psychiatrically ill parents should increase the chances of compliance and success with psychiatric treatment of suicidal youth.

Sometimes, the nature of the family conflict is more extreme, as in the case of physical or sexual abuse (Cohen-Sandler et al. 1982a, 1982b; Deykin et al. 1985; Green 1978; Hibbard et al. 1988; Roberts and Hawton 1980). The reporting of abuse is legally mandated. Additionally, for treatment purposes, it may be more appropriate to remove the child from the home than to try to treat the young suicidal patient in the context of such a toxic environment. In fact, failure to remove a suicidal child from an abusive or neglectful environment has been reported to be associated with an increased risk for repeated attempts (Cohen-Sandler et al. 1982a).

Perhaps the most important reason for family education and involvement is the crucial role of the family as a safety net for the patient. The clinician can train a parent to observe signs of a recurrence of psychiatric disorder (e.g., psychosis, affective symptoms) and can teach the parent how to respond when the patient might again begin to express suicidal thoughts. Such a repertoire of behaviors for the parent include empathic listening to their child, knowing when to re-contact the treating clinician (usually when the symptoms result in functional impairment), and when and how to obtain an involuntary commitment should the child appear to be a danger to him- or herself.

Restriction of the Availability of Lethal Agents

There is considerable evidence to suggest that the availability of firearms in the home increases the risk for suicide for the occupants (Brent et al. 1988b; Kellerman and Reay 1986; Markush and Bartolucci 1984). Therefore, parents of suicidal youth should be instructed to remove all firearms from the home. The availability of firearms appears to be a more significant risk factor than the accessibility, so that storage of the gun in a more "secure" fashion is probably not as protective as simply removing the gun from the home environment of the suicidal or at-risk adolescent (Brent et al. 1988).

Since the lethality of impulsive suicide attempts in adolescents appears to be related to the availability of lethal prescribed agents such as tricyclic antidepressants (Brent 1987), clinicians who prescribe such agents for children and adolescents should do so only for a clear indication of a psychiatric or schizophrenic disorder and should limit the quantity that is prescribed at any one time. If other household members have such agents prescribed, then these medications should be securely stored.

TREATMENTS FOR SUICIDAL YOUTH WITH PSYCHIATRIC DISORDERS

There have been few clinical trials to test the effectiveness of any type of intervention with psychiatrically ill children and adolescents. Therefore, we will make reference to relevant studies with adult populations and make recommendations for clinical practice, with the understanding that definitive information must await appropriate intervention studies in child and adolescent populations.

Since the majority of adolescent suicide attempters and completers are psychiatrically ill (Blumenthal and Kupfer 1988; Brent et al. 1986, 1988b; Crumley 1979; Pfeffer et al. 1979, 1980), it follows that treatment of the underlying psychiatric illness will reduce the risk for suicide and suicidal behavior in such patients. The most common disorders in suicide victims and suicide attempters are disorders of affect (unipolar and bipolar), substance abuse, and conduct; bulimia nervosa; and schizophrenia (Garfinkel and Garner 1982). Therefore, a review of the efficacy of pharmacologic and psychotherapeutic interventions for each of these disorders in this age group will be provided, and the relevant adult literature will be cited as well. In addition, because suicidal behavior appears to confer additional risk for subsequent suicidal behavior and suicide, interventions that specifically target suicidal behavior will be discussed.

Unipolar Depressive Disorder: Pharmacotherapy

Several studies suggest that antidepressant medication in prepubertal patients with major depression is effective. Such evidence includes response in an open treatment study (Puig-Antich et al. 1978), correlation of clinical response with antidepressant blood level (Geller et al. 1983, 1985; Preskorn et al. 1982, 1987; Puig-Antich et al. 1978, 1987), and superior efficacy over placebo in one double-blind placebo trial (Preskorn et al. 1987). However, the largest published double-blind placebo trial of antidepressant medication in prepubertal children showed the same response rate in the imipramine- and placebo-treated groups (Puig-Antich et al. 1987). Additionally, studies of prepubertal depressed children who received antidepressant medication and were evaluated in remission indicate the persistence of serious social impairment, albeit to a less severe degree than during the depressed state (Puig-Antich et al. 1985a, 1985b). The lack of strong evidence supporting the superiority of antidepressant medication over placebo, combined with the persistence of psychosocial deficits even on recovery, suggests that the optimum treatment of prepubertally depressed children must also include psychosocial interventions that target areas of psychosocial dysfunction.

Even less is known about antidepressant treatment in adolescents. An open trial of imipramine in adolescents with major depressive disorder found that only 44% responded to medication and that there was no relationship between clinical response and blood level (Ryan et al. 1986). In one clinical trial of adolescent inpatients with depression, Kramer and Feiguine (1981) found no advantage to the use of amitriptyline over placebo, although the sample size (10 subjects in each cell) precluded the detection of any but the largest of effect sizes. Ryan and Puig-Antich (1986) hypothesized several reasons for the failure to find a clinical response to tricyclic antidepressants in adolescents. First, high circulating sex steroid hormone levels may somehow inhibit the action of imipramine and other antidepressants. Second, the pattern of depression in adolescents and young adults is more of an "atypical" pattern (Quitkin et al. 1982) and therefore may respond preferentially to monoamine oxidase inhibitors (MAOIs) (Liebowitz et al. 1988). Third, a greater proportion of patients with early-onset affective illness may have an underlying bipolar illness (Strober and Carlson 1982), which may in turn be more refractory to tricyclic antidepressant treatment (Kupfer and Spiker 1981).

Bipolar Disorder

Bipolar illness is particularly important to diagnose and treat, given evidence that young patients with this disorder often go undiagnosed (Weller et al. 1986) and may be particularly vulnerable to suicide (Brent et al. 1988b; Otto, 1972; Welner et al. 1979). The clinician should carefully monitor for the onset in pharmacologically induced mania or mixed states in depressed children and adolescents being treated with antidepressants, given the relatively high proportion who will ultimately develop bipolar disorder (Strober and Carlson 1982).

Lithium is the pharmacologic treatment of choice (reviewed in Strober et al. 1988a). However, lithium resistance is not uncommon in in juvenile-onset bipolar patients and appears to be related to a positive family history, prepubertal onset, associated comorbid conduct disorder, attention-deficit disorder or substance abuse, and presentation in a mixed state or with rapid cycling (Himmelhoch and Garfinkel 1986; Strober et al. 1988b). One intervention that may benefit lithium-resistant bipolar youth (besides withdrawal from any substances of abuse) is the addition of carbamazepine to the treatment regimen (Himmelhoch and Garfinkel 1986). However, the efficacy of this regimen has not been demonstrated through any systematic clinical trials. It is also thought that bipolar depressed patients should be preferentially treated with MAOIs, rather than antidepressants (Ryan and Puig-Antich 1986). In fact, in adult bipolar depressed patients, there is some evidence to support the greater efficacy of MAOIs over tricyclic antidepressants (Himmelhoch et al. 1982; Kupfer and Spiker 1981). As is true of most psychiatric illnesses, it is likely that family support and psychoeducation will enhance medication compliance (Miklowitz et al. 1986), which is particularly critical when a young bipolar patient may be expected to adhere to a long-term regimen of daily lithium prophylaxis.

Substance Abuse

Although it is clear that there is a close relationship between substance abuse and suicidal behavior in adolescents, little is known about the optimal treatment of youthful substance abusers. However, a study of the program characteristics for the successful treatment of adolescent drug abusers indicates that several factors seem to predict good outcome for these patients (Friedman and Glickman 1986). These program characteristics included being a large, well-funded service, specializing in substance abuse, in which a large volume of adolescent clients are evaluated and treated by counselors with specialized experience in adolescent substance abuse. Additional programmatic characteristics associated with good outcome include the availability of ancillary services such as contraceptive counseling, vocational rehabilitation, and educational programs for school dropouts; the use of multiple therapeutic modalities; and client perceptions of the program as allowing for free expression and spontaneous action (Friedman and Glickman 1986). Studies of young adult substance abusers indicate that treatment of associated depressive conditions will improve outcome (Rounsaville et al. 1986). Similarly, there is evidence to support the efficacy of cognitively based treatment for substance abusers (Kosten et al. 1986). At a minimum, any substance-abusing adolescent must be detoxified and subsequently maintain abstinence from substance abuse to benefit from any other psychiatric intervention. Residential treatment coupled with attendance at self-help groups such as Alcoholics Anonymous or Narcotics Anonymous has been shown to decrease the rate of relapse (Grenier 1985).

Conduct Disorder

Conduct disorder is often comorbid with substance abuse and/or affective disorder (Puig-Antich 1982; Ryan et al. 1987). Therefore, despite the predominance of antisocial symptoms in a given patient, it is important not to neglect other related psychiatric conditions (e.g., depression or bipolar affective disorder). It is also important to re-member that youth remanded to adult correctional facilities have been reported to be at extremely high risk for suicide (Brown 1985). There-fore, the assessment of suicidality and the enforcement of strict suici-dal precautions for antisocial youth are particularly critical to the prevention of suicide.

Recently, certain psychosocial interventions have been reported to be effective in the treatment of oppositional and conduct-disor-dered youth (Kazdin et al. 1987a, 1987b). These approaches include altering the impulsive problem-solving style of these youngsters, teaching them to generate a greater number of and more socially appropriate alternatives, and helping parents to discipline their con-duct-disordered children more effectively (Kazdin et al. 1987a, 1987b).

Bulimia Nervosa

Follow-up studies of eating-disordered patients indicate that those with the bulimic subtype are at higher risk for suicide (Garfinkel and Garner 1982). It is unclear if this stems from the eating disorder per se, or whether the risk for suicide is increased due to the conditions that frequently co-occur in these bulimic patients: affective disorder, sub-stance abuse, and personality disorder (Garfinkel and Garner 1982). Therefore, it is important to diagnose and treat these comorbid condi-tions in addition to the serious and frequently socially impairing eating disorder.

Schizophrenia

Little has been written about the treatment of prepubertal and adoles-cent-age schizophrenic patients. However, it is clear that such patients are at high risk for suicide on follow-up (Otto 1972; Welner et al. 1979). In extrapolating from studies of young schizophrenic patients, those at highest risk are male patients who have had a chronic course with no return to a previously high level of premorbid functioning (Drake and Ehrlich 1985; Drake et al. 1984). Such patients are frequently dysphoric and hopeless about the loss of a bright future. Clinical studies indicate that higher than necessary doses of neuroleptics may contribute to these patients' sense of distress through the induction of akathisia (Marder et al. 1984). Furthermore, these side effects may even induce suicidal behavior or suicide (Drake and Ehrlich 1985; Shear et al. 1983). While previous studies have indicated that antidepressant treatment of dysphoric schizophrenic patients might lead to increased psychotic symptomatology (Prusoff et al. 1979), more recent work indicates that depressive symptoms in schizophrenic patients may be relieved by the addition of a tricyclic antidepressant to a regimen of neuroleptic medication without exacerbation of psychotic symptomatology (Siris et al. 1985).

TREATMENT MODALITIES AND APPROACHES FOR SUICIDE ATTEMPTERS AND SUICIDAL PATIENTS

The treatment of suicidal patients has two major components: the treatment of the underlying psychiatric disorder (as has been outlined above) and a psychoeducational approach that facilitates the patient's substitution of more adaptive behavior for suicidal responses when faced with stressful interpersonal crises. In this review of treatment approaches for suicide attempters and suicidal adolescents, we will describe the relevant psychosocial and pharmacotherapy studies of adult suicide attempters. This will be followed by a description of treatment approaches that have been successfully utilized in depressed, suicidal, or impulse-disordered patients.

Treatment Studies of Adult Suicide Attempters

Early studies suggest that those suicide attempters who self-select for treatment have a lower rate of suicide attempts than those who were not treated (Greer and Bagley 1971; Kennedy 1972). Although it is difficult to evaluate treatment effects when subjects have not been randomly assigned to treatment cells, the difference in outcome suggests that treatment may be helpful in preventing recidivism.

Several subsequent, more systematic treatment studies of suicide attempters employed random assignment of patients to "traditional" outpatient treatment, as compared to a more aggressive and flexible modality (e.g., telephone outreach, home visits). Although some of these studies reported that the experimental treatment program resulted in improved social functioning (Chowdhury et al. 1973; Hawton et al. 1981; Welu 1977), only one study demonstrated an effect of treatment on recidivism on a 4-month follow-up (Welu 1977).

Other investigators have used randomized clinical trials to study the efficacy of more focused psychotherapeutic interventions to decrease the recurrence of suicidal behavior. Gibbons et al. (1978) compared "task-centered" with traditional casework and found that on 12-month follow-up, while the task-centered group showed superior social adjustment, the two groups had similar rates of reattempts. In another study, psychiatrically hospitalized suicide attempters who had made at least two previous attempts were randomly assigned to either insight-oriented or cognitive-behavioral treatment (e.g., social skills, affect regulation) (Liberman and Eckman 1981). After a 24-month follow-up, there was no difference between the groups as far as actual suicide attempts. However, patients who received the cognitive-behavioral treatment showed better social adjustment and were less likely to have had suicidal plans. In summary, those treatment programs that have an active outreach component and target specific skills deficits frequently associated with suicidal behavior (see Hawton and Catalan 1987; Patsiokas and Clum 1985) appear to improve social functioning and may reduce the rates of suicidality on follow-up. The following discussion will detail the components of these targeted interventions that have been tested in depressed, impulsive, and/or suicidal youth. Particular attention will be devoted to cognitive, interpersonal problem solving, social skills, affect regulation, and family treatment approaches. A schematic outline describing the interaction of these different skills deficits and their impact on suicidality is depicted in Figure 1.

Cognitive Therapy

The clinical utility of cognitive therapy derives primarily from its successful application with depressed adult patients (Blackburn et al. 1981; Rush et al. 1977; Simons et al. 1984). In adult depressed populations, cognitive therapy may have some advantages over a 16-week course of pharmacotherapy, particularly for the treatment of suicidal patients. Patients treated with cognitive therapy show greater amelioration of hopelessness and suicidal ideation (Kovacs et al. 1981; Rush et al. 1977), greater compliance with outpatient treatment (Blackburn et al. 1981; Rush et al. 1977), and fewer relapses of depression (Kovacs et al. 1981; Simons et al. 1986).

Cognitive therapy has not yet been compared to medication in younger depressed populations. However, at least two clinical trials

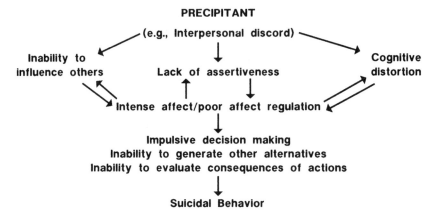

Figure 1. Pathways to suicidal behavior: prescriptions for psychosocial interventions. Reproduced from Brent and Kolko (1990) with permission from WB Saunders.

have indicated that depressed adolescents do benefit from this mode of treatment. Butler et al. (1980) found improvements in self-reported depression and self-concept relative to controls, although this was not corroborated by teacher report of academic performance and social adjustment. Reynolds and Coates (1986) found a greater reduction in clinician ratings of depression at follow-up among adolescents who received cognitive therapy than among adolescents who received relaxation training or no treatment. The adaptation of cognitive therapeutic techniques to adolescent patients has been elaborated by Bedrosian and Epstein (1984), who advocated an emphasis on monitoring of negative automatic thoughts through the use of diaries, and the challenge of negative cognitive distortions though collaborative behavioral experiments, distraction, and positive self-statements. In addition, Emery (1983) recommended the use of activity scheduling and the identification of rewards to encourage social participation. As is true with depressed adults, graded task assignments may enable the depressed adolescent to experience success in situations previously perceived as overly stressful. Clinical experience with suicidal adolescents has suggested that the cognitive distortions that are particularly important to overcome are those of dichotomous thinking, overgeneralization, selective abstraction, and pervasive pessimism. One way in which salient distortions are challenged is by arranging for the patient to confront a specific situation that has heretofore been avoided in light of a specific fear or concern (e.g., embarrassment, ostracism, rejection) and to instruct the patient to observe carefully the specific reactions that actually ensue. In many cases, patients are surprised to learn that they have been narrowly focusing on one or two reactions and that there are positive reactions that occur as well. Such an approach may be helpful, for example, in cases where a patient is excessively concerned about fitting into a group or refusing to engage in deviant group behavior.

While some clinicians have emphasized the use of certain techniques in the adaptation of cognitive therapy to adolescents, others have advocated a change in general approach. For example, derived from experience utilizing cognitive therapy to treat depressed adolescents, Wilkes and Rush (1988) noted that specific attention should be paid to the therapeutic alliance, the cognitive level of development of the adolescent, and the involvement of the family of origin in the assessment and treatment process. Specifically, the therapist should be attuned to the adolescent's potential ambivalence toward authority figures and therefore should focus on more action-oriented and concrete tasks in the assignment of homework. Finally, the involvement of the family is extremely important by use of such approaches as the dyadic mood monitor technique (Wilkes and Rush 1988).

Problem-Solving Skills Training

Whereas cognitive therapy usually attempts to alter existing cognitive distortions, problem solving often seeks to remediate cognitive deficits by teaching a systematic approach to social problems (Spivack and Shure 1982). The clinical objective of problem solving is to teach the person to adopt a more flexible approach to problems through a generalized series of skills: problem identification, generation of alternatives, response evaluation, decision making, implementation, and verification by testing the selected response (D'Zurilla and Goldfried 1971).

This approach derives empirical support from research showing that problem solving mediates the relationship between stress and depression in adults (Nezu et al. 1986), that suicidal individuals are restricted in their ability to develop new solutions to problems (Clum et al. 1979; McLeavy et al. 1987), and that depressed children show less effective techniques of problem solving than controls (Kaslow et al. 1983).

Problem-solving therapy has been shown to produce greater improvements in problem-solving ability and hopelessness than either cognitive or nondirective therapy in adult suicidal patients, although there were no differences between the treatment groups with regard to suicidality (Patsiokas and Clum 1985). Although these techniques have been incorporated into multimodal interventions for children, they have not been widely tested in suicidal patients (Butler et al. 1980; Petti and Wells 1980).

The problem-solving approach can often be introduced by asking patients to list alternate uses for common or mundane objects found in the office and then to evaluate the utility or efficiency of those applications that have been suggested. Following several of these training trials, a similar approach can be taken with a relatively simple but nonetheless personal concern that the patient has presented. Since some patients may "get stuck" by claiming to be unable to offer responses (e.g., "don't know," "nothing"), it may be advantageous to provide prompts or ask questions that encourage the patient to acknowledge and evaluate specific alternatives (e.g., "what about calling him on the phone," "writing a letter").

Social Skills Training

As noted above, many suicidal children and adolescents show marked difficulties in interpersonal relationships. In fact, conflict with parents or peers is a frequent precipitant for suicidal behavior. The motivation of the suicidal adolescent is often to influence a significant person with his or her social network. Therefore, it follows that the enhancement of social skills may reduce the chance of recidivism by decreasing the likelihood of conflict. In this way, suicidal patients can expand their repertoire of effective ways of influencing others beyond engaging in a suicidal behavior.

Social skills training has been an important and effective component of the treatment of depressed and suicidal adults (Bellack et al. 1981; Liberman and Eckman 1981) and children (Frame et al. 1982; Kolko 1986; Petti et al. 1980). However, aside from indirect support from one case study (Kolko 1986), there are no reports of the efficacy of social skills training on the reduction of suicidality.

Training has generally entailed providing systematic exposure to information and instructions about social behavior, modeling and behavioral rehearsal of targeted skills, and critical feedback regarding performance. Because suicidal adolescents frequently present with interpersonal difficulties, the clinician should assess the social skills deficits associated with these problems and help the patient devise appropriate coping strategies. Common targets include appropriate assertion and negotiation, expression of both positive and negative affects, and methods to get appropriate help from family and friends. Specific components of training could include a comprehensive review of both verbal behaviors (e.g., making clear requests, giving an explanation, suggesting what one does not like in a calm manner, suggesting an alternative) and nonverbal behaviors (e.g., eye contact, attention to body language, smiling, loudness, listening). It is important to encourage adolescent patients to practice these skills under naturalistic conditions, and to evaluate the patient's ability to monitor the impact of these skills on social outcome. Thus difficulties with assertion in response to instances involving family provocation may be remediated through a focused review of the patient's performance in these situations (e.g., "How do you usually act/react?"), followed by therapist modeling of appropriate alternative behaviors (e.g., saying you're angry, telling them why), patient role-playing or rehearsal using simulated family interactions, and performance feedback and discussion. Patients who seem more confident and competent in their ability to express their new skills then can be encouraged to apply them to in vivo situations, beginning with those that pose minimal challenge and proceeding toward more difficult encounters.

Affect Regulation

Hostility and irritability are prominent features of adolescent and young adult suicide attempters (Gispert et al. 1987; Hawton et al. 1982b; Weissman et al. 1973). The suicidal behavior is frequently impulsive and performed when the patient is angry or upset (Brent 1987; Hawton et al. 1982b; Linehan et al. 1986; Williams et al. 1977). In fact, many adolescents resort to suicidal behavior to express anger (Hawton et al. 1982c). Similar difficulties in affect regulation have been observed in aggressive, impulsive adolescents (a group whose characteristics overlap substantially with adolescent suicide attempters) (Gibbs 1981; Hawton et al. 1982b; Miller et al. 1982). Specific techniques of self-control training have been associated with reductions in hostility and aggression and concomitant increases in socially appropriate behavior (Feindler and Ecton 1986; Milan and Kolko 1985).

To heighten self-control, adolescents can be taught to identify when they are angry or upset, and then to use techniques such as progressive muscle relaxation or controlled breathing to help modulate intense emotions. Instruction in ways to relax specific muscle groups in which one experiences tension (e.g., neck, shoulders, jaw) is usually an easy, initial, and nonthreatening method for self-control of anxiety and related affective states. It is also an active coping strategy that can be practiced at home and implemented in brief during stressful situations. Other recommended techniques designed to enhance the appropriate expression of anger include identifying cues likely to elicit anger, learning to use positive coping self-statements to enhance and reinforce self-control, thinking ahead to the positive consequences of self-control, and practicing self-evaluation. Youthful patients frequently prefer to develop their own idiosyncratic expressions (e.g., "you're in control," "he can't hurt you") and suggest situations to which they would be willing to have them applied. Such control sets the stage for the deployment of other rational control strategies such as cognitive, problem-solving, and social skills techniques, described elsewhere in this chapter. Practice of these techniques and their application to real-life situations are essential to the success of this type of intervention.

Family-Based Treatment

The importance of mobilizing family involvement has already been stated. The components of family-based treatment likely to benefit depressed and suicidal adolescents include psychoeducation, feedback to parents, referral of parents for psychiatric treatment as necessary, conflict resolution, and increased efficacy of familial problem solving. Although there has been no test of the efficacy of parent-child conflict resolution on the suicidality of the identified patient, the intimate relationship between family conflict and suicidality makes it likely that this is a key area for intervention. One family-based treatment program designed to reduce family conflict has shown that teaching family members improved problem-solving and communication skills has resulted in decreased conflict and improved family functioning on follow-up (Robin 1979, 1981; Robin and Foster 1984). Accordingly, the entire family can be encouraged to replace specific types of aversive control activities (e.g., interruptions, put-downs, accusations) with more constructive options (e.g., self-disclosure, use of I-statements, active listening). These strategies reduce impulsive, hostile responding, while also serving to stimulate more reciprocal problem-solving efforts. Comparable approaches have been described in treatment programs for suicidal adolescents, but await empirical validation (Rotheram and Trautman, unpublished manuscript, 1986). However, preliminary results from this study suggest that a cognitive-behavioral approach that does not actively involve family members will have high drop-out rates (Trautman et al. 1987).

Pharmacotherapeutic Approaches to Recurrent Suicidal Behavior

Three randomized trials have examined the impact of pharmacotherapy on the prevention of suicide attempts among adult patients with recurrent suicidal behavior (Goldblatt and Schatzberg, Chapter 15, this volume). In the first study, depot injectable neuroleptic medication was found to be more effective than placebo in the reduction of the rate of attempted suicide on 6-month follow-up in 37 personality and nonaffectively disordered patients who had made at least four previous suicide attempts (Montgomery et al. 1979). These results are convergent with those of Soloff et al. (1986a), who have reported that patients with borderline personality disorder show improvement on low-dose haloperidol. These studies need to be replicated and extended to younger age groups to clarify the short- and long-term efficacy of neuroleptic mediation in the management of recurrent suicidal behavior.

On the other hand, antidepressant medications do not appear to be of benefit in the prevention of recurrent suicidal behavior in personality and nonaffectively disordered patients. Two studies have compared the efficacy of second-generation heterocyclic antidepressants to placebo in the prevention of recidivism in nonaffective patients with recurrent suicidal behavior, and both studies demonstrated that active treatment was no better than placebo (Hirsch et al. 1983; Montgomery et al. 1983). Moreover, in recurrently suicidal patients with borderline personality disorder, antidepressant medication may be contraindicated; amitriptyline was associated with a worsening of irritability and suicidality in adult borderline patients compared to placebo and haloperidol (Soloff et al. 1986b).

In summary, pharmacologic and psychosocial approaches that are likely to be effective in reducing the risk of suicidal behavior in depressed, impulsive, and/or suicidal youth include those that target the underlying psychiatric disorders and are based on a comprehensive assessment of cognitive, problem-solving, social skills; affect regulation; and family difficulties. Because suicidal adolescents are so diverse, treatment is best targeted to the particular deficits and problems of the individual patient and family. Blumenthal and Kupfer (1988) suggested that multiple interventions targeted at all the risk domains present is an effective strategy to prevent suicidal behavior. Hawton and Catalan (1987) described a problem-solving approach to suicide attempters that links the assessment of the precipitants and motivation for suicidal behavior to the type of treatment provided. For example, if the precipitant for the attempt was due to an interpersonal conflict within the family, then the attempter and the involved family members should be taught more adaptive ways for conflict resolution. Often, the attendant motivation of youthful suicide attempters is to gain attention or to express negative affect. When these motives are evident, Hawton and Catalan (1987) recommended that therapeutic efforts focus on teaching the attempter more adaptive means for eliciting attention from the social environment and more direct means for the expression of negative affect. Figure 1 illustrates a common constellation of deficits that may lead to suicidal behavior under stress. The remediation of these deficits may protect the attempter against future suicidality when under stress.

CONCLUSION

The proper identification, assessment, and treatment of psychiatric disorders in childhood and adolescence remain the basis for the prevention and amelioration of suicidality among youth. Additionally, it is important to assess those functional components of the patient's cognitions, social skills, affect regulation, and family environment that may contribute to suicidal risk. Treatment should follow from assessment and should target specific syndromes as well as functional deficits. General principles for treatment include aggressive outreach, availability of 24-hour clinical backup, use of the no-suicide contract with the patient and family, proper use of voluntary and involuntary hospitalization, formation of an alliance with the family, and removal of firearms from the home.

Currently, much of our limited knowledge about the efficacy of intervention to prevent suicidality in psychiatric patients is derived from work with adult populations (see Brent et al. 1988a). Replication, adaptation, and extension of previous work with suicidal adults to younger patient samples are required. Multicenter trials of psychosocial and somatic interventions are needed to determine which treatments are most effective in the amelioration and prevention of suicidality in psychiatrically disturbed children and adolescents.

REFERENCES

Asarnow JR, Carlson GA, Guthrie D: Coping strategies, self-perceptions, hopelessness, and perceived family environments in depressed and suicidal children. J Consult Clin Psychol 55:361–366, 1987

Baekeland F, Lundwall L: Dropping out of treatment: a critical review. Psychol Bull 82:738–783, 1975

Beck AT, Weissman A, Lester D, et al: The measurement of pessimism: the hopelessness scale. J Consult Clin Psychol 42:861–865, 1974

Beck AT, Beck R, Kovacs M: Classification of suicidal behaviors. I: Quantifying intent and medical lethality. Am J Psychiatry 132:285–287, 1975a

Beck AT, Kovacs M, Weissman A: Hopelessness and suicidal behavior: an overview. JAMA 234:1146–1149, 1975b

Beck AT, Weissman A, Kovacs M: Alcoholism, hopelessness and suicidal behavior. J Stud Alcohol 37:66–77, 1976

Beck AT, Steer RA, Kovacs M, et al: Hopelessness and eventual suicide: a 10-year prospective study of patients hospitalized with suicidal ideation. Am J Psychiatry 142:559–563, 1985

Bedrosian RC, Epstein N: Cognitive therapy of depressed and suicidal adolescents, in Suicide in the Young. Edited by Sudak HS, Ford AB, Rushforth NB. Boston, MA, John Wright, 1984, pp 345–366

Bellack A, Hersen M, Himmelhoch JM: Social skills training compared with pharmacotherapy and psychotherapy in the treatment of unipolar depression. Am J Psychiatry 138:1562–1567, 1981

Berlin IN: Suicide among American Indian adolescents: an overview. Suicide Life Threat Behav 17:218–232, 1987

Blackburn IM, Bishop S, Glen AIM, et al: The efficacy of cognitive therapy in depression: a treatment trial using cognitive therapy and pharmacotherapy, each alone and in combination. Br J Psychiatry 139:181–189, 1981

Blumenthal SJ: A guide to risk factors, assessment and treatment of the suicidal patient. Med Clin North Am 72:937–971, 1988

Blumenthal SJ, Kupfer DJ: Generalizable treatment strategies for suicidal behavior. Ann NY Acad Sci 487:327–340, 1986

Blumenthal SJ, Kupfer DJ: Overview of early detection and treatment strategies for suicidal behavior in young people. Journal of Youth and Adolescence 17:1–23, 1988

Boyd JH: The increasing rate of suicide by firearms. N Engl J Med 76:1240–1242, 1983

Boyd JH, Moscicki EK: Firearms and youth suicide. Am J Public Health 308:872–874, 1986

Brent DA: Over-representation of epileptics among a consecutive series of suicide attempters seen at a children's hospital, 1978–1983. J Am Acad Child Psychiatry 25:242–246, 1986

Brent DA: Correlates of medical lethality of suicide attempts in children and adolescents. J Am Acad Child Psychiatry 26:87–89, 1987

Brent DA, Kolko DJ: Suicide and suicidal behavior in children and adolescents, in Psychiatric Disorders in Children and Adolescents. Edited by Garfinkel BD, Carlson GA, Weller EB. Philadelphia, PA, WB Saunders, 1990, pp 372–391

Brent DA, Kalas R, Edelbrock C, et al: Psychopathology and its relationship to suicidal ideation in childhood and adolescence. Journal of the American Academy of Child Psychiatry 25:666–673, 1986

Brent DA, Perper JA, Allman C: Alcohol, firearms, and suicide among youth: temporal trends in Allegheny County, Pennsylvania, 1960–1983. JAMA 257:3369–3372, 1987a

Brent DA, Crumrine PK, Varma RP, et al: Phenobarbital treatment and major depressive disorder in children with epilepsy. Pediatrics 80:909–917, 1987b

Brent DA, Kupfer DJ, Bromet EJ, et al: The assessment and treatment of patients at risk for suicide, in American Psychiatric Press Review of Psychiatry, Vol 7. Edited by Francis AJ, Hales RE. Washington, DC, American Psychiatric Press, 1988a, pp 353–385

Brent DA, Perper JA, Goldstein CE, et al: Risk factors for adolescent suicide: a comparison of adolescent suicide victims with suicidal inpatients. Arch Gen Psychiatry 45:581–588, 1988b

Brown JW: Juvenile suicides in adult jails, in Report of the National Conference on Youth Suicide, June 19–20, 1985. Edited by Faderow N, Atman S, Thorne A. Washington, DC, Youth Suicide National Center, 1985, pp 69–76

Butler LF, Miezitis S, Friedman RJ, et al: The effect of two school-based intervention programs on depressive symptoms in preadolescent children. Am Ed Res J 17:111–119, 1980

Carlson GA, Cantwell DP: Suicidal behavior and depression in children and adolescents. Journal of the American Academy of Child Psychiatry 21:361–368, 1982

Centers for Disease Control: Suicide Surveillance 1970–1980. Atlanta, GA, U.S. Department of Health and Human Services, Public Health Service, Violent Epidemiology Branch, Center for Health Promotion and Education, 1985

Chia BH: Suicide on the Young of Singapore. Ann Acad Med Singapore 8:262–268, 1979

Chocquet M, Facy F, Davidson F: Suicide and attempted suicide among adolescents in France, in The Suicide Syndrome. Edited by Farmer RDT, Hirsch S. London, Croom Helm, 1980, pp 73–89

Chowdhury N, Hicks RC, Kreitman N: Evaluation of an after-care service for parasuicide (attempted suicide) patients. Soc Psychiatry 8:67–81, 1973

Clum GA, Patsiokas AT, Luscomb RL: Empirially based comprehensive treatment program for parasuicide. J Consult Clin Psychol 47:937–945, 1979

Cohen-Sandler R, Bermar AL, King RA: A follow-up study of hospitalized suicidal children. Journal of the American Academy of Child Psychiatry 21:398–403, 1982a

Cohen-Sandler R, Berman AL, King RA: Life stress and symptomatology: determinants of suicidal behavior in children. Journal of the American Academy of Child Psychiatry 21:178–186, 1982b

Coleman L: Suicide Clusters. Boston, MA, Faber & Faber, 1987

Crumley FE: Adolescent suicide attempts. JAMA 241:2404–2407, 1979

Deykin EY, Albert JJ, McNamara JJ: A pilot study of the effect of exposure to child abuse or neglect on adolescent suicidal behavior. Am J Psychiatry 142:1299–1303, 1985

Drake RE, Ehrlich J: Suicide attempts associated with akathisia. Am J Psychiatry 142:499–501, 1985

Drake RE, Gates C, Cotton PG, et al: Suicide among schizophrenics: who is at risk? J Nerv Ment Dis 172:613–617, 1984

Drye RC, Goulding RL, Goulding ME: No-suicide decisions: patient monitoring of suicidal risk. Am J Psychiatry 130:171–174, 1973

D'Zurilla TJ, Goldfried MR: Problem solving and behavior modification. J Abnorm Psychol 78:107–126, 1971

Emery PE: Adolescent depression and suicide. Adolescence 18:245–258, 1983

Feindler EL, Ection RB: Adolescent Anger Control: Cognitive Behavioral Techniques. Elmsford, NY, Pergamon, 1986

Frame C, Matson JL, Sonis WA, et al: Behavioral treatment of depression in a prepubertal child. J Behav Ther Exp Psychiatry 3:239–243, 1982

Frank E, Kupfer DJ: Psychotherapeutic approaches to the treatment of recurrent unipolar depression: work in progress. Psychopharmacol Bull 22:558–563, 1986

Frank E, Prien RF, Kupfer DJ, et al: Implications of noncompliance on research in affective disorders. Psychopharmacol Bull 21:37–42, 1985

Friedman AS, Glickman NW: Program characteristics for successful treatment of adolescent drug abuse. J Nerv Ment Dis 174:669–679, 1986

Friedman IM: Alcohol and unnatural deaths in San Francisco youths. Pediatrics 76:191–193, 1985

Friedman RC, Corn R, Hurt SW, et al: Family history of illness in the seriously suicidal adolescent: a life-cycle approach. Am J Orthopsychiatry 54:390–397, 1984

Garfinkel B, Froese A, Hood J: Suicide attempts in children and adolescents. Am J Psychiatry 139:1257–1261, 1982

Garfinkel PE, Garner DM: Anorexia Nervosa: A Multidimensional Perspective. New York, Brunner/Mazel, 1982, pp 40–57

Geller B, Perel JM, Knitter EF, et al: 1-Nortriptyline in major depressive disorder in children: response, steady-state plasma levels, predictive kinetics, and pharmacokinetics. Psychopharmacol Bull 19:62–65, 1983

Geller B, Cooper TB, Farooki ZQ, et al: Dose and plasma levels of nortriptyline and chlorpromazine in delusionally depressed adolescents and of nortriptyline in nondelusionally depressed adolescents. Am J Psychiatry 142:336–338, 1985

Gibbons JS, Butler J, Urwin P, et al: Evaluation of a social work service for self-poisoning patients. Br J Psychiatry 133:111–118, 1978

Gibbs JT: Depression and suicidal behavior among delinquent females. Journal of Youth and Adolescence 10:159–167, 1981

Gispert M, Davis MS, Marsh L, et al: Predictive factors in repeated suicide attempts by adolescents. Hosp Community Psychiatry 38:390–393, 1987

Goldacre M, Hawton K: Repetition of self-poisoning and subsequent death in adolescents who take overdoses. Br J Psychiatry 146:395–398, 1985

Goldberg EL: Depression and suicide ideation in the young adult. Am J Psychiatry 138:35–40, 1981

Goldney RD, Katsikitis M: Cohort analysis of suicide rates in Australia. Arch Gen Psychiatry 40:71–74, 1983

Gould MS, Shaffer D: The impact of suicide in television movies: evidence imitation. N Engl J Med 315:690–694, 1986

Gould MS, Shaffer D, Kaplan D: The characteristics of dropouts from a child psychiatry clinic. Journal of the American Academy of Child Psychiatry 3:316–328, 1985

Gould MS, Shaffer D, Kleinman M: The impact of suicide in television movies: replication and commentary. Presented at the American Academy of Suicidology, May 1987a

Gould MS, Wallenstein S, Kleinman M: Time-space clustering of teen suicide. Paper presented at the annual meeting of the American Academy of Child and Adolescent Psychiatry, Washington, DC, 1987b

Green AH: Self-destructive behavior in battered children. Am J Psychiatry 135:579–582, 1978

Greer S, Bagley C: Effect of psychiatric intervention in attempted suicide: a controlled study. Br Med J 1:310–312, 1971

Grenier C: Treatment effectiveness in an adolescent chemical dependency treatment program: a quasi-experimental design. Int J Addict 20:381–391, 1985

Haas GL, Glick FD, Spencer JH, et al: The patient, the family and compliance with posthospital treatment for affective disorders. Psychopharmacol Bull 22:999–1005, 1986

Harkavy-Friedman JM, Asnis GM, Boeck M, et al: Prevalence of specific suicidal behaviors in a high school sample. Am J Psychiatry 144:1203–1206, 1987

Hawton K, Catalan J: Attempted Suicide: A Practical Guide to Its Nature and Management, 2nd Edition. New York, Oxford University Press, 1987

Hawton K, Goldacre M: Hospital admissions for adverse effects of medicinal agents (mainly self-poisoning) among adolescents in the Oxford region. Br J Psychiatry 141:166–170, 1982

Hawton K, Bancroft J, Catalan J, et al: Domiciliary and out-patient treatment of self-poisoning patients by medical and non-medical staff. Psychol Med 11:169–177, 1981

Hawton K, O'Grady J, Osborn M, et al: Adolescents who take overdoses: their characteristics, problems and contacts with helping agencies. Br J Psychiatry 140:118–123, 1982a

Hawton K, Osborn M, O'Grady J, et al: Classification of adolescents who take overdoses. Br J Psychiatry 140:124–131, 1982b

Hawton K, Cole D, O'Grady J, et al: Motivational aspects of deliberate self-poisoning in adolescents. Br J Psychiatry 141:286–291, 1982c

Hellon CP, Solomon MI: Suicide and age in Alberta, Canada, 1951 to 1977: the changing profile. Arch Gen Psychiatry 37:505–510, 1980

Hibbard RA, Brack CJ, Rauchs, et al: Abuse, feelings, and health behaviors in a student population. Am J Dis Child 142:326–330, 1988

Himmelhoch JM, Garfinkel ME: Sources of lithium resistance in mixed mania. Psychopharmacol Bull 22:613–620, 1986

Himmelhoch JM, Fuchs CA, Symons BJ: A double-blind study of tranylcypromine treatment of major anergic depression. J Nerv Ment Dis 170:628–634, 1982

Hirsch SR, Walsh C, Draper R: The concept and efficacy of the treatment of parasuicide. Br J Clin Pharmacol (Suppl) 15:189s–194s, 1983

Hirschfeld R, Blumenthal S: Personality, life events, and other psychosocial factors in adolescent depression and suicide, in Suicide and Depression Among Adolescents and Young Adults. Edited by Klerman GL. Washington, DC, American Psychiatric Press, 1986, pp 213–253

Holinger PC, Offer D: Prediction of adolescent suicide: a population model. Am J Psychiatry 139:302–307, 1982

Kaminer Y, Robbins DR: Attempted suicide by insulin overdose in insulin-dependent diabetic adolescents. Pediatrics 81:526–528, 1988

Kaslow NJ, Tanenbaum RL, Abramson LY, et al: Problem-solving deficits and depressive symptoms among children. J Abnorm Child Psychol 11:497–502, 1983

Kazdin AE, French NHY, Unis AS, et al: Hopelessness, depression, and suicidal intent among psychiatrically disturbed inpatient children. J Consult Clin Psychol 51:504–510, 1983

Kazdin AE, Esveldt-Dawson K, French NH, et al: Effects of parent management training and problem-solving training combined in the treatment of antisocial child behavior. J Am Acad Child Adolesc Psychiatry 26:416–424, 1987a

Kazdin AE, Esveldt-Dawson K, French NH, et al: Problem-solving skills training and relationship therapy in the treatment of antisocial child behavior. J Consult Clin Psychol 55:76–85, 1987b

Kellerman AL, Reay DT: Protection or peril? An analysis of firearm-related deaths in the home. N Engl J Med 314:1557–1560, 1986

Kennedy P: Efficacy of a regional poisoning treatment centre in preventing further suicidal behavior. Br Med J 4:255–257, 1972

Klerman GL, Lavori PW, Rice J, et al: Birth-cohort trends in rates of major depressive disorder among relatives of patients with affective disorder. Arch Gen Psychiatry 42:689–693, 1985

Kolko DJ: Depression, in Behavior Therapy With Children and Adolescents: A Clinical Approach. Edited by Hersen M, VanHasselt VB. New York, John Wiley, 1986, pp 137–183

Kosky R: Childhood suicidal behavior. J Child Psychol Psychiatry 24:457–468, 1983

Kosky R: Incest: what do we really know about it? Aust N Z J Psychiatry 21:430–440, 1987

Kosky R, Silburn S, Zubrick S: Symptomatic depression and suicidal ideation: a comparative study with 628 children. J Nerv Ment Dis 174:523–528, 1986

Kosten TR, Rounsaville BJ, Kleber HD: A 2.5 year follow-up of depression, life crises, and treatment effects on abstinence among opioid addicts. Arch Gen Psychiatry 43:733–738, 1986

Kovacs M, Rush AJ, Beck A, et al: Depressed outpatients treated with cognitive therapy or pharmacotherapy: a one year follow-up. Arch Gen Psychiatry 38:33–39, 1981

Kramer A, Feiguine R: Clinical effects of amitriptyline in adolescent depression. Journal of the American Academy of Child Psychiatry 20:636–644, 1981

Kreitman N: Age and parasuicide (attempted suicide). Psychol Med 6:113–121, 1976

Kreitman N, Schreiber M: Parasuicide in young Edinburgh women, 1968–1975. Psychol Med 9:469–479, 1979

Kua EH, Tsoi WF: Suicide in the island of Singapore. Acta Psychiatr Scand 71:227–229, 1985

Kupfer DJ, Spiker DG: Refractory depression: prediction of non-response by clinical indicators. J Clin Psychiatry 42:307–312, 1981

Lester D: Preventive effect of strict handgun control laws on suicide rates (letter). Am J Psychiatry 140:1259, 1983

Lester D, Murrell ME: The influence of gun control laws on suicidal behavior. Am J Psychiatry 137:121–122, 1980

Liberman RP, Eckman T: Behavior therapy vs insight-oriented therapy for repeated suicide attempters. Arch Gen Psychiatry 38:1126–1130, 1981

Liebowitz MR, Quitkin FM, Stewart JW, et al: Antidepressant specificity in atypical depression. Arch Gen Psychiatry 45:129–138, 1988

Linehan MM, Chiles JA, Egan KJ, et al: Presenting problems of parasuicides versus suicide ideators and nonsuicidal psychiatric patients. J Consult Clin Psychol 54:880–881, 1986

Marder SR, Van Patten T, Mintz J, et al: Costs and benefits of two doses of fluphenazine. Arch Gen Psychiatry 41:1025–1029, 1984

Markush RE, Bartolucci AA: Firearms and suicide in the United States. Am J Public Health 74:123–127, 1984

Marzuk PM, Tierney H, Tardiff K, et al: Increased risk of suicide in persons with AIDS. JAMA 259:1333–1337, 1988

Matthews W, Barabas G: Suicide and epilepsy: a review of the literature. Psychosomatics 22:515–524, 1981

Mattsson A, Seese LR, Hawkins JW: Suicidal behavior as a child psychiatric emergency: clinical characteristics and follow-up results. Arch Gen Psychiatry 20:100–109, 1969

McAnarney ER: Adolescent and young adult suicide in the United States: a reflection of societal unrest? Adolescence 14:765–774, 1979

McIntire MS, Angle CR: The taxonomy of suicides as seen in poison control centers. Pediatr Clin North Am 17:697–706, 1970

McIntire MS, Angle CR, Wikoff RL, et al: Recurrent adolescent suicidal behavior. Pediatrics 60:605–608, 1977

McLeavey BC, Daly RJ, Murray CM, et al: Interpersonal problem-solving deficits in self-poisoning patients. Suicide Life Threat Behav 17:33–49, 1987

McManus M, Lerner H, Robbins D, et al: Assessment of borderline symptomatology in hospitalized adolescents. Journal of the American Academy of Child Psychiatry 23:685–694, 1984

Miklowitz DJ, Goldstein MJ, Nuecehterlein KH, et al: Expressed emotion, affective style, lithium compliance, and relapse in recent onset mania. Psychopharmacol Bull 22:628–632, 1986

Milan MA, Kolko DJ: Social skills training and complimentary strategies in anger control and the treatment of aggressive behavior, in Handbook of Social Skills Training and Research. Edited by L'Abate L, Milan MA, New York, John Wiley, 1985, pp 101–135

Miller ML, Chiles JA, Barnes VE: Suicide attempters within a delinquent population. J Consult Clin Psychol 50:491–498, 1982

Montgomery S, Montgomery D, Rani S, et al: Maintenance therapy in repeat suicidal behavior: a placebo controlled trial, in Proceedings of the 10th International Congress for Suicide Prevention and Crisis Intervention, Ottawa, Ontario, June 1979, pp 227–229

Montgomery SA, Roy D, Montgomery D: The prevention of recurrent suicidal acts. Br J Clin Pharmacol (Suppl) 15:183s–188s, 1983

Motto JA: Suicide prevention for high-risk persons who refuse treatment. Suicide Life Threat Behav 6:223–230, 1976

Murphy GE, Wetzel RD: Suicide risk by birth cohort in the United States, 1949 to 1974. Arch Gen Psychiatry 37:519–523,1980

Myers KM, Burke P, McCauley E: Suicidal behavior by hospitalized preadolescent children on a psychiatric unit. Journal of the American Academy of Child Psychiatry 24:474–480, 1985

Nezu AM, Nezu CM, Saraydaria L, et al: Social problem solving as a moderating variable between negative life stress and depressive symptoms. Cognitive Therapy and Research 10:489–498, 1986

O'Brien JP: Increase in suicide attempts by drug ingestion: the Boston experience, 1964–1974. Arch Gen Psychiatry 34:1165–1169, 1977

Orbach I, Feshback S, Carlson G, et al: Attraction and repulsion by life and death in suicidal and in normal children. J Consult Clin Psychol 51:661–670, 1983

Orbach I, Feshbach S, Carlson G, et al: Attitudes toward life and death in suicidal, normal, and chronically ill children: an extended replication. J Consult Clin Psychol 52:1020–1027, 1984

Orbach I, Rosenheim E, Hary E: Some aspects of cognitive functioning in suicidal children. J Am Acad Child Adolesc Psychiatry 20:181–185, 1987

Otto U: Suicidal acts by children and adolescents: a follow-up study. Acta Psychiatr Scand (Suppl) Vol 233, 1972

Patsiokas AT, Clum GA: Effects of psychotherapeutic strategies in the treatment of suicide attempters. Psychotherapy 22:281–289, 1985

Patterson GR: Families: Applications of Social Learning to Family Life. Champaign, IL, Research Press, 1975, pp 59–66

Paykel ES, Hallowell C, Dressler DM, et al: Treatment of suicide attempters: a descriptive study. Arch Gen Psychiatry 31:487–491, 1974

Perris C: A study of bipolar and unipolar recurrent depressive psychoses. Acta Psychiatr Scand (Suppl) 42:1–188, 1966

Petti TA, Wells K: Crisis treatment of a preadolescent who accidentally killed his twin. Am J Psychother 34:434–443, 1980

Petti TA, Bornstein M, Delameter A, et al: Evaluation and multimodality treatment of a depressed prepubertal girl. Journal of the American Academy of Child Psychiatry 19:690–702, 1980

Pfeffer CR: Interventions for suicidal children and their parents. Suicide Life Threat Behav 12:240–248, 1982

Pfeffer CR: The Suicidal Child. New York, Guilford Press, 1986

Pfeffer CR, Conte HR, Plutchik R, et al: Suicidal behavior in latency-age children. Journal of the American Academy of Child Psychiatry 18:679–692, 1979

Pfeffer CR, Conte HR, Plutchik R, et al: Suicidal behavior in latency-age children. Journal of the American Academy of Child Psychiatry 19:703–710, 1980

Pfeffer CR, Plutchik R, Mizruchi MS: Suicidal and assaultive behavior in children: classification, measurement, and interrelations. Am J Psychiatry 140:154–157, 1983

Pfeffer CR, Zuckerman S, Plutchik R, et al: Suicidal behavior in normal schoolchildren: a comparison with child psychiatric inpatients. Journal of the American Academy of Child Psychiatry 23:416–423, 1984

Pfeffer CR, Plutchik R, Mizruchi MS, et al: Suicidal behavior in child psychiatric inpatients and outpatients and in nonpatients. Am J Psychiatry 143:733–738, 1986

Pfeffer CR, Lipkins R, Plutchik R, et al: Normal children at risk for suicidal behavior: a two-year follow-up study. J Am Acad Child Adolesc Psychiatry 27:34–41, 1988

Phillips D: The influence of suggestion on suicide: substantive and theoretical implications of the Werther effect. American Sociological Review 39:340–354, 1974

Phillips DP, Carstensen LL: Clustering of teenage suicides after television news stories about suicide. N Engl J Med 315:685–689, 1986

Phillips DP, Paight DJ: The impact of televised movies about suicide. N Engl J Med 317:809–811, 1987

Pokorny AD: Characteristics of forty-four patients who subsequently committed suicide. Arch Gen Psychiatry 2:314–323, 1960

Preskorn SH, Weller E, Weller R: Depression in children: relationship between plasma imipramine levels and response. J Clin Psychiatry 43:450–453, 1982

Preskorn SH, Weller EB, Hughes CW, et al: Depression in prepubertal children: dexamethasone nonsuppression predicts differential response to imipramine vs. placebo. Psychophamacol Bull 23:128–133, 1987

Prusoff BA, Williams DH, Weissman MM, et al: Treatment of secondary depression in schizophrenia: a double-blind, placebo-controlled trial of amitriptyline added to perphenazine. Arch Gen Psychiatry 36:569–575, 1979

Puig-Antich J: Major depression and conduct disorder in prepuberty. Journal of the American Academy of Child Psychiatry 21:118–128, 1982

Puig-Antich J, Blau S, Marx N, et al: Prepubertal major depressive disorder: a pilot study. Journal of the American Academy of Child Psychiatry 17:695–707, 1978

Puig-Antich J, Lukens E, Davies M, et al: Psychosocial functioning in prepubertal major depressive disorders. I: Interpersonal relationships during the depressive episode. Arch Gen Psychiatry 42:500–507, 1985a

Puig-Antich J, Lukens E, Davies M, et al: Psychosocial functioning in prepubertal major depressive disorders. II: Interpersonal relationships after sustained recovery from affective episode. Arch Gen Psychiatry 42:511–517, 1985b

Puig-Antich J, Perel JM, Lupatkin W, et al: Imipramine in prepubertal major depressive disorders. Arch Gen Psychiatry 44:81–89, 1987

Quitkin FM, Schwartz D, Liebowitz MR, et al: Atypical depressives: a preliminary report of antidepressant response and sleep patterns. Psychopharmacol Bull 18:78–80, 1982

Reynolds WM, Coates KI: A comparison of cognitive-behavioral therapy and relaxation training for the treatment of depression in adolescents. J Consult Clin Psychol 54:653–660, 1986

Rich CL, Young D, Fowler RC: San Diego suicide study. I: Young vs old subjects. Arch Gen Psychiatry 43:577–582, 1986

Robins DR, Alessi NE: Depressive symptoms and suicidal behavior in adolescents. Am J Psychiatry 142:588–592, 1985

Robbins D, Conroy R: A cluster of adolescent suicide attempts: is suicide contagious? J Adolesc Health Care 3:253–255, 1983

Roberts J, Hawton K: Child abuse and attempted suicide. Br J Psychiatry 137:319–323, 1980

Robin AL: Problem-solving communication training: a behavioral approach to the treatment of parent-adolescent conflict. American Journal of Family Therapy 7:69–82, 1979

Robin AL: A controlled evaluation of problem-solving communication training with parent-adolescent conflict. Behavior Therapy 12:593–609, 1981

Robin AL, Foster SL: Problem-solving communication training: a behavioral-family systems approach to parent-adolescent conflict, in Adolescent Behavior Disorders: Foundations and Contemporary Concerns. Edited by Karoly P, Steffen J. Lexington, MA, DC Heath, 1984, pp 195–240

Robins LN: Suicide attempts in teen-aged medical patients, in Alcohol, Drug Abuse and Mental Health Administration Report of the Secretary's Task Force on Youth Suicide, Vol 4, Strategies for the Prevention of Youth Suicide (DHHS Publ No ADM-89-1624). Washington, DC, U.S. Government Printing Office, 1989, pp 94–114

Rosenthal PA, Rosenthal S, Doherty MB, et al: Suicidal thoughts and behaviors in depressed hospitalized preschoolers. Am J Psychother 40:201–212, 1986

Rotheram MJ: Evaluation of imminent danger for suicide among youth. Am J Orthopsychiatry 57:102–110, 1987

Rounsaville BJ, Kosten TR, Weissman MM, et al: Prognostic significance of psychopathology in treated opiate addicts: a 2.5 year follow-up study. Arch Gen Psychiatry 43:739–745, 1986

Roy A: Risk factors for suicide in psychiatric patients. Arch Gen Psychiatry 39:1089–1095, 1982

Rubenstein DH: Epidemic suicide among Micronesian adolescents. Soc Sci Med 17:657–665, 1983

Rush AJ, Beck AT, Kovacs M, et al: Comparative efficacy of cognitive therapy and pharmacotherapy in the treatment of depressed outpatients. Cognitive Therapy and Research 1:17–37, 1977

Ryan ND, Puig-Antich J: Affective illness in adolescence, in Psychiatry Update: American Psychiatric Association Annual Review, Vol 5. Edited by Frances AJ, Hales RE. Washington, DC, American Psychatric Press, 1986, pp 420–450

Ryan ND, Puig-Antich J, Cooper T, et al: Imipramine in adolescent major depression: plasma level and clinical response. Acta Psychiatr Scand 73:275–288, 1986

Ryan ND, Puig-Antich J, Ambrosini P, et al: The clinical picture of major depression in children and adolescents. Arch Gen Psychiatry 44:854–861, 1987

Salk L, Lipsitt LP, Sturner WQ, et al: Relationship of maternal and perinatal conditions to eventual adolescent suicide. Lancet 1:624–627, 1985

Sathyavathi K: Suicide among children in Bangalore. Indian J Pediatr 42:149–157, 1975

Shaffer D: Suicide in childhood and early adolescence. J Child Psychol Psychiatry 15:275–291, 1974

Shaffer D, Fisher P: The epidemiology of suicide in children and young adolescents. Journal of the American Academy of Child Psychiatry 20:545–565, 1981

Shaffer D, Gould M, Trautman P: Suicidal behavior in children and young adults. Paper presented at the Psychobiology of Suicidal Behavior Conference, New York, September 1985

Shafii M: Reply to JS Werry: handling threats in children and adolescents. Am J Psychiatry 143:1193–1194, 1986a

Shafii M: Psychological autopsy study of suicide in adolescents. Paper presented at the Child Depression Consortium, St. Louis, MO, October 1986b

Shafii M, Whittinghill R, Healy MH: The pediatric-psychiatric model for emergencies in child psychiatry: a study of 994 cases. Am J Psychiatry 136:1600–1601, 1979

Shafii M, Carrigan S, Whittinghill JR, et al: Psychological autopsy of completed suicide in children and adolescents. Am J Psychiatry 142:1061–1064, 1985

Shear MK, Frances A, Weiden P: Suicide associated with akathisia and depot fluphenazine treatment. J Clin Psychopharmacol 3:235–236, 1983

Shepherd D, Barracough BM: Suicide reporting: information or entertainment? Br J Psychiatry 132:283–287, 1978

Silanpaa M: Medico-social prognosis of children with epilepsy. Acta Paediatr Scand 62(suppl. 237):7–104, 1973

Simons AP, Garfield SL, Murphy GE: The process of change in cognitive therapy and pharmacotherapy for depression. Arch Gen Psychiatry 41:45–51, 1984

Simons AD, Murphy GE, Levine JL, et al: Cognitive therapy and pharmacotherapy for depression: sustained improvement over one year. Arch Gen Psychiatry 43:43–48, 1986

Sims M: Sex and age differences in suicide rates in a Canadian province: with particular reference to suicides by means of poison. Suicide Life Threat Behav 4:139–159, 1974

Siris SG, Rifkin A, Reardon GT, et al: A trial of adjunctive imipramine in post-psychotic depression. Psychopharmacol Bull 21:114–116, 1985

Smith K, Crawford S: Suicidal behavior among "normal" high school students (Fourth Annual Conference on Suicide of Adults and Youth, Topeka, KS, 1984). Suicide Life Threat Behav 16:313–325, 1986

Soloff PH, George A, Nathan RS: Paradoxical effects of amitriptyline border-line patients. Am J Psychiatry 143:1603–1605, 1986a

Soloff PH, George A, Nathan RS: Progress in pharmacotherapy of borderline disorders: a double-blind study of amitriptyline, haloperidol, and placebo. Arch Gen Psychiatry 43:691–697, 1986b

Spivack G, Shure M: The cognition of social adjustment: interpersonal cognitive problem-solving thinking, in Advances in Clinical Child Psychology, Vol 5. Edited by Lahey B, Kazdin AE. New York, Plenum, 1982, pp 323–372

Stanley EJ, Barter JT: Adolescent suicidal behavior. Am J Orthopsychiatry 40:87–96, 1970

Strayhorn JM Jr: Foundations of Clinical Psychiatry. Chicago, IL, Year Book Medical Publishers, 1982

Strober M, Carlson G: Bipolar illness in adolescents with major depression: clinical, genetic, and psychopharmacologic predictors in a three- to four-year prospective follow-up investigation. Arch Gen Psychiatry 39:549–555, 1982

Strober M, Hanna G, McCracken J: Bipolar disorder, in Handbook of Child Psychiatric Diagnosis. Edited by Last CG, Hersen M. New York, John Wiley, 1988a, pp 299–316

Strober M, Morrell W, Burroughs J, et al: A family study of bipolar I disorder in adolescents: early onset of systems linked to increased familial loading and lithium resistance. J Affective Disord 15:255–268, 1988b

Taylor EA, Stansfeld SA: Children who poison themselves. I: A clinical comparison with psychiatric controls. Br J Psychiatry 145:127–132, 1984a

Taylor EA, Stansfeld SA: Children who poison themselves. II: Prediction of attendance for treatment. Br J Psychiatry 145:132–135, 1984b

Tishler CL, McKenry PC: Parental negative self and adolescent suicide attempts. Journal of the American Academy of Child Psychiatry 21:404–408, 1982

Tishler CL, McKenry PC, Morgan KC: Adolescent suicide attempts: some significant factors. Suicide Life Threat Behav 11:86–92, 1981

Topol P, Reznikoff M: Perceived peer and family relationships, hopelessness and locus of control as factors in adolescent suicide attempts. Suicide Life Threat Behav 12:141–150, 1982

Trautman PD, Shaffer D: Treatment of child and adolescent suicide attempters, in Suicide in the Young. Edited by Sudak HS, Ford AB, Rushforth NB. Boston, MA, John Wright Publishing, 1984, pp 307–323

Trautman PD, Rotheram MJ, Chatlos C, et al: Differences among normal, psychiatrically disturbed and suicide attempting adolescent females. Paper presented at the American Academy of Child Psychiatry meeting, Toronto, Ontario, October 1984

Trautman PD, Lewin N, Krauskopf D: Home visits with noncompliant adolescent suicide attempters: a pilot study. Presented at the 34th Annual Meeting of the American Academy of Child and Adolescent Psychiatry, Washington, DC, October 24, 1987

Velez CN, Cohen P: Suicidal behavior and ideation in a community sample of children: maternal and youth reports. J Am Acad Child Adolesc Psychiatry 27:349–356, 1988

Ward JA, Fox J: A suicide epidemic on an Indian reserve. Canadian Psychiatric Association Journal 22:423–426, 1977

Weissman MM: The epidemiology of suicide attempts, 1960–1971. Arch Gen Psychiatry 30:737–746, 1974

Weissman MM, Paykel ES, Klerman GL: The depressed woman as mother. Soc Psychiatry 7:98–108, 1972

Weissman MM, Fox K, Klerman GL: Hostility and depression associated with suicide attempts. Am J Psychiatry 130:450–455, 1973

Weller RA, Weller EB, Tucker SG, et al: Mania in prepubertal children: underdiagnosed? J Affective Disord 11:151–154, 1986

Welner A, Welner Z, Fishman R: Psychiatric adolescent inpatients: eight to ten-year follow-up. Arch Gen Psychiatry 36:689–700, 1979

Welu TC: A follow-up program for suicide attempters: evaluation of effectiveness. Suicide Life Threat Behav 7:17–30, 1977

Wexler L, Weissman MM, Kasl SV: Suicide attempts 1970–1975: updating a United States study and comparisons with international trends. Br J Psychiatry 132:180–185, 1978

Wilkes TCR, Rush JR: Adaptations of cognitive therapy for depressed adolescents. J Am Acad Child Adolesc Psychiatry 27:381–386, 1988

Williams CL, Lyons CM: Family interaction and adolescent suicidal behavior: a preliminary investigation. Aust N Z J Psychiatry 10:234–252, 1976

Williams CL, Sale IM, Wignall AL: Correlates of impulsive suicidal behavior. Aust NZ J Psychiatry 85:323–325, 1977

Chapter 12

Suicide Among College Students: Assessment, Treatment, and Intervention

Allan J. Schwartz, Ph.D.
Leighton C. Whitaker, Ph.D.

SYSTEMATIC STUDY OF suicide among students at American colleges and universities now spans more than 50 years. Clinical reports such as case studies that address the assessment, management, and treatment of suicidal students have an even longer tradition. In the 1930s, suicide was the second leading cause of death among college students, leading Raphael et al. (1937) to address the problem. Raphael, then director of the mental health unit at the University of Michigan student health service, noted that three of five student deaths in the 1934–1935 academic year were suicides. In the context of the generally low mortality that characterized the student population, Raphael was particularly impressed by the high proportion of these deaths accounted for by suicide.

Raphael's epidemiologic sophistication, exemplified in this and several other reports on college mental health published between 1936 and 1944 (Raphael 1936a, 1936b; Raphael and Gordon 1938; Raphael and Himler 1944), led him to address not the rare event of completed suicide, but the considerably more frequent phenomenon of suicidality in this population. He explored the incidence of clinical concern about suicide among the students seen at the University of Michigan student mental health service during the 5-year period 1930–1931 through 1934–1935. It may well be that Raphael's emphasis on these less dramatic aspects of suicidality contributed to his report being virtually ignored in subsequent epidemiologic research. Had he proceeded in the fashion of Parnell (1951), who 14 years later reported on nine completed suicides among Oxford University students, he might well have precipitated a furor over suicide among American college students that matched the one precipitated in Great Britain.

Whatever the bases for the reception accorded Raphael's thoughtful and responsible report of suicidality among college students, the publications of Parnell (Parnell 1951; Parnell and Skottowe 1957) and other student health professionals in Great Britain during the 1950s and early 1960s (Carpenter 1959; Lyman 1961; Malleson 1954; Read 1954; Rook 1954, 1959; Still 1956) established the agenda that guided epidemiologic research on suicide among American college students during the latter half of this century. Two questions dominated: 1) Are suicide rates for students at American colleges and universities higher than for nonstudents; and 2) Are suicide rates for students at academically more competitive, selective, prestigious institutions higher than at institutions with less stringent academic standards and an academically more relaxed atmosphere (Arnstein 1986)? The British data suggested that, at institutions there, the answer to both questions was yes. (Apparently overlooked in the British studies was the hypothesis that an all-male student body, rather than an academically demanding setting, was the basis for elevated suicide rates at certain institutions.) The British findings appear to have influenced the reception given studies of American and Canadian institutions published in the 1950s, 1960s, and early 1970s that contradicted these conclusions (Braaten and Darling 1962; Parrish 1956, 1957; Peck and Schrut 1968, 1971; Sims and Ball 1973). Earlier reports that failed to support the extrapolation to American settings of the conclusions of British writers were apparently unknown (Diehl and Shepard 1939; Riggs and Terhune 1928). The findings that appeared to lend support to these assertions (Bruyn and Seiden 1965; Temby 1961) were the ones that impressed mental health professionals and established as bedrock realities conclusions that were either largely contradicted or ambiguously supported (cf. Ross 1969).

Since 1970 there has been a dramatic increase in the systematic collection of data on student suicides at American colleges and universities. Of the 567 student suicides reported, 400 (71%) have appeared in studies that have been published or conducted since that date. The epidemiology of attempted, threatened, and contemplated suicide among students has also received increased attention (Bernard and Bernard 1982; Mishara et al. 1976). Concurrently, the clinical issues of assessment, management, and treatment of suicidal and depressed students have received attention (Brown 1978; Hammen 1980; Miles 1977; Morgan 1981; Oliver and Burkham 1979; Rush et al. 1982). In this chapter, current empirical knowledge of the epidemiology of student suicide at American colleges and universities will be reviewed, and several other perspectives that also bear on the prevention of suicide in this population will be considered.

EPIDEMIOLOGY

In this section, we consider the evidence about whether suicide is more common among students at American colleges and universities than among their nonstudent peers. Several major issues will be reviewed: 1) the association between student suicide rates and the academic standards and/or prestige of the institution; 2) the principal methodological and technical issues associated with empirical research on student suicide; 3) the methods of suicide used by male and female college students; 4) a comparison of college students of each sex with United States national data; and 5) a review of student suicide rates in relation to students' sex and class standing; to the temporal variables of month of the year, day of the week, and time of day; and to prior contact with the campus mental health system and the presence of emotional distress or impairment. We conclude this section with a discussion of the suicidal continuum, including the incidence of attempted, threatened, and contemplated suicide and a review of how the incidence of depression may be related to suicidality in college students.

Student Versus Nonstudent Suicide

Figure 1 summarizes epidemiologic research on suicide at American colleges and universities. Twelve samples are shown: Vassar (Riggs and Terhune 1928), Michigan (Raphael et al. 1937), Yale (Fry and Rostow 1942, Parrish 1957), Harvard (Temby 1961), Berkeley (Bruyn and Seiden 1965), Cornell (Braaten and Darling, 1962), Los Angeles (Peck and Schrut 1968, 1971), Massachusetts-Amherst (Kraft 1980), South Dakota (Heinrichs 1980), the American College Health Association Mental Health Annual Program Survey (ACHA-MHAPS) (Schwartz and Reifler 1980, 1988), Big Ten (Bessai 1986), and California (Kagan 1988). Several of these samples (ACHA-MHAPS, Harvard, Los Angeles, Yale) are pooled samples representing the cumulative findings obtained during contiguous periods of study.

The standard mortality ratios (SMRs) displayed in Figure 1 were either reported in the relevant study or derived by comparing the suicide rate found for each of the 12 student samples with national, state, or local suicide rates during the period spanned by each study for persons of the same age, and matched for the proportion of men to

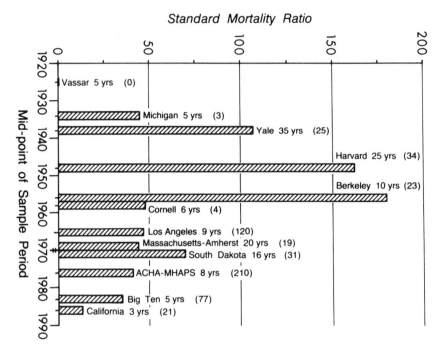

Figure 1. Twelve student suicide samples from American colleges and universities. The number of years spanned by each sample and, in parentheses, the number of suicides reported are also shown. Bars for each sample are located at the midpoint of the years spanned. References for samples: Vassar (Riggs and Terhune 1928), Michigan (Raphael et al. 1937), Yale (Parrish 1957), Harvard (Temby 1961), Berkeley (Bruyn and Seiden 1965), Cornell (Braaten and Darling 1962), Los Angeles (Peck and Schrut 1968, 1971), Massachusetts-Amherst (Kraft 1980), South Dakota (Heinrichs 1980), the American College Health Association Mental Health Annual Program Survey (ACHA-MHAPS) (Schwartz and Reifler 1980, 1988), Big Ten (Bessai 1986), and California (Kagan 1988).

women in the student sample. A mean SMR of 46 is obtained when these 12 samples are pooled, each sample being weighted by the number of student-years of risk it represents. Since an SMR less than 100 indicates a suicide rate for students that is lower than that for nonstudents, the cumulative empirical epidemiologic data on suicide among students at American colleges and universities strongly suggest that the suicide rate for students is about half the suicide rate for comparable groups of nonstudents. Of the total of 567 suicides reported, 485 (86%) are associated with a student suicide rate that is lower than the rate for nonstudents.

Further review of the SMR for each of the 12 samples shown in Figure 1 lends additional support to the inference that student suicide rates are lower than rates for nonstudents. Seven of the 12 samples reference the experience of a single institution (Berkeley, Cornell, Harvard, Massachusetts-Amherst, Michigan, Vassar, Yale). Of these seven studies, only the Berkeley and Harvard Studies suggest that student suicide rates are higher than the rate for nonstudents. While the number of suicides reported in the Vassar, Michigan, and Cornell samples is too small for the low SMR that each yields to be statistically significant, among the four remaining single-institution studies, two (Berkeley, Harvard) yield a significantly elevated student suicide rate, one (Massachusetts-Amherst) a significantly lower rate, and one (Yale) a virtually equal rate. All five multi-institution samples are associated with a significantly lower suicide rate for students (Big Ten; South Dakota; California; Los Angeles; ACHA-MHAPS). Thus, when considered on a sample-by-sample basis, for 9 of the 12 samples the suicide rate for students was lower than that for nonstudents. (For six of the eight samples where statistically significant differences were found, the suicide rate was lower for students.)

Academic Reputation

Bruyn and Seiden (1965), speaking of American colleges and universities, echoed the assertion first made by professionals studying student suicide in Great Britain that higher suicide rates for students were at least associated with, if not caused by, institutions having higher academic standards or prestige. Single-institution studies do not provide very strong support for this thesis. Among institutions that would popularly be regarded as highly prestigious, the Harvard and Berkeley studies reported student suicide rates that were significantly elevated, but Yale's study did not.

Some of the multi-institution samples showing significantly lower student suicide rates might also be regarded as consisting of institutions that lack the prestige or high academic standards that have been hypothesized to be associated with elevated student suicide rates. The California sample, for example, includes only the 19 state colleges, excluding all of the major universities, such as UCLA and Berkeley, in the California state system. The South Dakota sample may not include any campuses that would qualify as prestigious. Moreover, with only 31 suicides reported, it is unlikely that a strong test of the hypothesis could be undertaken with these data. The ACHA-MHAPS data include a sufficient number of suicides from adequately prestigious institutions (Chicago, Cornell, Dartmouth, Duke, Harvard, MIT, Princeton, and Yale) to support such a test. However, they have not been analyzed in this format. Peck and Schrut (1968), on the other hand, did subject their data to such an analysis. The campuses included in their sample forced them to confound age distribution, sex distribution, and campus size with prestige/academic standards, which they indexed by highest degree awarded (associate's, bachelor's, master's, doctorate). Nonetheless, Peck and Schrut were able to draw several instructive conclusions. First, they found evidence for the hypothesized association between institutional prestige and crude student suicide rates; that is, rates not adjusted for the sex and age distribution of the population at risk. More importantly, they found that it was not the high academic standards of these institutions but rather the elevated proportion of males enrolled there, and particularly males over 25, that was associated with elevated campus suicide rates.

Overall, the existing epidemiologic data fail to support the assertion that student suicide rates are higher at institutions usually regarded as more prestigious or as having very high academic standards. More clinically oriented reports also point to factors other than academic stress as the principal determinants of student suicide. Fry and Rostow (1942) reviewed 8 suicides and 17 suicide attempts by students at Yale. In their review, sexual concerns, significant psychiatric illness (schizophrenia, manic depression), acute emotional disturbance, family issues, and financial concerns were the prominent factors. Parrish (1957) reported virtually the same findings for his Yale sample. The extensive analysis of suicidality in 313 students seen at the University of Michigan mental health service found that "anxiety over school work" was the precipitating factor in only a modest minority (31%) of these cases. Among a nonpatient sample of more than 800 students, Bernard and Bernard (1982) found that while fully 9% of their predominantly undergraduate subjects reported having threatened or attempted suicide while enrolled in college, only 7% of these 75 persons described academic concerns as a significant factor in their suicide attempt.

Epidemiologic and clinical perspectives appear to converge. Together they indicate that academic concerns contribute only modestly to student suicidality, that institutional prestige or academic reputation does not affect student suicide rates in any powerful way, and that in those instances where it may appear to be associated with elevated student suicide rates, this apparent effect may well be an artifact of the demography of the population at risk; that is, a consequence of admission and selection factors, not of increased academic pressure.

Method of Suicide

We have already noted that the suicide rate for students is about half the rate for nonstudents. One factor that may be responsible for this finding is the degree to which college students have access to highly lethal methods of suicide relative to their nonstudent peers. We may consider access to methods as one aspect of the academic environment that can be managed with the goal of preventing student suicide.

Among the 12 samples described in Figure 1, five yield data on the method of suicide: Big Ten, Cornell, Harvard, Massachusetts-Amherst, and Yale. National data provide a standard with which these data for student suicides may be compared. These national data are routinely reported by sex and race, but not for specific age groups (National Center for Health Statistics 1960–1985). Accordingly, distributions based on these national data may conceal significant age-related distinctions. For this reason alone, inferences based on comparisons of student suicide data with these national standards may be erroneous. There are, however, other methodological details that should be considered.

With respect to national suicide statistics, both the major categories reported for methods of suicide and their associated subcategories have changed over the years, but these changes are both relatively minor and not particularly troublesome to manage when comparing data from different points in time (e.g., 1960 versus 1985). The principal concern in dealing with these differences is to ensure the comparability across time of the categories that are used. With respect to student suicides, the major issue is whether informal and official sources of data assign methods of suicide in a comparable fashion. No quantitative estimate exists for the potential disparity introduced by this feature. In any event, such a disparity will be smallest when comparisons of the method of suicide used by students and national samples are based on a relatively few inclusive categories. That is the approach employed here.

Over the 25-year period spanned by the six values used to determine the mean expected percentage, clear but modest trends are discernible in the prominence of some of the six categories. For white males, suicide by gas declined from about 12% of all suicides to about 9%; suicide by firearms and explosives increased from about 55% to about 65%. For white females, suicide by ingestion of a solid or liquid (i.e., "substances") declined from about 35% of all suicides to about 27%; suicide by gas increased from about 9% to about 12%. About 80% of the female student suicides reported in Table 1 occurred between 1980 and 1985. For the male student suicides, 44% occurred between 1980 and 1987, 11% between 1960 and 1979, and 45% between 1920 and 1960.

These methodological limitations provide one basis for caution in interpreting the data of Table 1. The paucity of the data, particularly

Table 1. Comparison of observed and expected distributions for method of suicide by college students

Method[a]	Males[b] (n = 124)				Females (n = 31)			
	Observed		Expected[c]		Observed		Expected[c]	
	n	%	n	%	n	%	n	%
Substances	21	16.9	9.3	7.5	10	32.3	9.8	31.6
Gas	17	13.7	13.0	10.5	5	16.1	3.5	11.3
Hanging	25	20.2	18.7	15.1	1	3.2	3.8	12.3
Firearms	40	32.3	74.0	59.7	6	19.4	10.0	32.3
Jumping	18	14.5	3.0	2.4	6	19.4	1.2	3.9
Other	3	2.4	6.0	4.8	3	9.7	2.7	8.7

[a]"Substances" includes suicide by use of any solid or liquid. "Gas" includes suicide by use of any gas; nationally 83% of these are by motor vehicle exhaust gas. "Hanging" includes suicide by hanging, strangulation, or suffocation, with 93% by hanging. "Firearms" includes suicide by use of firearms or explosives, with more than 99% by firearms. "Jumping" includes suicide by jumping from a high place, as contrasted with in front of a moving object, with 82% of the places being constructed structures. "Other" represents suicide by any other means, including drowning, electrocution, crashing a motor vehicle or aircraft, use of a cutting or piercing instrument (e.g., slashing wrists, stabbling), burns or fire, and extremes of cold.

[b]n observed versus n expected: $\chi^2 = 102$, 5 df, $P < .0001$. Cramers contingency coefficient C = .67.

[c]Expected number is derived from the expected percentage. Expected percentage is the mean proportion calculated from United States national data for white males and females of all ages for the years 1960, 1965, 1970, 1975, 1980, and 1985 (National Center for Health Statistics).

for female student suicide, is another. With these limitations in mind, however, the data suggest that the distribution of methods of suicide for male students is significantly different from that of nonstudents. The relationship between method and student versus nonstudent status is, moreover, not only highly significant but also quite strong, with about two-thirds of the variability in method being associated with student versus nonstudent status. Among males, students are more than twice as likely as nonstudents to use the less lethal method of substances and about half as likely to use the more lethal method of firearms. Jumping, accounting for only 2% to 3% of male suicides nationally, is six times as likely among students as nonstudents.

One can interpret these contrasting profiles for methods of student and nonstudent suicide in the following way. When compared with national data, there is an additional one-quarter to one-third of all male student suicides that would be expected to occur by use of the highly lethal method of firearms. This fraction of all male student suicides appears instead to be distributed among methods of marginally to significantly diminished lethality: jumping (12%), use of substances (9%), hanging (5%), and use of gas (3%). This altered pattern of methods of suicide might account for the comparatively lower suicide rate of male students in relation to their nonstudent age peers.

For females, the number of student suicides is too small to sustain a statistically meaningful comparison of the methods used by students and nonstudents. Descriptively, however, the use of substances, a method of relatively low lethality, is equally prominent for both female students and nonstudents (31% to 32%). Female student suicide by highly lethal firearms is 13% less than nonstudents, and hanging is 9% less for students. Jumping, however, is 16% higher and use of gas 5% higher. Overall, these contrasts in method of suicide might be expected to yield a more moderately diminished suicide rate for female students in relation to their nonstudent age peers.

Correlates of Student Suicide

Relatively few studies of student suicide provide the data required to test hypotheses relating the incidence of student suicide to variables that might guide campus suicide prevention programs. The goal of such analyses is to identify vulnerable groups or individuals within the student body and aspects of the academic environment that contribute to student suicide, either directly or through their interaction. Three samples yield student suicide rates specific to men and to women (Big Ten, California, Massachusetts-Amherst). As displayed in Table 2, all three studies show suicide rates for male students that are significantly lower than those for male nonstudents. Only one of

Table 2. College student suicides by sex

Sample	Males				Females			
	Suicides	Risk[a]	Rate	SMR[b]	Suicides	Risk[a]	Rate	SMR[b]
Massachusetts (1960–1979)	14	198,500	7.1	30*	5	137,800	3.6	65
Big Ten (1981–1985)	51	672,700	7.6	32*	25	573,100	4.4	84
California (1985–1987)	16	489,600	3.3	12*	5	530,400	0.9	13*
Total	81	1,360,800	6.0	25*	35	1,241,300	2.8	52*

Note. References for samples: Massachusetts (Kraft 1980), Big Ten (Bessai 1986), California (Kagan 1988).
[a]Risk measured in student-years.
[b]SMR = standard mortality ratio. The comparison group rate was derived from United States annual national suicide rates for 20- to 24-year-old white males and females, with proportions by sex matched to the sample population at risk.
*Difference between sample and comparison group significant at the .05 level.

the three, the California sample, shows a suicide rate for female students that is significantly lower.

It is tempting to infer from these findings that colleges and universities may be less hospitable environments for women students than for men. The data on methods of suicide suggest that any such disparity in benefit may arise from campus policies that limit students' access to firearms, a highly lethal method of suicide that, nationally, is the most common method for both sexes but is employed (again nationally) almost twice as often by men as by women. It would be this second feature that produces the greater benefit that appears to accrue to male students.

Institutional size was identified as a confounding variable in Peck and Schrut's (1968) study of academic standards and suicide rates. In the ACHA-MHAPS sample, this problem is minimized by the fact that nearly all of the participating institutions awarded doctoral degrees. Table 3 shows the suicide rates derived for institutions in each of four enrollment categories. There is no discernible trend in these rates as a function of enrollment nor a significant relation between enrollment and suicide rate. We give more extensive consideration to the issue of isolation versus connectedness as a determinant of student suicide in the second section of this chapter. For the moment, it appears that institutional size, as measured by full-time enrollment, does not have a systematic impact on this dynamic nor on other processes that may affect student suicide rates. The search for pathogenic influences related to institutional size will need to go beyond the crude index of full-time enrollment if it is to be fruitful.

Table 3.   College student suicide rates by size of institution

Full-time enrollment	Number of reports	Number of suicides	Student-years of risk	Suicide rate (per 100,000)[a]
0–7,999	48	18	201,100	10.3
8,000–14,999	21	14	215,700	6.5
15,000–19,999	25	35	437,600	8.0
20,000+	30	53	788,300	6.7
Total	124	120	1,642,700	7.3

[a] $\chi^2 = 1.61$, 3 df, NS.
Source.   American College Health Association Mental Health Annual Program Survey (Schwartz and Reifler 1980) for 1971–1972 through 1975–1976.

Class standing holds promise as a variable that might grossly identify stress points in the academic program. The Big Ten and Yale samples provide the incidence and risk data needed to assess the relation of incidence to class standing, although only in a tentative way. Neither study provides explicit information about the proportions by sex among graduate students, and the numbers of suicides for each level of class standing in the Yale study are so small that undergraduate classes must be pooled to provide a valid test of the observed proportions. Each sample individually shows no significant relationship between suicide and undergraduate versus graduate status. Even when the data are combined, as shown in Table 4, no significant relationship is found between suicide rate and class standing. While the frequently noted stress experienced by freshmen just entering college is not reflected in these data, this may be a confirmation of the effectiveness of programs specifically designed to facilitate their entry into undergraduate life.

A complementary approach to identifying times of heightened stress for students focuses on the month of the year. Heinrichs (1980) reported no significant difference in the distributions of student and nonstudent suicides, but did not provide specific monthly values for his sample of student suicides. Temby (1961) also gives inadequately

Table 4. Student suicide as a function of class standing

	Observed suicides			Risk (%)[a]	Expected suicides
	Yale	Big Ten	Total		
Freshman	2	9	11	18.9	17.80
Sophomore	7	12	19	16.9	15.85
Junior	2	13	15	17.7	16.68
Senior	4	12	16	17.7	16.68
All undergraduates	15	46	61	71.3[b]	67.00[b]
Graduate/ Professional	10	22	32	26.1	24.51
Other	—	1	1	2.6	2.48
Total	25	69	94	100.0	93.99[b]

Note. References for samples: Yale (Parrish 1957), Big Ten (Bessai 1986).
[a]Risk measured in student-years.
[b]Does not sum due to rounding error.

detailed information, but he noted that the pattern of student suicides did not conform qualitatively to the monthly distribution reported for national samples. The Big Ten and Yale studies do provide sufficiently detailed data, and these are displayed in Table 5 along with their combined monthly suicides. The monthly totals for observed suicides do not differ significantly from either chance or national values. It should be noted, however, that there is an emergent disproportion in student suicides for the months of January, March, and September, which have elevated proportions, and for June, July, and August, which have depressed proportions. If a total of 204 suicides (twice the number reported in the combined Yale and Big Ten samples) were distributed as these are, they would yield a statistically significant difference ($P = .01$) when compared with national proportions. Se-

Table 5. Student suicide as a function of month of the year

Month	Observed suicides			Expected suicides	
	Yale	Big Ten	Total	Chance[a]	National[b]
January	5	7	12	8.66	8.42
February	1	6	7	7.82	8.33
March	0	14	14	8.66	8.76
April	4	6	10	8.38	9.27
May	2	5	7	8.66	9.18
June	1	5	6	8.38	8.50
July	2	2	4	8.66	8.42
August	1	4	5	8.66	8.33
September	3	10	13	8.38	8.08
October	1	8	9	8.66	8.59
November	2	6	8	8.38	8.33
December	3	4	7	8.66	7.57
Total	25	77	102	101.96[c]	101.78[c]

Note. References for samples: Yale (Parrish 1957), Big Ten (Bessai 1986).
[a]Based on days per month for 365-day year. Versus total observed suicides: $\chi^2 = 12.92$, 11 df, NS.
[b]Based on United States annual national data as cited by Dublin (1963). Versus total observed suicides: $\chi^2 = 12.90$, 11 df, NS.
[c]Does not sum to 102 due to rounding error.

lective underreporting associated with the use of health service records for identifying student suicides would account for the June to August period. On the other hand, significantly elevated proportions for January, March, and September would appear to point to elements in the academic year that provoke student suicide. The stresses associated with the onset of the academic year, often noted clinically, may account for September; end-of-term examinations occur in January; and spring break is a feature of the academic calendar that often occurs in March, as do midterm examinations.

Using the coarse measure of time represented by a student's progress through the undergraduate years into graduate and professional study, no significant differential risk for suicide has been found or even suggested by existing data. Using the somewhat finer measure of months within the calendar and academic year, there are hints of significant factors that affect students at all levels of study. A third and still finer level of inquiry is represented by the days of the week (Table 6).

Only the Yale and South Dakota samples provide day-of-the-week data, and these are of somewhat limited value. First, they total only 56 suicides. Second, in the South Dakota sample, suicides were reported only as weekday (Monday–Thursday) or weekend (Friday–Sunday) events. Since Heinrichs (1980) obtained the incidence of both student and nonstudent suicide from the same governmental records, he was able to compare these two groups directly. He reported that students committed suicide significantly more frequently than non-

Table 6. Student suicide as a function of day of the week

	Observed suicides			
Portion of week	Yale[a]	South Dakota[b]	Total[c]	Chance
Weekdays (Monday–Thursday)	19	23	42	32
Weekend (Friday–Sunday)	6	8	14	24
Total	25	31	56	56

Note. References for samples: Yale (Parrish 1957), South Dakota (Heinrichs 1980).
[a]Versus chance: $\chi^2 = 3.63$, 1 df, $P < .10$.
[b]Versus chance: $\chi^2 = 3.70$, 1 df, $P < .10$.
[c]Versus chance: $\chi^2 = 7.29$, 1 df, $P < .01$.

students on weekdays. Cumulated data from diverse sources cannot be compared in this way.

Routine annual reports of national suicide data by day of the week first appeared in 1972. These are available, however, only for all ages and both sexes combined. The potential bias introduced by such pooling has already been addressed for other variables, and the same cautions obtain here. Analyses of these national data for the 6-year period 1980–1985 reveal relatively stable systematic variation in suicide rates by day of the week. As with monthly variations, deviations from chance (i.e., 14.3% per day) are small, less than 10% of the chance value (i.e., less than 1.4%), with the exception of Monday. Suicide rates decline monotonically from Monday (15.6%) through Saturday (13.6%), rising to 14.0% on Sunday.

Neither the Yale nor the South Dakota study alone reveals a statistically significant deviation from chance expectations for weekday versus weekend suicides, although each very nearly achieves significance. The combined data do show a statistically significant deviation from chance. This significant finding could be an artifact caused by selective underreporting. This possibility is raised by Parrish's (1957) use of health service records, which might be more likely to miss a weekend suicide. Heinrichs' (1980) data, however, are not subject to this bias, and his proportions closely parallel those reported by Parrish.

We next consider data on the proportion of student suicides who had had some contact with campus mental health services. Four samples provide these data: California, Harvard, Massachusetts-Amherst, and Yale. Table 7 summarizes these findings. On average, 36% of the total of 99 suicides reported in these four samples had had prior contact with campus mental health services.There is discernible variability in this proportion across the samples, although it fell just short of being statistically significant (χ^2 = 6.83, 3 df, .05 < P < .10).

If one views student contact with the campus mental health service as an opportunity for preventive intervention, then the fact that only a modest minority of student suicides had such contact is a source of concern. This fact underlines the need for such services to minimize all barriers to their voluntary use by students and to educate faculty, administrators, student affairs personnel, and residence hall staff, as well as students, about their existence and about referral processes.

A complementary perspective that considers usage rates for campus mental health facilities suggests that the proportion of student suicides having contact with these units is already fairly high. Usage rates vary widely across institutions (Schwartz and Reifler 1984). For individual campus medical-psychiatric facilities (i.e., men-

Table 7. Number and percentage of student suicides having had prior contact with campus mental health services

	California		Harvard		Massachusetts		Yale		Total	
	n	%	*n*	%	*n*	%	*n*	%	*n*	%
No prior contact	17	81	24	71	8	42	14	56	63	64
Prior contact	4	19	10	29	11	58	11	44	36	36
Total	21	100	34	100	19	100	25	100	99	100

Note. References for samples: California (Kagan 1988), Harvard (Temby 1961), Massachusetts (Kraft 1980), Yale (Parrish 1957).

tal health units affiliated with the campus health service), usage rates (per 1,000 students per year) vary from 15 to 200, with a mean ($\pm$SD) of 55 $\pm$ 15, or 5.5% of students annually. This indicates that the proportion of student suicides having contact with campus medical-psychiatric facilities (36%) is six to seven times as large as the proportion of all students using these facilities. Self-selection, referral processes, and related mechanisms may in fact already be working extremely well. Efforts to enhance further the likelihood that campus mental health services will have an opportunity to intervene with potential student suicides should, of course, be made. Realistically, however, the limits of prevention by tertiary intervention may have been reached.

Peck and Schrut (1971) contrasted completed suicides with students attempting, threatening, or contemplating suicide. Completed suicides were typically men and were not likely to call attention to themselves by a prior attempt or threat, nor by a sudden change of behavior, nor by notable inadequacy in their academic performance. Characterized by a lifelong pattern of isolation and withdrawal, they were also not likely to use campus mental health resources voluntarily. Rather, they received professional care when behaviors suggestive of psychotic levels of impairment precipitated an episode of inpatient treatment.

The inference by Peck and Schrut that, among students, psychosis was associated with completed suicide, but not with attempted, threatened, or contemplated suicide, is supported by other studies (Fry and Rostow 1942; Kraft 1980; Parrish 1957; Temby 1961). Psychosis is three times as likely to appear among student suicides as among students using campus mental health facilities. We have already noted that the mean usage rate for such facilities is about 55 per 1,000 students, making the prevalence of psychosis among the student population at risk about 1%. Psychosis, therefore, is 150 times more common among student suicides than among the student population at risk. No other characteristic of students so powerfully discriminates who among them is likely to suicide. Identifying and treating such students should be a priority in campus suicide prevention efforts.

Although the presence of psychosis identifies students at very high risk for suicide, 85% of student suicides will not be identified by this feature. Peck and Schrut (1971) provided perhaps the best descriptive approximation of the modal suicide. However, their small sample and atypical geographic context may limit the more general validity of their description. Perhaps more importantly, even a valid description of the modal suicide is not going to capture a large percentage of those students who do commit suicide (true positives) without also capturing a large proportion of all students (false positives).

An example of just this problem is the emphasis that has been given to depression as a harbinger or correlate of student suicide. Setting aside indications that depression may in fact discriminate those who will commit suicide from those who will attempt, threaten, or contemplate it, the prominence of depression is reflected not only in characterizations of student suicides, but also in estimates of its prevalence among both users of campus mental health services and the student population at risk. Estimates of the treated prevalence of diagnoses for which depression is a significant element are commonly reported as about 30% (Hersch et al. 1983; Stangler and Printz 1980; Walters 1970). Estimates of their prevalence in the population at risk are about half that value (Rimmer et al. 1982). Accordingly, even if depression is associated with a high proportion of student suicides (e.g., 60%), it is only twice as common among that minute fraction of students who both suicide and use campus mental health services as it is among those who are just users of the facilities, and just four times more common among student suicides than among students generally. In other words, the presence of depression can alert us to a higher proportion of impending student suicides (true positives) than the presence of psychosis, and it should be exploited as a warning sign. At the same time, depression is so common among students generally, as well as among those who use campus mental health facilities, that it cannot provide the precise focus we would ideally desire for either our primary prevention programs or our secondary and tertiary interventions.

Suicide, with a rate of about 8 per 100,000 students per year (50% males), and depression, with a rate of 15,000 per 100,000 students per year, anchor the ends of the suicidal continuum. These rates, however, are for all students, and we know that there are substantial differences between men and women in the prevalence of suicide and depression (Black and Winokur, Chapter 6, this volume). Table 8 summarizes data on rates of occurrence of eight points on the suicidal continuum, for each sex and for a coeducational student body that is 50% male.

In concluding this section, our goal is to provide a quantitative context for understanding the task of preventing student suicide. There are obviously troubling and troublesome events, like attempted suicide, whose frequency may be moderated by programs that focus on preventing completed suicide. Optimally, these programs also include interventions targeted at the problems and psychiatric disorders that correlate with suicidality in this population (e.g., depression, lack of social supports). In one respect, suicidality is like bad

Table 8. Annual rates of events on the suicidal continuum among students

Event	Males	Females	Coed campus (sex ratio = 1/1)
Suicide	12	4	8
Attempted suicide	96	230	163
Serious	22	20	21
Moderate	30	74	52
Gesture	44	136	90
Threatened suicide	140	580	360
Contemplated suicide	480	800	640
Depression	10,400	19,600	15,000
Acute	1,400	1,600	1,500
Diagnosable	9,000	18,000	13,500
Use of campus mental health services			
Medical-psychiatric[a]	4,400	6,600	5,500

Note. All rates are per 100,000 per year. Reports by Bloom (1970) and Winer et al. (1973) contributed to the value for use of campus-wide mental health resources. Kagan's (1988) report, the American College Health Association Mental Health Annual Program Survey data (Schwartz and Reifler 1980, 1988), the classic study by Schneidman and Farberow (1961), and more recent publications (Bernard and Bernard 1982; Mishara et al. 1976) were employed in establishing values for attempted, threatened, and contemplated suicide.
[a]Medical-psychiatric facilities are mental health units affiliated with the campus student health service.

weather. The low pressure system that brings overcast skies and moderate rain for days on end contains many hundreds of times the energy of the hurricane that wreaks havoc on the landscape in a few hours. We live well enough with overcast skies, perhaps grumbling a little; we are intensely mobilized by word of an approaching hurricane. Our responses to depression and suicide in college settings are similar.

In the concluding section of this chapter, we address the prevention of student suicide from clinical, social, developmental, and administrative perspectives. In doing so, we are behaving in the manner of the meteorologist: pointing out hints of approaching inclement weather, offering suggestions about how to cope with it, and suggesting accounts of a phenomenon over which we may have rather little control.

CLINICAL AND CAMPUS INTERVENTIONS

In this section of the chapter, we focus on clinical and community interventions to prevent student suicide. Special challenges to the college campus, developmental issues, risk factors, crisis and support networks, emergency and hospital readiness, principles of psychotherapy, administrative considerations, and what to do after an actual suicide will be discussed.

The Campus as Community

Structural aspects of the college or university such as the psychological ambience of the campus can influence the occurrence of student suicides. At its worst, the university is a cold and impersonal place where students feel that they are treated like mere numbers. At its best, the university is a humane environment, a sensitive, encouraging community of people interested in each other's well-being, and one that offers highly accessible student services and resources for interpersonal and academic assistance. The campus community best suited for preventing student suicide provides an atmosphere of warm and interested acceptance and maintains strong networks and linkages within its milieu.

Even the most sensitive, informed, and well-prepared university is faced with major challenges if the prevention of student suicide is one of its priorities. Psychiatrically ill, emotionally handicapped, and other vulnerable students will gain admission to the university if their academic qualifications are adequate, if only because they are protected by Section 504 of the Federal Rehabilitation Act of 1973 (Pavela 1985), which prohibits discrimination against emotionally as well as physically handicapped persons on the basis of their handicaps per se. Similarly, the presence of a mental disorder, whether preexisting or emerging after admission, may not be sufficient grounds for dismissal. As many as 15% of all student suicides will occur among those students who are burdened by such emotional handicaps.

One major impediment to the campus community functioning as a caring environment for these and other students is the transient nature of university life. Attending college requires that undergraduates break away from their families and hometowns, graduate students from their former institutions. The academic calendar has interludes when students, particularly undergraduates, are expected to leave the campus. Students who are not able to progress smoothly along the path to graduation must contend with additional disruptions and transitional adjustments: they flunk out, take leaves of absence, fail courses, and get out of step with their classmates. At some large state universities, as little as one-fourth of an entering class may actually graduate together.

Institutional programs designed to support students in contending with these tasks, particularly campus mental health services, are limited by the institution's general financial constraints and by the perceived relationship between such programs and the institution's principal mission, the pursuit of its academic programs. The provision of campus mental health services, or the development of the campus into a supportive or therapeutic community, tends to be viewed as outside the major mission of the institution. Too often it is the occurrence of a suicide on campus that stimulates the belated enhancement of mental health resources and services.

It is the conjunction of these factors—the presence of particularly vulnerable students located in a population experiencing developmental stressors, the inevitability of significant challenges confronting a transient student population, and the necessary limitations on the resources that can be devoted to supporting students—that makes the prevention of student suicide as an institutional goal particularly difficult to achieve.

Developmental Issues

What is known of the concerns of students who attempt and complete suicide indicates that often they have been unable to meet normative developmental challenges for their age group and circumstances. An understanding of these challenges provides insight into the experience of students who, faltering in their efforts to master these challenges, become at risk for suicide, and leads to more effective identification, intervention, and prevention of student suicide.

Entering college represents an important developmental milestone for young people. Students who leave home to attend college are separating from family, friends, and familiar surroundings to become part of a relatively unknown and typically more demanding environment. Previously experienced feelings of being loved and accepted at home may seem extremely remote and irreplaceable in the college or university setting. When great differences exist between the student's hometown life and the culture of the university, there is an enhanced probability of a more traumatic adjustment. Separation fears may aggravate doubts about one's self-worth, identity confusion, and feelings of shame about being dependent and homesick. Not all students run unabashed to the campus mailroom in search of comforting letters and "care packages" from home. Many students react with a thinly veiled bravado, attempting to quell their fears by showing how much alcohol they can consume or how much they can rebel against authority, or acting as though everything is fine when it is not. Campus friends may be too new or too defensive themselves to serve as confidants. The shock of leaving home may be especially great for those students who cannot return home for holidays or during breaks in the academic calendar. Additionally, higher academic standards at the university as compared to the student's high school may contribute to increased stress.

From a developmental point of view, immaturity and impulsivity are major risk factors for suicidal behavior. Students who are not ready for college because of emotional immaturity are out of step with their peers and may be traumatized by their failures to meet the challenges of normative developmental hurdles. Consequent losses of self-esteem, due to academic and social failures, and lack of peer support, due to falling farther behind their classmates, may stimulate or intensify suicidal inclinations in these students. Impulsivity, which often accompanies immaturity, is likely to increase self-destructiveness in depressed adolescents.

Students at Risk

Although epidemiologic studies have delineated one small subgroup of students at particularly high risk for suicide (i.e., those with psychotic disorders), 85% of student suicides are not among this group. Indeed, it is unlikely that any very precise method will emerge in the near-term future for identifying the majority of student suicides. Necessarily, therefore, determining suicidal risk will involve a broad array of relatively imprecise indices.

When assessing which students are at highest risk for suicidal behavior, the clinician should consider five dimensions: epidemiologic, developmental, cultural, social, and clinical. Each of these contributes risk factors for suicidal behavior, especially when considered in combination (Blumenthal 1988; Blumenthal and Kupfer 1986). Groups of students particularly at risk are males, high-risk takers, substance abusers, students without social supports, foreign students, students who have low self-esteem, impulsive and immature students, and depressed, psychotic, and schizophrenic students (Blumenthal, Chapter 26, this volume).

As noted in the first section of this chapter, male students, in comparison with female students, are a primary high-risk group. Yet men in our society, including college student men, may fear seeking psychological help more than women (Whitaker 1987). Significantly, campus mental health service utilization rates are half again as high for women as for men. These gender differences in morbidity rates and mental health service utilization may in part be accounted for by the machismo orientation of men (Whitaker 1987), which vaunts daring, destructiveness, and drugs while stigmatizing admission of fear and emotional neediness. Many of the behaviors cultivated in the machismo orientation—for example, driving under the influence of alcohol (Selzer 1980); various forms of substance abuse (Rivinus 1988); and the possession of guns and other lethal weapons—are at least indirectly self-destructive and may readily lead to suicidal behavior (Farberow 1980), whether deliberate or "accidental." The role of firearms in suicide, particularly for males, has already been described (Table 1).

College students who use psychoactive drugs, including alcohol, are more often involved in traffic violations (Nicholi 1985) and drunken driving (i.e., life-threatening behaviors), whether or not labeled suicidal or homicidal. The vast majority of life-threatening behaviors in college and university-age persons involve alcohol and other drug use, reckless driving, and outright suicide threats and actions, singly or in combination. Unfortunately, the students who are most likely to engage in death-defying behavior may be the least likely to value personal sensitivity and to seek the help of a psychotherapist. Since men are generally less likely to make explicit suicide threats and less likely to ask for help, it is important to reach these high-risk students through special channels, such as a "men's studies" curriculum and substance abuse programs, as well as by encouraging counseling and psychotherapy.

A second important risk group are those students who are severely estranged from their families, either geographically or emotionally. Foreign students, especially when they are from a very different culture, may find it especially difficult to form relationships with other students (Earls et al., Chapter 21, this volume). Additionally, foreign students who come from cultures that are not oriented to psychological services and who may be reluctant to draw on resources outside of the family may feel especially stigmatized by any association with counseling or psychotherapy. In some cases, academic failure represents a disgrace for which suicide may seem a fit punishment. Although there is great heterogeneity among foreign students, universities that provide special programs and group activities for foreign students may help reduce suicidal behavior. Foreign student advisors who warmly accept and take an interest in their students, providing them with social support and positive nurturance, may help prevent acute emotional distress in these students.

Students who are emotionally estranged from their families are especially vulnerable to adverse experiences on campus since they cannot turn to their families for emotional support and for reassurance that they are worthwhile and valued persons. These students may be difficult to identify and to approach diplomatically. Many, however, can be reached through faculty and academic advisors, and primary care physicians and nurses.

Another group of students at risk are those who never find, or find and then lose, a meaningful and appreciated position among their peers or professors at the university. These young people have extremely low self-esteem and lack the daily emotional support they need. Social isolation on the campus is a factor in many student suicide attempts. For example, a scenario of suicidal despair may quickly overwhelm the student who is rejected after having invested all of his or her energies in a romantic relationship while neglecting other friendships. Such a student may have been academically successful and content at school until the crisis occurred. At that time, without friends to share feelings with, the student may feel humiliated, alone, and emotionally devastated.

From a clinical viewpoint, psychotic students are at greatest risk for suicide. Students who are schizophrenic or exhibiting schizophreniform symptoms tend to be inaccessible, at least initially, for clinical assessment, making prevention of suicide difficult with this group. Depressed students, however, will include a larger number of suicides, and they are also at increased risk, if only moderately so.

Crisis and Support Networks

Given the diverse characteristics of students at elevated risk for suicide and the fact that 65% of student suicides have had no prior contact with campus health services (Table 7), it is evident that health services staff cannot simply wait in their offices for opportunities to assess students clinically. Prevention of suicide on campus is dependent on the early identification of students at risk and on providing them with support and assistance from a broad array of university resources. Dashef (1984) emphasized the need for an active suicide intervention program by campus mental health services. In addition to highly accessible clinical programs, an active crisis intervention service requires sensitive and comprehensive alerting, referral, and support networks.

Systematic social networks are required both to detect early warning signs of suicidal behavior and to support the student's referral into treatment. These systems include residence hall advisors, deans, faculty, security staff, peer networks, and health services and counseling staffs. Clearly, any member of the university community may be a valuable resource for identifying the need for special attention to particular students. Contrary to some notions that suicidal persons do not want people to help them, such attention is often much appreciated, especially when it is given with sensitivity and with concern for confidentiality and the student's self-esteem.

Negative or avoidant attitudes on the part of university members toward suicidal students may impede recognition of signs of distress. People may not want to acknowledge a student's disturbance for fear that they may have to become involved in the crisis situation. In addition, the student's distress may resonate in uncomfortable ways with another person's depression and despair. Empathizing with suicidal persons means getting in touch with one's own capacity for distress, and that may be personally threatening. Prevention strategies need to address these avoidant attitudes, which may otherwise result in community members minimizing a student's suicide risk and need for help.

Training in specific methods of intervention is essential for those persons involved in alert and support networks. For example, orientation of resident advisors should always include training on how to be responsive and effective in a mental health crisis such as a suicide threat or attempt. Additionally, since suicidal students may be resistant to seeking professional help, residence hall advisors and other university staff should be taught how to facilitate a referral for psychotherapy (Boswinkel 1986) as well as how to obtain emergency help in a crisis situation.

Since most suicidal students will not permanently leave the university community, and because community support is so vital to any kind of treatment progress, resident advisors, faculty, and university professional staff should be encouraged to take a continuing interest in the student after the crisis has passed. The student should learn that favorable attention and support can be obtained without being in an emotional crisis.

Sometimes the most important and effective part of an alert and support network consists of one or two people with whom the student has formed a relationship. Entreaties to suicidal students by deans, faculty, and mental health professionals may all fail while an appeal from a close friend may be quickly effective. The suicidal person may be testing, often unwittingly, to determine whether others "really care" enough to persist in efforts to help them.

A male student who had successfully referred other students to the university's mental health services suffered some major upsets in his own life connected with family illness and death. Generous with his time and support for other students, even his closest friends could not persuade him to get professional help. His friends persisted valiantly, and he came for assistance to the health service, admitting that he had been feeling extremely depressed and suicidal. During the process of psychotherapy, it became evident that this student held a double standard, one learned during his childhood when he felt it necessary to subdue his own emotional needs in favor of attending to those of a parent. He expressed gratitude that other students had overcome his resistance and his unwitting testing of their caring about him.

Emergency and Hospital Readiness

Identifying students at risk, understanding the developmental and circumstantial source of student stress, grasping the character of the suicidal student's experience, and alerting appropriate personnel are steps that ideally lead to the provision of effective care. To achieve this outcome, appropriate professional resources must be available.

To be adequately responsive to suicidal and other crises, the university should have available at least the following four mental health service components: 1) skilled interviewers, 2) an emergency after-hours on-call service, 3) immediate access to a hospital emergency unit complete with attending psychiatrist, and 4) ready access to a psychiatric inpatient unit.

The on-call service should be in effect 24 hours a day when the university is in session, and it should be made easily available to anyone in the university community who feels the need to make contact, either to get help for themselves or to communicate information about other people's suicidal behavior. The mental health service should be immediately responsive. A university walk-in clinic (Hersch and Lathan 1985; Johnson et al. 1980; Love 1983) can help guarantee immediate attention to disturbed students who would not be inclined to make regular appointments. However, suicidal students detected in this setting should be carefully evaluated, and a thorough follow-up plan should be constructed. If initial evaluation suggests the likelihood of lethal behavior, the student should be constantly supervised and/or hospitalized until further evaluation and treatment can be undertaken. If the university does not have its own hospital or associated department of psychiatry, special arrangements should be made with a local hospital to guarantee access to immediate emergency evaluation and hospitalization.

Parents or other family members will often be contacted soon after a serious suicide attempt. In these instances, parents should be encouraged and supported to reassume a maximum degree of responsibility for the student, including decisions about providers of future care and continuation of enrollment. A high level of parental involvement is particularly important when the student is a minor. The university mental health service should ensure that these matters are addressed. If the student plans to return to active status at the university, a mental health services staff member should follow the student in the hospital and make sure that the transition back to campus goes well. Discharge from the hospital should never occur before there is a carefully thought out and well-orchestrated follow-up plan that should include advance notification to the university mental health service that the student will return to campus.

While patient confidentiality should be preserved as much as possible, lack of communication between the hospital staff and the university mental health service may severely jeopardize the student's successful return to campus life. A bi-directional flow of information should occur so that both agencies can obtain a complete and accurate picture of the student's suicide risk and treatment needs.

Psychotherapy and Other Treatments

Fortunately, only 1% to 2% of the students who contemplate suicide actually commit suicide (Table 8). However, substantial numbers of students may become suicidal. For many of them, prevention will require effective psychotherapeutic intervention.

The vast majority of seriously suicidal students will need to understand and to learn how to cope with those pressures and conflicts that have driven them toward suicide. Psychotherapy is an excellent means of helping to prevent student suicide (Whitaker 1987), especially in terms of reversing depressive transformations by altering the cognitive distortions, low self-esteem, and social withdrawal that can occur, even in the face of strong social and academic supports.

> A male graduate student decided to suicide and came close to dying. Afterward, he exclaimed that he was convinced that he ought to die because he didn't deserve the strong emotional support he had been getting from a professor and fellow students. His reasoning was based

on an assumption that he had never been able to question, that his abusive father had been right about his son not deserving better treatment. Thus the supportive male figures around him could be written off as exercising bad judgment about his worth. Psychotherapy was helpful in rectifying this depressive cognitive distortion.

The therapist needs ample opportunity to develop with the student an understanding of the underlying reasons and precipitants for the suicidal crisis. This means exploring the combined influences of the student's personality development, interpersonal relationships, and the circumstances that may have provoked suicidal behavior. Since suicidal students have often experienced great difficulty in communicating with adults, failure to establish an alliance with "expert" adults may result in even more frustration and anger, and in a proclivity toward various kinds of self-damaging behaviors.

In summary, there are several vital steps in psychotherapy with suicidal students. First, the therapist must actively and empathetically enter into the student's frame of reference, which generally has become quite constricted. The therapist should not attempt to undo the depressive or psychotic transformation by giving commonsense advice or "pep talks," because this may further alienate the student. Second, the therapist should help the student to modify false but often rigidly held assumptions about the self by helping the student to see alternatives to the previous "only logical solution" of suicide. Third, the therapist should provide sufficiently intensive and sustained psychotherapy. The process of psychotherapy must occur at sufficiently frequent intervals and for a long enough time to establish the necessary trust and understanding. Brief psychotherapy may be both inadequate and counterproductive in cases of severe, long-term depression and suicidal behavior. Limiting such a student to a few weekly sessions may result in a suicide threat or attempt being seen as the only legitimate way to obtain the needed attention.

Resource limitations and other academic priorities prevent many universities from providing longer-term psychotherapy. Therefore, the university mental health service needs to be able to refer students to outside psychotherapists and to develop the needed referral skills (Medalie 1987). When referring suicidal students, the outside therapist should be contacted and urged to maintain a communication link with the university mental health service so that both can be alerted quickly in case of further suicidal behavior.

The use of antidepressant medication may be indicated for depressed and suicidal persons concurrent with treatment directed to the underlying psychiatric disorder. However, prescribed drugs must be administered with caution and must be carefully supervised because they may be used in suicide attempts (Rivinus 1988). For example, Kathol and Henn (1983) have shown that tricyclic antidepressants were used in about 50% of potentially lethal overdoses. Since college students predominantly use pills in their suicide attempts, and because their access to prescription drugs is high, it is vital to monitor the use of any psychotropic medication, particularly antidepressants. Specifically, medication should be prescribed only following a thorough clinical evaluation by a psychiatrist. The psychiatrist should confer with the student's psychotherapist and prescribe only small amounts of medication at one time. Prescribing psychiatrists should carefully elicit a history of psychoactive drug use for nonmedical reasons (Nicholi 1985). This precaution will help to prevent cross-medication, overmedication, and drug abuse. All treatment staff should be especially alert to alcohol and other drug abuse in their patients, particularly for their potential use in suicide attempts and other self-destructive behavior. Yet even seemingly strict precautions may be inadequate.

A female university student, who was intent on suicide, gathered together a combination of her brother's sleeping pills and her own antidepressant medication and took enough of these drugs, together with a couple of alcoholic drinks, to render her unconscious overnight. In retrospect, it seemed as though her therapist or the prescribing psychiatrist might have picked up on her drug-taking proclivities, including her drinking tendencies, but the student had been quite evasive.

Administrative Considerations

Earlier we noted that such institutional realities as competing priorities and limited resources made the prevention of student suicide in the university setting a difficult goal to achieve. Administrative considerations introduce other sets of competing principles that can also impede the prevention of student suicide.

Students who are experiencing a life-threatening crisis present special administrative as well as clinical challenges. Medicolegal considerations make it especially important in these cases to keep detailed notes, including developments that in some cases involve communications with people besides the student. At the same time, therapeutic considerations require as much confidentiality as possible. These two conflicting needs are resolved, theoretically at least, by a "need to know" policy. That is, information is not communicated by the mental health service to anyone not assisting in reducing the threat to life. In practice, carrying out this policy requires considerable judgment and sensitivity; decisions often have to be made on short notice and in ambiguous circumstances. Ineffective resolution of this conflict can lead the carefully cultivated alert and support network, and the student body generally, to lose confidence in the campus mental health service's commitment to the well-being of suicidal (and any other) students. If that service is perceived as being motivated by institutional or legal concerns, rather than therapeutic ones, it will be ignored and avoided by the very persons it depends on to fulfill its role in suicide prevention and by its other student clientele.

Students whose emotional problems interfere with their ability to succeed academically or to conform to standards of community behavior can involve the campus mental health service in this dilemma. Such students may elect to leave the university for "health reasons." A so-called health withdrawal or medical leave permits the student to leave the university without academic disadvantage in that no failing grades will appear on the transcript. A more controversial procedure is needed when the student resists taking a medical leave of absence. Dismissing students with mental disorders is fraught with complex concerns, including their protection under Section 504 of the 1973 Rehabilitation Act (Pavela 1985) and the administrative policies of the university. One recourse is to dismiss students on disciplinary or academic grounds if there has been highly disruptive or severely disturbed behavior, rather than to place the university's mental health staff in the position of deciding whether emotional disturbance per se should result in a medical withdrawal. Students actually faced with the possibility of disciplinary dismissal may then opt for a health withdrawal. Hopefully, even though quite disturbed, a student might be amenable to psychiatric treatment while continuing as a student. These and other considerations need to be explored (Whitaker 1986a, 1986b) by the deans, mental health staff, and other college and university health practitioners at the university.

A related context gives rise to a similar predicament. Students who have been on mental health leaves of absence may be required to have a readmission interview with the director of mental health services, or his or her designee, and to provide a letter from their treating therapist indicating readiness to return to school. Letters from outside mental health professionals who have been treating students are usually overly optimistic, and students often return prematurely (Gift and Southwick 1988). Such optimism may be based on a period of successful adaptation outside of the university, which is translated into an expectation of the student's success at the university (where pressures and demands are usually greater). The student's goal, sometimes pursued at the urging of parents and not reflecting the student's self-assessment, is to gain readmission. The university's goal is to ensure that, on readmission, the student will experience success, not a second failure, and that the university community will not be subjected to the stress and trauma imposed by a suicide, a suicide attempt, an episode of bizarre behavior, or the presence of a depressed and marginally functional student. It is costly to have irate parents demanding to know why the institution is subjecting their child to the experience of living with a suicidal, "crazy" roommate.

Probably the best policy in these matters is to meet with the student and discuss the university's desire that he or she be ready enough to succeed on returning rather than have another discouraging experience at the university. The dean of students and the director of mental health services should agree on the exact approach and speak with the student accordingly. Engaging the student in reflecting on his or her readiness to return to campus based on the student's own longer-term self-interest may contribute to a choice of postponing reentry.

The Aftermath of Suicide on Campus

A completed suicide on campus combines the already devastating effects of a premature death with many other serious sequelae. First of all, as in the reaction to any death, survivors tend initially to deny the event and to become numb. Additionally, when a death by suicide occurs, there are likely to be strong feelings of guilt, remorse, anger, and despair connected with beliefs that not everything possible was done to prevent the tragedy. These feelings can be so painful that special strategies may be required to help elicit them from survivors of a suicide, including ventilating feelings within a supportive group atmosphere as well as in individual therapy. In the case of an actual suicide, there is an even greater need for help in acknowledging what has happened, in grieving, and, quite importantly, in determining what can be done to help suicidal people in the future (Ruben, Chapter 23, this volume).

Suicide also poses the problem of stigma at the university. Various religions consider suicide a sin, and many people feel considerable discomfort and hostility toward the suicidal person and/or those persons who were closest to the victim. Questions like "Why didn't you do more to prevent it?" are inevitable, whether spoken out loud or not. There is something especially stigmatizing when a person commits suicide, particularly when that person is a student who had an entire adult life ahead. Who drove the student to suicide? Who overlooked the suicidial risk? Who was the student trying to punish, to condemn for not caring? Questions like these exist in the survivors' minds and they need to be addressed, at least implicitly if not explicitly.

The suicidal death, like a death from natural causes, should be announced (barring objection from the student's family) by the university through its president or another high-ranking official, so that the university community can discuss the suicidal death openly, thereby helping community members to acknowledge and work through the tragedy. In this way, the university president constructively encourages enhanced communication rather than implicitly reinforcing denial. The university's mental health service staff also needs to discuss the suicide and its circumstances in a case conference format so that treatment and services can be improved for others in the university community. Group discussion formats for students, in addition to individual counseling or psychotherapy sessions, should be made available. When the student who suicided has been treated by the mental health service, obtaining the opinions of an outside consultant may be particularly valuable in helping to disentangle and process staff reactions in constructive ways.

Ultimately, the most constructive response to the aftermath of a suicide is to "do something about the suicide" both through the grieving process and by implementing steps to help prevent further tragedies of this kind on campus. These actions can promote a more caring and responsive community atmosphere so that alternatives to suicide can be identified by students before self-destructive acts occur.

SUMMARY

While there has been much speculation about increased rates of suicide among college students, in fact the suicide rate for students at American colleges and universities appears to be about half that of their nonstudent age-mates, and there appears to be no relationship between the prestige or academic standards of colleges and universities and student suicide rates. Earlier representations of student suicide rates as being higher than those of nonstudents and as being positively correlated with academic standards were based on flawed analyses, biased interpretations and reporting, and inaccurate inferences. Concern about the use of health service records and other informal (i.e., nongovernmental) sources of data about student suicide, while warranted, has been exaggerated. Informal sources appear to underestimate the incidence of student suicide by about 30% when compared with official governmental sources. Both sources support the finding that the suicide rate for students is lower than for nonstudents. The restriction of access by students to the highly lethal method of suicide represented by firearms, a restriction that may be an intended feature of the campus environment, may be the principal factor yielding reduced student suicide rates. This feature would be likely to have a greater potential impact on suicide by males than by females, a possibility that is supported when student suicide data are analyzed separately for each sex. Institutional size and class standing are unrelated to student suicide rates, but other features of academic life may be correlated with student suicide. There is suggestive evidence that, within the calendar (or academic) year, September, January, and March are times of increased risk for students relative to nonstudents. Weekdays (Monday through Thursday) are more definitively times of increased risk for students, and the midnight to 6 A.M. period may be associated with elevated suicide rates, but whether this is true for students only is not known. Factors associated with individual students also appear correlated with suicide. The presence of psychosis in a student increases the risk of suicide by that student by a factor of 150 over baseline student rates. If a student is depressed and has contact with a campus medical-psychiatric facility, risk is increased by a factor of 12. If depression is absent, contact with a medical-psychiatric facility represents a sixfold increase in risk. A depressed student who does not have contact with such a facility has a twofold increase in risk.

These findings suggest that opportunities for suicide prevention in the university setting exist in two complementary areas: 1) modification of those structural aspects of the university environment that stimulate or intensify suicidality and that facilitate suicidal acts, and 2) identification and treatment of students at risk for suicide. The first area includes limiting access to highly lethal methods of suicide such as firearms and sites for jumping, modifying curricular and other features to modulate student stress, and instituting programs designed to aid students in the successful mastery of those challenges they must inevitably confront. The second area includes implementing postadmission health history and other screening devices that can aid in the identification of intrinsically vulnerable students, enhancing the campus community's ability to recognize students at risk for suicide and to direct them to appropriate sources of support and care, and making effective professional services readily available.

The implementation of these mechanisms functions best in a university environment characterized by sensitivity to others and an interest in their well-being, by widespread understanding of students' normative development and the implications of their student circumstances, and by insight into the experience of the suicidal student. Within this environment, there should be a well-coordinated and comprehensive network of persons who can identify students in crisis, alerting appropriate institutional personnel and directing such students to appropriate sources of care. This network would include student peers and family and university personnel at all levels and in all spheres of university life. There should be adequately comprehensive professional mental health services available to this network and the students it serves. Minimally these services would include clinically skilled campus-based interviewers, a 24-hour emergency on-call service, an immediately available hospital-based psychiatric emergency unit, and ready access to a psychiatric inpatient facility. Ideally, there would also be a capacity for providing comprehensive psychotherapeutic treatment that is geographically and financially accessible to students.

Effective functioning of any program of secondary and tertiary intervention will inevitably require astute management of the conflicting priorities represented by medicolegal, institutional, and therapeutic perspectives. Similarly, primary prevention initiatives will encounter the tension between educational and therapeutic values and the constraints imposed by limited institutional financial resources. Whatever balance is struck among these competing priorities, neither primary prevention nor secondary and tertiary intervention will prevent all student suicides. When one occurs, public announcement of this event by a high-level university administrator should be used to undo denial, stimulate the process of grieving by the university community, and legitimate constructive consideration of enhanced prevention efforts. The campus mental health service may need to play a facilitative role in these processes, both clinically and administratively.

In conclusion, the task of future research about suicide among college students is to confirm and elaborate on the hypothesis-generating findings presented in this chapter and to assess the effectiveness of preventive initiatives. The best strategies for achieving these goals are the development of cooperative multi-institution designs employing standard reporting conventions and the analysis of suicide data derived from governmental sources.

REFERENCES

Arnstein RL: The place of college health services in preventing suicide and affective disorders, in Suicide and Depression Among Adolescents and Young Adults. Edited by Klerman GL. Washington, DC, American Psychiatric Press, 1986, pp 337–361

Bernard JL, Bernard ML: Factors related to suicidal behavior among college students and the impact of institutional response. Journal of College Student Personnel 23:409–413, 1982

Bessai J: College student suicides: a demographic profile. Paper presented at the annual meeting of the American Psychological Association, Washington, DC, August 1986

Bloom BL: Characteristics of campus community mental health programs in Western United States—1969. J Am Coll Health Assoc 18:196–200, 1970

Blumenthal SJ: Suicide: a guide to risk factors, assessment and treatment of suicidal patients. Med Clin North Am 72:937–971, 1988

Blumenthal SJ: Kupfer DJ: Generalizable treatment strategies for suicidal behavior. Ann NY Acad Sci 487:327–340, 1986

Boswinkel J: The college resident assistant (RA) and the fine art of referral for psychotherapy. Journal of College Student Psychotherapy 1:53–62, 1986

Braaten LJ, Darling CD: Suicidal tendencies among college students. Psychiatr Q 36:665–692, 1962

Brown BM: Depressed college students and tricyclic antidepressant therapy. J Am Coll Health Assoc 27:79–83, 1978

Bruyn HB, Seiden RH: Student suicide: fact or fancy? J Am Coll Health Assoc 14:69–77, 1965

Carpenter RG: Statistical analysis of suicide and other mortality rates of students. British Journal of Preventive and Social Medicine 13:163–174, 1959

Dashef SS: Active suicide intervention by a campus mental health service: operation and rationale. J Am Coll Health 33:118–122, 1984

Diehl HS, Shepard CE: The Health of College Students. Washington, DC, American Council on Education, 1939

Dublin LI: Suicide. New York, Ronald Press, 1963

Farberow NL (ed): The Many Faces of Suicide: Indirect Self-Destructive Behavior. New York, McGraw-Hill, 1980

Fry CC, Rostow EG: Mental Health in College. New York, Commonwealth Fund, 1942

Gift TE, Southwick WH: Premature return to school following a psychotic episode. J Am Coll Health 36:289–292, 1988

Hammen CL: Depression in college students: beyond the Beck Depression Inventory. J Consult Clin Psychol 48:126–128, 1980

Heinrichs EH: Suicide in the young: demographic data of college-age students in a rural state. J Am Coll Health Assoc 28:236–237, 1980

Hersch JB, Lathan C: The mental health walk-in clinic: the University of Massachusetts experience. J Am Coll Health 34:15–17, 1985

Hersch JB, Nazario NS, Backus BA: DSM-III and the college mental health setting: the University of Massachusetts experience. J Am Coll Health 31:247–252, 1983

Johnson NJ, Whitaker LC, Porter G: The development and efficacy of a university mental health service walk-in clinic. J Am Coll Health Assoc 28:269–271, 1980

Kagan D: A survey of student suicide 1984-85 through 1986-87. Long Beach, CA, The California State University, Office of the Chancellor, March 3, 1988

Kathol RG, Henn FA: Tricyclics: the most common agent in potentially lethal overdoses. J Nerv Ment Dis 171:250–252, 1983

Kraft DP: Student suicides during a twenty-year period at a state university campus. J Am Coll Health Assoc 28:258–262, 1980

Love RL: A walk-in clinic in a university mental health service: some preliminary findings. J Am Coll Health 31:224–225, 1983

Lyman JL: Student suicide at Oxford University. Student Medicine 10:218–234, 1961

Malleson N: The distressed student. Lancet 1:824–825, 1954

Medalie JD: Psychotherapy referral as a therapeutic goal of college counseling. Journal College Student Psychotherapy 1:83–103, 1987

Miles CP: Conditions predisposing to suicide: a review. J Nerv Ment Dis 164:231–246, 1977

Mishara BL, Baker AH, Mishara TT: The frequency of suicide attempts: a retrospective approach applied to college students. Am J Psychiatry 133:841–844, 1976

Morgan HG: Management of suicidal behaviour. Br J Psychiatry 138: 259–260, 1981

National Center for Health Statistics: Vital Statistics of the United States, Vol II, Mortality, P&A (annual vol for 1960, 1965, 1970, 1975, 1980, 1985). Washington, DC, U.S. Government Printing Office

Nicholi AM: Characteristics of college students who use psychoactive drugs for nonmedical reasons. J Am Coll Health 33:189–192, 1985

Oliver JM, Burkham R: Depression in university students: duration, relation to calendar time, prevalence, and demographic correlates. J Abnorm Psychol 88:667–670, 1979

Parnell RW: Mortality and prolonged illness among Oxford undergraduates. Lancet 1:731–733, 1951

Parnell RW, Skottowe I: Towards preventing suicide. Lancet 1:206–208, 1957

Parrish HM: Causes of death among college students: study of 209 deaths at Yale University. Public Health Rep 71:1081–1085, 1956

Parrish HM: Epidemiology of suicide among college students. Yale J Biol Med 29:585–595, 1957

Pavela G: The Dismissal of Students with Mental Disorders: Legal Issues, Policy Considerations and Alternative Responses. Asheville, NC, College Administration Publishers, 1985

Peck M, Schrut A: Suicide among college students, in Proceedings: Fourth International Conference for Suicide Prevention, Los Angeles, California, October 18–21, 1967. Edited by Farberow NL. Los Angeles, CA, International Association for Suicide Prevention, 1968, pp 356–359

Peck ML, Schrut A: Suicidal behavior among college students. HSMHA Health Report 86:149–156, 1971

Raphael T: Four years of student mental-hygiene work at the University of Michigan. Mental Hygiene 20:218–231, 1936a

Raphael T: The place and possibilities of the mental hygiene approach on the college level. Am J Psychiatry 92:855–876, 1936b

Raphael T, Gordon MA: Psychoses among college students. Am J Psychiatry 95:659–675, 1938

Raphael T, Himler LE: Schizophrenia and paranoid psychoses among college students. Am J Psychiatry 100:443–451, 1944

Raphael T, Power SH, Berridge WL; The question of suicide as a problem in college mental hygiene. Am J Orthopsychiatry 7:1–14, 1937

Read JC: The mental health of undergraduates in England: report on first 18 months of psychiatric service for students at London School of Economics. Lancet 1:822–824, 1954

Riggs AF, Terhune WB: The mental health of college women. Mental Hygiene 12:559–568, 1928

Rimmer J, Halikas JA, Shuckit MA: Prevalence and incidence of psychiatric illness in college students: a four year prospective study. J Am Coll Health Assoc 30:207–211, 1982

Rivinus TM: Alcohol and other substance abuse in college students. Journal of College Student Psychotherapy 2:3–4, 1988

Rook A: An investigation into the longevity of Cambridge sportsmen. Br Med J 1:773–777, 1954

Rook A: Student suicides. Br Med J 1:599–603, 1959

Ross M: Suicide among college students. Am J Psychiatry 126:220–225, 1969

Rush AJ, Beck AT, Kovacs M, et al: Comparison of the effects of cognitive therapy and pharmacotherapy on hopelessness and self-concept. Am J Psychiatry 139:862–866, 1982

Schneidman ES, Farberow NL: Statistical comparisons between attempted and committed suicides, in The Cry for Help. Edited by Farberow NL, Schneidman ES. New York, McGraw-Hill, 1961, pp 19–47

Schwartz AJ, Reifler CB: Suicide among American college and university students from 1970–71 through 1975–76. J Am Coll Health Assoc 28:205–210, 1980

Schwartz AJ, Reifler CB: Quantitative aspects of college mental health: usage rates, prevalence and incidence, suicide. Psychiatric Annals 14:681–688, 1984

Schwartz A, Reifler CB: College student suicide in the United States: incidence data and prospects for demonstrating the efficacy of preventative programs. J Am Coll Health 37:53–59, 1988

Selzer ML: The accident process and drunken driving as indirect self-destructive activity, in the Many Faces of Suicide: Indirect Self-Destructive Behavior. Edited by Farberow NL. New York, McGraw-Hill, 1980, pp 284–299

Sims L, Ball MJ: Suicide among university students. J Am Coll Health Assoc 21:336–338, 1973

Stangler RS, Printz AM: DSM-III: psychiatric diagnosis in a university population. Am J Psychiatry 137:937–940, 1980

Still RJ: The prevention of psychological illness among students. Leeds University Quarterly 9:1–3, 1956

Temby WD: Suicide, in Emotional Problems of the Student. Edited by Blaine GB, McArthur CC. New York, Appleton-Century-Crofts, 1961, pp 133–152

Walters OS: Prevalence of diagnosed emotional disorders in university students. J Am Coll Health Assoc 18:204–209, 1970

Whitaker LC: Psychotherapy as opportunity to prevent college student suicide. Journal of College Student Psychotherapy 1:71–88, 1986a

Whitaker LC (ed): Special symposium papers: voices and boundaries in college mental health. Journal of College Student Psychotherapy 1:1–85, 1986b

Whitaker LC: Macho and morbidity: the emotional need vs. fear dilemma in men. Journal of College Student Psychotherapy 1:33–47, 1987

Winer JA, Dinello FA, Pasca A, et al: University mental health services in Illinois. J Am Coll Health Assoc 22:138–142, 1973

Chapter 13

Geriatric Suicidal Behavior: Assessment and Treatment

Nancy J. Osgood, Ph.D.
Samuel Thielman, M.D., Ph.D.

SUICIDE IS A VERY serious problem among the old, particularly for those 65 years and older. Compared to younger individuals, the old openly communicate their suicidal intent less frequently, use more violent and lethal means, and less often attempt suicide as a means to gain attention or to cry for help. All of these factors increase the risk of death from suicide for older people. The suicide rate of the old (65+) is 50% higher than that of the young. In 1987, United States suicide rates were 12.7 per 100,000 for the nation, 12.9 for those 15 to 24 years old, and 21.7 for those 65 and over (National Center for Health Statistics 1987). For elderly white men, who historically have had the highest rate, it was 46.1. Thus the highest rates of suicide by age are found not among the young, as many in our society believe, but among the elderly (65+). This observation has been true as long as official suicide data have been kept by the United States government, and is accurate for most other countries as well (Shulman 1978).

In a national study of suicide in long-term care facilities, Osgood and Brant (unpublished) found the rate of overt suicide among institutionalized elderly to be 15.8 per 100,000 compared to the rate of 19.2 for the community elderly. When deaths from overt suicide and intentional life-threatening behaviors—such as refusing to eat or drink, refusing medications, or eating foreign objects—were combined, the calculated rate of such behavior was 94.9 per 100,000, a rate more than four times higher than the reported rate of overt suicide for the community elderly (Osgood and Brant, unpublished).

Risk Factors for Suicide in the Elderly

Careful assessment must begin with a knowledge of risk factors of suicide, since these provide a basis for estimating the likelihood of suicide attempts in patients in whom the likelihood of suicide is uncertain. Prediction of dangerousness in psychiatry is notoriously unreliable, and generalizations made about large population groups may not apply in individual cases. Nonetheless, our understanding of the epidemiology of suicide in late life provides a beginning for clinical assessment.

Age, Gender, and Ethnicity. Some older adults are more "at risk" of committing suicide than others. White males and the very old (75+) are the highest risk for suicide. The National Center for Health Statistics (1987) reported that there were 34.8 reported suicides for every 100,000 males from 65 to 74 years of age in 1987. The rate escalated to 57.1 among men 75 to 84 years old. For men over 85, the rate rose to 66.9. Male rates of suicide increase and peak in old age; female rates increase until middle age (mid-40s to mid-50s) and decline thereafter. Female suicide rates are generally lower than those for males at all ages, and particularly so in old age. Investigations of both suicide and attempted suicide have shown that relatively more males as a group use violent and lethal methods such as firearms, hanging, and jumping more frequently; females usually prefer less violent techniques such as poisoning and suffocation (McIntosh and Santos 1985–1986). While suicide rates for whites in the United States increase with age and peak with old age, those for nonwhites peak in young adulthood (generally in the 20s or early 30s) and decline thereafter. Nonwhite elderly suicide rates are low, particularly in late life, and have remained so over time. Among the major American ethnic groups, white men have the highest suicide rate; however, suicide among nonwhite men has dramatically increased in the last decade (Manton et al. 1987; McIntosh 1985). Additionally, specific racial-ethnic group differences can be found (McIntosh 1985).

Social Isolation. A number of investigations have shown that social isolation and suicide are significantly related, and at least one study has shown that suicide decreases with the number of inhabitants in a dwelling (Maris 1981). Some have suggested that beyond simply isolation, change in the *state* of isolation may be important, and consequently people who had recently moved into a situation where they were living by themselves or people who have, for whatever reason, been separated from those with whom they had previously lived would be at special risk. Since older people often live by themselves, isolation can be a particularly lethal situation for depressed or psychotic individuals.

Marital Status, Recent Bereavement, and Family Support. Mortality from suicide increases following loss of a spouse. Kaprio et al. (1987) found an excess of mortality from violent causes to be especially common in the first year following the death of a spouse, and, in fact, there was some degree of increased mortality during the entire period of the study. Suicide following widowhood was greater than expected among men for the entire 12-year period of one study, and was increased in the first 6 months of widowhood for both men and women (Helsing et al. 1982). Thus patients, particularly older men, who have been bereaved recently should be considered to be at particularly high risk for suicide. The elderly male widower is the most emotionally and socially isolated. He has fewer relatives and kin living nearby, participates less with family and friends, and is less involved in formal organizations and the community. Elderly living in urban areas, particularly low-income transient areas in central cities, are more at risk than are those living in rural areas.

Previous Attempts. Older individuals, particularly men, who have attempted suicide have a much higher rate of successful completion of suicide. In one study, older men with a history of a prior suicide attempt had a rate 20 times that of younger individuals (Shulman 1978). Patients should therefore be carefully questioned as to whether they have made any prior attempts to kill themselves.

Health Status. The association between suicide and physical debility has been known for many years (Shulman 1978). In a study of completed suicide among elderly individuals, concern about health was determined to be the single most common reason for suicide where a reason could be determined (Copeland 1987). Indeed, Blazer et al. (1986) predicted that physical health problems and apprehension about the accessibility of health care will be an increasing problem as public assistance for older people lessens. Thus careful assessment of physical health status, particularly the patient's own concern about physical health, is quite important. Patients with chronic pain, with significant impairment of activities of daily living, with an organic mental disorder, and/or with a marked reduction in their previous activities because of health impairment should be considered particularly at risk.

Mental Health and Suicide in Later Life. Some, although not all, mental disorders have a greater incidence of death from suicide than the general population (see Black and Winokur, Chapter 6, this volume). Higher mortality from suicide is associated with depression (Coryell 1981; Martin et al. 1985), schizophrenia, alcohol dependence (Blazer 1982; Osgood 1987), and organic brain syndrome (Pokorny 1964). Given this association, it is important to identify and treat underlying mental disorders in elderly patients with suicidal ideation.

Suicide Rates Among the Institutionalized Elderly. Suicide rates calculated for the institutionalized elderly (Osgood and Brant, unpublished) revealed higher rates of suicide for males than for females and higher rates for Caucasians than for non-Caucasians. Osgood et al. (1988–1989) found that, in the institutionalized elderly population, males are more likely than females to engage in overt suicidal behavior, such as wrist slashing and hanging. The "old old" (75+) are more likely than the "young old" (60–74) or those under 60 to engage in indirect life-threatening behaviors, such as refusing to eat or drink, than in overt suicidal acts. Nevertheless, the "old old" are the most likely to die from their suicidal behavior.

Depression

Psychological factors play a crucial part in late-life suicide. The elderly suffer many losses, including loss of health; impaired vision and hearing; loss of mobility; financial loss; loss of home and possessions; loss of independence; cognitive loss and mental impairment; and loss of social roles in work, family, and the community. These losses result in stress at a time in life when the individual is least able to resist and cope with stress. These losses and the stress suffered from them often result in feelings of loneliness, depression, and despair (Miller 1979; Osgood 1985). Many older individuals experience a deep sense of emptiness and meaninglessness and lose all motivation for working, playing, and even living. Those who have suffered severe loss and are socially and emotionally isolated often feel rejected and dejected, unwanted, unneeded, and unloved. Their self-esteem suffers, and they view themselves as inadequate and inferior.

Three major psychological factors have been recognized as characterizing depression and suicide among the aged: haplessness, helplessness, and hopelessness. Lowered self-concept and self-esteem contribute to the unhappiness and self-hatred of the aged (Pavkov

1982). Seligman (1975) defined helplessness as a state in which individuals experience an inability to control significant life events and suggested that it is the core of all depression. The aged are most susceptible to feelings of helplessness, according to Seligman, because they have experienced the greatest loss of control. Schulz (1976) similarly argued that loss of job, income, physical health, work, and childbearing roles results in increased helplessness and depression in the aged. Karl Menninger (1938) characterized suicides of the elderly as a result of the wish to die, emphasizing hopelessness as a major contributing factor. Farber (1968) similarly conceived of suicide among the aged as a desperate response to hopeless and intolerable life situations. Those who have analyzed suicide notes of individuals of various ages have found that the elderly express a sense of hopelessness and "psychologial exhaustion" in their notes (Cath 1965; Farberow and Shneidman 1970). They are tired of life and tired of living. They have just given up.

Other factors that increase vulnerability to suicide—many of them secondary to depression—include alcoholism, bereavement, diagnosis of cancer or other terminal illness, a major move, or a serious argument or flare-up with a family member or friend.

Depressive symptoms occur in somewhere between 30% and 65% of individuals over the age of 60 (La Rue et al. 1985). Although depressive *symptoms* are quite common, major depression and dysthymic disorder actually occur at a lower rate among elderly individuals than among the general population (Myers et al. 1984). Nonetheless, major depression and dysthymic disorder are among the most common mental disorders of later life (Blazer et al. 1987). Diagnosing major depression in the geriatric population presents special challenges. Vegetative symptoms of depression such as insomnia, anergia, and loss of appetite may be difficult to ascribe to depression, since they may be symptoms of other medical illnesses or, as in the case of insomnia, may be a problem symptomatic of physiological changes in late life (Kales and Kales 1984). Consequently, cognitive symptoms of depression—such as hopelessness, worthlessness, guilt, preoccupation with death, predominance of depressed mood, diurnal variation in mood, lack of reactivity, and prior history of affective disorder—take on particular importance in older patients. Biologic markers for depression, particularly the dexamethasone suppression test and the thyrotropin-releasing hormone stimulation test have been extensively evaluated for their clinical utility in diagnosing depression. Although these diagnostic tools are of some use in clinical practice (Davis 1985), their use in elderly populations, particularly in patients who are demented, is controversial (Thielman and Blazer 1987).

Because DSM-III-R (American Psychiatric Association 1987) criteria may be problematic in older patients, the use of diagnostic instruments designed specifically for the elderly may be useful in the clinical evaluation. Several instruments have been assessed to determine their clinical usefulness in the older age group (Gallagher 1986). The Beck Depression Inventory (BDI), although not designed specifically for use in the elderly, has been found to diagnose depression accurately in this age group (Gallagher and Thompson 1983). A modified version of the BDI, the Geriatric Depression Scale (Yesavage and Brink 1983), is particularly useful because it eliminates somatically oriented questions and employs an easy-to-understand yes-no answer format rather than the 4-point answer scale of the BDI.

Older patients presenting with depressive symptoms should be carefully screened for the presence of dementia; depression may be the earliest presenting symptom of dementia in this age group. Even among experienced clinicians, the depression of early dementia may be misdiagnosed as being simply depression (Reding et al. 1985). Because of the difficulty in differentiating depression and dementia, patients in whom dementia is suspected should undergo a thorough evaluation for dementia (Table 1).

A small group of patients with depression alone exhibit cognitive deficits that remit when the depression is treated (McAllister and Price 1982; McAllister et al. 1982). This condition, termed *pseudodementia*, received a tremendous amount of attention during the late 1970s and early 1980s, although in recent years the concept has come under closer scrutiny (Folstein and McHugh 1978; McAllister 1983; Shraberg 1978). If depression exists in a person who has cognitive deficits, obviously the depression should be treated. If the deficit goes away, so much the better. The problem with the notion of pseudodementia has been that the concept is fuzzy. (Sometimes the term is used to describe patients with "poor effort" mistakes on the mental status exam who are clearly not demented. At other times, it is used to describe clear-cut cognitive deficits that disappear when the depression is treated.) Further, the criteria often said to distinguish between pseudodementia and dementia (e.g., preoccupation with memory loss, poor effort responses, apparent recent onset) do not actually distinguish very well between depressed demented patients and depressed only patients.

Psychotically depressed patients present a particularly high suicide risk (Roose et al. 1983); therefore patients in whom depression is suspected should be carefully questioned about the presence of command auditory hallucinations. Because patients are sometimes guarded in their answers about hallucinations, the examiner should approach the issue with tact and empathy.

Table 1. Assessment for dementia in the depressed patient

History
   Patient interview
     Is the patient aware of memory loss?
     Is the patient "defensive" about possibility of memory loss?
     Does the patient get lost easily?
     Does the patient have new trouble managing monetary affairs?
     Did the patient's social withdrawal precede the depressive symptoms?
     If the patient still works, was there a decline in occupational functioning
       that preceded the onset of depressive symptoms?

   Family interview (above questions *plus*):
     Does the patient have difficulty finding words?
     Does the patient repeat questions?
     Is the current presentation of depression consistent with previous
       episodes of depression (if the patient has a history of depression)?
     Has there been a recent change in the patient's personality beyond social
       withdrawal (uncharacteristic accusations, uncharacteristic cursing or
       deprecating of others, accusations of stealing when missing items are
       lost)?

Clinical examination
   Blood pressure, pulse
   Fundoscopic examination
   Structured cognitive examination such as the Mini Mental State
     Examination,[a] the Blessed Dementia Scale,[b] the Neurobehavioral Mental
     Status Examination, the Mattis Dementia Scale[c]
   Neurological examination
   Referral for neuropsychological testing if cognitive testing indicates a deficit

Laboratory and radiological examination
   Complete blood count
   Urinalysis
   Chest X-ray (if not recently done)
   Serum chemistry profile
   Sedimentation rate
   Serum vitamin B-12 and folate determinations
   Thyroid function test
   Fluorescent trepohemal antibody absorption test
   Electroencephalogram
   Computed tomography scan of head with contrast, or magnetic resonance
     imaging if computed tomography scan is negative and multi-infarct
     dementia is suspected

[a]Folstein et al. (1975).
[b]Blessed et al. (1968).
[c]Mattis (1976).

Elderly patients in whom suicidal ideation is suspected, depressed or otherwise, should be questioned directly about suicidality. A common initial approach is to ask if the patient has ever felt life was not worth living. If the answer is yes, the interviewer should inquire directly about suicidal thoughts. If the patient has had such thoughts, the interviewer should ask whether the patient has plans. Since patients who are the most serious about committing suicide may deny both frank suicidal ideas as well as plans, the interviewer should consider not only the patient's explicit statements but also the patient's guardedness, indirect communications, and the family or care giver's assessment of suicide potential.

Dementia

Dementia is the most common mental disorder of late life, and patients with "organic brain syndrome" have significantly higher rates of suicide than the general population (Pokorny 1964). Patients depressed early in the course of dementia may express suicidal ideas. The diagnosis of dementia is usually made by confirming with neuropsychological testing a deficit elicited by careful clinical screening. When patients are found to have an irreversible dementia (as is usually the case), psychiatric involvement need not (and should not) stop. Reifler et al. (1986) noted, however, that even patients who have untreatable dementias often, when depressed, respond to treatment with antidepressants. They reported that 85% of the depressed demented patients treated in their series responded to medical treatment for depression with improvement in mood, lessening of vegetative symptoms, and improvement in activities of daily living. Thus patients with depression and dementia, many of whom express suicidal ideas, should be treated for their depression with the assurance that they may experience amelioration of their clinical condition.

Substance Abuse

Although drug abuse is an uncommon problem in older people, alcohol abuse is, next to cognitive impairment, the most common diagnosable mental disorder of later life. Older alcoholics have a higher suicide rate than nonalcoholics (Schuckit and Pastor 1979). Since alcohol abuse is often not a presenting complaint, specific information should be elicited from every patient with depressive or suicidal ideation to determine whether alcohol may be a part of the clinical picture. Alcohol abuse may be particularly difficult to diagnose in older people for several reasons. The amount of alcohol needed to produce intoxication is lower in the aged because of increased sensitivity of the central nervous system to alcohol and because of an increase in the percentage of lean body mass (which produces a concomitant decrease in the volume of distribution of alcohol).

Since the usual criteria for alcohol abuse are strongly related to social functioning, they are most relevant to younger, employed individuals and do not account for the different social styles of older adults. Thus they tend to underestimate the degree of impairment in the older alcoholic (Stern and Kastenbaum 1984).

A spouse, child, or other care giver should be interviewed in conjunction with the patient so that specific questions can be asked about alcohol consumption, work history, alcohol-associated decline and social functioning, and any change in prior drinking habits. The medical history, physical exam, and laboratory examination—including complete blood count (CBC), serum metabolic screen (SMA-18), GGT, serum magnesium, blood alcohol level, serum amylase, and urinalysis—may reveal medical conditions that point to a history of chronic alcohol use (e.g., cirrhosis, aspiration pneumonia, chronic pancreatitis, gonadal atrophy, megaloblastic anemia, unexplained cardiomyopathy, broad-based gait, polyneuritis, unexplained constipation or diarrhea, seizures, tremulousness or hallucinations following cessation of drinking).

TREATMENT

The Decision to Hospitalize

Once suicidality has been determined, the next question must be whether or not to hospitalize the older patient. This decision should be based on several criteria: 1) the seriousness of the intent, 2) the current location of the patient, 3) the potential for lethality, and 4) patient cooperation.

Seriousness of Intent. Because older patients express suicidal ideation less often than younger patients, and because they are most likely to complete suicide successfully when they attempt it, all elderly patients expressing suicidal ideas should be taken very seriously. In the absence of convincing evidence to the contrary, one should assume that the external environment will be insufficient to manage a suicidal patient, and the patient should be hospitalized.

Location of the Patient. Most suicides of elderly people occur at home (Copeland 1987). Although elderly people living with others may, of course, attempt suicide, an attempt is more likely when the patient is alone. Suicidal elderly patients who live alone should not be left in their isolated state. If caring family members will take the patient in, and if the patient appears to be reassured by family involvement and agrees not to commit suicide, hospitalization may be avoided. Suicidal patients without clear intent who live in personal care or nursing homes may also be amenable to treatment within that setting. Patients who have clear-cut intent, however, should be hospitalized.

Potential for Lethality. Older people tend to use violent means to kill themselves. In one study (Copeland 1987), gunshot wounds accounted for 37% of deaths by suicide in this age group. Other means of death include drug overdose (22%), asphyxia by hanging or drowning (22%), and blunt trauma (from falls or walking in front of moving vehicles) (11%) (Copeland 1987). Because of the great efficiency with which many older suicidal patients complete suicide, careful questioning of suicidal patients and their families is required. For patients who have access to firearms, strict instructions must be given to family members to see that guns are removed from the home, even if the patient has expressed no desire to implement suicide by this means. Other ways of committing suicide are more difficult to guard against, since many implements that may be used for asphyxiation (belts, plastic bags) and overdose (common household medicines such as acetaminophen or aspirin) are ubiquitous. Further, if a patient wants to jump to his or her death or walk in front of a moving vehicle, there is virtually no way to prevent death apart from hospitalization. Thus serious expressions of suicidal ideation in the elderly must be evaluated with the awareness that older people often attempt suicide in ways that are difficult to reverse once implemented, and consequently, virtually all elderly patients who express suicidal intent should be hospitalized in a psychiatric facility equipped to prevent suicide attempts.

Patient Cooperation. Patient cooperation is a most significant factor in the decision whether or not to hospitalize. Patients who have expressed suicidal ideas who respond to the reassurance of the therapist and the concern of family members may be amenable to management as outpatients, as long as they do not have to stay alone and are able to express suicidal ideas to a care giver. Patients with suicidal ideas who are guarded or skeptical about clinical interventions and who are unable to receive family support are much more likely to require hospitalization.

Psychopharmacology

In addition to psychosocial methods of treatment, antidepressants should be used to treat the suicidal patient who is depressed if the patient is not immediately suicidal and if the medication can be administered by a responsible care giver or on an inpatient unit. Cyclic antidepressants and monoamine oxidase inhibitors (MAOIs) are both effective and safe pharmacological treatments in otherwise healthy older people. However, administering antidepressants to older patients does require that certain precautions be observed.

Antidepressant Therapy. Although tricyclic antidepressants are a mainstay in the psychiatric treatment of depression, they present particular problems in older suicidal patients because of the increased incidence of untoward side effects in older patients and also because they may be lethal in overdose.

Standard tricyclic antidepressants all produce anticholinergic side effects (dry mouth, constipation, urinary hesitancy or retention, tachycardia, delirium, hallucinosis, and blurred vision), and these effects are more pronounced and disturbing to elderly than younger individuals. Older people with dry mouth may suffer from increased caries, demineralization of teeth, and decreased taste acuity. Constipation is common in sedentary older patients and, if untreated, may lead to symptoms that are interpreted as somatization, such as bloating, belching, flatus, faintness, and anxiety. Thus patients on tricyclics should be taken seriously when they complain of abdominal complaints, and the offending medication discontinued if response to improved diet and mild laxatives is ineffective. Untreated constipation can lead to fecal impaction, stercoral ulcer, and anal fissures. Likewise, urinary retention may lead to overflow incontinence, which is often mistaken for incontinence of neurological origin. The delirium and hallucinosis of the tricyclics, especially in otherwise debilitated or demented elderly patients, may be attributed to "organic brain syndrome" or dementia, and left untreated.

Very careful thought should be given to the possibility of overdose with these medicatons. Lethal overdoses have occurred following ingestion of as little as 5 g of imipramine 5000 (about 30 days' worth for a patient receiving 150 mg daily) (Driesbach 1983). Certain antidepressant medications such as trazodone and fluoxetine are apparently safer in overdose than the tricyclic antidepressants and therefore may be preferable for first-line treatment of depression in some cases for suicidal outpatients.

In older patients, the general rule for pharmacological treatment is "start low and go slow." Although newer antidepressants appear to have certain advantages in older patients, it is prudent to begin with an established drug with a low incidence of side effects (such as desipramine) at a dose of 10 to 25 mg daily, increasing the dose gradually until the patient is receiving 75 to 150 mg daily. If the patient cannot tolerate the anticholinergic side effects of the tricyclic antidepressants, trazodone or fluoxetine would be appropriate treatments. If orthostatic hypotension is a problem for the patient, nortriptyline is an appropriate alternative initial drug. MAOIs are also suitable for treatment of depressed suicidal older patients, as long as treatment can be overseen by a care giver, and the patient does not develop ambulatory instability from the effect of the MAOIs on vascular tone.

Electroconvulsive Therapy

In the acutely suicidal patient, electroconvulsive therapy is probably the treatment of choice. Despite frequent adverse publicity, electroconvulsive therapy remains one of the most effective treatments in the psychiatric armamentarium, provided it is used to treat appropriate disorders under appropriate conditions. When electroconvulsive therapy is used to treat major depression, it results in more rapid improvement and shorter hospital stays than tricyclic antidepressant therapy (Markowitz et al. 1987). In the suicidal elderly patient with melancholia or psychotic depression, electroconvulsive therapy may well be the treatment of choice. For older patients, as for younger patients, unilateral electroconvulsive therapy with brief pulse-wave stimulus is the preferred means of treatment, since unilateral electroconvulsive therapy tends to have substantially less cognitive toxicity than bilateral electroconvulsive therapy (Weiner et al. 1984).

Electroconvulsive therapy is generally regarded as a safe treatment in older patients. Data from younger patients attest to electroconvulsive therapy's safety in comparison to tricyclic antidepressants, although similar studies have not been done in the elderly. Despite its relative safety, complications from electroconvulsive therapy in older patients can be significant, particularly if patients are medically ill or if they continue to take psychotropic medications during this treatment. In one series, complications were particularly frequent in the oldest old, and included such conditions as high blood pressure following stimulation, hypotension, persistent tachycardia, falls, and pneumonia (Burke et al. 1987). Thus one must carefully assess older patients who are candidates for electroconvulsive therapy to ensure that the possibility of complications minimized. Appropriate steps would be discontinuing all psychotropic medications prior to treatment (although occasionally in a severely delusional or agitated patient, this is not possible); employing appropriate pre-electroconvulsive therapy evaluations, such as electroencephalogram (EEG) or computed tomography (CT) scan of the head, CBC, SMA-18, urinalysis, and spine films; and carefully weighing the potential anesthesia risk by using a standard risk measurement scheme. In all cases, the attending psychiatrist should seek anesthesiology consultation, monitor the patient's

EEG, electrocardiogram (EKG), and blood pressure during the treatment, and provide posttreatment observation to protect the patient against problems associated with post-ictal delirium, falls, or aspiration. Careful, systematic assessment of the patient's mental and physical status during the course of electroconvulsive therapy is required so that treatment can be truncated if problems begin to emerge.

Psychotherapy

Several forms of psychotherapy may be used with the depressed elderly, including insight-oriented, behavioral, cognitive, supportive, and milieu therapy (see Kahn, Chapter 16; Weishaar and Beck, Chapter 17, this volume). "Psychodynamic therapies are based on theories of personality that emphasize the dynamic interplay of the physiological substrate of the individual and the social forces of the environment as mediated by inner psychological states" (Storandt 1983, p. 19). The theories of Freud, Jung, and Adler form the basis for most psychotherapy. They focused on the importance of symbols, images, and dreams and emphasized the role of unconscious feelings, impulses, and emotions in determining unconscious moods and behaviors.

The major goal of psychodynamic psychotherapy is to give the patient insight into disturbing behaviors and feelings (Gotestam 1980). The emphasis in psychotherapy is on experiencing, as opposed to understanding in an intellectual sense. Psychotherapy is "therapeutic communication." The therapist must determine why the patient is thinking, feeling, and acting in a particular manner at a particular time (Verwoerdt 1976).

Bibring (1954) outlined five major uses of psychotherapy: 1) suggestion, in the form of hypnosis or some form of including ideas, impulse, and emotions to facilitate emotional expression, gain insight, or help the patient face reality and deal with problems; 2) abreaction, or emotional discharge of damned-up tensions through emotionally charged verbalizations; 3) manipulation of the patient's ideas and emotions through mobilizing various emotional systems; 4) clarification of issues and emotions; and 5) insight, or conscious understanding and interpretation of unconscious material, thoughts, and emotions. Verwoerdt (1976) described the following techniques of psychotherapy: nonverbal communication, empathy, optimistic attitude, hope and reassurance, preservation of dignity, and management of maladaptive defenses. The most common psychotherapeutic technique used by psychiatrists is psychodynamic psychotherapy. The same general principles and goals guide both individual and group psychotherapy.

Freud felt that the elderly would be poor candidates for psychotherapy; however, more recent clinical and empirical observations challenged Freud's position (Brink 1979; Gallagher 1981; Gallagher and Thompson 1982; Levy et al. 1980; Zung 1980). The first published report on psychotherapy with the elderly was by Martin and De Gruchy in 1930. However, as Lawton (1976) pointed out, there is very limited literature on the effects of psychotherapy on depressed elderly patients. Group psychotherapy may also be a very helpful treatment for elderly patients. Group psychotherapy was first successfully used with the elderly in 1950 by Silver. Wolff (1963), Stein (1959), and others have reported favorable changes using group psychotherapy with older depressed patients. In this section the focus is on individual psychotherapy. For a very detailed discussion and review of the literature on several types of psychotherapy conducted with depressed elderly individuals, the reader is referred to Gotestam (1980).

Insight-oriented psychotherapy, influenced by the work of Freud, is based largely on psychoanalytic principles and involves the therapist heavily in treatment. The therapist acts as a facilitator and interprets feelings and behavior. Early memories are reactivated to mobilize feelings associated with them. The expression of fears, anxieties, doubt, guilt, and other emotions is encouraged by the therapist. Unconscious and repressed emotions are brought to the level of consciousness so that they may be recognized, squarely faced, and dealt with in a positive way. Insight is achieved when the patient can recognize the nature and cause of his or her particular problem or maladaptive defense(s) and can recognize a reasonable solution or alternative response that is more adaptive. According to Verwoerdt (1976), "through intrapsychic alterations the ego emerges as a more mature and effective mental agency" (p. 136). Insight-oriented psychotherapy aims to strengthen the ego and eliminate anxiety and depression.

Freud discouraged the use of insight therapy with individuals over 45, claiming that "after 45 the patient's character would be too inflexible to make the necessary personality changes which were brought about by increased insight" (in Gotestam 1980, p. 786). However, Goldfarb (Goldfarb and Turner 1953), a psychoanalytic therapist, developed a form of brief psychodynamic therapy in which rigidity and increased dependency of the elderly are used as therapeutic tools. Goldfarb advocated a technique in which the therapist takes on the role of parent to allow the client to attain gratification for emotional needs and to build high self-esteem. The therapist, seen as a "protective parent," becomes a "significant other" who can provide help and hope to the dependent elder. The older client is allowed to "defeat" the parent, which is a way to help the client gain strength. Godbole and Verinis (1974) and Rechtschatten (1959) also reported success with this approach. This type of therapy requires the therapist to take an active role in directing therapy, providing guidance and reassurance and actively intervening in the patient's life.

Behavioral psychotherapy, guided by the principles of classical conditioning (Pavlov 1955) and operant conditioning (Skinner 1936), has also been used effectively to relieve late-life depression. Behaviorists view depression and other mental health problems as learned behaviors. According to behaviorists, the focus of therapy should be on the particular overt problem behavior or thought pattern, not on the internal subjective experience for the client. Changing the principles by which such behavior is learned can effectively change or eliminate the problem behavior or negative thought pattern.

Classical conditioning is "the learning process by which neutral cues (or stimuli) become associated with emotional reactions" (Edinberg 1985, p. 170). Two classical conditioning techniques, systematic desensitization and relaxation, are frequently used with the elderly to diminish anxiety. The older adult must be trained to relax. Patients can be taught to associate the feelings of being relaxed with cue words such as "calm." Elderly patients can also be taught "successive relaxation techniques" (Jacobson 1938), in which various muscle groups in the body are systematically relaxed.

Operant conditioning techniques, also referred to as behavior modification, are based on the premise that "maladaptive behaviors can be altered by manipulating stimulus variables or reinforcements" (Whanger 1980, p. 457). Use of positive or negative reinforcements, extinction procedures, and token economies have all proven effective with older adults. Gallagher and Thompson (1982) reported reduced depression in elderly subjects who had been treated with behavioral psychotherapy. Gallagher (1981) reported reduced depression in elderly clients after they received supportive group psychotherapy and behavioral therapy. Mishara and Kastenbaum (1973) found that living in a token economy, in which positive behaviors are rewarded by tokens that may be exchanged for food, cigarettes, and privileges and negative behaviors are discouraged through loss of tokens, significantly reduced the incidence of suicidal behavior among hospitalized elderly veterans.

One of the most popular current psychotherapies, cognitive or cognitive-behavioral therapy, is grounded in the theories and concepts proposed by Aaron Beck and his colleagues at the University of Pennsylvania (see Weishaar and Beck, Chapter 17, this volume). Beck (1967) proposed a cognitive theory to explain the etiology of reactive depression. According to Beck, "central to the pathogenesis of depression are the individual's attitudes toward self, the social environment, and the future" (quoted in Blazer 1982, p. 80). Individuals who have negative views about themselves and the world around them and who regard themselves as unworthy, undesirable, or useless are especially vulnerable to reactive depression when confronted with a stressful event or life crisis. According to Beck, "the affective response is determined by the way an individual structures his experiences. Thus, if an individual's conceptualization of the situation has an unpleasant context, he will experience a corresponding unpleasant affective response" (qtd. in Blazer 1982, p. 81).

Beck used three concepts to explain depression: 1) negative "cognitive triad," which encompasses negative perceptions of self, present situations, and the future; 2) underlying beliefs or "schemas," developed out of past experiences, which determine how an individual interprets situations and events; and 3) "cognitive errors" in logic and information processing that support negative (depressive) self-concepts. According to this theory, feelings of hopelessness and worthlessness lead to depression (Weishaar and Beck, Chapter 17, this volume).

Cognitive therapy emphasizes the patient's internal experiences —thoughts, wishes, and attitudes—rather than focusing exclusively on overt behavior. The aim of cognitive therapy for the elderly patient is to change negative thoughts or cognitions and distorted perceptions that reinforce negative self-concepts and lead to depressed feelings. Cognitive restructuring of events and situations, in which more positive interpretations are substituted, is a major goal of cognitive therapy.

Cognitive therapy with older patients involves uncovering and identifying negative thoughts; teaching patients how to identify negative thoughts and self-statements that lead to depression and how to examine the evidence for or against such thoughts; and changing patients' attitudes and negative world view so they begin to develop more reality-oriented and more adaptive interpretations of reality. The focus is on present-day problems, and the therapist takes an active role in teaching the patient problem-solving and coping skills. Feelings of mastery and pleasurable experiences are encouraged. The therapist also helps patients identify underlying negative themes that lead to negative cognitions. In the elderly, several such themes may be present such as "I'm too old to change," "old people are not good for anything," and "if only some situation would change, I would not be depressed."

Cognitive therapy has demonstrated its effectiveness in reducing late-life depression. Gallagher and Thompson (1983) reported on their study of 30 patients 55 and over who were diagnosed as suffering from major depressive disorders. Subjects were divided into three treatment groups: the first group received cognitive therapy, the second group received behavioral therapy, and the third group were treated with brief psychotherapy. Gallagher and Thompson found the greatest improvements in depression (assessed using four different scales designed to measure depression) for those subjects receiving behavioral and cognitive psychotherapy. Haley (1983) and Steuer (1982) also reported on the effectiveness of cognitive therapy in reducing depression in elderly clients. All of these therapies may be effective in reducing suicidal feelings, impulses, and behaviors in older patients.

Reminiscence and Life Review Therapy

Reminiscence may be defined as "the act, process, or fact of recalling or remembering the past" (Butler 1964, p. 266). When reminiscing, one is remembering past life events, experiences, people, and places. The activity can be mental or verbal. One may recall thoughts or feelings, even smells or sounds, connected with the past. Thoughts of the past may emerge as "stray, seemingly insignificant thoughts about self or may become continuous" (Butler 1971, p. 49). Reminiscence may produce nostalgia, pleasure, an idealized past, or mild regret. On the other hand, it may lead to anxiety, guilt, depression, or despair: "Memory pains us and shames us and entertains us and serves the sense of self and its continuity" (Butler 1964, p. 266).

The term *life review* has gained wide recognition through the writings of Dr. Robert Butler, former director of the National Institute on Aging. Life review encompasses reminiscence, but includes much more. In a life review, one does not just remember the past, one analyzes, evaluates, restructures, and reconstructs past life events and experiences and their meanings to arrive at a better understanding of one's life. The process puts the past into coherent order and proper perspective in light of present values, attitudes, and life experiences. The life review—more common in late life but apparent in all life stages—is thus an active process of personality reorganization. Birren (1964) described it as "setting one's house in order." During life review, the elderly "integrate life as it has been lived in relation to how it might have been lived" (p. 275).

Freud referred to neurotic illnesses as "diseases of reminiscence" (Qtd. in Butler 1963, p. 523), suggesting the therapeutic value of remembering and the psychopathology of repressing, forgetting, or removing memories from conscious awareness. In the same vein, Butler (1963) noted that "recovering important memories is a basic ingredient of the curative process in psychoanalysis and necessary for change" (p. 525). In this view, reminiscence and life review are a natural form of personal psychotherapy. Jung (1934) suggested that the life review helps to reduce psychic tension and restore psychic balance and is necessary to personality development. To achieve integrity over despair, Erikson (1950) noted that older individuals must review their lives and determine whether they were inevitable, meaningful, and worthy. If they accept their lives and feel they have done all they could and do not wish anything different, they will achieve integrity over despair and gain wisdom.

Empirical findings confirm the therapeutic value of reminiscence and life review for older adults suffering from depression. Based on clinical data collected from a large-scale study of human aging conducted at the National Institute of Mental Health from 1955 to 1961, Butler (1980-1981) reported several examples of positive personal change in subjects after they engaged in reminiscence and life review. The therapeutic benefits ranged from a better ability to cope with aging and death to greatly improved relations with family members. From his clinical observations, Butler concluded that "people get much out of the opportunity to express thoughts and feelings to someone willing to listen" (p. 37). In his study of 24 white males aged 65 and over, Lewis (1971) found that reminiscence is positively related to maintaining self-concept, especially in times of pervasive stress. He found that reminiscence helps one get through various life crises, particularly the loss of a spouse. A more recent study of 91 subjects between the ages of 58 and 98 by Romaniuk and Romaniuk (1981) concluded that "interpersonal reminiscence appears to be a pleasant activity and is essentially a method of bolstering self-esteem during the course of social interactions. Apparently, self-esteem is maintained through recollections which demonstrate current personal worth and utility or past worth" (p. 68).

Life review therapy is defined by Lewis and Butler (1974) as a psychoanalytically oriented action process in which the therapist does not initiate a process but rather "taps into an already ongoing self-analysis and participates in it with the older person" (p. 166). In their view, the major purpose of a psychotherapeutic intervention through life review is "to make it more conscious, deliberate, and efficient" (p. 166). The technique is an effective way to get the elderly to do necessary developmental work of late life, primarily achieving integrity over despair and coming to terms with death. Life review therapy helps the elderly put their pasts into perspective in the light of present events, values, and attitudes. It allows them to experience and acknowledge important emotions and to integrate them into the self, which is essential for healthy functioning. The intervention strategy can be used to help reduce loneliness, enhance self-esteem, increase morale, and extend cognitive functioning (Reedy and Birren 1980). By helping elderly individuals bring past events back to mind and to relive, reexperience, and savor them, therapists can aid them in identifying and mitigating real guilt, in exorcising problematic child-hood identifications, in resolving intense earlier conflicts, in reconcil-ing family relationships, and in transmitting knowledge and values to others (Pincus 1970). In addition, such therapy can help older persons integrate the aging experience into the entire life process and see death as a natural part of life.

By carefully listening as the older person relates and reconstructs the past by telling a life story, the therapist can begin to see and understand critical issues and unresolved conflicts, feelings of guilt over past mistakes or wrongdoings, concerns over inability as a parent, and other fears, anxieties, and doubts. The degree of emotion with which certain past events or people are recalled provides a clue as to the nature and intensity of feelings about them. Nuances and slips of the tongue can provide clues about self-image, the amount of stress the patient is experiencing, and the types of relationships the person hopes to foster. Listening intently to the patient also provides the opportunity to form an interpersonal bond with the older person and to reawaken the person's interests (Butler 1961). Moreover, a sensitive listening can help elderly patients put past events in proper perspective and turn the life review into "a positive attempt to recon-cile life, to confront real guilt, and to find meaning in their lives, especially in the presence of acceptance and support from others" (Lewis and Butler 1974, p. 169).

Lewis and Butler (1974) outlined three steps in life review ther-apy: recording of a detailed life history, careful observation, and systematic eliciting of memories. To elicit memories, the individual is encouraged to write or tape an autobiography or detailed personal life history. Individuals are encouraged to focus on a particular person, life event, or time period of significance. Life review therapy tech-niques include pilgrimages to important places from the past; re-unions (church, class, family); genealogy construction; and the use of memorabilia (scrapbooks, photo albums, old letters).

It is particularly important that the therapist who chooses life review therapy as an intervention technique to help the troubled older person be an effective listener and be able to use the skills of explora-tion, focusing, and probing to help the individual order the past as a coherent whole (Pincus 1970). The objective should be to help the troubled older person to achieve a sense of meaning and to maintain integrity over despair, thereby decreasing the risk of suicide. By reducing feelings of despair, the risk of suicide is greatly reduced also.

Creative Arts Therapy

The use of dance, song, and visual arts in religious and magical ways to cure physical or emotional ills dates back to antiquity. Aristotle recognized the value of dramatic play for relaxation "as a medicine" and noted the value of tragedy as catharsis because it allows for the "purgation of emotions" (Courtney 1968, p. 10). Greek tragedies encouraged the expression of such emotions as pity and fear as the actors (and audience) identified with characters.

During the 20th century there has been dramatic growth in and acceptance of the use of creative arts or expressive therapy with the sick. Creative arts therapies are closely allied with and have been greatly influenced by psychoanalysis and humanistic psychology. Both Freud (1955) and Jung (1964) recognized the therapeutic value of the drawing or painting of dreams, which are experienced as visual images and difficult to express in words.

The arts allow for creative expression, development of personal insight, and self-awareness. Similarly, spontaneity, flexibility, and originality resulting from the creative process are encouraged through the use of creative therapy. Art—whether in music, visual media, drama, or dance—is naturally therapeutic. Often the creative process enables a person to uncover aspects of the self that are blocked from conscious sight. The arts provide a means of expanding the consciousness, of naturally becoming more aware of one's self, particularly of the connection between mind and body. It forces us to become more in tune with our senses (sight, hearing, touch) and our bodies. The arts also provide a means to achieve an identity. The search for identity, one's sense of who one is and where one stands, has always led to music, art, and drama.

Dwedney (1977), Landgarten (1981), Weiss (1984), and others have effectively used the visual arts as therapy with the elderly. Art therapy has proven to be particularly effective for chronic pain patients. The expression of pain and the accompanying feelings of anger, rage, guilt, or sorrow through artwork permits catharsis and leads to successful management of the feeling (Landgarten 1981). Many elderly experience feelings of depression, and artwork is one method of working through such feelings. Such feelings expressed through art can be shared and discussed with positive results. These individuals can obtain therapeutic benefits by examining their own feelings and emotions as expressed in concrete form in artworks.

Many practitioners have used music therapy effectively with the elderly. Music therapy has been used with older people as an outlet for creative expression, as a vehicle to invoke powerful emotions, and as an aid in grief work and in dealing with the experience of death and dying. It naturally encourages group participation and, as such, has reportedly alleviated feelings of loneliness, hopelessness, depression, and despair in elderly participants.

Specifically, music therapy has been used to address a number of different problems of the elderly. Kartman (1980) used music therapy with elderly patients in long-term–care facilities to help alleviate depression and stress. Olson (1984) found that exposure to player piano music resulted in improved life satisfaction and feelings of well-being for elderly subjects. Bright (1985) emphasized the role of music in combating the loneliness, isolation, and depression of older people. Further, music is useful in psychotherapy with the old. Through its strong powers of association and memory-evoking properties, music can help to bring past and present feelings and emotions to the surface so they can be expressed and dealt with.

As a therapeutic technique, creative dramatics has its roots in dramatic play and is closely related to psychodrama. Psychodrama grew out of Jacob Moreno's experience with Viennese children at play. Derived from the Greek terms *psyche*, meaning mind or soul, and *dramein*, meaning to do or to act, psychodrama refers to the expressing or acting out of thoughts and emotions through speech, gestures, and movement (Duke 1974). In psychodrama, individuals play roles and create parts; the emphasis is on spontaneity, creativity, action, process, self-disclosure, risk taking, and the here-and-now. The individual acts out unconscious thoughts, feelings, and impulses to recapitulate unsolved problems and to experience catharsis. The group drama encourages empathy as the players identify with one another. Like psychodrama, creative dramatics involves the creation of role, role-playing, improvisation, and expression of thoughts, feelings, and emotions through verbal and nonverbal means of communication.

In the last decade, creative dramatics has been used increasingly with the elderly. From data she collected on the effects of drama on the elderly, Gray (1974) cited the following as major benefits: opportunity to be of service to others, increased self-confidence resulting from successful memorization and good performance, communication and social interaction skills developed through the group experience, and the emotional outlet provided by the experience. Burger (1980) demonstrated that the elderly who participate in the creative drama experience begin to communicate and see themselves as useful again; life takes on a new meaning. Davis (1985) reported that "drama helps older adults integrate their thoughts, words, actions, and emotions through original improvisation in which they draw on their life experience" (p. 315). Based on analysis of quantitative and qualitative data, Clark and Osgood (1985) concluded that participation in applied theater decreases loneliness and increases life satisfaction; in addition, those who engage in the drama activities see themselves as younger than those who do not.

Dance as a form of therapeutic intervention has its basis in the development of the modern dance and has been used successfully with older adults. Zandt and Lorenzen (1985), who have used dance with seniors, found that it helped people relax, reduced stress, and provided tranquility. Older dancers said they felt less lonely, less depressed, and more self-assured as a result of their dancing. Garnet (1974) has effectively used movement sequences that employ rhythmic use of swings, twists, stretches, pulls, and pushes to meet physical needs and to stimulate somatic and psychological feelings of comfort, ease, and humor in elderly subjects. Fersh (1981) concluded that dance or movement therapy with the elderly can be an enlightening experience that can inspire the therapist and clients to face life and death with love and energy.

Creative arts offer the older adult choice. In creative art activities, the individual chooses the medium (e.g., clay, wood), chooses the colors and textures, and chooses what to make and how to make it. The art object is personalized. So, too, in dance and drama: the individual decides what to say or do and in what manner. Choice builds pride, confidence, self-esteem, and a sense of control to offset the negative psychological effects of loss. Through participating in creative activities, older adults come to view themselves as active, vital, useful human beings.

Additionally, the arts are inspirational, infusing the older adult with a spirit or zest for life and hope for the future. Creative therapy is a valuable means of releasing fear, doubt, guilt, and grief and of decreasing hopelessness—emotions that plague many potentially suicidal elderly. Creative therapy also provides a positive experience of participation in a social group, with accompanying feelings of acceptance, belonging, positive self-esteem and self-concept, personal competence, mastery, and accomplishment. As such, the arts represent a major technique for reducing suicidal risk in older adults.

Family and Support Group Therapy

Blazer (1980) noted that "decreased social support may be of more importance in the increased prevalence of depression in late life than personality style, and intrapsychic conflicts or genetic predisposition" (p. 261). Social support encompasses interpersonal communication and interaction, protective feedback, love and understanding, caring and concern, affection and companionship, financial assistance, respect, and acceptance. Social support is usually provided by family members and kin, close friends, and neighbors. Such support can also be provided by a support group comprised of individuals who are facing the same problems and have the same needs and concerns. Family therapy and support group therapy are two major supportive therapies that can effectively reduce depression and suicidal behavior in older individuals.

In 1965 Shanas and Streib published an important collection of writings reaffirming the importance of the family to elders and pointing out that older people need to be viewed in the social context of their family (Herr and Weakland 1979). Since that time, numerous geriatric psychiatrists, geropsychologists, social workers, and others who counsel older people have recognized the numerous benefits of family therapy for older adults who suffer from depression and other age-related problems (Brody 1966; Brody and Spark 1966; Richman 1986).

The family is held together by bonds of love and affection. The major function of the family is to provide companionship among members, physical necessities, maintenance of motivation and morale, and continuing communication and patterns of interaction (Murray et al. 1980). The family is likely to be the individual's major strength and defense against the problems and crises of daily living. According to Bengtson and Treas (1980), families contribute to the mental health and well-being of members in two important ways: first, by providing a support system that offers love and affection, financial assistance, needed services, assistance with tasks,and other forms of strength and help; and, second by influencing self-concept through social interactions, communication, and evaluations of role performance.

The elderly are particularly dependent on the family for support. Weiss (1976) noted that support is especially important in times of crisis, transition, and stress. Many older adults face the transition of widowhood or retirement. Others face the loss of physical health and mobility or income, status, and power. Family support in the form of love and understanding, caring and concern, affection and companionship, and acceptance is vital to the older individual. The family can aid the older member by "helping him/her to mature; become more adaptive, integrated, and open to his/her experiences; and to finding meaning in his/her situation" (Murray et al. 1980, p. 52). The family, according to Caplan (1976), functions as a collector and disseminator of information, a feedback guidance system, a source of ideology, a guide and mediator in problem solving, a source of mutual aid, a haven for rest and recuperation, a reference and control group, a source and validator of identity, and a place for emotional expression. As such, the family represents the major force for mediating the negative effects of stress and loss on older individuals.

Family therapy can play a major role in suicide prevention. According to Richman (1986), the major goal of family therapy is to release the healing forces each family possesses and help the family become a self-help group. The therapist is a catalyst who functions to remove barriers to continued growth and development, individuation, caring, and cohesion. Herr and Weakland (1979) advocated a similar approach in which the family therapist works with troubled family members to identify and define the problem, decide on solutions, and set realistic family goals; the therapist also mobilizes the family system to solve the problem and reach the goals set.

According to Blazer (1982), the therapist working with families who have a depressed elderly member must evaluate the following elements of the family system: past and present psychological state of individual family members; family structure, including location, roles, and boundaries; type, quantity, and quality of interactions; family atmosphere or "ambience"; family values, especially values regarding mental health and the role of the elderly and aging; type, extent, availability, and accessibility of support; and the level of internal family unit stress.

Blazer (1982) pointed out that frequent, high-quality interactions among family members have a positive impact on the older depressed member. Similarly, a family that values older members as useful and productive and includes them in activities, discussions, and decisions offers a more positive environment than one that devalues age and perceives older members as a useless burden and bother. Blazer (1980) identified four "intangible supports" that are particularly important for the depressed family member: a dependable social network, social participation or interaction, belongingness, and intimacy.

Blazer (1982) offers several suggestions to those treating the family of a depressed older adult. First, he recommends that the family be taught the nature of depression in late life and the risk of suicide. He also suggests that they learn how to read warning signs and know the clues to depression and suicide. He advocates that practitioners carefully explain the nature of the illness and assure family members that comments made by the depressed elder should not be taken personally. The practitioner can instruct family members on how to communicate with the depressed elder and encourage positive interactions. Finally, Blazer suggests that family members be encouraged to express and discuss their feelings openly.

Support groups are also a helpful intervention for suicidal patients. The principle of mutual aid or joint struggle against common problems underlies the development of mutual help or support groups. Support groups are patterned after the family or small community and are expressive in nature. They offer members understanding and acceptance as unique personalities with both good and bad qualities, with both strengths and weaknesses. They offer a place where emotions can be freely expressed and where recognition, status, and security are offered. Most support groups are established by and for individuals who are stigmatized, either for a short time or permanently (Traunstein and Steinman 1973). For example, widows may feel they are "misfits," "marginals," or "fifth wheels" in a couple-oriented society. The very word *widow* has negative connotations and carries a stigma for many women. In a support group, these individuals can find acceptance among others suffering the same plight. When everyone shares the same stigma, one finds acceptance; feelings of isolation and marginality are reduced.

In a support group, the members 1) learn by their participation in developing and evaluating a social microcosm; 2) learn by giving and receiving feedback; 3) have the unique opportunity to be both helpers and helpees; and 4) learn by the consensual validation of multiple perspectives (Bednar and Kaul 1978). As noted by Yalom (1970) and Burnside (1978), the group offers opportunities for people to confront feelings of alienation by providing for free expression of feelings and experiences with group members who are "in the same boat." Participating in a support group can instill hope in members who see others successfully coping with similar problems or life experiences (Yalom 1970).

In the last decade, the popularity of support groups has greatly increased. Currently, support groups exist for widows and widowers, Alzheimer's victims and their family care givers, cancer patients, heart patients, arthritics, and depressed elderly dealing with the problems of grief, loss, and aging, among others. Those working with support groups have noted the many positive effects of such groups on the elderly. Burnside (1978) described her success with groups of grievers, claiming that such groups help the members by facilitating adjustment to the loss of a spouse and preventing subsequent problems. Positive effects were reported by Hiltz (1977), who started a program for widows in 1970. Weekly discussion groups were successful in alleviating feelings of loneliness and providing assurance that the widow was not unique, that others had similar problems. Members of the group cited emotional support as the major benefit obtained from participation. Someone to listen and give sympathy were the benefits most valued by the widows.

Petty et al. (1976) organized support groups for elderly arthritic individuals. Most of these individuals were experiencing moderate depression in adjusting to the aging process. Participation in a support group decreased feelings of loneliness, depression, and unhappiness; increased knowledge of physical functioning; and resulted in better communication with family and friends and a desire to be more actively involved in life. The members also came to feel that their frustration and problems were "normal" and a part of aging. They made new friends and learned how to use community resources more effectively through their participation in the group.

Clinicians working with the depressed, suicidal geriatric patient should be aware of the various support groups in their community and should consider recommending them to the patient. Certain characteristics of the group should be considered. Based on his experience with groups, Lowy (1967) cited three important factors in effective group work: authority, structure, and language. The group must have a clear sense of goals and purposes, and there must be some clear-cut form of leadership. The members must speak a common language and share common symbols and meanings. The group's structure must provide a basis for relating and accomplishing group goals. A certain format or standard procedure and use of a common language will serve to provide such a structure.

Environmental Manipulation

The belief that the environment affects health and disease has a long history. The Hippocratic writings note the direct causal relationship between changes of seasons, risings and settings of the sun, wind and temperature patterns, and other elements of the physical environment and the state of physical health and disease in humans. During the 18th century, some social reformers advocated exposure to an optimum physical environment as a means of alleviating mental illness. Influenced by such early ideas, many recent students of physical and mental health have argued that human behavior must be studied in the context of the physical and social environment in which the individual lives and functions. Ittelson (1970) pointed out that the environment surrounds and enfolds the individual.

The field of social ecology may be defined as "the study of the impacts of the physical and social environments on human beings" (Moos 1974). Researchers concerned with the relationship between human behavior and the physical-social environment have produced a rich body of literature that confirms the importance of the physical and social environment in which the individual lives and functions to his or her optimum physical and mental health (Moos 1976). The quality of the environment is important to satisfying the needs of older persons; for an individual to develop his or her full potential, therefore, successful interaction and adaptation to the environment are necessary.

In the process of aging, alterations occur in varying degrees from one person to another and at one time or another. The need for maintenance of good health, self-determination, dignity, freedom of choice, appropriate sensory stimulation, physical activity, social interaction, meaningful activity, and social status all contribute to a sense of control and mastery within the environment; these needs are continuous and necessary to some degree throughout life (Beck et al. 1984).

Because the environment is such an important factor in the health and overall well-being of individuals, Kiernat (1982) called it "the hidden modality" in rehabilitation programs. Researchers in the field of aging have demonstrated an even greater influence of the physical and social environment on the health and behavior of the elderly, who are more dependent for support on their immediate surroundings (Lawton 1980).

The institutionalized elderly, who are the most vulnerable due to functional deficits and lack of other social support, are the most dependent on their immediate environment (George 1980) and often are able to exercise less control over their environments and activities than are the elderly in the community. However, it should be recognized that the impact of the environment is tempered by the personal life space of the individual.

According to Bengtson (1978), the three social-psychological needs of older people are connectedness, effectance, and identity. Connectedness refers to the need to be a part of the social setting and social group, the feeling of belonging. Effectance refers to a sense of control over one's life and one's environment and the ability to make choices and influence change. Identity is a personal sense of one's place in the world and of one's unique qualities as a human being. The environment in which the older individual lives largely determines to what extent these three needs are met. The environment also has a major impact on the physical and cognitive functioning of the older person and on that person's physical and mental health.

An individual's behavior is shaped, facilitated, or constricted by the environment (Lawton 1980). Environments may be conducive to challenge and stimulation or they may promote relaxation. The environment can provide needed challenge, stimulation, and supports necessary for optimum functioning and positive mental health. Individuals can use the physical environment to engage in activities, accomplish tasks, or influence other people.

Lawton's (1977) environmental docility hypothesis states that the lower the individual's capabilities relative to the environment, the more salient are the impacts of environmental demands (Faletti 1986). Thus the less competent and more debilitated the older adult, the greater the effect of the environment on the person's overall functioning. Lawton and Nahemow (1973) suggested that the demands or "press" of the environment must be congruent with the skills and capacities of the older individual for effective behavior to occur. Too much demand will result in fear, stress, and anxiety; too little demand results in boredom, lethargy, and sensory and cognitive deprivation. Efforts to improve competence, enhance independence, and improve affective state should match the competencies of the older person with the demands of the person's environment.

Kahana (1974) presented a congruence model in which she characterized the optimal environment as one that provides maximal congruence between individual needs and environmental press. When such an optimal person-environment "fit" occurs, a high level of individual well-being is the outcome. Research findings support Kahana's model. Studies of the institutionalized aged have confirmed that person-environment congruence and an institutional environment that fosters autonomy, personalized care, and social integration result in higher morale and better adjustment of residents (Bennett 1963; Coe 1965; Kahana et al. 1980).

Lindsley (1964) and Beyer and Nierstraz (1967) described a "prosthetic environment" in which various physical aids and supports are available to increase mobility and prevent falls and injuries in the elderly. Prosthetic environments also include sensory stimulation devices and aids to reduce disorientation, such as large calendars and reality boards with the day, month, year, and other information. A prosthetic environment is designed to compensate for various physical, cognitive, and sensory losses, which are experienced by an older individual, and to enhance physical and mental competence, individuality, independence, and personal autonomy.

Most studies of the impact of environment on physical and mental health of older adults have been conducted in institutions. Certain key elements of the environment have been identified as exerting a major inflence on quality of life and morale. In his study of environmental factors that influence quality of care in nursing homes, Tobin (1974) placed nursing homes on a continuum of resource-rich to resource-poor on three dimensions: organizational, social service system, and health service system. On the organizational dimension, resource-rich facilities tended to be corporately owned and required extra charges. On the social service system dimension, the resource-rich facilities tended to be nonurban, to be located in affluent areas, and to have a large number of private paying patients. On the third dimension, health service system, the resource-rich facilities tended to have more residents who were referred by a physician or hospital and more residents whose care was reimbursed by Medicare. Tobin also found a significant difference between resource-rich and resource-poor facilities in his measure of quality of care. Of the residents in resource-rich facilities, 95%—as compared with only 40% in resource-poor facilities—felt that their needs were met. Presumably, higher-cost facilities will be able to provide more and better quality resources for residents. Osgood and Brant (unpublished) found that suicidal behavior was significantly less likely to occur in high-cost institutions than in those charging less for care.

Size is one facility characteristic that has been shown to affect patient outcomes. The early work of Greenwald and Linn (1971) suggested that as homes for the aged increase in size, patient satisfaction, activity, and communication decline. In another well-known study of the effect of size on patient outcomes and quality of care, Curry and Ratliff (1973), who studied 26 licensed proprietary homes in Ohio, found that residents in small facilities were less isolated and more sociable than those in larger facilities. Residents in smaller homes had more friends in homes, more monthly contacts with those friends, and more total monthly contacts with relatives and family. Osgood and Brant (unpublished) also found size to be a major predictor of suicidal behavior. Larger facilities were significantly more likely to experience suicides than were smaller facilities.

Personal space needs are of prime importance in maintaining the individual's integrity. Although information related to the personal space needs of the elderly is limited, Louis (1981) found that intrusion into any patient's personal behavior space may weaken the individual's defense and may result in anger, refusal of procedures, or silence. These responses can be detrimental to the elderly, who, as Louis affirmed, have fewer resources to counter such weakened defenses. Although the environment influences the actions of persons of all ages, its impact is more clearly evident on older people whose competencies and coping mechanisms are reduced by illness or disability.

Privacy has been identified as another important factor influencing patient outcomes. Koncelik (1976) reported differences in behavior of nursing home residents as a function of the amount of privacy available. The author found that the residents who perceived they had more privacy were better adjusted than those who perceived they had less privacy. When Lawton (1977) surveyed elderly residents of long-term–care facilities, he found that approximately 50% of those sharing rooms desired a private room. Almost all researchers agree that the attainment of privacy is essential to maintaining positive self-regard, self-reflection, and autonomy and to providing emotional release in the institutionalized elderly (Louis 1981; Tate 1980; Windley and Scheidt 1980). Privacy is essential for suicidal patients who suffer from low self-esteem and feelings of hopelessness and helplessness. A suicidal watch may be necessary for such patients, but some degree of privacy and personal autonomy is still important for the patient.

Mishara and Kastenbaum (1973) examined the impact of changed environment on intentional suicidal behavior of 40 residents in the medical unit of a large state hospital. They were interested in finding out whether or not enriching the environment would alter suicidal behavior. Subjects were divided into three groups: 1) those living in a token economy, in which desirable behaviors were rewarded by tokens that could be exchanged for cigarettes, candy, permission to leave, and other privileges, and undesirable behaviors were punished by not rewarding with tokens or by taking back tokens; 2) those on an enrichment ward, which was cheerier and offered more activities and social stimulation and more personal choice regarding food and personal grooming; and 3) those living on a traditional custodial care ward. After 9 months on one of the three wards, residents' behavior was systematically observed and recorded by trained observers for 7 days. Observations were done using a self-injurious behavior observation scale developed by Mishara and Kastenbaum. Analysis of results confirmed that the nature and quality of the environment has a significant influence on level of suicidal behavior of residents. Residents of the token economy and enrichment wards engaged in significantly less suicidal behavior than did those living on traditional custodial care wards. Mishara and Kastenbaum concluded that those who live in "better" environments engage in fewer suicidal behaviors.

More attention has been directed toward the effect of social environment on health and well-being than toward the physical environment. The physical environment refers to the "built" environment and encompasses space, objects, architecture, physical design features, and the outdoor grounds. The physical environment can exert a powerful influence on social relationships, quality of daily life, and physical and mental health of residents. Several elements of the physical environment can be designed to enhance mental and physical functioning and to promote independence and autonomy. To compensate for visual impairments that accompany the aging process, lighting should be low-glare and colors should be bright and cheery and varied from room to room and unit to unit to help in orientation. To compensate for auditory changes, background noise should be kept at a minimum and conversation should be clear and louder, if necessary. Music can also enhance the physical environment and is pleasant to the ears. Physical aids such as signs, calendars, large-face clocks, and reality orientation boards can be used to make the environment more understandable, predictable, and less confusing, and can compensate for memory loss and confusion, which characterize many older adults. Comfort needs can be met by controlling air temperature and air quality, eliminating drafts, and providing comfortable furniture appropriate to the physical condition of the older individual. Privacy can be facilitated by designing private rooms, doors that lock, and small private spaces. Safety features include wheelchair ramps, pull bars, absence of steps, nonslip flooring, lower-level cabinets, and other such features. Finally, the physical environment contributes to the aesthetic beauty we all need. Landscaping, gardening, fountains, pictures, artwork, and plants can all be used to beautify the environment. The use of colors, lighting, and music can also contribute to the aesthetics. Pets may also be introduced as therapeutic aids. Pets add joy to life and often become companions to love and care for. Pets may, in fact, have effects on the mood of elderly patients, helping to relieve depression and improving physical health (Corson et al. 1977; Cuszak and Smith 1984; Katchner 1982; Mugford and M'Comisky 1975).

Based on studies of the institutionalized elderly, it appears that to prevent suicide among the institutionalized aged, facilities should provide for the individual's needs for freedom of choice and personal autonomy, privacy, and personal space. Facilities should also provide an enriched and supportive environment that includes appropriate and necessary physical design and safety features; well-trained and caring staff members who recognize the uniqueness and individuality of each older adult and treat him or her with dignity and respect; and a variety of recreational, social, and health-related services and resources. Whenever possible, family members and care givers working with the community elderly should also ensure the provision of such an environment for their loved ones/clients. Clinicians working with the suicidal geriatric patient should work with family members, social workers, and other care givers to increase community involvement and support for the suicidal patient. Table 2 provides an overview of psychosocial treatments for depression in late life.

Table 2. Psychosocial treatments for depression and suicidal behavior in older adults

Psychotherapy	Family therapy
Individual	Support group therapy
Group	Environmental manipulation
Insight-oriented	Pets and plants
Behavioral	Music
Cognitive	Prosthetic devices
Reminiscence therapy	Freedom, privacy, and
Creative arts therapy	independence-enhancing features
Drama	
Dance	
Music	
Art	

CONCLUSION

The role of the physician or other gatekeeper in recognizing and treating the suicidal geriatric patient cannot be overemphasized. Early recognition of depression and other underlying mental disorders is essential to suicide prevention in this age group. Awareness of major demographic factors (e.g., age, gender, race) that put an older adult at risk is important. Treatment should be specific to the mental disorder involved and should also include other supportive therapies. Effective treatments might include psychopharmacology, electroconvulsive therapy, psychotherapy, reminiscence therapy, creative arts therapy, family therapy, support group therapy, environmental manipulation, and various other forms of therapy.

REFERENCES

American Psychiatric Association: Diagnostic and Statistical Manual of Mental Disorders, 3rd Edition, Revised. Washington, DC, American Psychiatric Association, 1987

Beck AT (ed): Depression: Clinical, Experimental, and Theoretical Aspects. New York, Harper & Row, 1967

Beck CM, Rawlins RP, Williams SR (eds): Mental Health-Psychiatric Nursing: A Holistic Life-cycle Approach. St. Louis, MO, CV Mosby, 1984

Bednar R, Kaul T: Experimental group research: current perspectives, in Handbook of Psychotherapy and Behavior Change: An Empirical Analysis. Edited by Garfield S, Bergin A. New York, John Wiley, 1978, pp 769–816

Bengtson VL: The aged and their social needs, in Psychosocial Needs of the Aged: A Health Care Perspective. Edited by Seymour E. Los Angeles, CA,University of Southern California Press, 1978

Bengtson VL, Treas J: The changing family context of mental health and aging, in Handbook of Mental Health and Aging. Edited by Birren JE, Sloane RB. Englewood Cliffs, NJ, Prentice-Hall, 1980, pp 400–429

Bennett R: The meaning of institutional life. Gerontologist 3:117–125, 1963

Beyer GH, Nierstraz FHJ: Housing the Aged in Western Countries. New York, Elsevier, 1967

Bibring E: Psychoanalysis and the dynamic psychotherapies. J Am Psychoanal Assoc 2:745–770, 1954

Birren JE (ed): The Psychology of Aging. Englewood Cliffs, NJ, Prentice-Hall, 1964

Blazer D (ed): Social Supports and Mortality in a Community Population. Chapel Hill, NC, University of North Carolina Press, 1980

Blazer D (ed): Depression in Late Life. St. Louis, CV Mosby, 1982

Blazer DG, Bachar JR, Manton KG: Suicide in late life: review and commentary. J Am Geriatr Soc 34:519–525, 1986

Blazer D, Hughes DC, George LK: The epidemiology of depression in an elderly community population. Gerontologist 27:281–287, 1987

Blessed G, Tomlinson BE, Roth M: The association between quantitative measures of demential and of senile change in the cerebral grey matter of elderly subjects. Br J Psychiatry 114:797–811, 1968

Bright R (ed): Music in Geriatric Care, 2nd Edition. New York, Alfred Publishing, 1985

Brink T: Geriatric Psychotherapy. New York, Human Sciences Press, 1979

Brody EH: The aging family. Gerontologist 6:201–206, 1966

Brody EH, Spark GM: Institutionalization of the aged: a family crisis. Fam Process 5:76–90, 1966

Burger I (ed): Creative Drama for Senior Adults: A Program for Dynamic Living in Retirement. Wilton, CT, Morehouse-Barlow, 1980

Burke WJ, Rubin EH, Zorumski CF, et al: The safety of ECT in geriatric psychiatry. J Am Geriatr Soc 35:516–521, 1987

Burnside IM (ed): Working with the Elderly: Group Processes and Techniques. North Scituate, MA, Duxbury Press, 1978

Butler RN: Re-awakening interest. Nursing Homes 10:8–19, 1961

Butler RN: Recall in retrospection. J Am Geriatr Soc 11:523–529, 1963

Butler RN: The life review: an interpretation of reminiscence in the aged, in New Thoughts on Old Age. Edited by Kastenbaum R. New York, Springer, 1964, pp 265–280

Butler RN: Age: the life review. Psychology Today 5:49–51, 89, 108, 1971

Butler RN: The life review: an unrecognized bonanza. Int J Aging Hum Dev 12:35–38, 1980–1981

Caplan G: The family as a support system, in Support Systems and Mutual Help: Multidisciplinary Exploration. Edited by Caplan G, Killilea M. New York, Grune & Stratton, 1976, pp 19–36

Cath SH: Discussion notes, in Geriatric Psychiatry: Grief, Loss and Emotional Disorders in the Aging Process. Edited by Berezin MA, Cath SJH. New York, International Universities Press, 1965, pp 128–129

Clark P, Osgood NJ (eds): Seniors on Stage: The Impact of Applied Theater Techniques on the Elderly. New York, Praeger, 1985

Coe R: Self-conception and institutionalization, in Older People and Their Social World. Edited by Rose AM, Peterson WA. Philadelphia, PA, FA Davis, 1965, pp 225–244

Copeland AR: Suicide among the elderly: the Metro-Dade County experience, 1981–83. Med Sci Law 27:32–36, 1987

Corson SA, Corson EO, Gwynne PH, et al: Pet dogs as nonverbal communication links in hospital psychiatry. Compr Psychiatry 18:61–72, 1977

Coryell W: Diagnosis-specific mortality: primary unipolar depression and Briquet's syndrome (somatization disorder). Arch Gen Psychiatry 38:939–942, 1981

Courtney B (ed): Play, Drama, and Thought. New York, Drama Book Publishers, 1968

Curry TJ, Ratliff BW: The effects of nursing home size on resident isolation and life satisfaction. Gerontologist 13:295–298, 1973

Cuszack O, Smith E (eds): Pets and the Elderly: The Therapeutic Bond. New York, Haworth Press, 1984

Davis BW: The impact of creative drama training on psychological states of older adults: an exploratory study. Gerontologist 25:315–321, 1985

Driesbach RH (ed): Handbook of Poisoning: Prevention, Diagnosis, and Therapy. Los Altos, CA, Lange Medical Publications, 1983

Duke C (ed): Creative Dramatics and English Teaching. Urbana, IL, National Council of Teachers of English, 1974

Dwedney I: An art therapy program for geriatric patients, in Art Therapy in Theory and Practice, 2nd Edition. Edited by Ulman E, Dachinger P. New York, Schocken Books, 1977

Edinberg M (ed): Mental Health Practice With the Elderly. Englewood Cliffs, NJ, Prentice-Hall, 1985

Erikson E (ed): Childhood and Society. New York, WW Norton, 1950

Faletti MV: Environmental impact on mental health and functioning in nursing homes: implications for research and public policy, in Mental Illness in Nursing Homes: Agenda for Research (DHHS Publ No. ADM-86-1459). Edited by Harper MS, Lebowitz BD. Rockville, MD, Division of Clinical Research, National Institute of Mental Health, 1986

Farber ML (ed): Theory of Suicide. New York, Funk & Wagnalls, 1968

Farberow NL, Shneidman ES: Suicide and age, in The Psychology of Suicide. Edited by Shneidman ES, Farberow NL, Litman RE. New York, Science House, 1970, pp 164–174

Fersh I: Dance/movement therapy: a holistic approach to working with the elderly. Activities, Adaptation, and Aging, 2 (Fall):21–30, 1981

Folstein MF, McHugh PR: Dementia syndrome of depression in Alzheimer's disease: senile dementia and related disorders. Aging 7:87–93, 1978

Folstein M, Folstein SF, McHugh PR: Mini-mental state: practical method for grading for cognitive state of patients for the clinician. J Psychiatr Res 12:189–198, 1975

Freud S (ed): Origin and Development of Psychoanalysis. Chicago, IL, Regenery-Gateway, 1955

Gallagher D: Behavioral group therapy with elderly depressives: an experimental study, in Behavioral Group Therapy, Vol 3. Edited by Upper D, Ross S. Champaign, IL, Research Press, 1981, pp 187–224

Gallagher D: Assessment of depression by interview methods and psychiatric rating scales, in Handbook for Clinical Memory Assessment of Older Adults. Edited by Poon LW. Washington, DC, American Psychological Association, 1986, pp 202–212

Gallagher D, Thompson L: The treatment of major depressive disorders in older outpatients with brief psychotherapies. Psychotherapy: Theory, Research and Practice 19:482–490, 1982

Gallagher D, Thompson L: Effectiveness of psychotherapy for both endogenous and nonendogenous depression in older adult outpatients. J Gerontol 38:707–712, 1983

Garnet ED: A movement therapy for older people. Dance Therapy: Focus on Dance 7:59–61, 1974

George LK (ed): Role Transitions in Later Life. Monterey, CA, Brooks/Cole, 1980

Godbole A, Verinis JS: Brief psychotherapy in the treatment of emotional disorders in physically ill geriatric patients. Gerontologist 14:143–148, 1974

Goldfarb AI, Turner H: Psychotherapy of aged persons, II: utilization and effectiveness of "brief" therapy. Am J Psychiatry 109:916–921, 1953

Gotestam KG: Behavior and dynamic psychotherapy with the elderly, in Handbook of Mental Health and Aging. Edited by Birren JE, Sloane RB. Englewood Cliffs, NJ, Prentice-Hall, 1980

Gray P (ed): Dramatics for the Elderly: A Guide for Residential Care and Senior Centers. New York, Teachers College, Columbia University, 1974

Greenwald SR, Linn MW: Intercorrelations of data on nursing homes. Gerontologist 11:337–340, 1971

Haley WE: Behavioral self-management: application to a case of agitation in an elderly chronic psychiatric patient. Clinical Gerontologist 1:45–52, 1983

Helsing KJ, Comstock GW, Szklo M: Causes of death in a widowed population. Am J Epidemiol 116:524–532, 1982

Herr JJ, Weakland JH (eds): Counseling Elders and Their Families: Practical Techniques for Applied Gerontology. New York, Springer, 1979

Hiltz SR (ed): Creating Community Services for Widows: A Pilot Project. Port Washington, NY, Kennikat Press, 1977

Ittelson WH: Their perception of the large-scale environment. Paper presented to the New York Academy of Sciences, New York, April 1970

Jacobson E: Progressive Relaxation: A Physiological and Clinical Investigation of Muscular States and Their Significance in Psychology and Medical Practice, 2nd Edition. Chicago, IL, University of Chicago Press, 1938

Jung CG (ed): Modern Man in Search of a Soul. New York, Harcourt Brace, 1934

Jung CG (ed): Man and His Symbols. Garden City, NY, Doubleday, 1964

Kahana E: Matching environments to needs of the aged: a conceptual scheme, in Late Life: Recent Developments in the Sociology of Aging. Edited by Gubrium J. Springfield, IL, Charles C Thomas, 1974

Kahana E, Liang J, Felton BJ: Alternative models of person-environment fit: prediction of morale in three homes for the aged. J Gerontol 35:584–595, 1980

Kales A, Kales JD (eds): Evaluation and Treatment of Insomnia. New York, Oxford University Press, 1984

Kaprio J, Koskenvuo M, Rita H: Mortality after bereavement: a prospective study of 95,647 widowed persons. Am J Public Health 77:283–287, 1987

Kartman LL: The power of music with patients in a nursing home. Activities, Adaptations, and Aging 1:9–15, 1980

Katchner AH: Are companion animals good for your health? Aging, September/October, 1982, pp 331–332

Kiernat JM: Environment: the hidden modality. Physical and Occupational Therapy in Geriatrics 2:3–12, 1982

Koncelik JA (ed): Designing the Open Nursing Home. Stroudsberg, PA, Dowden, Hutchinson, & Ross, 1976

La Rue A, Dessonville C, Jarvik L: Aging and mental disorders, in Handbook of the Psychology of Aging. Edited by Birren JE, Schaie KW. New York, Van Nostrand Reinhold, 1985, pp 664–702

Landgarten HD (ed): Clinical Art Therapy: A Comprehensive Guide. New York, Brunner/Mazel, 1981

Lawton MP: Geropsychological knowledge as a background for psychotherapy with older people. J Geriatr Psychiatry 9:221–233, 1976

Lawton MP: The impact of the environment on aging and behavior, in Handbook of the Psychology of Aging. Edited by Birren JE, Schaie KW. New York, Van Nostrand Reinhold, 1977, pp 290–298

Lawton MP (ed): Environment and Aging. Monterey, CA, Brooks/Cole, 1980

Lawton MP, Nahemow L: Ecology and the aging process, in The Psychology of Adult Development and Aging. Edited by Eisdorfer C, Lawton MP. Washington, DC, American Psychological Association, 1973

Levy S, Derogatis L, Gallagher D, et al: Intervention with older adults, in Aging in the 1980s: Psychological Issues. Edited by Poon LW. Washington, DC, American Psychological Association, 1980, pp 41–61

Lewis CN: Reminiscing and self-concept in old age. J Gerontol 26:240–243, 1971

Lewis MI, Butler RN: Life-review therapy: putting memories to work in individual and group psychotherapy. Geriatrics 29:165–173, 1974

Lindsley OR: Geriatric behavioral prosthetics, in New Thoughts on Old Age. Edited by Kastenbaum R. New York, Springer, 1964, pp 41–60

Louis M: Personal space boundary needs of elderly persons: an empirical study. Journal of Gerontological Nursing 7:395–400, 1981

Lowy L: Roadblocks in group work practice with older people: a framework for analysis. Gerontologist 7:109–113, 1967

Manton KG, Blazer DG, Woodbury MA: Suicide in middle age and later life: sex and race specific life table and cohort analyses. J Gerontol 42:219–227, 1987

Maris RW (ed): Pathways to Suicide: A Survey of Self-Destructive Behaviors. Baltimore, MD, Johns Hopkins University Press, 1981

Markowitz J, Brown R, Sweeney J, et al: Reduced length and cost of hospital stay for major depression in patients treated with ECT. Am J Psychiatry 144:1025–1029, 1987

Martin LJ, De Gruchy C (eds): Salvaging Old Age. New York, Macmillan, 1930

Martin RL, Cloninger CR, Guze SB, et al: Mortality in a follow-up of 500 psychiatric outpatients. II: Cause specific mortality. Arch Gen Psychiatry 42:58–66, 1985

Mattis S: Mental status examination for organic mental syndrome in the elderly patient, in Geriatric Psychiatry: A Handbook for Psychiatrists and

Primary Care Physicians. Edited by Bellak L, Karasu TB. New York, Grune & Stratton, 1976, pp 77–121

McAllister TW: Overview: pseudodementia. Am J Psychiatry 140:528–533, 1983

McAllister TW, Price TR: Severe depressive pseudodementia with and without dementia. Am J Psychiatry 139:626–629, 1982

McAllister TW, Ferrell RB, Price TR, et al: The dexamethasone suppression test in two patients with severe depressive pseudodementia. Am J Psychiatry 139:479–481, 1982

McIntosh JL: Suicide among minority elderly. Paper presented at the annual meeting of the Gerontological Society of America, 1985

McIntosh JL, Santos JF: Methods of suicide by age: sex and race differences among the young and old. Int J Aging Hum Dev 22:123–139, 1985–1986

Menninger K (ed): Man Against Himself. New York, Harcourt Brace World, 1938

Miller M (ed): Suicide After Sixty: The Final Alternative. New York, Springer, 1979

Mishara BL, Kastenbaum R: Self-injurious behavior and environmental change in the institutionalized elderly. Int J Aging Hum Dev 4:133–145, 1973

Moos R (ed): Evaluating Treatment Environments: A Social Ecological Approach. New York, John Wiley, 1974

Moos R (ed): Evaluating Treatment Environments: A Social Ecological Approach. New York, John Wiley, 1976

Mugford RA, M'Comisky JG: Some recent work on the psychotherapeutic value of cage birds with old people, in Pet Animals and Society. Edited by Anderson RS. London, Balilliere Tindall, 1975

Murray R, Huelskoetter M, O'Driscoll D (eds): The Nursing Process in Later Maturity. Englewood Cliffs, NJ, Prentice-Hall, 1980

Myers JK, Weissman MM, Tischler GL, et al: Six-month prevalence of psychiatric disorders in three communities 1980 to 1982. Arch Gen Psychiatry 41:959–967, 1984

National Center for Health Statistics: Advance report of final mortality statistics 1983. NCHS Monthly Vital Statistics Report, 34 (6, Suppl 2), 1985. Hyattsville, MD, U.S. Department of Health and Human Services, 1987

Olson BK: Player piano music as therapy for the elderly. Journal of Music Therapy 21:35–44, 1984

Osgood N (ed): Suicide in the Elderly: A Practitioners Guide to Diagnosis and Mental Health Intervention. Rockville, MD, Aspen, 1985

Osgood NJ: The alcohol/suicide connection in late life. Postgrad Med 81:379–384, 1987

Osgood NJ, Brant BA, Lipman A: Patterns of suicidal behavior in long-term care facilities: a preliminary report on an ongoing study. Omega 19:69–78, 1988–1989

Pavkov J: Suicide in the elderly. Ohio's Health 34:21–28, 1982

Pavlov IP: Selected Works. Edited by Gibbons J. Translated by Belsky S. Moscow, Foreign Languages Publishing House, 1955

Petty BJ, Moeller TP, Campbell RZ: Support groups for elderly persons in the community. Gerontologist 16:522–528, 1976

Pincus A: Reminiscence in aging and its implications for social work practice. Social Work 15:47–53, 1970

Pokorny AD: Suicide rates in various psychiatric disorders. J Nerv Ment Dis 139:499–506, 1964

Rechtschatten A: Psychotherapy with geriatric patients: a review of the literature. J Gerontol 14:73, 1959

Reding M, Haycox J, Blass J: Depression in patients referred to a dementia clinic: a three-year prospective study. Arch Neurol 42:894–896, 1985

Reedy MN, Birren JE: Life review through guided autobiography. Paper presented at the annual meeting of the American Psychological Association, Montreal, Canada, September 1980

Reifler BV, Larson E, Teri L, et al: Dementia of the Alzheimer's type and depression. J Am Geriatr Soc 34:855–859, 1986

Richman J (ed): Family Therapy for Suicidal People. New York, Springer, 1986

Romaniuk M, Romaniuk J: Looking back: an analysis of reminiscence functions and triggers. Exp Aging Res 7:477–489, 1981

Roose SP, Glassman AH, Walsh BT, et al: Depression, delusions, and suicide. Am J Psychiatry 140:1159–1162, 1983

Schuckit MA, Pastor PA: Alcohol related psychopathology in the aged, in Psychopathology of Aging. Edited by Kaplan OJ. New York, Academic, 1979, pp 211–228

Schulz R: Effects of control and predictability on the physical and psychological well-being of the institutionalized aged. J Pers Soc Psychol 33:563–573, 1976

Seligman MEP (ed): Helplessness: On Depression, Development, and Death. San Francisco, CA, WH Freeman, 1975

Shanas E, Streib G (eds): Social Structure and the Family: Generational Relations. Englewood Cliffs, NJ, Prentice-Hall, 1965

Shraberg D: The myth of pseudodementia: depression and the aging brain. Am J Psychiatry 135:601–603, 1978

Shulman K: Suicide and parasuicide in old age: a review. Age Ageing 7:201–209, 1978

Silver A: Group psychotherapy with senile psychotic patients. Geriatrics 5:147–150, 1950

Skinner BF (ed): Behavior of Organisms. New York, Appleton-Century-Crofts, 1936

Stein A: Group psychotherapy in a general hospital: principles and practice. Paper presented at the annual meeting of the American Group Psychotherapy Association, New York, January 1959

Stern D, Kastenbaum R: Alcohol use and abuse in old age, in Geriatric Mental

Health. Edited by Abrahams JP, Crooks V. Orlando, FL, Grune & Stratton, 1984

Steuer J: Psychotherapy for depressed elders, in Depression in Late Life. Edited by Blazer DG. St. Louis, MO, CV Mosby, 1982, pp 195–220

Storandt M: Counseling and Therapy With Older Adults. Boston, MA, Little, Brown, 1983

Tate JW: The need for personal space in institutions for the elderly. Journal of Gerontological Nursing 6:439–449, 1980

Thielman SB, Blazer DG: Depression and Dementia, in Dementia. Edited by Pitt B. New York, Churchill Livingstone, 1987, pp 251–264

Tobin SS: How nursing homes vary. Gerontologist 14:516–519, 1974

Traunstein DM, Steinman R: Voluntary self-help organizations: an exploratory study. Journal of Voluntary Action Research 2:230–239, 1973

Verwoerdt A (ed): Clinical Geropsychiatry. Baltimore, MD, Williams & Wilkins, 1976

Weiner RD, Rogers HJ, Welch CA, et al: ECT stimulus parameters and electrode placement: relevance to therapeutic and adverse effects, in Basic Mechanisms. Edited by Lerer B, Weiner RD, Belmaker RH. London, John Libbey & Co, 1984, pp 139–147

Weiss JC (ed): Expressive Therapy With Elders and the Disabled: Touching the Heart of Life. New York, Haworth Press, 1984

Weiss RS: Transition states and other stressful situations: their nature and programs for their management, in Support Systems and Mutual Help: Multidisciplinary Explorations. Edited by Caplan G, Killilea M. New York, Grune & Stratton, 1976, pp 213–232

Whanger AD: Treatment within the institution, in Handbook of Geriatric Psychiatry. Edited by Busse EW, Blazer DG. New York, Van Nostrand Reinhold, 1980, pp 453–472

Windley PG, Scheidt RJ: Person-environment dialectics: implications for competent functioning in old age, in Aging in the 1980s: Psychological Issues. Edited by Poon LW. Washington, DC, American Psychological Association, 1980, pp 407–432

Wolff K: Individual psychotherapy with geriatric patients. Diseases of the Nervous System 24:688–691, 1963

Yalom ID (ed): The Theory and Practice of Group Psychotherapy. New York, Basic Books, 1970

Yesavage JA, Brink TL: Development and validation of a geriatric depression screening scale: a preliminary report. J Psychiatr Res 17:37–49, 1983

Zandt SV, Lorenzen L: You're not too old to dance: creative movement and older adults. Activities, Adaptation, and Aging 6:121–130, 1985

Zung W: Affective disorders, in Handbook of Geratric Psychiatry. Edited by Busse E, Blazer DG. New York, Van Nostrand Reinhold, 1980, p 353

Chapter 14

Crisis Management of the Suicidal Patient

Brian B. Doyle, M.D.

CRISIS INTERVENTION WITH THE ACUTELY SUICIDAL PATIENT

Few situations so tax the clinician as intervening with an acutely suicidal patient. The encounter has an unusual intensity and emotional charge. The stakes, a person's life, are high, but that is common in clinical medicine. However, instead of being the clinician's ally, suicidal patients are potentially the instrument of their own destruction. That, too, is common; many patients have self-destructive patterns of smoking or drinking or nonadherence to necessary medical regimens. In daily practice, the clinician can and does address self-destructive issues. When a patient is acutely suicidal, however, those issues leap to the forefront; it is not at all "business as usual." Dealing with acute suicidal patients brings other professional work to a halt, provokes anxiety, and demands the clinician's total involvement.

The suicidal patient is in crisis, uncertain whether to live or die. Clinicians may underestimate how much time and energy is required to manage a suicidal patient appropriately. During the crisis period, and often longer, the clinician is on the line. The clinician must blend enough compassion so that the suicidal person experiences the clinician as an ally and enough detachment so that the clinician is not overwhelmed by his or her own responses to the patient's pain. No matter how minor or severe an attempt, the suicidal person is in pain, desperate, and feeling that there are no other options. A patient who is sad and overwhelmed is a comparatively straightforward case for the clinician. All too often, however, the suicidal patient is extremely difficult: provocative, ambivalent, openly hostile, or passive-aggressive and vengeful. These specific features alienate the doctor, threatening professional equilibrium. Frequently, the clinician may be a late and reluctant actor in the drama of the patient's life, swept up in issues long preceding the involvement and over which the clinician has little control. Indeed, the central assumption of the clinician's work, to prolong and enhance life, is under covert or direct attack. The conditions exist for a power struggle that the patient can always "win" by committing suicide. Patients who are determined to kill themselves may eventually do so, regardless of medical safeguards and psychiatric precautions. However, the clinician's task is to help relieve the patient's pain and detoxify the acute situation while providing treatment and interventions that will diminish lethality. The clinician needs to form a strong therapeutic bond with the suicidal patient, permitting the despairing person to weigh options and to explore the sources of difficulty and stress. Additionally, the clinician must provide hope. Such an intervention is a delicate and difficult task (Blumenthal 1988).

The clinician's first job is to manage his or her own feelings generated by the crisis situation and not to be driven by discomfort. The clinician can act out in a variety of ways, from failing to inquire about suicidality with an obviously upset or depressed person ("It sounds bad, but surely you're not *suicidal*."); by fleeing from the subject when the patient brings it up ("Uh-huh. And how is your appetite?"); by actively colluding with the patient's wish to commit suicide ("Sounds like there isn't any reason for you to live."); or by openly or covertly directing the patient to die ("Why don't you do it *right* the next time!") (Rosen 1985). In our society, as a method to influence, force, and manipulate the attitudes and behaviors of others, the threat of suicide has no peer (Schneidman 1967).

The suicidal person usually goes through the stages of crisis specified by Caplan (1963): increased tension, unpleasant affect and disorganized behavior, cognitive confusion, inability to resolve conflict, further use of more maladaptive and emergency approaches to problem solving, and perceptual distortion, confusion, and disorganization. The patient's mounting agitation, anxiety, anger, feelings of worthlessness, and inadequacy contribute to the increasing appeal of suicide as an option. The suicidal person turns increasingly to magical thinking and fantasy with the failure of rational cognition to present satisfying alternatives. The empathetic clinician responds to the patient's distress, just as a tuning fork resonates if it is on the same wavelength as another that is struck (Doyle 1986a). The clinician's emotional responses provide valuable clues to the patient's emotional state. The clinician's experience of anxiety, anger, sadness, or confusion may reflect the patient's internal milieu and suggest areas for exploration and intervention. Is the patient having those feelings? If so, how and why are they so intense? Rather than avoiding or denying feelings, the clinician uses them to form hypotheses about the patient that deserve further investigation.

Crisis theory provides other practical pointers for managing the suicidal patient. The clinician must be flexible about schedule. It must be possible to see a patient on little notice, for longer and more frequently than usual (Wekstein 1979). Being active and confident are essential characteristics for the clinician. This is not accomplished by acting omnipotent or omniscient, but by systematic intervention and education with the patient and family. The crisis becomes a set of problems that can be sorted out, explored, and ultimately resolved. Such a process enables patients to mobilize and use their own resources and adaptive functions.

Resourcefulness is a key quality in clinicians dealing with suicidal patients. If one approach does not work, then another must be constructed; if that does not work, then another plan must be formulated, and so on. The therapist's resourcefulness and persistence are critical because of the transitory and episodic nature of intense suicidal feelings in most patients (Mintz 1971). This kind of persistence and problem solving with the patient often averts disaster.

The clinician who is treating a suicidal patient can usefully remember that this is a seriously, perhaps terminally, ill person. An estimate for the mortality of major depression is 15% by suicide (Guze and Robins 1970). Additionally, there are many other persons who kill themselves who suffer from other psychiatric disorders or who are undergoing overwhelming personal crises. Clinicians cannot save all terminally ill patients; some will die whether they have leukemia or a major depression. As with any potentially terminally ill patient, there are important interventions the clinician can undertake. But to keep therapeutic expectations reasonable, the physician must also temper the fantasy that if the clinician does just the right thing, this person will live.

INTERVENING WITH THE SUICIDAL PATIENT

The principles of working with the suicidal patient come from crisis intervention theory as proposed by Parad and Caplan (1960). In summary, the basic components of intervention include 1) identifying the precipitant(s); 2) encouraging the patient to acknowledge, tolerate, and bear the painful affects aroused by the crisis; and 3) specifying and implementing a plan of action.

Establishing and Maintaining Contact

Continuous contact is essential for a successful intervention with the suicidal patient. This is relatively easy to accomplish if the patient is in the clinician's office. It is much more difficult when the patient is on the other end of a telephone line or, worse, in a dangerous physical setting such as on a window ledge. The clinician should make every effort to interview the patient alone and in private, providing the patient with a safe place to ventilate emotions without feeling exposed or humiliated. It is particularly important to interview the patient alone before speaking with the family. This communicates to the patient that the clinician is interested foremost in the patient's views and experiences.

In some instances, when accompanied by friends or relatives, the patient may be so disorganized or upset that it is ineffective to meet alone. It may be more sensible for the clinician to begin the interview with the patient and accompanying person present and then to meet with the patient alone as the patient becomes more comfortable (Wekstein 1979).

The initial approach to the patient sets the framework for subsequent interaction. It should communicate to the patient that the clinician is committed to understanding the patient respectfully and easing distress. On first encountering any patient, clinicians should promptly identify themselves and their role. This can help to put the patient at ease. Preferably, clinicians should begin by addressing patients by their last name, with the prefix Mr., Mrs., or Ms. Even with adolescents, it is preferable to begin by using the patient's last name, unless the patient specifically requests otherwise (Wekstein 1979). Some clinicians prefer to ask the patient what name to use. Generally, it is preferable to use the patient's last name because it implies respect and does not infantilize the patient, given that the patient is calling you "Dr." The clinician can also attend to simple comforts (e.g., a cup of coffee, food, facial tissues). Attention to such concrete details may help ease the patient's distress and facilitate the therapeutic alliance. The principal objective of this first session is to decrease the patient's sense of aloneness. If the patient is feeling alienated from everyone, then the first goal is to forge a link with the clinician. From the start, the effort is to promote reconnections between the patient and the crucial people in the patient's life, especially those with whom the patient has long-term relationships. Is there someone the patient would like to see or to talk to? How can that person be reached? If not available in person, can this person be contacted by telephone? If the patient rejects the clinician's overtures, warm persistence is necessary. Sometimes the patient will test the clinician's commitment by sarcastic or contemptuous rebuff. Systematic, determined, caring efforts can almost always break through a patient's cynical or despairing facade (Litman and Farberow 1961). Generally, once a patient has responded to any appeal or suggestion by the clinician, even in the smallest way, then the patient is engaged in the therapeutic process (Victoroff 1983).

Another aspect of setting the basic framework for the therapeutic interaction is to inform the patient about the extent of the confidentiality of your discussion. Most clinicians feel that the usual rules for confidentiality do not apply when working with a suicidal patient. Assuring the patient that your session will be totally confidential unduly restricts the clinician and may make the patient more vulnerable. Of course, the patient should know that the clinician will respect privacy and convey only the information necessary to others to ensure the desired result; details are often superfluous. In an empathetic· manner, the clinician should inform the patient that the suicide wish will be shared with whoever needs to know because the clinician wants the patient to live. Some practitioners insist on the therapeutic efficacy of complete mutual respect and trust expressed by unqualified privacy of patient communications: confidentiality should not be breached under any conditions (Wekstein 1979). While being respectful of this principle, most clinicians feel that therapists must be able to recognize their own limitations, including their need to include others in the evaluation and treatment of a suicidal person in crisis.

Investigating Suicidality

Once the clinician has engaged the patient and a working relationship has begun, a more complete investigation of the suicidal state can occur. Suicidal behavior must be understood in the context of the patient's life. While it has self-destructive aspects, it is also the patient's attempt to resolve a crisis situation. The clinician must attempt to determine what the problem is and why it is causing such despair. What is the person trying so hard to change, and why does the person feel so hopeless about changing it? These questions facilitate the clinician's inquiry; the attempt to understand the suicidal state helps make the patient feel supported (Mintz 1971).

Certain medical traditions facilitate this process. First, there is the physician's medical authority. The clinician traditionally investigates thoroughly that which is avoided in ordinary social interchange. As in assessing any medical problem, the clinician's investigation of a patient's suicidality begins with a history of the present illness: What hurts now? How is the patient feeling? What are the precipitants?

When did the patient start feeling this way? The clinician should look particularly for losses, including external ones such as the loss of significant persons in the patient's life by separation, divorce, or death. These precipitating life events can also be the loss of a job or of one's health. More important, losses need to be assessed for their internal impact; what do they mean to the patient? The patient's loss of self-esteem or of hope for the future can be far more devastating than loss of material possessions or even of significant others. What makes the suicidal feelings worse? What has the patient tried for relief; does anything help? This question is particularly important in assessing drug use, including alcohol. Alcohol and other drug use almost always increases suicidal potential and destabilizes the clinical situation. Is there any person who helps the patient feel better, and is that person available right now? Under what conditions does the patient want to continue living? Is there some time limit? Similarly, is the desire to live dependent on a particular event, such as the threatened loss of a loved one?

How concerned is the patient that he or she will act on the suicidal impulses? Here the clinician enlists the patient in helping to predict his or her own dangerousness. The patient may find such inquiries offensive or cynical: "What do you mean, *how* suicidal am I? You're the doctor!" The clinician needs to persist gently but specifically: "Yes, but what do you think the chances are that you will actually act on your impulses? Are they close to 100%? 50%? 1%?" When the clinician conveys thoughtful empathic concern, patients will often specify the degree of their suicidality. Often surprising, the results are useful; a totally despairing person may predict little likelihood of action, and another patient may be calm because of certainty that the plans will be carried out. (For a more complete discussion of the suicide interview, see Hendren, Chapter 10, this volume.)

Next, the clinician should investigate the potential lethality of the suicide method the patient is considering. Lethality is a combination of intrinsic dangerousness and availability of a method. Many have been prevented from shooting themselves by lack of ready access to a gun; conversely, increasing suicide rates in the United States are in part due to the greater availability of firearms (Boyd 1983). Thus the suicide risk is greater in an angry, impulsive adolescent with ready access to a loaded handgun than it is for a profoundly depressed middle-aged person with no firearms and a nonlethal supply of medication.

> An 81-year-old woman, hospitalized for her second serious overdose of psychotropic medication in 6 months, defiantly stated her continuing wish to die. A former judge, she was single and beset with multiple chronic medical problems. She had judged for herself that her allotted

80-year life span was over. Yet, as clearly, she would use no "ugly" or "messy" way to end her life; there would be no wrist-slashings with broken intravenous bottles, no jumping out of hospital windows, and so on. Without access to pills, she was safe in the general hospital. Vigilance on the part of the hospital staff was necessary to ensure that she not get access to lethal amounts of medication.

Numerous studies have shown that suicidality correlates strongly with how hopeless the patient feels (Beck et al. 1985; Fawcett et al. 1987; Hendin 1986). Hopelessness may represent a specific cognitive vulnerability in times of decompensation—in the words of Beck et al. (1985), "the activation of specific cognitive schemes organized in a matrix of negative expectations." The reoccurrence or persistence of hopelessness over time appears to result in a higher likelihood of suicide (Beck et al. 1985). Hopelessness can be measured clinically through a patient's responses to a Hopelessness Scale (Beck et al. 1974; Minkoff et al. 1973) or to the pessimism item of the Beck Depression Inventory (Beck et al. 1961).

As part of the assessment, the clinician must investigate the patient's current behaviors as well as the patient's feelings. Clues to seriousness of suicidal intent include giving away precious things (e.g., old letters, mementos, prized objects), taking out a new or additional life insurance policy, making a will or revising an existing one, or writing goodbye letters (Bhatia et al. 1986).

A depressed 75-year-old chronically ill woman sent to friends Christmas packages containing special possessions of hers with notes that she wanted the friends to have the objects because they "would specially appreciate them." Two days after Christmas she was found dead of carbon monoxide poisoning in her car in the garage.

In addition to inquiring about current thoughts, feelings, and behavior in determining the history of present illness, the clinician should also investigate the past medical and psychiatric history. A pattern of previous attempts, especially obviously lethal ones, significantly increases the likelihood of eventual death by suicide (Ettlinger 1964).

A family history of suicide increases the likelihood of suicide in 7% to 14% of those attempting suicide for varied reasons (Adam 1985). In some families it seems more related to cultural or imitative factors than to a specific genetic predisposition. Once the instinctive taboo against killing oneself is violated, this can become part of the family's identity. Debate continues about the relationship of affective illness in families to suicide. Murphy and Wetzel (1982) found that attempted suicides with a diagnosis of primary affective disorder, for example, had a family history of suicidal behavior less often than those with a diagnosis of personality disorder. Conversely, Egeland and Sussex (1985), in a cohort of Old Order Amish over a 100-year period, found that 92% of 26 cases of suicide were diagnosed with major affective disorders. Further, the suicides clustered in four primary pedigrees that followed the distribution of affective disorders in these kinship lines.

Thus the data that emerge from the investigation with the patient enables the clinician to make decisions about clinical management. A careful, thorough, diagnostic investigation conveys to the patient that the clinician is interested and competent and is not overwhelmed by the crisis situation. The patient's fear of total devastation by the crisis is replaced and restructured as a set of problems that can be managed and solved. The patient experiences the clinician's kindly concern and systematic intervention as "defusing an explosive" (Wekstein 1979), helping to decrease the affective charge.

Once the clinician has accumulated information about the patient, a framework is needed for ordering the data and predicting suicide risk. Adam (1985) reviewed suicide prediction instruments, noting that while many scales are valid, they are not clearly useful. Noting the "intractable problem of predicting infrequent events," Murphy (1983) emphasized the varying suicidality of the individual at different times. Motto et al. (1985) developed a risk scale for suicide with 14 key variables, each having numerical scales for varying weights (Table 1).

A useful scale for evaluating suicidal patients is the SAD PERSONS Scale, the acronym rising from the 10 categories rated (Patterson et al. 1983). Table 2 summarizes the features of the scale. Unfortunately, the scale does not register the degree of the patient's hopelessness, which would provide a very important additional measure. On the basis of the total score, Patterson et al. (1983) recommended guidelines for action (Table 3). These authors prudently advocated use of the scale only as a helpful guideline. They stressed the importance of clinical judgment, especially in the presence of certain other factors not specified in the scale. One such critical factor is the quality of the doctor-patient relationship.

Building the Alliance

The clinician's primary resource with the suicidal patient is their relationship. This may be a new alliance, as when a patient comes to the emergency room physician, or it may be in the context of a long-standing relationship, as when a psychiatrist meets with a chronically troubled person during the course of ongoing treatment. The clinician's stance needs to be one of steady hopefulness. Even the

Table 1. Risk factors for suicide

Risk factor	Highest risk of suicide
1. Age	Older people (> age 50)
2. Occupation	Executive; administrator; professional; owner of business; semiskilled worker
3. Sexual orientation	Bisexual (sexually active); homosexual (not sexually active)
4. Financial resources	Higher income; unemployed
5. Threat of significant financial loss	Yes
6. Special stress, unique to subject	Yes
7. Change of weight	Weight gain or loss of > 10%
8. Ideas of persecution or reference	Moderate or severe
9. Intensity of present suicidal impulses	Moderate or severe
10. Seriousness of intent to die, if attempt made	Unequivocal; ambivalent, but weighed toward suicide
11. Previous psychiatric hospitalizations	Several hospitalizations
12. Results of previous efforts to obtain help	Unsatisfactory or varied
13. Emotional disorder in family	Depression, alcoholism
14. Interviewer's reaction to person	Neutral or negative

Source. Adapted from Motto JA, Heilbron DC, Juster RP: Development of a clinical instrument to estimate suicidal risk. Am J Psychiatry 142:680–686. Copyright 1985, The American Psychiatric Association. Reprinted by permission.

most suicidal patient is ambivalent about the act; as long as the patient is talking, the patient is living, and some intervention is possible. Even if the patient's life circumstances are desperate and the odds overwhelming, the physician has rational bases for hope: one cannot predict the future, and who knows what options will develop? Are there treatments that have not been pursued?

Table 2.   The SAD PERSONS Scale for assessing the risk of suicide

Sex	1 if patient is male, 0 if female
Age	1 if patient is 19 or younger or 45 or older
Depression	1 if present
Previous attempt	1 if present
Ethanol abuse	1 if present
Rational thinking loss	1 if patient is psychotic for any reason (schizophrenia, affective illness, organic brain syndrome)
Social supports lacking	1 if these are lacking, especially with recent loss of a significant other
Organized plan	1 if plan made and method lethal
No spouse	1 if divorced, widowed, separated, or single
Sickness	1 especially if chronic, debilitating, severe

Note.   The total score ranges from 0 (very little risk) to 10 (very high risk).
Source.   From Patterson WM, Dohn HH, Bird J, Patterson GA: Evaluation of suicidal patients: the SAD PERSONS Scale. Psychosomatics 24:343–349, 1983, used with permission.

Table 3.   Guidelines for action with the SAD PERSONS scale

Total points	Proposed clinical action
0 to 2	Send home with follow-up
3 to 4	Close follow-up; consider hospitalization
5 to 6	Strongly consider hospitalization, depending on confidence in the follow-up arrangement
7 to 10	Hospitalize or commit

Source.   From Patterson WM, Dohn HH, Bird J, Patterson GA: Evaluation of suicidal patients: the SAD PERSONS Scale. Psychosomatics 24:343–349, 1983, used with permission.

The patient often sees suicide as the only way out. Some patients may be seeking peace or relief from despair through suicide. At times, the clinician may feel overwhelmed by the patient's life situation and may be hard-pressed to find a basis for hope. While the patient's life situation may sound terrible and the despair seems understandable, it may be ill-founded. In a high proportion of cases, the suicidal patient is upset and depressed; his or her judgment is clouded and thinking confused. Hardly a reliable or objective reporter, the patient is in no position to make a rational assessment of whether to commit suicide. The clinician maneuvers to keep the patient considering the situation without forcing the patient's hand and to help secure the patient's active voluntary collaboration in the treatment process. However, this is possible only when the clinician is truly available and not feeling overwhelmed or angry (Victoroff 1983). At times, as Maltsberger and Buie (1974) pointed out, the clinician may become frustrated and experience hatred toward the patient.

Sometimes the use of humor can help facilitate the therapeutic relationship. At times the clinician may be able to use humor to good effect. A clinician negotiating with a suicidal teenager knew he was an ardent football fan; he reminded the youth that if he killed himself he'd miss knowing the results of the National Football League playoffs! The boy responded with a laugh and was able thereafter to collaborate better in his treatment (Wekstein 1979).

A clinician may gently remind a patient established in treatment that committing suicide means that the patient will miss his or her next appointment. This observation shocks with its simplicity and truth, and the patient may respond favorably to its half-humorous, half-serious nature. Humor recasts the situation and nudges the patient to see it freshly. However, there is a serious danger that a patient can misinterpret a humorous remark as a dismissal or as sarcasm. Humor is probably best used when the clinical situation, while not settled, is in the process of resolving successfully; it is *not* an effective last resort and should be used carefully and competently by the clinician (Victoroff 1983).

Contracting With the Patient

The clinician and patient must come to an agreement about their relationship. The patient must understand fully the nature, extent, and limits of the assistance the clinician offers. Providing magical solutions for often intractable problems is unrealistic, but the clinician can emphasize a willingness to listen actively and to "be with" the patient during this crisis (Morgan 1979). The patient agrees only not to act on suicidal impulses before the next contact with the clinician and to come at the appointed time. The patient further agrees that the clinician will be contacted should there be a temptation to act on the suicidal impulses. The patient agrees also to give to others any potentially lethal agents, such as guns, pills, and alcohol or other drugs. In turn, the clinician promises to continue to be available and to work on developing a treatment program that has a reasonable chance of providing the patient with relief. Being available is just that; the patient needs to know where the clinician is and must have ready access to the clinician. Being continuously available is burdensome, and the clinician must be direct about needs for respite and the mechanisms for coverage. Patient and clinician alike need names and telephone numbers to cover any contingencies in a crisis, including such details as the names of friends and relatives, car license numbers, and so on (Mintz 1961).

Others must be involved in this contracting process. It is always wise to function with key other persons in the patient's life. While respecting the privacy of the bond to the patient, the clinician needs to include other people in the treatment plan. Family and friends of the patient can provide corroborative or alternative information about the patient and are necessary allies in managing a suicidal patient out of the hospital. Additionally, it is to these people that the patient will return after the crisis is over. Family, friends, neighbors, employers, and clergy can be part of the supportive network (Murphy and Wetzel 1982). For example, they are essential in ensuring that the patient does not have access to a lethal amount of medication, to alcohol or other drugs, or to another method of self-destruction. Of course, the clinician must separately assess the reliability of these individuals; they may be trustworthy and extremely helpful, or unconsciously or actively malevolent (Litman and Farberow 1961).

> A schizophrenic patient who was an avid gun collector and marksman became suicidal after hospital discharge when his voices recurred and his energy flagged. His psychiatrist emphasized that to make it possible for the patient to stay out of the hospital, as he and the family wished, all guns (and there were many) had to be removed from the house. The family and patient agreed. Five days later the patient shot himself to death in his bedroom. At the inquiry that followed, the family members revealed that they had removed all the guns except for a brace of ornamental pistols, which they considered harmless.

Any agreement between the patient and the clinician cannot be implemented effectively without the active collaboration of family, whether that be the patient's biological relatives or a network of friends (Wekstein 1979).

To move from exploring and negotiating the crisis situation to implementing a treatment plan, the clinician must ensure that there is a real agreement with the patient, not a pseudo-agreement. This is another reason for involving in the decision making others who know the patient. They can help the clinician decide if the patient is truly cooperating.

There is no avoiding this step. At times, a patient may seem to agree to a treatment plan, but only because he or she is tired of the discussion and has secretly opted for suicide. The patient may neither like nor trust the clinician sufficiently to level with him or her. In such instances, the clinician must attend to his or her own inner promptings and confront the patient. The process has to begin again until there is either a genuine agreement between the clinician and the patient or the recognition that such an agreement is not currently possible. If the clinician cannot count on the patient's cooperation, then he or she must secure the patient's safety until the situation can be reassessed.

Implementing a Plan

When a real agreement has been made between the doctor and patient, the clinician can then proceed with a plan that should always include the following elements (Blumenthal 1988):

1. *Supervise.* The patient is not to be left alone, ever. Vigilance must be exercised even if the patient is to be hospitalized or transferred from one facility to another. Tensions naturally ease once a plan has been agreed on. However, a patient can get lost in the transitions between phases of a treatment program.
2. *Restrict access to method.* The patient is to have no access to a potentially lethal method.
3. *Restrict and monitor medications.* If medication is used, the clinician must ensure that the patient has access only to sublethal doses. Many of the antidepressants, for example, are toxic. They are fatal in overdose, and surprisingly small doses are sufficient to kill people. The total amount of any drug available to the patient should be less than 1 g. Since that is often only a few days' supply, it may cause annoyance about the need for frequent trips to the pharmacy. An alternate plan is to dispense a larger amount to a responsible family member who will administer daily doses. However, this presupposes that the clinician has a good working relationship with that person.

If the clinician cannot make an agreement with the patient that ensures safety until the next therapeutic contact, then the patient must be voluntarily or involuntarily hospitalized. The clinician must know the procedures involved and have the means and persons available in advance. Commitment procedures differ from locale to locale. More specific and rigorous criteria for commitment have become commonplace in response to what was viewed by some as arbitrary past procedures. The clinician may feel somewhat hopeless about what will happen once the patient sent for commitment has been retained for the mandatory 48 hours. However justified the reservations, the clinician must still press for commitment if it is indicated. Such purposeful action shows patients that they are being taken seriously. It is also important for medicolegal reasons. Additionally, longer periods of continued commitment are possible if the patient meets certain criteria. Physician certification and arbitration by a judge is usually required for this procedure.

Additionally, the clinician must be resourceful in finding ways to mobilize people to help implement the treatment plan. Being direct with family members or others who have accompanied the patient is often necessary; they can take courage from the clinician's convictions. Often, faced with a cadre of determined helpers, the patient's resistance will crumble and he or she will be better able to cooperate. If family or friends are not available, then the police can be requested to help. Much as they dislike the task, they will usually comply if the clinician is firm and clear and lets them know the adverse public consequences if they refuse to help and the patient commits suicide.

Even if the patient is cooperative, finding resources to help may at times test the resourcefulness of the clinician.

> On a Sunday morning, a suicidal woman in rural Newfoundland telephoned the resident on call at the Boston psychiatric hospital where she had been hospitalized some years before. She was alone and despairing, with no friends or family nearby, no psychiatrists or other physician, no community mental health center or hospital. As a last resort, the doctor suggested that the Royal Canadian Mounted Police (RCMP), the "Mounties," be called on to help. There was a RCMP station nearby, and the patient responded well to the instructions to go there. Many hours later she called to report that the Mounties had been sympathetic and receptive, that they had helped her contact some relatives, and she now had the strength to go on.

Clinicians must also attend to their own needs and should enlist resorces on their own behalf, not just for the patient. Contending with a suicidal patient is taxing and demanding. Whatever the clinician's practice setting—whether it be as a team member in a suicide prevention center, a physician in an outpatient setting, an emergency room doctor, or a psychiatrist in an office or hospital—having consultants, collaborators, and supervisors is essential in the management of a suicidal patient. A consultant may suggest resolutions to impasses that develop (Schneidman 1967). Consultation also provides some protection if there should be any legal action against the clinician.

Clinicians must also carefully document their thoughts and actions. Writing up the interaction with the patient clarifies the clinician's thinking as well as provides essential documentation if there should be subsequent legal action. Especially when the circumstances are confusing and complex and when the patient is ambivalent, it is necessary to provide an accurate record. Although courts do not expect clinicians to predict a patient's course, they do expect that the clinician considered the case fully, provided adequate treatment, and documented all aspects of the clinical care. Unfortunately, the clinician's recollection or oral description of his or her thinking is both insufficient and unconvincing; full documentation is required (see Amchin et al., Chapter 24; Ruben, Chapter 23, this volume). The following is a hypothetical note:

> The patient is intensely suicidal but has agreed to contact me before acting on his impulses. Family members, aware of the danger, have promised to contact me promptly if they have increased concern. Family also agrees to monitor medications; his wife has been consistent and reliable about this in the past. She is still actively sympathetic to her husband, although concerned with the effect his despair is having on the children. He has been hospitalized at X Hospital before, did not like it and does not want to return. The doctor on call at X says that the patient does not sound sufficiently suicidal to admit. I have reviewed the case with my consultant, Dr. Y, who agreed with my assessment and urged telephone contact with patient and family before the next scheduled visit in 48 hours. The patient and family have my telephone number and schedule for the next 2 days; further, they have the schedule and telephone number of Dr. A, who is on call for me this evening.

Dealing with the suicidal patient requires that the clinician actively investigate, plan, and develop resources. If the patient's prospects are grim, the clinician can exemplify the kindliness and caring that make the prospect of living worthwhile. If the patient can find some relief in the experience with the clinician, then there is hope for that in relationships with other people. When the clinician manages the crisis effectively, it is remarkable how much progress a patient can make in a short time.

CARING FOR THE SUICIDAL PATIENT IN SPECIFIC SETTINGS

The Primary Care Setting

Studies have repeatedly shown that most persons who commit suicide have seen their primary care physician within hours to a few months before their death, and that most suicidal persons will talk about their fears, plans, and impulses if the clinician asks directly (Heimburger 1980; Mintz 1971; Rockwell and Pepitone-Rockwell 1978; Wekstein 1979). Estimates are that the average physician encounters six suicidal patients a year and has 10 to 12 completed suicides over the course of a medical career (Litman 1970). Family physicians who consider the well-being of all family members their clinical responsibility need particularly to remember that suicide occurs between people. Wishes to hurt, punish, or escape from a significant other are often behind suicidal impulses.

It is problematic that suicidal patients in primary care settings often touch on their suicidal preoccupations indirectly, if at all. The physician may be preoccupied with a variety of physical complaints in a patient who makes no reference to suicidal thoughts or feelings. There are several clinical presentations requiring investigation for suicidal thoughts and impulses: when there are numerous physical complaints without organic basis; when the patient is alcoholic; or when the physical complaints are suggestive of depression (e.g., lethargy, insomnia, anorexia, difficulty concentrating, headache, constipation/diarrhea, feeling slowed down, lack of libido). The clinician can proceed knowing that the typical patient finds relief in the inquiry (Doyle 1986b; Usdin and Lewis 1979). Often the primary care physician is the first one to have contact with the suicidal person. The primary care physician may have had a long-standing relationship with the patient around nonpsychiatric medical problems. The comfort in that relationship can help the patient discuss concerns about suicide (Ruben 1979).

The primary care physician needs to be alert to the possibility of suicide in teenagers and in children as well as in adults. Although teenagers are often reticent with adults about their inner life, they will respond to direct inquiry, and they can be reliable reporters of their suicidal potential (Robbins and Alessi 1985). Adolescents at particular risk are those with major depressive illness (Robbins and Alessi 1985), a history of drug abuse (usually multiple; usually marijuana, alcohol, and cocaine) (Fowler et al. 1986), chronic rage (Gispert et al. 1987), a history of having been abused or neglected as children (Deykin et al. 1985; Shafii et al. 1985), or some combination of these factors (Blumenthal 1988). Adolescents are the only group of Americans who have not improved their health status in the past 30 years. More than 77% of adolescent deaths are currently caused by accidents, suicide, and homicide. Although it is difficult for primary care clinicians to go beyond traditional medicine, they must address the social, psychological, behavioral, and environmental factors that underline current morbidity and mortality in our youth (Blum 1987).

Considering that younger children can be suicidal is a relatively new development for American psychiatrists, much less primary care physicians. However, children have suicidal impulses, and they act on them (Renshaw 1981). In one study of schoolchildren who were not psychiatric patients, almost 12% had suicidal thoughts, and 3% took suicidal action (Pfeffer et al. 1982). A complicating factor in children is that suicidal behavior may reflect impulsivity more than it does severe depression (Carlson and Cantwell 1982). The usual signs of depression may be missing in a youngster at risk.

A major problem in primary care settings is underrecognition and undertreatment of depression (Doyle 1986b; Waltzer 1979). In Murphy's (1975b) study of 49 persons who had seen their internist 6 months or less before their suicide, more than two-thirds of the patients had histories of suicide attempts or threats; only two-fifths of the physicians knew about those histories. The great majority of the patients were depressed, yet few were diagnosed as such and only a very few were recognized as suicidal. A physician's lack of interest in or hostility toward the suicidal person has often contributed to patient despair and, on occasion, has been linked directly to the patient's death (Victoroff 1983). Continuing difficulties include lack of physician agreement about the severity of depression, leading to markedly different treatments (Fisch et al. 1981). A heartening change is the increasing requirement for board certification in family practice, general internal medicine, and pediatrics that trainees master the necessary knowledge and skills to recognize and treat the depressed patient (Linn and Yager 1984; Schurman et al. 1985). This goes beyond treating suicidality to having a more full view of the doctor-patient relationship, recognizing and managing such issues as physician overidentification or excessive patient dependency (Siomopoulos 1986).

The primary care physician who recognizes and investigates the suicidal patient should do so according to the framework presented earlier. The treatment plan rests on several variables, of which the degree of danger of suicide is only one. Also important are the clinician's interest and experience in treating such patients, the number of such persons already in the physician's practice, and the availability of psychiatric resources. The suicidal patient whom the primary care physician elects to treat will usually have low to moderate risk. This will commonly involve suicide precautions at home (e.g., making sure no lethal methods are available), some combination of psychotherapy and pharmacotherapy, and reevaluation of the plan within 2 weeks (Mintz 1966). Ensuring continuity of care with a specific next appointment is mandatory. The amount of potentially lethal medication that the primary care physician prescribes is a major focus for concern; in Murphy's (1975a) study of 32 deaths by drug overdose, more than half had received a prescription for a lethal amount of the toxic substance within a week of their dying. Primary care physicians should consider carefully which patients they choose to treat and document their information and decision-making process, both for optimal patient care and to defend against the danger of future adverse legal action (Bhatia et al. 1986; Schwartz 1987). Continual availability and vigilance are the key qualities of the primary care physician in these circumstances. Having a psychiatrist as consultant to review the treatment and monitor the primary care physician's reactions is often helpful (Doyle 1986b; Mintz 1971).

Primary care physicians need not explore in depth the suicidal potential of every depressed or otherwise upset patient. They may recognize their own inadequacy or unwillingness in this area. They must, however, recognize such problems and refer such patients for psychiatric treatment in the context of their continued availability for general medical care (Waltzer 1979).

Psychiatric Outpatient Settings

The great majority of patients who commit suicide are psychiatrically ill and are often treated in psychiatric outpatient settings. Many of the safeguards and backup persons and systems available in emergency rooms or inpatient units elsewhere are often missing in this setting.

The psychiatrist in outpatient practice needs to be especially alert for and trained to deal with suicidal patients. A study of suicides among persons with and without psychiatric contacts found significant differences between the two populations. Psychiatric patients with high suicide risk were almost equally female or male and had a median age of 42 years; a high proportion were divorced or widowed and unemployed or retired. Persons diagnosed as alcohol abusers or as having affective psychosis, depressive neurosis, and schizophrenia were especially at risk (Kraft and Babigian 1976). Suicide of the identified psychiatric patient resulted in a significantly higher risk of suicide in remaining relatives. Further, first-degree relatives of psychiatric patients (schizophrenic or bipolar illness) have a higher rate of suicide than do nonpsychiatric controls. The male relatives have a higher rate than do female relatives (Tsuang 1983).

Although depressed patients are a natural focus for concern, clinicians need to be particularly alert for suicide in schizophrenic patients. An estimated 1 in 10 schizophrenic patients commits suicide (Miles 1977), resulting in a suicide rate 20 times that of the normal population (Osmond and Hoffer 1978). Schizophrenic patients who commit suicide are more often men; they tend to be young, never married, non-Protestant, and white. They tend not to communicate their suicidal intent directly, and they use highly lethal methods. Finally, there is often *not* a stressful life event associated with their suicides (Breier and Astrachan 1984).

The psychiatrist needs to heighten concern when any outpatient spirals downward, becoming increasingly hopeless and isolated and feeling that the clinician is his or her only friend. A subtle shift to more malignant despair in the patient's talk or behavior must be investigated. Particularly worrisome are actively hostile fantasies centering around death or fantasies or dreams that show that the patient consciously or unconsciously sees death or suicide as an idyllic, satisfying, or fulfilling solution to life's difficulties. The affective message of the patient's dreams is important; look especially for increasingly violent manifest content, for dreams replete with themes of death and dying or of giving up or surrendering, or for increasingly morbid content (Mintz 1961). A sudden shift to seeming peace or quietude without good reason may be the only sign that the patient has "solved" the conflicts by deciding definitely to die. Critical is the period of initial home visits from the hospital and the first few months following discharge from the hospital. For many outpatients there is a "last straw," whether it is the loss of a job, divorce papers being filed or being final, an anniversary reaction, or the clinician's going on vacation.

The fundamental principles of managing the acutely suicidal person in outpatient psychiatric practice are the same as elsewhere. The message is one of hope, reminding the patient that feelings change, that suicidal feelings must not be acted on, and that the psychiatrist cannot help the patient if the patient is dead. The clinician always needs to work in concert with others, with a combination of family members, friends of the patient, consultants, and psychiatric peers. As nowhere else in clinical practice, alertness to countertransferential feelings is essential. The clinician seeks to remain available but not overwhelmed, neither surprised nor discouraged by the patient's status, neither casual nor fatalistic in outlook.

At times the psychiatrist may feel that the patient's suicidal feelings are also serving as a powerful manipulative lever. Then the function served by the feelings in the treatment must be acknowledged and dealt with directly. Intrusive behavior during a suicidal crisis, such as the patient's barraging the clinician with telephone calls, requires understanding and confrontation as well as limit setting (Halperin 1979). Clinicians must attend to the number and severity of suicidal patients in their practice. At times, if they lose the necessary compassionate detachment, they must responsibly transfer the patient to another clinician. This should clearly *not* be because the patient is hopeless or the clinician has given up, but because the practitioner does not have the necessary resources and is arranging for the suicidal person to get the help needed (Wekstein 1979). Occasionally a concerned person, whether a relative or another physician or therapist, will call for advice concerning someone's suicidal talk or behavior. Offering advice constitutes accepting clinical responsibility. Judging on the basis of often fragmentary information is difficult, and it is usually better to err on the side of caution.

At times the clinician decides that hospitalization is in the patient's best interest. Patients and family members may object strenuously, citing threats to job or livelihood, loss of government clearance, disgrace and humiliation in the eyes of neighbors and relatives, and so on. The clinician must be firm; the relatives who enthusiastically oppose hospitalization may just as energetically sue the clinician for malpractice if the patient does not enter the hospital and does commit suicide. The clinician in this bind should urge a consultation. If that fails, the clinician should send a certified letter to an appropriate family member or enlist help from a community agency or both (Wekstein 1979). It is rare for a patient or family or both to persist in opposing the clinician who is reasonable, concerned, and consistent in presenting the logic and data behind the recommendations.

In the case when the clinician sends a suicidal patient to the hospital, he or she must ensure that the patient is transported safely, accompanied by alert guardians. Further, the clinician must supply the receiving medical-psychiatric team with specific information concerning history, treatment program, issues precipitating the need for hospitalization, and medications—name, type, dosage, and amount that the patient may have ingested, in the event of overdose.

In some circumstances, a patient may overdose or make a suicide attempt and then relent, calling the clinician. Alternately, a relative or friend may find the patient and call. In such instances, the clinician directs the caller to summon an ambulance and gathers whatever specific information about the attempt possible. In patients who are conscious, vomiting should be induced by taking ipecac or by stimulating the back of the throat (Wekstein 1979).

The Suicidal Patient in the Emergency Room

Psychiatric patients who present to emergency rooms of general hospitals are an especially high-risk group for suicide. In one study, the suicide rate of such patients was more than seven times the age and sex-adjusted rate for the general population but similar to that of other clinical psychiatric populations (Hillard et al. 1983). As emergency rooms have increasingly become the "poor man's family doctor" during the last two decades, visits to general hospitals for psychiatric emergencies have tripled (Zonana 1973). Although large numbers of patients with suicide attempts are brought to emergency rooms, the services provided for them vary markedly (Monto et al. 1975).

Drug overdoses account for a high proportion of contemporary suicide attempts leading to emergency room visits (Weissman 1974). Self-inflicted gunshot wounds are also numerous; more than 15,000 Americans kill themselves annually by this method, and many more attempt it (Conn et al. 1984). Regardless of the heterogeneity of presenting problems and services available, estimates are that 90% to 95% of patients brought to the emergency rooms and intensive care units will survive their suicide attempt (Victoroff 1983).

Emergency Room Staff. Emergency room medical and nursing staff usually intervene rapidly and effectively with desperately ill patients. However, they may find themselves outraged by the suicidal patient who tries to thwart their efforts or who actively resists lifesaving treatment. Often the emergency room staff must contend with complex general medical problems while having little to no information from the patient, family, or referring physician or, all too often, misinformation (Guzzardi 1984). Such patients consume inordinate amounts of time and attention from the whole staff, often triggering adverse reactions (Victoroff 1983). Patients who self-inflict gunshot wounds or are otherwise violent or potentially violent particularly rouse staff anger. Use of guns in suicide attempts results in health care providers making omissions in history taking, such as for alcohol consumption; in treatment, such as not seeking psychiatric consultation; and follow-up, such as not recommending psychiatric care after discharge. The nurses and doctors tend to minimize the seriousness of the suicidal act or express judgmental attitudes; they see the injury as personal weakness rather than as a serious indication of emotional illness (Conn et al. 1984). Sometimes emergency room staffers vent their negative feelings on the patient, rationalizing harsh treatment as a deterrent to future self-destructive acts. The more painful the experience, however, the more convinced the patient may be that he or she has expiated guilt, or that the medical profession is profoundly unworthy of trust (Victoroff 1983).

The procedures for the emergency room treatment of the suicidal patient with self-inflicted trauma or overdose are clear (Guzzardi 1984). Goldfrank et al. (1982) presented a standard protocol for managing the overdose patient, which can be modified according to the specific substance ingested (Figure 1).

Of more concern here is the psychological management of the patient, which must begin with psychological management of the

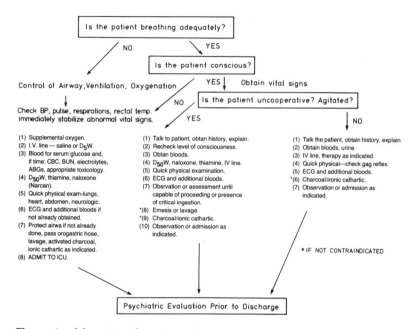

Figure 1. Managing the poisoned or overdosed adult patient without specific toxic syndromes. The principles demonstrated in this algorithm form the basis for management of the poisoned and overdosed patient. The management protocols may appear to be aggressive, but we usually operate under the supposition that the history is less than reliable and the unknown or mixed ingestion is potentially dangerous. BP = blood pressure. IV = intravenous. CBC = complete blood count. BUN = blood urea nitrogen. ABG = arterial blood gas; ECG = electrocardiogram. ICU = intensive care unit. (From Goldfrank LR, Flomenbaum NE, Weisman RS: General management of the poisoned and overdosed patient, in Goldfrank LR: Toxicologic Emergencies: A Comprehensive Handbook in Problem Solving, 2nd Ed. New York, Appleton-Century-Crofts, 1982, used with permission.)

staff. They need well-established protocols for psychiatric emergencies, including lists of resources, outlines of procedure, and telephone numbers of available consultants and helpers (Victoroff 1983). These are especially important when working with the patient who is potentially or actually violent. To decrease that potential, the emergency room clinician needs to avoid or diminish the adversarial aspect of the relationship. Havens (1980) proposed using language that counters the patient's tendency to place responsibility for his or her own fear and anger onto others, the defense mechanism known as projection. With dangerous patients, Jacobs (1983) noted, the clinician must direct remarks "out there" at the threatening figures (such as police), not "in here" at the doctor-patient relationship. The clinician must talk about the emotion-arousing persons specifically (while not in their presence) and convey feelings similar to those the patient may have; for example, "The police don't give anyone a chance these days—four of them to one of you!" Avoid direct confrontation with the patient; stand to the side and minimize eye contact. The clinician should never turn his or her back on the violent patient and should always be closer to the door. The suicidal patient in the emergency room setting should always be supervised and accompanied, even to the bathroom. Tragedies have occurred when patients have asked to go to the bathroom and have subsequently hung themselves with their belt or cut themselves with a scalpel they took from their room.

Medication and nonchemical restraints may be necessary with the violent suicidal patient. Before using any medications, the clinician must try to distinguish between a "functional" and an organic disorder. Psychotic patients respond well to a flexible dose strategy of high-potency antipsychotics (Ericksen et al. 1976). Most patients will respond to one to four intramuscular injections of 2.5 to 10 mg each of haloperidol (for a total of 10 to 20 mg), given at 30-minute to 1-hour intervals. Absorption is rapid, with peak blood levels at 20 minutes postinjection. Intramuscular or intravenous sodium amytal is an effective alternative at dosages of 200 to 500 mg.

Occasionally physical restraints are necessary; procedures for their use should be explicit (Table 4). There should be adequate staff present. Ideally, five persons should be available to administer full physical restraints: one for each limb and one for the head. (Remember, patients can bite.) If the patient will not comply with this procedure, he or she should be placed on a hospital stretcher and the limbs restrained. Once secured, the patient should remain accompanied and the restraints checked frequently for adequate circulation. Afterward, the staff need to review the specifics of the incident, to document the rationale in the chart, and to amend their procedures as necessary (Jacobs 1983).

With all suicidal patients, the emergency room staff must seek psychiatric consultation, preferably with the consultant coming to the emergency room in person. To protect physicians and staff, all procedures and thinking must be documented in the event of subsequent legal action (Julavits 1983).

The Psychiatrist and the Suicidal Emergency Room Patient. The emergency psychiatrist comes into a complex social field when attempting to help the suicidal patient. He or she must contend not only with the patient's ambivalence or hostility but also with the emergency room staff's often negative feelings about psychiatry in general and difficult suicidal patients in particular. The psychiatrist orches-

Table 4.   Protocol for application of restraints

---

1. There should be a doctor's orders to restrain a patient. This need only be in verbal form owing to the emergency nature of the situation.

2. The on-line staff (paraprofessionals, nurses, social workers, psychologists) should be delegated the authority for making the decision when a patient needs to be restrained.

3. Security and/or police should be contacted prior to the application of restraints. It is helpful to have either panic buttons installed or a secret code so that staff members can dial Operator in the presence of patient. A code such as "Please ask Doctor Blue to come to the emergency room" is more than adequate.

4. There should be adequate personnel present. Ideally there should be five people, one for each limb and one person to give orders (and/or hold the patient's head). There should always be a minimum of two people present.

5. If there are not adequate staff available, do the following:
   A. Allow the patient to leave and then contact the local police.
   B. Ask for immediate assistance of police to help with the patient.

6. Explain to security and/or police the indications for restraints and the importance of teamwork.

7. Attempt voluntary application of restraints by saying to the patient, "We would like you to lie down on the stretcher so that we can restrain you for your own protection," or "You seem to be out of control—we want to protect you and others from getting hurt."

8. Do not bargain with the patient. If the patient does not respond in a brief time to your voluntary request, ask hospital security to place the patient onto a stretcher. If security is not available, use other staff members.

9. Once the patient is on the stretcher, begin application of restraints.

10. The patient should be gently grabbed and placed on his or her back with one arm extended above his or her head and one arm at his or her side.

11. The sex and role of staff present when restraints are being applied should be considered in relation to the patient's problem; for example, try to have a woman present when a young woman is out of control and needs restraint.

12. After application of restraints, the patient must not be left alone. One staff member should be assigned to talk to the patient about his or her feelings and explain the purpose of the restraints.

13. Restraints should be checked for proper application—that is, for adequate circulation to limbs.

Table 4.   Protocol for application of restraints, *continued*

---

14. The doctor should make decisions about medication—dosages and frequency.

15. Restraints should be checked every 15 minutes.

16. Allow time for a debriefing period after the situation is over for staff, police, security, and so on.
    A. Ask people what their reactions were to a particular patient.
    B. Could the situation have been handled differently?
    C. What went wrong and what went right?
    D. How can everybody work together better as a team?

17. Documentation:
    A. Indication for using restraints; for example, presence of self-destructive behavior.
    B. Prior attempts at less restrictive alternatives, such as verbal communication.

18. Hints for avoiding injury:
    A. Keep a safe distance.
    B. Expect the unpredictable.
    C. Never turn your back on the patient.
    D. Watch out for the head—remember, patients can bite.
    E. Remove any sharp objects from the examination room.

Source.   From Jacobs D: Evaluation and management of the violent patient in emergency settings. Psychiatr Clin North Am 6:259–269, 1983, used with permission.

trates a complex team made up of other mental health professionals and emergency room medical staff (Barton 1983). He or she has to be active while acknowledging and tolerating often intense negative feelings and countertransference. Fear and anger are often realistic; the psychiatrist has to contain those feelings and proceed carefully and thoughtfully (McCarthy 1983; Victoroff 1983). Just as the emergency room physician must keep in mind the possibility of psychosocial as well as biologic factors influencing the etiology of behavior in patients, so must the psychiatrist include organic factors in the assessment. Fauman (1983) presented a schema for adequately evaluating organic mental disorders in the suicidal patient (Figure 2). Additionally, the psychiatric consultant must be especially aware of procedures and techniques for dealing with patients who may be or are violent (Jacobs 1983).

Once the assessment is complete, the emergency psychiatrist needs to make an effective disposition. In one study of suicide at-

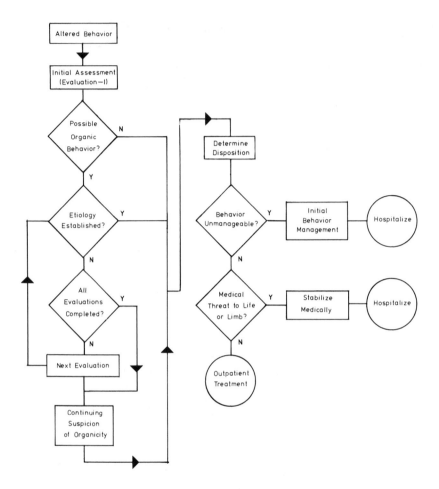

Figure 2. Flow chart for the emergency psychiatric evaluation of organic mental disorders.
(From Fauman MA: The emergency psychiatric evaluation of organic mental disorders. Psychiatr Clin North Am 6:233-257, 1983, used with permission)

tempters, 9% required medical intensive care hospitalization, 44% had psychiatric hospitalization, 38% were referred for outpatient psychiatric care, and 8% had no further treatment (Paykel et al. 1974). Often the crucial question in this setting is whether or not to hospitalize the patient. Key clinical variables in this study were the previous history, the characteristics of the attempt, the patient's motivation, and the mental status. Less important were the patient's sociodemographic characteristics, living circumstances, or emotional impact on the clinician. One useful schema emphasizes positive criteria for hospitalization, not thinking of it as a sole or last resort (Friedman 1983). According to these criteria, there are three purposes for which the hospital has special resources and is particularly helpful: protection, diagnosis, and treatment. Does the patient need protection? One should consider the patient's dangerousness to him- or herself or to others. Severe psychopathology makes compliance with an outpatient program unlikely or impossible. What is the patient's need for disengagement from a noxious environment? Are there special diagnostic needs? These can involve nonpsychiatric medical problems requiring hospital studies (e.g., computed tomography scans, neurological or other laboratory tests). Patients who present diagnostic puzzles may require 24-hour observation by unbiased observers. Are there special treatment needs that the hospital resources can best provide? These may include the psychiatric needs of medical or surgical patients, or medical treatments in emotionally fragile psychiatric patients. The hospital may be preferable in situations where close monitoring, medical support, or enforced compliance is called for. Regressed or acting-out patients whose behavior indicates a need for therapeutic containment may do better in a hospital whether or not they are acutely suicidal. The hospital therapeutic milieu, with its multimodal treatment team and investigations, can effectively stimulate change for patients with ingrained characterological problems.

However, in most cases, hospitalization is difficult; it is even more so if the patient is unwilling. The effective psychiatric emergency clinician knows about other resources and possibilities and how to mobilize them. This includes staying in contact with the referring clinician, whether psychiatrist, nonpsychiatric physician, or other mental health professional. That clinical alliance may help secure needed hospitalization or ease developing an alternate plan. The psychiatrist who works well with nonpsychiatric hospital physicians has more flexibility in ensuring thorough investigation of biologic aspects of the patient's symptoms and in arranging a treatment plan (McCarthy 1983).

Problems in Referral. Effecting a safe transition from the emergency room to another site for further treatment is another danger point. The clinician has to be alert to the patient's continuing safety, whether the disturbed person is going to the medical intensive care unit, a psychiatric ward or hospital, or home with follow-up plans. Even if a patient is staying within the general hospital, there must be transmission of information about the patient's dangerousness, either verbal or with a note attached to the chart (Victoroff 1983).

Various studies show drop-out rates of 30% to 60% in patients referred for outpatient care following a suicide attempt (Goldney

1975). Delay in instituting the treatment program is a major contributor to drop-out. This is especially true when hospital services do not coordinate well with follow-up or when the emergency room staff have been unsympathetic, both situations that are all too common (Ramon et al. 1975). The effective clinician must know community, family, and medical resources and how to integrate them on behalf of the patient. It is now possible to study and improve this process in more detail. Members of one quality assurance committee studied rates of referral failures for potentially suicidal patients seen in the psychiatry section of a university hospital's emergency room (Knesper 1982). Of a group of 290 patients with moderately to extremely severe suicidal potential, rates of failure were 24% within the university hospital system and 33% outside that system. A special statistical procedure, outlier analysis, identified clinicians whose referral rates differed significantly from their peers. The methods of clinicians who more effectively transferred patients were identified and transmitted to those with substandard performance, resulting in changes for the better.

Legal Considerations. In attending to the needs of the patient, clinicians must concern themselves with providing proper medical care; any legal questions will center on whether the care was appropriate and within the state of the art (see Amchin et al., Chapter 24, this volume; Julavits 1983). A hospital with emergency care facilities must provide service to emergency patients, regardless of the patient's financial or other resources. Psychiatrists or other physicians with special experience should evaluate such patients, and hospitals lacking these resources are responsible to refer suicidal patients to sources of such individuals or services. The emergency room staff should take precautions for the safety of the patient, hospital staff, and other patients before, during, and after active diagnostic and treatment efforts. Often effective, informed consent to treatment is unavailable from the suicidal patient, and the clinician must still proceed. In such situations, consent is best obtained from the next of kin. Generally, minors can be treated in emergency situations with implied parental consent, but it is always advisable to notify parents or next of kin if a minor's legal status is uncertain. Whenever possible, detailed written consent to treatment is advisable; if not, there should be documentation in the chart of whatever the patient agrees to. Generally, the prudent course is medically to stabilize the patient, whether or not the patient willingly agrees to treatment.

Documentation of the patient's diagnosis, treatment, and disposition is essential, including the status of informed consent, explanations of any delays in examination or diagnosis, conditions calling for restraint, and consultations and medications. Given the often intensely private and emotionally painful nature of psychiatric emergencies, the clinician must attend carefully to the patient's confidentiality, whether an adult or a minor. Some clinical situations, such as gunshot wounds, are required by law to be reported to the state. The duty of confidentiality is not absolute (e.g., when the clinician needs to protect the welfare of the patient who is suicidal).

One should carefully document the exceptional patient who is competent, not committable, and who leaves against medical advice. If there is concern about the patient's well-being, it is advisable to contact the next of kin.

Reasons for discharge should also be documented. If there is any question about the appropriateness of a patient's discharge, the clinician should treat the patient conservatively. When in doubt, it is useful to consult another psychiatrist and document both the consultation and the clinical thinking about discharge.

The physician-patient relationship established in the emergency room means that the physician must keep informed about the patient and administer to his or her needs until a transfer is complete to another clinician or to another institution (Julavits 1983).

Medical and Surgical Services of General Hospitals

Staff members on the medical and surgical services of general hospitals have a sizeable task in the standard medical management of their patients. They understand that patients on their services are distressed in reaction to hospitalization and illness. Yet some medical and surgical patients are severely troubled emotionally. Some of them are suicidal; some commit suicide in the hospital. Such patients may be at risk because their suicidality is unrecognized or is minimized when it has been recognized. Staff alertness is absolutely necessary. Among patients who are a particular cause for concern are those with a psychiatric illness, especially affective disorders, and those with an organic deficit in central nervous system (CNS) function (Kellner et al. 1985). When there is global impairment, such CNS deficits are easy to detect. More insidious and potentially more lethal are the subtle deficiencies and interferences that cloud thinking and distort judgment (Himmelhoch 1987).

In the general hospital, suicidal patients are cared for by a team comprised of the attending physician, the house officer, one or more nurses, and a consulting psychiatrist. Some one person must be in charge of interventions with the suicidal patient.

Greater staff awareness of the potential problem and better interdisciplinary cooperation may contribute to a pattern of decreasing suicides in this setting. Pisetsky and Brown (1979) studied one group of medical and surgical patients who committed suicide and found that they tended to be older, married, and suffering from a chronic illness (five malignancies, six CNS syndromes, three cardiac cases, one burn, and one osteomyelitis). Many had several medical illnesses and tended to be chronically dependent patients who feared hospital discharge.

In one study of deaths by suicide of general hospital patients with malignant neoplasms, hematopoietic malignancies accounted for a disproportionately large number of suicides in patients under 45 years of age, whereas the malignancies of the larynx and pharynx accounted for a disproportionately large number of suicides in older patients (Farberow et al. 1963).

In Glickman's (1980) study of patients who attempted suicide on the nonpsychiatric services of a general hospital, three-quarters were in one of the following three groups: 1) those admitted following a suicide attempt who were agitated and not effectively tranquilized, 2) those with poor medical prognoses, and 3) those in delirium tremens (DTs) who were not adequately sedated. Patients with DTs who attempted suicide did so within 24 hours of the onset of their delirium. A high index of suspicion for this condition and prompt intervention when it occurs are important suicide prevention techniques (Farberow et al. 1963).

Several studies documented death by jumping out of the window, a particularly frequent method of committing suicide in this setting (Brown and Pisetsky 1960; Friedman and Cancellieri 1958; Glickman 1980; Pisetsky and Brown 1979; Pollack 1957). Reich and Kelly (1976) attributed the comparative success of the Peter Bent Brigham Hospital (*no* successful suicides in 70,404 medical and surgical admissions from 1967–1976) at least in part to the fact that the hospital is housed in a group of low buildings. Ensuring that windows are secure (e.g., access is blocked, panes are of shatterproof or impenetrable material) may be the simplest and most effective suicide prevention technique with the general hospital patient.

Patients hospitalized after drug overdose on the intensive care unit (ICU) of a general hospital are a natural focus for concern. Their numbers are increasing. In one study at the Massachusetts General Hospital, they accounted for 5% of admissions to the ICU (Stern et al. 1984). The mean age of this population was 33 years, with men slightly more often involved than women. Almost all (99%) of the patients survived their hospitalization; 45% admitted to having had suicidal intent. Those patients not considered suicidal tended to be substance abusers; in follow-up they had other overdoses and high mortality. The majority of the patients had received psychiatric treatment, had been regular users of alcohol, and had made previous suicide attempts. Character pathology, with abundant impulsivity and a history of drug and alcohol abuse, was more common than a DSM-III-R (American Psychiatric Association 1987) Axis I diagnosis of major affective disorder in most of these patients. This population presents special problems in terms of follow-up, since the same character pathology contributing to their overdosing interferes with their adhering to a treatment program.

Implementing Suicidal Precautions. Alertness to the possibility of suicidal risk is necessary with hospital patients, from the first inquiry regarding an available bed to when the person is discharged. All hospital staff should be aware of the issue. Generally, the nurses can usually best detect suicidal feelings and behavior on a continuous daily basis. They can alert house officers and attending physicians, implement existing nursing guidelines, and recommend a psychiatric consultation (Victoroff 1983). Nurses in the emergency room or the ICU can easily forewarn their counterparts on medical and surgical services, if necessary with a conspicuous sticker or code note on the patient's chart.

Victoroff (1983) has comprehensively detailed administrative policies regarding the patient who is suicidal, homicidal, or both (see Appendix II). Many precautions can be built into the hospital environment. Unremarkable in themselves, precautions such as screened unbreakable windows, shielded electrical outlets, covered pipes and ventilation grids, open closets and light plastic hangers reduce the possibility of suicide in the hospital setting. Stairwells need to be protected so that patients cannot jump from strategic points. Precautions should be taken so that patients cannot get access to ventilating shafts and elevator ducts. Fixtures such as horizontal rods or clothes hooks from which a patient might string a noose should be made of material that will not suspend someone's weight or that will break away from the supporting walls.

Once identified as suicidal, patients should not have access to any of the following: glass utensils; nail files or clippers; perfume; electrical equipment; razors; cigarette lighters; scissors; any alcohol-containing beverages; soda cans; hangers; plastic bags; glass mirrors; and any kind of knife, gun, or hook.

With the patient identified and the external environment stripped of dangerous objects or features, attention can turn to exploring and improving the patient's internal environment: the suicidal feelings. Here a thoughtful, warm, and hopeful attitude on the part of hospital staff is essential. An understanding and sympathetic listener, a gentle and appropriate gesture of reassurance such as holding a patient's hand, are simple measures that can be lifesaving.

Similarly, the clinician can attend to the patient's vulnerability by clearly and thoughtfully explaining diagnostic and treatment procedures and by orienting confused patients. It is useful to show that suicidal feelings are taken seriously and that the clinician is doing everything possible to safeguard the patient. This means ensuring that the suicidal patient is never left alone, either in the hospital room or during diagnostic or treatment procedures. Having another person available for security reasons is essential; this may be a psychiatric technician, trained nurse, or a responsible (and carefully screened) family member or friend. Patients must be protected at least temporarily from persons who may inflame or upset them further, even if those persons are close family members.

Sometimes protecting patients from their impulses and providing extra interpersonal support will suffice. At other times, other methods, such as physical restraints and psychotropic medications, are necessary. Another controversial but effective method is electroconvulsive therapy (ECT). This treatment often helps suicidal patients whose complicating medical illnesses render using antidepressants difficult to impossible. ECT is indicated when the clinician cannot wait the weeks necessary for antidepressants to work, or when a patient is dangerously suicidal (e.g., with a combination of distorted or delusional thinking and *no* psychomotor retardation). When patients are so depressed that they are barely eating or moving, this is another indication for ECT. Clinicians considering restraints, psychotropic medications, or ECT will usually want to work closely with a consultation-liaison psychiatrist.

Psychiatric and Other Consultation. Suicidal patients should routinely have a psychiatric consultation; this should be standard hospital policy for patients on the wards, in the emergency room, and in the ICU. While nonpsychiatric physicians vary widely in their willingness to consult and follow hospital policy, activism on the part of the nurses should ensure that suicidal patients are seen in consultation by a psychiatrist. Patients with organic brain syndromes, alcoholic patients and other drug abusers, and persons who have previously attempted suicide are also standard candidates for psychiatric consultation. The medical and nursing staff should tell the patient that the psychiatric consultant will conduct an interview, that this is hospital policy, and that the patient is neither "crazy" nor a hopeless case.

The psychiatric consultant should respond quickly to the request and contact the consultee to ascertain what question is being asked and by whom (Schiff and Pilot 1959). The consultant should review the chart, talk with nursing and house officer staff as well as with the attending physician, and examine the patient. In a prompt and concise note, the consultant should summarize the history and current mental and physical status and specify appropriate psychiatric diagnoses using the terminology of DSM-III-R (Garrick and Stotland 1982). The note should specify the interplay of psychological, social and biological variables. The psychiatric consultant should also recommend further investigations as well as management techniques. The consulting psychiatrist should state exactly how suicidal or homicidal he thinks the patient is and the consequences of that assessment: recommendations for medication; restraints; transfer to another service (psychiatry) or another facility; and the advisibility of involvement of other services such as social workers, religious persons, attorneys, or court officials. The psychiatric consultant should offer to assist in the process of committing the patient to another setting if that proves necessary. The consultant should indicate his or her ongoing availability, including phone numbers, and specify the provisions for coverage in his or her absence (Hackett and Stern 1987).

In hospitals without psychiatric consultants, other mental health specialists often assess suicide risk and review options, developing a more effective and collaborative relationship with the patient. Often the nurses will have access to their full- or part-time specially trained psychiatric nurse consultant or staff member from the psychiatry service. Some hospitals have a sophisticated team approach to consultation around such issues, with the psychiatrist working with the social workers, nurse, and other professionals on an ongoing basis.

When trained mental health specialists are not available, the physician must consult other medical colleagues; they can often defuse complicated and anxiety-arousing situations and provide alternate options. In addition, peer consultation provides protection to the responsible clinician should later events result in a lawsuit. Good medical care and prudent protection against legal actions both dictate that clinicians caring for the suicidal patient thoroughly document not just their plans and actions but also their rationale.

Involving others naturally includes hospital administration, both for the specifics of an individual case and for general guidelines and procedures. (See Appendix II for a set of administrative guidelines for patients who are suicidal or homicidal.)

Covert Forms of Suicidal Behavior.   There are covert as well as obvious forms of suicidal behavior (Kellner et al. 1985). One pattern of presentation is refusal of medical treatment in patients who are chronically or seriously ill (or both). Given the rising numbers of patients with chronic and serious illnesses, advancing age, and multiple personal losses, one can anticipate more persons who will consider suicide an appealing option. Often they may view suicide as a "rational" source of relief for their distress, and noncompliance with recommended treatment is a likely suicide method. Chronic dialysis patients often meet this description. However, one study found that in most cases the patient's wish for suicide was not as rational as the patient claimed; usually multiple factors, some potentially correctable, resulted in serious emotional conflicts and in suicidal feelings and acts (Abram et al. 1971). In any chronically or seriously ill patient who is suicidal, the central question is whether a potentially treatable psychiatric condition, such as an affective disorder or an organic brain disorder, is contributing to suicidal behavior.

Another form of covertly suicidal behavior is seen in some patients who are considered uncooperative or "problem" patients. Nelson and Farberow (1982) developed a scale to measure "indirect self-destructive behavior" in chronically ill medical patients. These behaviors included abusing the treatment program; conflicts with the medical staff; and eating, drinking, or smoking inappropriately. These behaviors may be more acceptable to such patients than overtly suicidal acts. However, a downward spiral occurs; an increasingly angry and rejecting staff ignores or rebuffs the patient, who then escalates the noxious and self-destructive behaviors. Groves (1978) developed guidelines for patients who display "unconsciously self-murderous behaviors." Included among them were those patients he described as "hateful." Among his recommendations for treatment of these patients was first to recognize the limits of the health care system, and second to work diligently as long as possible to preserve the patient. Finally, he urged that clinicians get psychiatric consultation to determine whether the patient has a treatable depression.

Forensic Concerns. A general hospital can be held to a high standard of care in suicide prevention. In defending against negligent action brought against them, the staff of one general hospital in which a patient committed suicide claimed that the hospital should not be held liable because it had no special facilities for mental patients. In rejecting this argument, the court held that the hospital staff took responsibility in accepting (and not referring) the patient. If a patient shows suicidal tendencies, the fact that the patient is admitted for some other problem and is not on a psychiatric service is irrelevant (Waltzer 1979).

The Psychiatric Inpatient Unit

The highest concentration of suicidal patients is among persons hospitalized on psychiatric inpatient units. The best hospital precaution is the combination of a responsive, well-trained staff and lack of access to lethal methods of committing suicide. As in other treatment settings, the patient's developing a trusting relationship with the clinician is essential. The capacity of psychiatric staff to foster a strong positive countertransference, while minimizing access to self-destructive means, explains the low rate of suicide among psychiatric inpatients. This requires the clear designation of a primary clinician to manage the treatment program and a smoothly functioning hospital team to reach out to the patient from the moment of admission. The primary clinician and hospital team must also work with the family members from the time of admission. It is essential to ease the distress of relatives as well as of patients to improve communication among family members and to involve them in planning for the treatment program after the patient is discharged.

Admission. The process of admission to the psychiatric inpatient service is critical. Just as hospital staff in emergency rooms, ICUs, and medical and surgical services can forget about the psychological needs of suicidal patients in their zeal to treat "real" disease, so can psychiatric inpatient staff neglect diagnosis and treatment of nonpsychiatric medical illness in their patients. Admission screening should include a thorough physical as well as mental examination, full personal and social history from the patient and significant others, and routine laboratory tests, including serologic tests for syphilis and acquired immune deficiency syndrome. Up to 50% of patients admitted to one psychiatric unit had medical illnesses directly related to their psychiatric presentations (Comstock 1983). Medical conditions including anemias, liver or pancreatic disease, multiple pulmonary emboli, chronic infections (including CNS tuberculosis), early organic brain syndromes and other physical illnesses may be responsible for psychological symptoms. Specific medical therapies will be necessary to treat nonpsychiatric organic illness and deficit conditions such as dehydration, malnutrition, and electrolytic imbalance (Harris and Myers 1968).

Implementing Suicide Precautions. Security policies for suicidal patients vary widely from one extreme to another. In a tight security prison, suicidal inmates may be locked naked in empty, padded cells; in an entirely open hospital, few precautions are possible (Harris and Myers 1968). Neither extreme is ideal, and striking the right balance between supervision and autonomy is a clinical art. In general, the open-door policy adopted by many hospitals has been associated with reduced suicide rates. Any open ward, however, should have within it an area where observation can be intense, where nursing staff are concentrated, and where physical security is tight (Morgan 1979). While precautions for this area resemble those described previously for the medical or surgical setting, some points deserve emphasis. Suicidal patients should be under direct observation at all times. They may not even have access to the usual privacy measures for the toilet. Restraints, if necessary, are optimal when the patient is in a bed with a mattress rather than on a stretcher, except as a brief expedient. Since soft restraints are unreliable and may occlude circulation, padded leather extremity cuffs are the best method of securing the patient. Nursing staff should attend scrupulously to the circulatory and excretory needs of restrained patients, documenting them every 15 minutes (Comstock 1983).

There need to be clear policy guidelines for advancing the patient's degree of autonomy as the staff decide the patient is less suicidal and impulsive. Victoroff (1983) (see Appendix II) has detailed prudent measures concerning many aspects of this clinical problem.

Treatment Issues. The treatment program needs to be multimodal, a combination of appropriate psychotropic and other medications and additional psychological and social interventions. Individual, group, and family psychotherapeutic efforts usually supplement the other's effect (Blumenthal 1988).

ECT is an option, long neglected because of reaction to previously indiscriminate use. Responsible clinicians are again using it with acutely suicidal patients, especially when it is unsafe to wait the necessary weeks for antidepressant drugs to take hold (Morgan 1979), or for the seriously psychotic patient whom the staff cannot keep from sustained attempts to commit suicide (Gerson and Bassuk 1980; National Institute of Mental Health 1985).

The staff need to be alert at particularly critical junctions of the patient's hospitalization; classic examples include the early days of hospitalization and the transition back to daily life after discharge. A particularly dangerous discharge occurs when the staff and patient disagree about the indications, and the patient feels pushed out prematurely. In Morgan's (1979) study, half of the patients who committed suicide did so after a confrontation in which they insisted they could not manage outside the hospital. Such confrontations are risky but at times necessary. The staff always need to guard against the concept of the ward as a magic island where the patient is safe from the demands of a hostile outside world.

Specialized Psychiatric Units: Emergency Intensive Care. In addition to the conventional psychiatric units in general and psychiatric hospitals, there are some highly specialized ones providing emergency intensive care (Comstock 1983). Aiming at an ultrashort stay, such as 72 hours, these units emphasize multidisciplinary approaches that minimize inpatient regression, accelerate treatment planning, rapidly involve the support system, and definitively resolve the current stress (Gerson and Bassuk 1980). For some patients, they may produce better results than do conventional units, especially when coupled with good follow-up programs (Herz et al. 1977). While economical in their use of hospital time, they are expensive because of increased staffing needs. The central conflict in such units is that between the need to protect dangerous patients from themselves and others, and the push from staff to resolve the current stress definitively. Active and intensive work with family and follow-up agencies needs to be undertaken, and staff members must communicate clearly with each other and with those outside the hospital. Given the levels of stress, it is hardly surprising that staff turnover is high, with the average staff person staying about 2 years. This parallels with experience on medical and surgical ICUs. Although the stress is severe, specific role definitions, attention to staff safety, frequent meetings to share views and feelings, and optimistic and vigorous leadership can mitigate its worst effects (Comstock 1983).

Problem Patients: Borderline Personality Disorder. All suicidal patients are challenging but some are more so. Patients with a borderline personality organization cause conflicts and cross-currents of intense feelings in treatment settings. Their intense object hunger, strongly dysphoric mood, object and ego splitting, and impulsive behavior make them formidably difficult when they are suicidal. Staff members need promptly to identify such patients as borderline, contain their negative reactions, and work on restoring the patient's usual levels of coping based on the "reintegrative strength of transference gratifications" (Comstock 1983, p. 310). The goal is to generate a stable outpatient treatment alliance or mend if possible a disruption in an existing therapeutic program. Short-term hospitalization often serves this goal best.

When a Psychiatric Inpatient Commits Suicide. Suicides do occur, and when they do the staff must be able to document that the patient was thoroughly evaluated and that hospital personnel demonstrated skill and good judgment, providing reasonable care and attention for the patient's safety. Having developed a good relationship with the patient's family prior to the suicide maximizes the possibility that all concerned will negotiate their painful reactions responsibly. The staff need to deal with their feelings separately, usually in special meetings that allow them to ventilate, share concerns, identify weaknesses in treatment programs and facilities, and plan for the future (Harris and Myers 1968).

Summary

Caring for the acutely suicidal patient is a challenge for the clinician in all treatment settings. The work should build on the clear conceptual framework of crisis intervention theory discussed in this chapter. It requires integrity and courage in the clinician, who must communicate directly and honestly with the patient about painful issues and stand by his or her convictions in the face of challenges by the patient; family members; members of the hospital staff; and legal, adminstrative, policy, and other personnel. In Himmelhoch's (1987) words, "involvement is the essence of psychotherapy in suicide management" (p. 45).

Although the work with suicidal patients over the life cycle is stressful, it can be deeply gratifying. Although emotionally intense, when the work is successful it carries with it the certainty that the clinician has saved a life.

References

Abram HS, Moore G, Westervelt FB: Suicidal behavior in chronic dialysis patients. Am J Psychiatry 127:1199–1204, 1971

Adam KS: Attempted suicide. Psychiatr Clin North Am 8:183–201, 1985

American Psychiatric Association: Diagnostic and Statistical Manual of Mental Disorders, 3rd Edition, Revised. Washington, DC, American Psychiatric Association, 1987

Barton GM: Psychiatric staff and the emergency department: roles, responsibilities and reciprocation. Psychiatr Clin North Am 6:317–323, 1983

Beck AT, Ward CH, Mendelson M, et al: An inventory for measuring depression. Arch Gen Psychiatry 4:561–571, 1961

Beck AT, Weissman A, Leste D, et al: The measurement of pessimism: the Hopelessness Scale. J Consult Clin Psychol 42:861–865, 1974

Beck AT, Steer RA, Kovacs M, et al: Hopelessness and eventual suicide: a 10-year prospective study of patients hospitalized with suicidal ideation. Am J Psychiatry 142:559–563, 1985

Bhatia SC, Khan MH, Sharma A: Suicide risk evaluation and management. Am Fam Physician 34:167–174, 1986

Blum R: Contemporary threats to adolescent health in the United States. JAMA 257:3390–3395, 1987

Blumenthal SJ: A guide to risk factors, assessment and treatment of the suicidal patient. Med Clin North Am 72:937–971, 1988

Boyd JH: The increasing rate of suicide by firearms. N Engl J Med 308:872–874, 1983

Breier A, Astrachan BM: Characterization of schizophrenic patients who commit suicide. Am J Psychiatry 141:206–209, 1984

Brown W, Pisetsky JE: Suicidal behavior in a general hospital. Am J Med 29:307–315, 1960

Caplan G: Emotion crises. The Encyclopedia of Mental Health 3:521–532, 1963

Carlson GA, Cantwell DP: Suicidal behavior and depression in children and adolescents. Journal of the American Academy of Child Psychiatry 21:361–368, 1982

Comstock BS: Psychiatric emergency intensive care. Psychiatr Clin North Am 6:305–316, 1983

Conn LM, Rudnick BF, Lion JR: Psychiatric care for persons with self-inflicted gunshot wounds. Am J Psychiatry 141:261–263, 1984

Deykin EY, Alpert JJ, McNamara JJ: A pilot study on the effect of exposure to child abuse or neglect on adolescent suicidal behavior. Am J Psychiatry 142:1299–1303, 1985

Doyle BB: Anxiety (Monograph #80, AAFP Self Study), Kansas City, MO, American Academy of Family Physicians, 1986a

Doyle BB: Depression (Monograph #84, AAFP Self Study). Kansas City, MO, American Academy of Family Physicians, 1986b

Egeland JA, Sussex JN: Suicide and family loading for affective disorders. JAMA 254:915–918, 1985

Ericksen SE, Hurt SN, Davis JM: Dosage of antipsychotic drugs. N Engl J Med 294:1296–1297, 1976

Ettlinger RW: Suicides in a group of patients who had previously attempted suicide. Acta Psychiatr Scand 40:363–378, 1964

Farberow NL, Schneidman ES, Leonard CV: Suicide among general medical and surgical hospital patients with malignant neoplasm. Bulletin of the Veterans Administration MB-9:1–11, 1963

Fauman MA: The emergency psychiatric evaluation of organic mental disorders. Psychiatr Clin North Am 6:233–257, 1983

Fawcett J, Scheftner W, Clark D, et al: Clinical predictors of suicide in patients with major affective disorders: a controlled prospective study. Am J Psychiatry 144:35–40, 1987

Fisch HU, Hammond KR, Joyce CR, et al: An experimental study of the clinical judgment of general physicians in evaluating and prescribing for depression. Br J Psychiatry 138:100–109, 1981

Fowler RC, Rich CL, Young D: San Diego suicide study, II: substance abuse in young cases. Arch Gen Psychiatry 43:962–965, 1986

Friedman JH, Cancellieri R: Suicidal risk in a municipal general hospital. Diseases of the Nervous System 19:556–560, 1958

Friedman RS: Hospital treatment of psychiatric emergencies. Psychiatr Clin North Am 6:293–303, 1983

Garrick T, Stotland N: How to write a psychiatric consultation. Am J Psychiatry 139:849–855, 1982

Gerson S, Bassuk CL: Psychiatric emergencies: an overview. Am J Psychiatry 137:1–11, 1980

Gispert M, Davis MS, Marsh L, et al: Predictive factors in repeated suicide attempts by adolescents. Hosp Community Psychiatry 38:390–393, 1987

Glickman LS: Psychiatric Consultation in the General Hospital. New York, Marcel Dekker, 1980, pp 181–182

Goldfrank LR, Flomenbaum NE, Weisman R: General management of the poisoned and overdosed patient, in Toxicologic Emergencies: A Comprehensive Handbook in Problem Solving, 2nd Edition. Edited by Goldfrank LR. New York, Appleton-Century-Crofts, 1982

Goldney RD: Out-patient follow-up of those who have attempted suicide: fact or fantasy? Aust N Z J Psychiatry 9:111–113, 1975

Groves JE: Taking care of the hateful patient. N Engl J Med 298:883–887, 1978

Guze S, Robins E: Suicide and primary affective disorder. Br J Psychiatry 117:437–483, 1970

Guzzardi LJ: Role of the emergency physician in treatment of the poisoned patient. Emerg Med Clin North Am 2:3–13, 1984

Hackett TP, Stern TA: Suicide and other disruptive states, in Massachusetts General Hospital Handbook of General Hospital Psychiatry, 2nd Edition. Edited by Hackett TP, Cassem NH. Littleton, MA, PSG Publishing, 1987, pp 268–296

Halperin DA: Psychodynamic strategies with outpatients, in Suicide: Theory and Clinical Aspects. Edited by Hankoff LD, Einsidler B. Littleton, MA, PSG Publishing, 1979, pp 363–372

Harris JR, Myers JM: Hospital management of the suicidal patient, in Suicide Behaviors, Diagnosis and Management. Edited by Resnick HLP. Boston, Little, Brown, 1968, pp 297–305

Havens L: Explorations in the uses of language in psychotherapy: counter-projective statements. Contemporary Psychoanalysis 16:53–67, 1980

Heimburger L: Facts about suicide: how knowledgeable is the primary care physician? Missouri Medicine, June 1980, pp 295–298

Hendin H: Suicide: a review of new directions in research. Hosp Community Psychiatry 37:148–154, 1986

Herz MI, Endicott J, Spitzer RL: Brief hospitalization: two-year follow-up. Am J Psychiatry 134:502–507, 1977

Hillard J, Ramm D, Zung W, et al: Suicide in a psychiatric emergency room population. Am J Psychiatry 140:459–462, 1983

Himmelhoch J: Lest treatment abet suicide. J Clin Psychiatry (Suppl) 48:44–54, 1987

Jacobs D: Evaluation and management of the violent patient in emergency settings. Psychiatr Clin North Am 6:259–269, 1983

Julavits WF: Legal issues in emergency psychiatry. Psychiatr Clin North Am 6:335–345, 1983

Kellner CH, Best CL, Roberts JM, et al: Self-destructive behavior in hospital-ized medical and surgical patients. Psychiatr Clin North Am 8:279–289, 1985

Knesper D: A study of referral failures for potentially suicidal patients: a method of medical care evaluation. Hosp Community Psychiatry 33:49–52, 1982

Kraft DP, Babigian HM: Suicide by persons with and without psychiatric contacts. Arch Gen Psychiatry 33:209–215, 1976

Linn LS, Yager J: Recognition of depression and anxiety by primary physi-cians. Psychosomatics 25:593–600, 1984

Litman RE: Management of suicidal patients in medical practice, in The Psychology of Suicide. Edited by Schneidman ES. New York, Science House, 1970, pp 112–119

Litman RE, Farberow NL: Emergency evaluation of self-destructive potential-ity, in The Cry for Help. Edited by Farberow NL, Schneidman ES. New York, McGraw-Hill, 1961, pp 48–59

Maltsberger JT, Buie D: Countertransference hate in the treatment of suicidal patients. Arch Gen Psychiatry 30:625–633, 1974

McCarthy EA: Resolution of the psychiatric emergency in the emergency department. Psychiatr Clin North Am 6:281–292, 1983

Miles CP: Conditions predisposing to suicide: a review. J Nerv Ment Dis 164:231–246, 1977

Minkoff K, Bergman E, Beck AT, et al: Hopelessness, depression, and at-tempted suicide. Am J Psychiatry 130:455–459, 1973

Mintz RS: Psychotherapy of the suicidal patient. Am J Psychother 15:348–367, 1961

Mintz RS: Some practical procedures in the management of suicidal persons. Am J Orthopsychiatry 36:896–903, 1966

Mintz RS: Basic considerations in the psychotherapy of the depressed suicidal patient. Am J Psychother 25:56–73, 1971

Monto A, Ross C, Heymann G, et al: A survey of hospital services for suicidal persons. Suicide 5:169–176, 1975

Morgan HG: Death Wishes? The Understanding and Management of Deliber-ate Self Harm. New York, John Wiley, 1979

Motto JA, Heilbron DC, Juster RP: Development of a clinical instrument to estimate suicidal risk. Am J Psychiatry 142:680–686, 1985

Murphy GE: The physician's responsibility for suicide, I: an error of commis-sion. Ann Intern Med 82:301–304, 1975a

Murphy GE: The physician's responsibility for suicide, II: errors of omission. Ann Intern Med 82:305–309, 1975b

Murphy GE: On suicide prediction and prevention. Arch Gen Psychiatry 40:343–344, 1983

Murphy GE, Wetzel RD: Family history of suicidal behavior among suicide attempters. J Nerv Ment Dis 170:86–90, 1982

National Institute of Mental Health: Electroconvulsive Therapy Consensus

Development Conference Statement 5 #11, Washington, DC, National Institute of Mental Health, 1985

Nelson F, Farberow NL: The development of an indirect self-destructive behaviour scale for use with chronically ill medical patients. Int J Soc Psychiatry 28:5–14, 1982

Osmond H, Hoffer A: Schizophrenia and suicide. Orthomolecular Psychiatry 7:57–67, 1978

Parad HJ, Caplan G: A framework for studying families in crisis. Social Work 5:3–15, 1960

Patterson WM, Dohn HH, Bird J, et al: Evaluation of suicidal patients: the SAD PERSONS Scale. Psychosomatics 24:343–349, 1983

Paykel E, Hallowell C, Dressler D, et al: Treatment of suicide attempters: a descriptive study. Arch Gen Psychiatry 31:487–491, 1974

Pfeffer P: Suicidal thoughts and behavior among school children. Journal of American Academy of Child Psychiatry 21:564, 1982

Pisetsky JE, Brown W: The general hospital patient, in Suicide: Theory and Clinical Aspects. Edited by Hankoff LD, Einsidler B. Littleton, MA, PSG Publishing, 1979, pp 279–297

Pollack S: Suicide in a general hospital, in Clues to Suicide. Edited by Schneidman ES, Farberow NL. New York, McGraw-Hill, 1957, pp 148–162

Ramon S, Bancroft JHJ, Skrimshire AM: Attitudes toward self-poisoning among physicians and nurses in a general hospital. Br J Psychiatry 127:257–264, 1975

Reich P, Kelly M: Suicide attempts by hospitalized medical and surgical patients. N Engl J Med 294:298–301, 1976

Renshaw DC: Suicide in children. American Family Physician 24:123–127, 1981

Robbins DR, Alessi NE: Depressive symptoms and suicidal behavior in adolescents. Am J Psychiatry 142:588–592, 1985

Rockwell DA, Pepitone-Rockwell F: The suicidal patient. J Fam Pract 7:1207–1213, 1978

Rosen DH: View from the bridge. JAMA 254:3314, 1985

Ruben HL: Managing suicidal behavior. JAMA 241:282–284, 1979

Schiff S, Pilot M: An approach to psychiatric consultation in the general hospital. Arch Gen Psychiatry 1:349–357, 1959

Schneidman E (ed): Crisis, disaster and suicide: theory and therapy, in Essays in Self-Destruction. New York, Science House, 1967, pp 380–398

Schurman RA, Kramer PD, Mitchell JB: The hidden mental network: the treatment of mental illness by nonpsychiatrist physicians. Arch Gen Psychiatry 42:89–94, 1985

Schwartz HI: Legal and ethical pitfalls in family practice psychiatry. American Family Physician 35:103–108, 1987

Shafii M, Carrigan S, Whittinghill JR, et al: Psychological autopsy of completed suicide in children and adolescents. Am J Psychiatry 142:1061–1064, 1985

Siomopoulos V: Psychiatric iatrogenic disorders. American Family Physician 34:111–116, 1986

Stern TA, Mulley AG, Thibault GE: Life-threatening drug overdose. JAMA 251:1983–1985, 1984

Tsuang MT: Risk of suicide in the relatives of schizophrenics, manics, depressives, and controls. J Clin Psychiatry 44:396–400, 1983

Usdin G, Lewis JM: The physician and the suicidal patient, in Psychiatry in General Medical Practice. Edited by Usdin G, Lewis JM. New York, McGraw-Hill, 1979, pp 458–474

Victoroff VM: The Suicidal Patient: Recognition, Intervention, Management. Oradell, NJ, Medical Economics Books, 1983

Waltzer H: The medical practitioner, in Suicide: Theory and Clinical Aspects. Edited by Hankoff LD, Einsidler B. Littleton, MA, PSG Publishing, 1979, pp 122–126

Weissman M: The epidemiology of suicide attempts 1960 to 1971. Arch Gen Psychiatry 30:737–746, 1974

Wekstein L: Handbook of Suicidology: Principles, Problems, and Practice. New York, Brunner/Mazel, 1979

Zonana H, Henisz JE, Levine M: Psychiatric emergency services a decade later. Psychiatr Med 4:273–290, 1973

Chapter 15

Somatic Treatment of the Adult Suicidal Patient: A Brief Survey

Mark J. Goldblatt, MBBCH
Alan F. Schatzberg, M.D.

THROUGHOUT HISTORY, THE magnitude and power of death by suicide has challenged psychiatrists, sociologists, and philosophers. Durkheim's (1897/1951) seminal work drew attention to the extent of suicidal thought and behavior. While most scholars emphasize the sociological aspects of his work, few have recognized that his observations parallel contemporary views that suicidal behavior and ideation occur in association with many psychiatric conditions. Durkheim wrote that: "no psychopathic state bears a regular and indisputable relation to suicide" (p. 81). In 1936, Zilboorg reported that persons suffering from depressive psychoses, compulsive neuroses, and schizophrenia committed suicide. He concluded that "there is no clinical entity recognized in psychiatry that is immune to the suicidal drive" (p. 282). Zilboorg viewed suicide as a "reaction of a developmental nature which is universal and common to the mentally sick of all types and probably also to many so-called normal persons" (p. 289).

Other contributors to this volume review risk factors for suicide (Adam, Chapter 3; Black and Winokur, Chapter 6; Winchel et al. Chapter 4) and specific psychotherapeutic interventions with adult suicidal patients (Kahn, Chapter 16; Weishaar and Beck, Chapter 17). In this chapter, we will emphasize somatic treatments that can be effective with adult suicidal patients and describe the biological rationale and underpinnings of these interventions.

Biochemistry of Suicidal Behavior: Implications for Treatment

In recent years increasing attention has been paid to the psycho-biology of suicide, with particular emphasis on the examination of two neurotransmitters—serotonin and dopamine—and the hypothal-amic-pituitary-adrenal (HPA) axis. This research has pointed to a number of biochemical features that may be common to the seemingly disparate group of psychiatric disorders that have higher incidences of suicide associated with them, and may provide the basis for devel-oping specific treatment approaches for some suicidal patients (for a more detailed discussion, see Winchel et al., Chapter 4, this volume).

The role for serotonin as a unifying clue to suicidal behavior stems originally from studies by Åsberg et al. (1976), who reported an association between suicidal behavior and low levels of cerebrospinal fluid (CSF) 5-hydroxyindoleacetic acid (5-HIAA) in depressed pa-tients. These observations have been replicated and expanded by reports that violent types of suicide in particular were associated with low CSF 5-HIAA levels (Traskman et al. 1981). In addition, markedly impulsive character-disordered patients have been shown to have low CSF 5-HIAA levels (Linnoila et al. 1983). Additionally, levels of 5-HIAA have been shown to be lower in the brains of completed suicides (Beskow et al. 1976).

In recent years, investigators have also explored tritiated impra-mine binding in platelets as a model for serotonin receptor function. Several groups have reported decreased imipramine binding in the platelets of depressed patients (Paul et al. 1981), particularly those with psychotic features. Meltzer et al. (1981) reported decreased sero-tonin transport in depressed patients.

Mann et al. (1986) reported a significant increase in the mean number of serotonin-2 receptors (and beta-adrenergic) binding in the frontal cortices of suicide victims. This research supports the hypoth-esis that suicide completed by violent methods is associated with altered presynaptic serotonin receptor activity that has generated compensatory up-regulation of the postsynaptic serotonin receptor sites. In addition, there may be a concomitant increase in postsynaptic noradrenergic activity. In this study, decreased norepinephrine and serotonin levels were implicated as contributing factors in suicidal behavior.

Furthermore, when hospitalized patients with severe major de-pressive disorder are treated with antidepressant drugs and electro-convulsive therapy (ECT), tritiated imipramine binding sites are in-creased, but this may be unrelated to clinical response (Wagner et al. 1987). Zimelidine, a serotonin uptake inhibitor, has been reported to have more effect on reducing suicidal thoughts than amitriptyline in the early stages of treatment, further suggesting that serotonin may play a primary role in this behavior (Montgomery et al. 1981a).

Over the past decade, considerable evidence has emerged pointing to the key role of serotonin systems in mediating alcoholic behavior. In rats that are genetically bred to consume alcohol, consumption is decreased by the administration of L-tryptophan or serotonin reuptake blockers, but not by norepinephrine reuptake blockers—that is, tricyclic antidepressants (TCAs) (Zabik et al. 1985). In heavy social drinkers, treatment with serotonin reuptake blockers results in a small, but statistically significant decrease in alcohol consumption (Sellers et al. 1981). These effects are not due to nausea or other nonspecific reactions. Taken together, these data suggest that serotonin may also play an important role in alcoholism. Thus serotonin could be a common underpinning to suicidality in both depressed and alcoholic patients, and serotonin reuptake blockers could play a role not only in treating alcoholic patients but also in treating depressive patients with a history of alcohol abuse.

A number of studies have pointed to the curious coupling of serotonin and dopamine systems in various regions of the brain. High-order correlations between CSF homovanillic acid (HVA) and 5-HIAA in depressed patients have been reported in several studies (Åberg-Wistedt et al. 1985). The role of dopamine in suicidal character-disordered patients has been inferred from studies on the use of dopamine receptor blockers to decrease suicidal behavior in such patients. In 1981, Montgomery and Montgomery reported on the use of flupenthixol, a dopamine receptor blocker, in patients with personality disorders (mainly borderline or histrionic) who had a history of multiple suicide attempts. They raised the possibility that the effect of reducing suicidal behavior in personality disorders is mediated via the dopamine system. They also noted lower levels of CSF HVA, the metabolite of dopamine, in depressed patients with a history of suicidal acts. More recently, Soloff and colleagues (1986) reported that haloperidol decreased suicidality in borderline patients. Thus, blocking postsynaptic dopamine receptors appears helpful in decreasing suicidality in character-disordered patients.

The HPA axis has been a major focus of research in depressive disorders. Elevated 24-hour urinary free cortisol (UFC) and dexamethasone nonsuppression are not uncommon features of depressed patients. A number of years ago, suicidal behavior was reported to be associated with elevated 24-hour urinary 17-ketosteroids, an observation that has recently been confirmed by others (Bunney and Fawcett 1965; Fawcett et al. 1987). Nemeroff and colleagues (1988) have reported decreased corticotropin-releasing factor (CRF) receptor activity in the brains of suicide victims, suggesting that elevated levels of CRF may play a role in suicidality in depression. Cortisol and dexamethasone have been reported to decrease serotonin or 5-HIAA levels in the frontal cortex of rats, perhaps by stimulating alternate synthetic pathways (Green and Curzon 1968). Conversely, enhanced postsynaptic serotonin activity or sensitivity has been implicated in increased cortisol levels in depressed patients. These data suggest that cortisol and serotonin may be intimately tied to one another, particularly in suicidal depressive patients.

In depressed subjects, cortisol levels are highest in those with psychotic features, (Schatzberg et al. 1983b), a subgroup that has been reported to be at increased risk for completing suicide. Our group, and others, have reported that psychotic depressive patients demonstrate not only extremely elevated plasma cortisol levels but also high plasma dopamine levels (Rothschild et al. 1987). Others have reported generally higher levels CSF HVA and 5-HIAA in psychotic depressive patients (Ågren and Terenius 1985), although low HVA and 5-HIAA levels have been reported in a subgroup of older psychotic depressive patients with suicidal ideation (Brown et al. 1987). Glucocorticoids have been reported to increase plasma dopamine and HVA levels in normal control subjects, again pointing to possible negative consequences of hypercortisolemia (Rothschild et al. 1984; Wolkowitz et al. 1985). The role of elevated HVA or 5-HIAA levels in suicidal behavior in psychotic depressive patients has not been well studied, but findings to date suggest that low or high extremes in levels of serotonin or dopamine (i.e., low 5-HIAA/HVA or high 5-HIAA levels) may each play a role in different suicidal psychiatric patients.

TREATMENT PRINCIPLES

Interventions with suicidal patients are based on an understanding of the risk factors for suicide, a set of general management principles, and the treatment of associated psychiatric disorders. After a diagnosis has been made, a treatment plan can be effected, one that often includes both somatic and psychotherapeutic treatments.

General Management Approaches

All patients undergoing psychiatric evaluation need to be assessed as to the presence of suicidal ideation and/or plans. This assessment should take place within the context of the psychiatric interview, with special emphasis not only on the presence or absence of suicidal ideation but also on the patient's overall psychopathology and personality structure, and the extent and quality of social and interpersonal support. Aspects of the general principles of assessment have been described in other chapters of this volume (see Blumenthal, Chapter 26; Doyle, Chapter 14; Hendren, Chapter 10, this volume).

In determining risk for suicide, the following factors in the patient's history and presentation are particularly important:

1. Extent of a current plan or thoughts about hurting oneself
2. Overall psychopathology—psychotic depression, unipolar and bipolar depression with hopelessness, schizophrenia with command hallucinations, and substance abusers while intoxicated
3. Strength of social supports
4. History of past suicide attempts and their outcomes
5. Current stressors, including degree of losses
6. Availability of means to follow through with suicidal plans
7. Quality of the therapeutic alliance between the patient and clinician
8. Strength of alliance between the patient's family and the treating clinician
9. Degree of patient's communication about his or her depression, dysphoria, and suicidality

The clinician's primary concern, once a substantial risk for suicide has been determined, is how to ensure the patient's safety. Crisis intervention techniques have been discussed at length elsewhere in this volume (see Doyle, Chapter 14, this volume). However, it is appropriate to underscore here that if there is any concern about dangerousness, it is generally better to hospitalize the patient, at least briefly, so that the clinical situation may at least be followed in a safe, structured setting. Intensive treatment can be initiated under supervision. Furthermore, an enlarged treatment team, consisting of ward staff, admitting physician, administrator, and family therapist, can participate in the evaluation and share parts of the decision making or, at least, part of the anxiety that goes hand in hand in dealing with these stressful crises.

However, it should be kept in mind that hospital resources are both limited and costly. Forced hospitalization can be traumatic and frightening to the unwilling patient and can destroy the therapeutic alliance that the clinician is attempting to build. Patients also enjoy the right to participate in their treatment planning and as such should be included as much as possible in determining the lines of safety and structure necessary for their short- and long-term needs. In the end, the clinician is often faced with the dilemma of when to hospitalize and how much risk to take. Clinical skill and experience are often the main guides for solving this dilemma, but unfortunately are not totally infallible despite the best intentions.

Somatic Therapy

In general, somatic therapies for the adult suicidal patient should be aimed at treating symptoms of the underlying, primary condition. However, when treating the suicidal patient, the potential lethality of the specific medication needs to be respected. In this context, the physician needs to avoid merely handing patients prescriptions, but rather to place the somatic treatment in the context of the overall educational and treatment approach to the illness. Medication should be delivered in the context of a positive physician-patient relationship, one that includes mutual respect and conveys a sense of hopefulness. The clinician should not expect to dissuade patients of their hopelessness; rather the clinician must win the patient's cooperation to undergo, and stick with, treatment. This requires a supportive approach and the building of a working alliance. The clinician's expression of his or her hopefulness that the patient will respond to treatment is an important element in dealing with suicidal patients.

For the physician to balance adequate treatment with an avoidance of oversupplying patients with dangerous amounts of medication, a careful approach should be developed. This begins with a careful review of the adequacy of previous medication trials vis-à-vis dosage, duration, clinical response, and the patient's history of compliance. The physician should attempt to follow a plan of prescribing relatively small total amounts, while ensuring adequate daily doses and allowing for periodic increases. For example, patients started on imipramine could receive 50 mg per day for 3 days, and then 75 mg for 4 days. The patient should receive a 1-week supply at their initial appointment, to cover the amount of medication needed, including dosage increase. In the face of no side effects, dosage should be increased weekly until the patient demonstrates a persistent clinical response, or until maximum levels are obtained. Again, adequate supplies to ensure this must be prescribed. If the prescribing physician is concerned about the possibility that the patient may misuse the medications, then limited amounts (e.g., a 3-day supply) can be prescribed. However, in this type of situation, hospitalization will probably be required to ensure safety and adequate treatment. Once treatment has begun, all efforts should be expended to ensure a full trial and to prevent undertreatment. Once again, hospitalization may be necessary if a patient is noncompliant or cannot tolerate a full trial of medication because of side effects.

Prevention of suicidal behavior depends on the appropriate treatment of the underlying psychiatric disorders. Specific considerations of somatic treatments of depression, delusional depression, schizophrenia, alcoholism, and borderline personality disorder will be considered.

Depression. The National Institute of Mental Health Collaborative Study of Depression revealed that a substantial undertreatment of depressed patients was common, even in academic settings; the generally low dosages of treatment and the variability of treatment regimens were attributable to individual medical practitioners' decision making (Keller et al. 1986). Earlier, we reported that less than half of the medication trials that "refractory" depressed patients received had been adequate in dosage or duration (Schatzberg et al. 1983a).

Generally, the pharmacologic treatment of seriously depressed patients begins with a TCA, although recently serotonin reuptake blockers have become increasingly popular. If patients are not responding to TCA medication, the clinician must assess whether an adequate trial has been achieved. The response to TCAs is often slower than one might hope. Trials as long as 4+ weeks must be undertaken with adequate doses. Indeed, in their review of a series of studies on TCAs in depressed patients, Quitkin et al. (1984) concluded that relatively few patients demonstrate significant improvement after only 2 weeks of therapy, and many require as long as 6 weeks to respond.

If only a limited clinical response is noted with TCAs after 6 weeks, the physician should consider increasing the dosage; some patients rapidly metabolize medication and may require higher doses to respond. Plasma levels may be helpful for adjusting the dosage of TCAs or for determining the adequacy of a trial. For nortriptyline, a curvilinear relationship has been described, with a critical range of 50 to 150 ng/ml representing a "therapeutic window"; levels above and below are frequently associated with poorer responses (Åsberg et al. 1971). In endogenously depressed patients, Glassman et al. (1977) have reported a sigmoidal relationship between response and imipramine plus desipramine levels, clinical response increasing with plasma levels up to 250 ng/ml, then leveling off thereafter.

For some patients, adding lithium carbonate or cytomel (T3) can increase the likelihood of a clinical response. Lithium has been argued to act through increasing serotonergic function. Although the mechanism of action of T3 potentiation of TCAs is unclear at this time, it may be related to its facilitating receptor adaptation, or as a treatment of subtle forms of thyroid dysfunction, presenting as clinical depression. If these additions are not effective, the physician is faced with the option of either changing the class of drug or moving on to ECT.

The TCAs act primarily by blocking the reuptake of norepinephrine rather than serotonin. Clomipramine is an exception, exerting considerable effect on blocking serotonin reuptake, and thus may prove to be a useful alternative treatment for suicidal patients. This has not been well studied, nor is the drug readily available in the United States at the present time.

Fluoxetine is one of a new group of antidepressant drugs that selectively inhibits the reuptake of serotonin. Its side effect profile is generally more favorable than that of TCAs; it appears to facilitate weight loss and does not potentiate seizures in humans. Fluoxetine has a long half-life and appears relatively safe when taken in overdose. Because it is new to the market, broader clinical use will be needed to delineate this medication's side effect profile and safety limits more fully. However, data from Reimherr et al. (1984) point to its being particularly effective in patients who have failed on TCAs. Suicidality has not been well studied as a predictor, but since depressive patients who suicide often have a chronic course, one might expect that fluoxetine and related drugs may become treatments of choice in suicidal depressive patients. As noted above, zimelidine was reported in one study to be more effective in decreasing suicidal behavior than was amitriptyline (Montgomery et al. 1981a). Trazodone has mixed reuptake and receptor blocking effects on serotonin function and is another alternative in the treatment of depressed patients. It too is less lethal when taken in overdose.

Monoamine oxidase inhibitors (MAOIs) block the intraneuronal action of monoamine oxidase (MAO), the enzyme that degrades various neurotransmitters, including norepinephrine, dopamine, and serotonin. MAOIs have been reported to be particularly effective in refractory patients, hysteroid dysphoric patients, and those with atypical depression, and offer a major alternative in severely ill refractory patients. Clinicians frequently worry that suicidal patients might kill themselves by going off their diets or using proscribed agents. We have seldom seen this. Generally, even suicidal patients are frightened by the potential pain and sequelae of hypertensive reactions, such that this becomes an unattractive method of self-harm. Rather, MAOIs are often very effective for some suicidal depressive patients and should be strongly considered. If there is concern about the patient's compliance, clinicians may choose to hospitalize patients briefly while beginning treatment with MAOIs. In the United States, phenelzine and tranylcypromine are the two most commonly used MAOIs. Phenelzine is more calming and anxiolytic; tranylcypromine is more stimulating. Isocarboxazid is similar to phenelzine in its pharmacologic profile.

ECT has generally been shown to be the most broadly effective treatment of depression, with response rates of approximately 80%. ECT should be strongly considered for any seriously depressed patients who have failed to respond to other treatments, or for those with delusions. In patients with compromised physical states due to anorexia or psychosis and in cases of pronounced suicidal ideation or behavior, ECT should be considered early in treatment.

Delusional Depression. Suicide risk is five times higher in delusional versus nondelusional depressions. Robins (1986) reported that 19% of 134 subjects who committed suicide had also been psychotic, a finding that has been confirmed by others. Roose et al. (1983) found that delusionally depressed patients were five times more likely to commit suicide than nondelusionally depressed patients. In our experience, these patients are among the most difficult to treat; they hide the degree of their cognitive disturbance, become frozen or distant, and are difficult to assess for true suicidal risk. Clinicians should be wary in accepting any assurances about control of suicidal behavior in a delusionally depressed patient.

Several groups have now suggested that increased activity of dopamine may play a role in delusional depression (Åberg-Wistedt et al. 1985; Rothschild et al. 1987). These patients respond better to neuroleptic-TCA treatment or to ECT than to TCAs alone (Avery and Lubrano 1979; Spiker et al. 1981). Better responses to the combination of neuroleptic and TCA versus the TCA alone do not appear to reflect the increased plasma levels of either the TCA or the neuroleptic. Responsivity of this condition to other antidepressants (e.g., fluoxetine, trazodone, or phenelzine) or to combinations of these agents with antipsychotics has not been well studied.

Schizophrenia. Although schizophrenic disorders are primarily considered to involve difficulties with cognition and thinking, rather than with mood, suicide is a serious and unfortunately common complication of this disorder. More than 20% of patients hospitalized for schizophrenia will attempt suicide at some time. The majority of schizophrenic suicides occur in outpatients, usually soon after discharge from the hospital.

Some schizophrenic patients who suicide demonstrate increased agitation or psychosis at the time of committing suicide. In this subgroup, adequate treatment with antipsychotic medication is essential. The consensus in the literature is that suicidal schizophrenic patients are more likely to be depressed than nonsuicidal schizophrenic patients. However, it is often difficult to distinguish depression from the "negative symptoms of schizophrenia." Initially it was believed that antidepressant treatment of the symptoms resulted in an exacerbation of the schizophrenic condition. However, more recent studies have argued that some of these symptoms respond to treatment with TCAs, or alprazolam, and that these agents are considered worth a trial. Trazodone has been reported to be less likely to promote psychotic decompensation than are other antidepressants. In severe cases, ECT and lithium carbonate can also be considered.

Early studies aimed at trying to separate the impact of adequate antipsychotic treatment of schizophrenic patients from concomitantly occurring depression suggested that neuroleptics, in particular depot preparations, gave rise to severe depressive moods and therefore facilitated suicide (De Alarcon and Carney 1969). Later studies contradicted this finding (Niturad and Nicholschi-Oproiu 1978). There have, however, been reports of two patients who attempted suicide to relieve severe akathisia (Shear et al. 1983). Thus picking the "right" drug for schizophrenic patients may be less relevant than developing effective approaches to side effects. It is important to obtain a detailed drug history from the patient, family, and past care givers, clarifying which drugs the patient has received and how he or she has responded to them.

Thioridazine is approved by the Federal Drug Administration for use in moderate to marked depression with anxiety or agitation. However, there is no evidence that any neuroleptic is generally superior to standard antidepressants for the treatment of depression. Thioridazine should probably be avoided in sexually active young males because of its sexual side effects. There is also no evidence that daily dosages greater than 15 mg of haloperidol or 400 mg of chlorpromazine are more effective than are lower dosages. Thus lower rather than higher dosages should be tried first.

If a patient dislikes the first few doses of a particular antipsychotic, some physicians advocate trying one or two others to see if the patient would feel less distressed and would be more cooperative with the treatment. If a patient does not begin to improve on an adequate dose of antipsychotic, a different antipsychotic drug can be tried. However, in the absence of undesirable side effects, it is difficult to be sure whether a shift to a different drug, at more or less equivalent doses, will actually be more effective than continuing the original drug for a longer period at higher dosages. Pragmatically, 2+ weeks without response in a markedly psychotic patient and 5 to 6 weeks in a patient with milder symptoms generally speaks toward some sort of change in medication regimen. Shifting the chemical class of antipsychotic would be a reasonable strategy, but this has not been well studied. Clozapine, an atypical neuroleptic, does offer an alternative treatment for patients who have failed on standard neuroleptics. The addition of a different class of drug, such as lithium or a TCA, can sometimes be effective. Depot preparations ensure compliance in patients who are not responding, especially those who do not seem to be responding to adequate doses.

The risk of tardive dyskinesia in particular makes the long-term use of these drugs worrisome. It is currently not possible to predict which patients will develop tardive dyskinesia. However, the best available data suggest a rate of development of dyskinesia of about 3% to 4% over the first 4 or 5 years of exposure. Elderly women and patients with affective disorders appear at greater risk than do schizophrenic patients (Gardos and Casey 1984).

In summary, suicide is a real risk in schizophrenic patients. The condition is debilitating, and the patient is easily demoralized by the cycles of decompensation and recompensation. However, interventions aimed at reducing psychosis and alleviating distress and depressive or other negative symptoms should help to decrease the likelihood of untoward outcomes.

Alcoholism. Alcoholism and drug abuse are commonly associated with suicide (see Flavin et al., Chapter 8, this volume). The lifetime risk for suicide is 1% in the general population and approximately 15% for those with alcoholism. Alcohol increases the risk for suicidal behavior for both alcoholic and nonalcoholic populations, being associated with 50% of all suicides and 5% to 27% of suicides in alcoholics (Robins et al. 1984).

Alcoholics can suffer from other psychiatric illnesses as well that also are associated with an increased risk of suicide. Depression is particularly common. There are at least three types of depression that are associated with alcoholism (Ciraulo and Jaffe 1981). First, there is the direct toxic effect of alcohol. Second, there is a withdrawal-related depression, which is probably time-limited (1 to 3 weeks) and generally clears, irrespective of treatment. TCAs appear to help the physiological symptoms that accompany this withdrawal (Wilson et al. 1970). Third, there seems to be a familial form of affective dysregulation, which can manifest itself as sociopathy, depression, or alcoholism. A common question has been whether some alcoholics drink to deal with an underlying depressive disorder, a question likely to be debated for quite some time.

Serotonin represents a possible link between alcoholism and depression. For example, as indicated above, L-tryptophan lowers alcohol consumption in genetically bred strains of mice, an effect that can be produced by serotonin reuptake blockers (e.g., zimelidine). Sellers et al. (1981) reported that serotonin reuptake blockers reduce alcohol consumption in heavy drinkers. Moreover, Weingartner et al. (1983) reported that zimelidine, a relatively specific serotonin reuptake blocker, attenuates the impairing effects of ethanol on learning and memory. Thus serotonin activity may provide a link between suicidality in alcoholic and depressed patients. Prospective studies on serotonin reuptake blockers as a treatment for suicidal alcoholics seem reasonable, as does this approach on a clinical basis. This is in no way a substitute for treatment programs aimed at abstinence. Rather, the use of serotonin reuptake blockers should only be included in an overall approach to this serious problem.

    Borderline Personality Disorder. Borderline personality disorder is characterized by impulsivity, unstable and intense interpersonal relationships, inappropriate and intense anger, identity disturbance, affective instability, self-destructive acts, and a chronic sense of emptiness. Generally, patients with borderline personality disorder are not marked responders to psychopharmacological treatments; however, medication may alleviate certain key symptoms.

    Montgomery et al. (1981b) treated 58 personality disorder patients with mianserin or placebo and noted no significant reduction in the number of suicidal acts during the 6-month treatment period. However, in a flupenthixol versus placebo double-blind study, there was a significant reduction over placebo in the number of suicidal acts in the patients treated with flupenthixol at 4, 5, and 6 months (Montgomery et al. 1979). Although various underlying mechanisms are probably involved, flupenthixol's effect on dopamine systems may be inferred to be involved in decreasing suicidal behavior in personality disorders.

    Soloff et al. (1986) reported that haloperidol produced significant improvement on a broad spectrum of symptom patterns, including depression, anxiety, hostility, paranoid ideation, and psychoticism in borderline patients. In contrast, amitriptyline was found to be minimally effective, with some improvement noted in areas of depressive content. On a composite measure of overall symptom severity, haloperidol was found to be superior to both amitriptyline and placebo, with no difference noted between amitriptyline and placebo. Goldberg et al. (1986) also reported a therapeutic benefit from thiothixene over placebo in treating some selected symptoms of borderline personality disorder. Significant drug-placebo differences were found on illusions, ideas of reference, psychoticism, obsessive-compulsive symptoms, and phobic anxiety, but not on depression. The mean daily dosage was lower than that used in schizophrenic outpatients. Although at least two studies have indicated that phenothiazines are helpful in reducing suicidal and other symptoms in borderline patients, there is still much debate about how and whether to use them. Gunderson (1986) noted that neuroleptics should be reserved for borderline patients who present with sustained and severe symptoms of the kind described above (i.e., illusions, ideas of reference, and psychoticism). For borderline patients without these symptoms, or those in whom symptoms are acute, reactive, or nonsevere, drugs are less likely to be useful and may present unnecessary risks of harmful side effects. This area requires further study.

Two other treatment strategies that may be helpful in patients with borderline personality disorder are MAOIs and anticonvulsants. The MAOIs may be most useful in treating anxiety with related depression in patients with personality disorders. As noted above, phenelzine has been shown to be efficacious in patients with hysteroid dysphoria and those with atypical depressions with pronounced anxiety. Cowdry and Gardner (1986) noted that carbamazepine was effective in decreasing the self-destructive behavior of borderline patients when compared to other drug regimens. However, self-destructive behaviors in this group were by no means eliminated. Still, further studies on this approach appear warranted.

CONCLUSION

The suicidal patient represents a challenge to the practitioner. Treatment must begin with a careful assessment of the patient's condition and suicidal potential. Thereafter, an organized approach to treating the underlying condition can be undertaken. This approach should include psychotherapeutic interventions and the prescription of appropriate medications in adequate trials (both in time and amount of drug). Biologic and psychopharmacologic studies suggest that serotonin reuptake blockers and TCAs may prove particularly helpful for alcoholic and depressed patients with suicidal behavior, and that neuroleptics may have an important place in treating patients with schizophrenia, borderline personality disorder, and psychotic depression. These pharmacological treatments should be administered in conjunction with psychotherapeutic and environmental interventions, which are discussed in other chapters in this volume.

REFERENCES

Åberg-Wistedt A, Wistedt B, Bertilsson L: Higher CSF levels of HVA and 5-HIAA in delusional compared to nondelusional depression. Arch Gen Psychiatry 42:925–926, 1985

Ågren H, Terenius L: Hallucinations in patients with major depression: interactions between CSF monoaminergic and endorphinergic indices. J Affective Disord 9:25–34, 1985

Åsberg M, Cronholm B, Sjoquist F, et al: Relationship between plasma level and therapeutic effect of nortriptyline. Br Med J 7:331–334, 1971

Åsberg M, Traskman L, Thoren P: 5-HIAA in the cerebrospinal fluid: a biochemical suicide predictor? Arch Gen Psychiatry 33:1193–1197, 1976

Avery D, Lubrano A: Depression treated with imipramine and ECT: the De Carolis study reconsidered. Am J Psychiatry 136:559–562, 1979

Beskow J, Gottfries CG, Roos BE, et al: Determination of monoamine and monoamine metabolites in the human brain: postmortem studies in a group of suicides and in a control group. Acta Psychiatr Scand 53:7–20, 1976

Brown RP, Keilip J, et al: CSF monoamine and depressive subtypes. New Research Program and Abstracts, 140th Annual Meeting of the American Psychiatric Association, Chicago IL, May 1987, p 28 (NR11)

Bunney WE Jr, Fawcett JA: Possibility of a biochemical test for suicidal potential. Arch Gen Psychiatry 13:232–239, 1965

Ciraulo DA, Jaffe JH: Tricyclic antidepressants in the treatment of depression associated with alcoholism. J Clin Psychopharmacol 1:146–150, 1981

Cowdry RW, Gardner DC: Pharmacotherapy of borderline personality disorder. Arch Gen Psychiatry 45:111–119, 1986

De Alarcon R, Carney MW: Severe depressive mood changes following slow-release intramuscular fluphenazine injection. Br Med J 3:564–567, 1969

Durkheim E: Suicide. Glencoe, IL, Free Press, 1897/1951

Fawcett JA, Scheftner WA, Fogg L, et al: Acute versus long-term clinical predictors of suicide, in 1987 CME Syllabus and Proceedings Summary, 140th Annual Meeting of the American Psychiatric Association, Chicago, IL, May 1987, pp 206–207

Gardos G, Casey D: Tardive Dyskinesia and Affective Disorders. Washington DC, American Psychiatric Press, 1984

Glassman AH, Perel JM, Shostak M: Clinical implications of imipramine plasma levels for depressive illness. Arch Gen Psychiatry 34:197–204, 1977

Goldberg SC, Schulz SC, Schulz PM, et al: Borderline and schizotypal personality disorders treated with low-dose thiothixene vs placebo. Arch Gen Psychiatry 43:680–686, 1986

Green AR, Curzon G: Decrease of 5-hydroxytryptamine in the brain provoked by hydrocortisone and its prevention by allopurinol. Nature 220:1095–1097, 1968

Gunderson JG: Pharmacotherapy for patients with borderline personality disorder. Arch Gen Psychiatry 43:698–700, 1986

Keller MB, Lavori PW, Klerman GL, et al: Low levels and lack of predictors of somatotherapy received by depressed patients. Arch Gen Psychiatry 43:458–466, 1986

Linnoila M, Virkkunen M, Scheinin M, et al: Low cerebrospinal fluid 5-hydroxyindoleacetic acid concentration differentiates impulsive from non-impulsive violent behavior. Life Sci 33:2609–2614, 1983

Mann JJ, Stanley M, McBride PA: Increased serotonin[2] and beta-adrenergic receptor binding in the frontal cortices of suicide victims. Arch Gen Psychiatry 43:954–959, 1986

Meltzer HY, Arora RC, Baber R: Serotonin uptake in blood platelets of psychiatric patients. Arch Gen Psychiatry 38:1322–1326, 1981

Montgomery SA, et al: Maintenance therapy in repeat suicidal behavior: a placebo controlled trial. Proceedings of the 10th International Congress for Suicide Prevention, Ottawa, 1979, pp 227–229

Montgomery SA, McAuley R, Rani SJ, et al: A double-blind comparison of zimelidine and amitriptyline in endogenous depression. Acta Psychiatr Scand (Suppl) 290:314–327, 1981a

Montgomery D, Roy D, Montgomery S: Mianserin in the prophylaxis of suicidal behavior: a double blind placebo controlled trial. Proceedings of the XI International Congress of Suicide Prevention, Paris, 1981b

Nemeroff CB, Owens MJ, Bissette G, et al: Reduced corticotropin releasing factor binding sites in the frontal cortex of suicide victims. Arch Gen Psychiatry 45:577–579, 1988

Niturad A, Nicholschi-Oproiu L: Suicidal risk in the treatment of outpatient schizophrenics with long-acting neuroleptics. Aggressologie 19:145–148, 1978

Paul SM, Rehavi M, Skolnick P, et al: Depressed patients have decreased binding of tritiated imipramine to platelet serotonin "transporter." Arch Gen Psychiatry 38:1315–1317, 1981

Quitkin FM, Rabkin JG, Ross D, et al: Duration of antidepressant drug treatment: what is an adequate trial? Arch Gen Psychiatry 41:238–245, 1984

Reimherr FW, Wood DR, Byerley B, et al: Characteristics of responders to fluoxetine. Psychopharmacol Bull 20:70–72, 1984

Robins E: Psychosis and suicide. Biol Psychiatry 21:665–672, 1986

Robins LN, Helzer JE, Weissman MM, et al: Lifetime prevalence of specific psychiatric disorders in three sites. Arch Gen Psychiatry 41:947–958, 1984

Roose SP, Glassman AH, Walsh TB, et al: Depression, delusions and suicide. Am J Psychiatry 140:1159–1162, 1983

Rothschild AJ, Langlais PJ, Schatzberg AF, et al: Dexamethasone increases plasma free dopamine in man. J Psychiatr Res 18:217–223, 1984

Rothschild AJ, Schatzberg AF, Langlais PJ, et al: Psychotic and nonpsychotic depressions: I. Comparison of plasma catecholamines and cortisol measures. Psychiatry Res 20:143–153, 1987

Schatzberg AF, Cole JO, Cohen BM, et al: Survey of depressed patients who have failed to respond to treatment, in The Affective Disorders. Edited by Davis JM, Maas JW. Washington, DC, American Psychiatric Press, 1983a, pp 73–85

Schatzberg AF, Orsulak PJ, Rothschild AJ, et al: Platelet MAO activity and the dexamethasone suppression test in depressed patients. Am J Psychiatry 140:1231–1233, 1983b

Sellers EM, Naranjo CA, Peachey JE: Drugs to decrease alcohol consumption. N Engl J Med 305:1255–1262, 1981

Shear M, Frances A, Weiden P: Suicide associated with akathisia and depot fluphenazine treatment. J Clin Psychopharmacol 3:235–236, 1983

Soloff PH, George A, Nathan S, et al: Progress in pharmacotherapy of borderline disorders: a double-blind study of amitriptyline, haloperidol and placebo. Arch Gen Psychiatry 43:691–700, 1986

Spiker DG, Hanin I, Cofsky J, et al: Pharmacological treatment of delusional depressives. Psychopharmacol Bull 17:201–202, 1981

Traskman L, Åsberg M, Bertilsson LJ, et al: Monoamine metabolites in CSF and suicidal behavior. Arch Gen Psychiatry 38:631–636, 1981

Wagner A, Åberg-Wistedt A, Bertilsson L: Effects of antidepressant treatments on platelet tritiated imipramine binding in major depressive disorder. Arch Gen Psychiatry 44:870–877, 1987

Weingartner H, Buchsbaum MS, Linnoila M: Zimelidine effects on memory impairments produced by ethanol. Life Sci 33:2159–2163, 1983

Wilson IC, Alltop LB, Riley L: Tofranil in the treatment of postalcoholic depressions. Psychosomatics 11:488–494, 1970

Wolkowitz OM, Sutton ME, Doran AR, et al: Dexamethasone increases plasma HVA but not MHPG in normal humans. Psychiatry Res 16:101–109, 1985

Zabik JE, Binkerd K, Roache JD: Serotonin and ethanol aversion in the rat, in Research Advances in New Psychopharmacological Treatments for Alcoholism. Edited by Naranjo CA, Sellers EM. Amsterdam, Elsevier Science Publishers, 1985, pp 87–101

Zilboorg G: Differential diagnostic types of suicide. Archives of Neurology and Psychiatry 35:270–291, 1936

Chapter 16

Principles of Psychotherapy With Suicidal Patients

Alvin Kahn, M.D.

Macbeth: Canst thou not minister to a mind diseas'd,
Pluck from the memory of a rooted sorrow,
Raze out the written troubles of the brain,
And with some sweet oblivious antidote
Cleanse the stuff'd bosom of that perilous stuff
Which weighs upon the heart?
Doctor: Therein the patient
Must minister to himself.
Macbeth: Throw physic to the dogs; I'll none of it.

Anamnesis and sharing of pain denied; possible medication not offered; the opportunity to enter into a helping alliance refused: the stage was set for Lady Macbeth's suicide.

The challenge of psychotherapeutic work with the suicidal patient taxes the full range of the therapist's intellectual and emotional resources. To enhance clinical sturdiness and gain a wiser therapeutic perspective, the historical evolution of theories of suicidality will be reviewed. These considerations lead naturally to a heightened awareness of the importance of the therapeutic alliance in clinical approaches to suicidality. The therapist's part of this alliance demands a lively sense and knowledge of the dynamics common to narcissistic injury and the narcissistically vulnerable ego. It is not rage and depression alone that must regularly be addressed in therapy, but underlying dispositions to envy, rivalry, and jealously. Implicit in these affective dispositions are just those cognitive distortions that figure largely in suicidal deliberations and that tend to enhance feelings of hopelessness and helplessness. In this chapter, manifestations of these issues at different stages in the life cycle will be discussed, and their contribution in specific conditions, such as alcoholism and severe physical illness, will be highlighted, where they serve to illuminate the workings of the helping alliance. Aspects of countertransference are woven throughout this examination of psychotherapy under the threat of suicide. A more explicit elaboration of salient countertransference issues concludes this chapter.

HISTORICAL PERSPECTIVE

There is no grand unified theory of suicidality. Over the years, many loosely coupled variables have been examined and correlated with suicide rates: age, sex, marital status, religion, nationality, cultural and economic background, occupation, family history, medical and psychiatric histories, season, climate, and rural in contrast to urban living conditions (see Buda and Tsuang, Chapter 2, this volume). Complementing this list of external conditions of the individual, there is an even lengthier accounting of possible internal dynamics that predispose to suicide (see Adam, Chapter 3, this volume). Abraham (1924) and Freud (1957) emphasized the turning of aggression onto the internalized lost object. Klein (1975) attributed self-destructiveness to an elaboration of primitive persecutory fantasies in which the motive for suicide is ridding one's self of bad objects, at the same time protecting and preserving the good. For Horney (1950), suicide was the result of painful awareness of the gulf between idealized and actual self, or a final burst of rage from previously self-effacing individuals, or, lastly, the ultimate fate of those resigned mortals who, in their search for freedom from conflict, become so detached and isolated that life is no longer felt to be worth living. Menninger (1938) articulated his well-known triad: suicide expresses the wish to kill, the wish to be killed, and the wish to die. Sullivan (1956) and others observed motivations of punishing others, hopes of rebirth, dreams of reunion with loved ones, and desperate attempts to ward off the dangers of psychosis or of murder.

More recently, Kernberg (1984) identified three types of self-destructive patients: those who attempt to reestablish control over a chaotic inner world, those whose narcissism impels them to proclaim superiority over death or triumph over their therapist, and those laboring under bizarre psychotic fantasies or impelled to suicide by the urgings of auditory hallucinations. Finally, Kohut (1978) drew attention to the expression of narcissistic rage and the intolerance to feelings of shame that figure largely in the self-destructiveness of severely disturbed patients. Augmenting these dynamics is the loss of narcissistic cathexis of the self as a whole, or of parts of the body-self, that would otherwise serve as a buffer against self-directed rage.

There have also been attempts to tease out a genetic basis for suicidality (see Kety, Chapter 5, this volume; Ranier 1984) and to determine what disturbances in neurochemical balance may have significance for self-destructiveness (see Winchel et al., Chapter 4, this volume; van Praag et al. 1986). Despite all these varied theoretical considerations, the key to the *deterrence* of suicide is more clearly apparent in the sociological studies that have followed since the time of Durkheim's (1897/1951) significant work. Implicitly or explicitly, the importance of interpersonal connectedness comes to the fore. Durkheim emphasized that the degree of integration of the individual with society, the connectedness with others, was directly correlated with the unlikelihood of suicide. He was also aware of oppressive connections, so that he could distinguish those situations where relatedness entails the loss of a helping relationship, and the individual self feels so depleted or enslaved that suicide is the result. Later investigators such as Henry and Short (1986) and Gibbs and Martin (1964) directed attention to the importance of the narcissistic parameters of connectedness: they addressed considerations of status and the significance of transients in status determination for vulnerability to suicide. Other writers stressed the importance of social isolation as perhaps the most telling variable in studying suicide in school-age and college-age populations (Reece 1967; Seiden 1966). Sociologists have also proposed that the lower rates of completed suicide among women may reflect their inclination to put greater value on making and sustaining relationships. In this light, the higher incidence of women among suicide attempters may be testimony to the relationship-seeking nature of many such attempts.

The essence of this interpersonal component in the prevention of suicide was lyrically expressed by John Davidson (Peterson 1972) before Durkheim's (1897/1951) work appeared:

But now that refuge of despair is shut
For other lives have twined themselves with mine.

ALLIANCE AND COUNTERALLIANCE

Thirty years ago, in a small private psychiatric hospital north of Boston, a young man was admitted in the throes of an acute psychosis that had developed during a trip with his family to Malaya. Along with auditory hallucinations, he was deluded that he would melt into a pool of water if he dared to urinate. His physician sat with him, relatively helpless to engage in any continuous dialogue. Then, somewhere out of this morass of mutual despair, the thought emerged and was expressed that what the patient needed most was an ally. The acute psychosis ultimately abated, and the young man went on to pass through subsequent episodes of schizoaffective psychosis, of mania and depression, of hypochondriasis, and finally of bouts of alcoholism, until he finally was able to manage a fairly trouble-free and steady existence, working as a respected and valued counselor at an alcoholism clinic. In one of his recent letters to the therapist of 30 years ago, he expressed his gratitude for the one saving recollection he had of that earlier troubled time: the acknowledgment of both his worth and his plight in the observed need for an ally, which had registered through the confusion of his psychosis, and stayed with him during difficult years.

Human connectedness assumes most critical importance when the issue of suicide is under consideration. Even therapists who have had none or few suicides in their clinical experience have had frequent encounters with individuals who, in misery and great distress, are dissuaded from ending their lives only by thoughts of those children, parents, and friends with whom they are positively bonded. Another testimony to the efficacy of relatedness in thwarting suicidal intent can be found implicitly in Thomas Browne's observation that it is not in the power of the strongest to deprive us of death; it is our own ambivalence that deters—and the positive side of that ambivalence is most often supported by connection to others and not by self-love alone (Browne 1928).

Professionalism enters with the attempt to clarify, discriminate, and understand the cognitive, affective, and dynamic aspects of these helping relationships. They partake of both the merging and oppositional aspects of the ego, but are more truly congruent with what is genuinely autonomous. Suicidal patients can be temporarily rescued from peril by positive and even negative transferences that arise with varying swiftness in the course of therapy. As these intensify, or dissolve, or meet with frustration, the strength and sturdiness of the underlying therapeutic alliance—the helping alliance—carries the day and makes the difference between success or disaster in treatment.

The therapeutic alliance is a bonding between that healthy core of ego that resides in all patients, no matter how sick or despairing, and the engaged helping ego of the therapist. In the patient's co-alliance there is a wish to cope with self and the external world, a wish to grow that has its origins in earliest childhood, and some modicum of hope that is the residual of past positive experiences. On the therapist's side, what we may term the counteralliance (Kahn 1982a, 1982b, 1984) is compounded of sound technical and theoretical knowledge, affective flexibility, and the ability to allow the patient to impact on the therapist, and remain neutral to pathology while responsive and caring to the person. The counteralliance is seasoned by experience, which makes the efforts of those younger clinicians who are most often confronted with suicide even more paradoxically challenging. But if not so born, one can learn to become a "menschenkenner" if cognitive confusion can be tolerated and human pain shared and endured.

The feelings of helplessness and hopelessness that are common to many at a suicidal impasse reflect not only a sense of failure in self-reliance but a lack of faith that one can rely on others. A person's first ally is a parental figure, whose positive and involved attitude is hopefully (in the fullest sense) internalized. The first helplessness is not a failure of self-reliance, but of the trust that one can rely on another. It is not uncommon to find oneself tending unconsciously to replicate poor early caring by slipping into an attitude of distanced, attenuated concern for a patient. Recognizing this as a countertransference phenomenon and not simply a realistic response to the unpleasant or "boring" aspects of the patient illuminates an entire field of therapeutic work. To the extent that therapists idealize their own parents, or hold parents above serious reproach, a blind spot exists that is hazardous to treatment. On the other hand, clarifying such countertransference responses and appropriate communication of the dynamic issues involved to the patient is one of the most powerful methods that, in dissolving a transference, builds and fortifies a genuine alliance.

Direct alliance-building help is also given in therapy by clarifying the behavior of others for the patient. A middle-aged man, driven to desperation by the flirtation of his wife with a teenage boy, felt significant relief when the actually psychotic nature of her behavior was translated for him. He could see her own need for help behind what had seemed to him to be only rejecting vengefulness. Nothing defuses rage as effectively as a new perspective.

Patients need to feel that the therapist is on their side. There are patients who, after a difficult, torturous course of therapy, can account for the salutary outcome only by observing that no matter what, they felt the therapist was on their side. One must always be alert in the therapeutic process to the subtle underminings that are not infrequently perpetrated on children under the guise of "special" care and concern: such as the boy who was allowed to mark up and deface the walls of his own room, because he was "creative," while his sisters were enjoined against such destructive activity. His later self-harming behavior was a shock to his parents, who innocently believed they could in no way have contributed so directly to his pathology, who believed that they had always been devoted to his best interests.

A much deeper aspect of the problem of "side taking" probably has its roots in evolutionary biological forces. Just as the species could not well survive if there were not strong forces opposed to destroying the young—identification with one's babies and displacement of aggression outward from the family—so there is a deep inhibition in all against unbridled aggression toward the mother. Unhappy children whine, or act overtly self-destructive, rather than bite or otherwise attack the mother. They learn early to take *her* side instead of their own. Many individuals grow up with the general expectation that no one really would be on their side and can gain strength only by their devoted affiliation with others. In any dispute, they are invariably the losers, since it is always two against one: themselves and the other allied against themselves. One malignant example of this is in the high suicide rate among those Vietnam veterans who are so committed to their comrades who were killed that they feel no right to be survivors. By way of contrast, manipulators are frequently people who feel that only by emotional fascism can they force anyone to side with their interests even temporarily.

The fine structure of establishing therapeutic rapport requires attention to how the communications of the therapist are received by the patient. Hungry individuals may be so starved for good feeding that they swallow anything that is told them; others are so fearful of malign influence that they nod assent while ignoring and rejecting any ideas that are different from their own, unable to take in the sweet or nourishing that the therapist offers and separate it from the chaff. Many, for whom all relationships are competitive, are constantly assessing who is smarter, who is superior, and are unable to conceive that there is such a thing as "time out" when competitors put aside their rivalry to share refreshment. For such, alliance means only humiliation or triumph. It can be of value to ask directly who, in the patient's past—a relative, neighbor, teacher, camp counselor, friend —has been helpful or perceived as an ally. Any preexistent models for a helping relationship are worthy of reawakening. For many individuals, none exist.

COMMON DYNAMIC ISSUES: ENVY AND RIVALRY

These finer issues in establishing working alliances illuminate problems that are central to the common dynamics of many suicidal individuals and that are relevant in all matters pertaining to self-esteem and object relations. Reviewing some of these basic aspects of human pathology has the same value as repeated practice of a Bach two-part invention: it ensures a more deft therapeutic touch and helps one from getting lost in the more difficult passages.

The affective conditions associated with suicide that are most amenable to ordinary psychotherapeutic intervention are depression and, to a lesser extent, anxiety and panic states. The simple clarification of diagnosis in these instances can itself be helpful to the extent that the patient feels heard and understood. In depression associated with patent loss or defeat, the path of therapy has a natural course, so much so that even laypersons can be of great assistance to friends bereaved or confronted with failure. A higher level of sophistication can discern another frame of reference contributing to malignancy in depression and phobia: beneath both, sustaining and contributing to them, are the disposition to envy, the disposition to rivalry, and the blending of both of these that constitutes jealousy.

Some degree of envy and jealousy resides in all of us, and in small doses they act as the salt and pepper of life, giving tang and impetus to our existence. We can in this respect cite the preacher of Ecclesiastes: "I see that all effort and all achievement spring from men's mutual jealousy." In larger amounts, however, envy and jealousy make life unpalatable. They produce only misery.

When troublesome envy and rivalry can be identified, clarified, and appropriately confronted, the patient's ego has an intrapsychic issue that is almost always experienced as dystonic, as a problem and challenge to be worked through. While it is customary and appropriate to maintain an open mind about the dynamics of each new patient, scientific objectivity does not mean a posture of assumed ignorance. It can be hazardous to feel one has the leisure to let all dynamics slowly unfold and use assumed ignorance as a pretext for aloofness in therapy. More timely intervention and confrontation can provide the patient not only with the feeling of being more deeply understood but also with the hope that there are solutions that have not yet been considered. In this regard, alertness to hints of these underlying issues can open the way for swifter appropriate intervention and a more certain therapeutic engagement.

Envy and rivalry are *prima facie* narcissistic affects. Their intensity and power are in inverse proportion to autonomous ego and its prime affect of objective curiosity. Both are testimony to an ego not satisfied with itself, unformed, wanting more structure. Envy arises out of abandonment and has within it the wish to be someone other than who one is, to enhance worth by affiliation and attachment, if not by outright fusion with someone else. It tends toward the illusory recreation of the original idealized mother-child unit, where all is supposedly free of conflict. Like all illusions, this is compounded of fragments of reality—those early times that were indeed blissful—and intense wishful distortion that one can regain this state. The illusion is supported by aspects of current reality that are to a degree congruent with it. For example, the appearance of freedom from conflict assumed and envied in the rich, the beautiful, or the famous. Many seemingly crazy love affairs are supported by the illusion that the loved man or woman, in that person's apparent freedom and vitality, is free of guilt and that this absolution will be granted to the lover entwined with him or her. On a larger social scale, some cults offer this same false promise that salvation is to be had on earth by devotion to a charismatic leader. When such bondings are made, the weak self tries to draw strength and identity from fusing with another. When the bondings are threatened, the pain of illusory loss of self can be so great that suicide is the outcome—in a religious colony in Guyana, or in an Elvira Madigan adolescent love affair. Knowing that the lover is envied in this latter kind of love relationship can be of vital importance in easing the pain of its loss and resolution. Knowing that beneath all is an attempt to avoid conflict opens the possibility of facing the growing ego with the challenge of psychological weightlifting: of bearing and coping with greater degrees of conflict, rather than seeking illusory escape in a weightless world.

Rivalry, like envy, seeks to define the self, but by oppositional rather than affiliative means. That it is part of narcissism is apparent in its black-and-white character: one triumphs and erases the rival, or is faced with total defeat and nothingness. Just as envy unrequited by bonding leads to overvaluation of the envied object, and corresponding devaluation of the self, rivalry feels that the self cannot exist if the other has any existence at all. Both affects tamper with reality; both do not recognize limitation, time, or growth. To the extent that the clinician is dealing with an immature ego in a suicidal patient, it is essential to understand that these are the considerations that frame the patient's world, and that they derive a reality sense from having indeed been true in infancy.

The feelings of worthlessness so rife in suicidal persons are too often attributed principally to past conditions of rejection and unlove. Herein may lie a poor reality-sense of the therapist. Not having mastered issues of envy, rivalry, and jealousy is, in fact, a good reason to feel inferior: it *is* inferior, insofar as the mass of relatively well-functioning individuals, who can maintain friendships and bear the onerous conditions that any employment entails, must have come to better terms with these matters. Paradoxically, it is enormously reassuring to some despairing individuals to acknowledge that they are indeed inferior in a way, but have a task before them that, if others have been able to deal with, they can too. Every individual has to learn to play the cards dealt, even if deficient in face cards and honors: enviously ogling what others may possess accomplishes little, and upsetting the card table is still avoiding the game.

In this respect it is well to bear in mind the desirable evolution of envy and rivalry toward true love and viable competition. The affiliative vector moves toward finding the good in lovers and competitors. The oppositional moves toward joy in the difference between man and woman, discrimination in relationships with others, and appreciation and respect for one's colleagues. One comes to live in a world where perhaps reality is colored by emotion, rather than a more purely emotional world lightly tinted by realistic considerations.

AUTONOMY

At this point we may review those criteria that distinguish the autonomous ego from the symbiotic. It is advantageous to underline the goal that one strives for in all therapies: a self-reliant, reality-oriented ego. But most especially is this so when suicide looms as a possibility. A firm sense of autonomy helps direct the therapist to what is healthy in the patient and to maintain an appropriate perspective of the therapist's role, with all its limitations, in the process that unfolds. It is just this sense of limitation and proportion that is most at variance with the narcissistic and symbiotic parts of the self that recognize no boundaries and see all interaction in all-or-nothing, black-and-white terms. What are felonies for the immature ego are often parking violations for the adult self.

The therapist requires a fine sense of what a patient can bear to determine when to hazard outpatient treatment or when hospitalization is necessary. One needs an awareness of when his or her limits are taxed, and consultation is required. The clinician must always be alert to unrealistic hopes of rescue and unrealistic self-condemnation when conscientious and well-informed efforts are to no avail.

The autonomous ego also has a realistic sense and understands that all acute distress has its season, that the deepest grief and most intense rages abate. We strive to allow considered reflection to play its part in the patient's suicidal deliberations. A middle-aged woman who was partially dissuaded from killing herself when she heard she had terminal lung cancer, was later grateful that, because of an unsuccessful attempt, she had an opportunity to say goodbye to her children, parents, and friends, and die with more dignity. An enormously decent man, dying of acquired immune deficiency syndrome, had made his goodbyes. In his last therapy hour he expressed the wish to be able to walk alone down a beach in New England that he loved, unaccompanied by the usual relatives who were there to support him should he stagger and fall in the water. When this idea of suicide was gently questioned, he reminded himself of his daughter, and his unwillingness to leave her with an even greater burden than she already had. He died peacefully a week later.

The therapist's autonomous ego has the strength to bear pain. It does not need to shut off dismaying or frightening communication prematurely. It does not find pseudo-strength in recourse to moralistic pronouncements when patients disclose truly unsavory aspects of themselves—their nastiness, meanness, sadism, hurtfulness, vindictiveness. It is an aspect of autonomy to tolerate the patient's inherently self-destructive wishes for revenge. The therapist may remind the patient that if revenge they must, they could attempt it with more discrimination and reflection than can be found in the ordinary, impulse-ridden case. The clinician's posture of autonomy toward human ugliness is that of the scientist with curiosity toward emotional puzzles, rather than that of the moralist making easy condemnations. When therapists lapse into moralistic attitudes, they may at times betray their own symbiotic need to enhance their self-esteem at the expense of another's. To the extent that the therapist mistrusts his or her own rage, or hate, or anger, there is pressure to externalize on the patient, where one can always find a ready nidus of reality. Therapeutic judgment is thus compromised. Suicide may appear a danger when none exists, or actual peril may be denied. The ability of the autonomous ego to tolerate appropriate regression in the service of reading another's emotional reality is one of the most vital tools in any therapy.

Autonomy can relate in an appropriate way. It can engage in truly helpful partnerships. Part of the binding forces in these relationships are mutually shared values. In this respect, the therapist need feel no hesitancy to express to the patient a bias on the side of life, questioning the value of suicide, and a devotion to the work of problem solving, which requires more of the self than the simplistic considerations of the patient's narcissistic ego may care to entertain. At the same time, different views and contrary attitudes of the patient must be respected. The clinician need not, in the face of frustration, regress to what Glover (1955) aptly characterized as the despairing therapist's equivalent of the highwayman's formula: "Your cooperation, or your life!"

Autonomy makes use of both head and heart. Derivatives from the symbiotic aspects of the self find their way into the mature self, wedded to intellect in the form of intuition and to affect in the form of empathy. But intuition and empathy cannot be regarded as ends in themselves—alone, they have never saved anyone. Intuition and empathy are the therapist's *tools*, to be employed in the process of engaging, understanding, and conveying valuable perspective and strength to the patient.

NARCISSISTIC INJURY

Most significant for present considerations is the response of the autonomous ego to loss and to injury to its healthy self-esteem. Instead of simple rage and helplessness, a gamut of responses are available: moderated disappointment, anger, tolerable guilt, disgust, a wish to understand, and, most important of all, genuine grief and sadness, which is so hard for the narcissistic ego to endure. Having experienced genuine comforting in the past, the autonomous ego tries to comfort itself. Therapists who meet repeated frustration in attempting to comfort their patients in pain forget that comfort must first come from the self to itself, in true compassion (which is not quite the same as feeling sorry for oneself). Yet patients who hate themselves for their own self-pity need to be reminded that any sustained comfort can come only from themselves, to their own self. Much hate that leads to suicidal ideas stems from the inability of people to forgive themselves for having cared and having made themselves vulnerable. The mature ego can risk injury and acknowledge its own mortality. It is capable of genuinely caring for another for who they really are, with limitations and failings. To an extent, one must learn to submit graciously to be another's victim if one is to have any enduring relationships at all. Bearing grief and being able to mourn is synonymous with digesting reality, coming to terms with it, returning after a loss to resume life in it. The adult ego seeks restitution, but may ultimately have to settle for being sadder and, hopefully, wiser.

When disappointment threatens an envious bond, or dissatisfaction a rivalrous one, very different dynamics are observed. The disruption takes place within a self-object system and not simply between two separate, although related, individuals. The trauma is experienced internally as well as externally. Because of this, the pain of narcissistic injury is always greater. The feeling that part of the self is lost or damaged, perhaps beyond retrieval or repair, makes matters more desperate. It may seem easier to eliminate a damaged ego as not worthy of rescue than bear the full measure of grief that looms in the background. Many unhappy love relationships owe their persistence to this need to avoid the full depth of disappointment in the other, and consequent loss of hope for an ideal in the other and in the self.

Undisturbed, the attachment between symbiotically bound individuals may appear tranquil. With stress, and a moving apart consequent to actual or threatened separation, the narcissistic affects spring into view, much as the lines of force between two magnets sprinkled with iron filings. Envy and jealousy are object-seeking affects, as Modell (1980) has observed, and are most energetically present when the object system is transiently disturbed. Once more included in the orbit of the envied person, the envier is tranquil. Having reestablished the position of favorite, the jealous person is more at peace. Assured of some fairly defined status in a competitive hierarchy, the rivalrous person more easily tolerates his or her position.

Should events proceed in a contrary manner, there is a further breakdown of integrity, and specific urges arise with great force. Envious bonds disturbed by disappointment and by loss give rise to intense hunger, to strong oral cravings that may be expressed directly as such or find their way into greedy desire for material objects or insatiable sexual activity. It is as if the self, in feeling part of its soul-substance missing, must thrash about to replenish the loss. A more benign and common example of this is in the enhanced appetite so commonly experienced after funerals. Some despairing patients, unable to take sustained comfort from anything the therapist says, are able to relax and take heart when the simple matter of their longing for a real feeding is clarified. In others, orality laced with destructiveness finds expression in all manner of lethal ingestions and poisonings.

Rivalrous and jealous bonds that are broken are succeeded by blind rage and hate. The oppositional origin of these feelings is frequently evidenced in powerful defiance: defiance of reason, of kindly intervention, of all attempts at helpfulness. This is particularly so in adolescence. Injured persons feel as if they are asked to "say uncle" in a mortal wrestling match. They would just as soon destroy themselves along with others than submit to what is felt to be intolerable humiliation. Again, identifying defiance as such, and respecting it while acknowledging the pain of actual humiliation, returns to the patient a small but vital atom of self-possession.

Hate, like love, is a compound of fusing and oppositional forces. But in hate, the oppositional wish is to erase and destroy utterly. The mangled affiliative wish is to bind oneself to another by sadism and hurting: as if the only path open to have the satisfaction that one's life matters, that one has not been diminished to nothingness, is by the infliction of pain. This is akin to vengefulness and might be seen as a degenerate form of an appeal to empathy. The patient attempts to reconstitute the original entity by making both parties equally miserable, and so united in the company that misery is supposed to enjoy (Kahn 1984). Hate must be called by its true name. Too often it is euphemistically softened in description and spoken of as anger. It is qualitatively not the same. Anger can still see the good in the object; hate looks for and finds the evil. When a patient feels that *hate* is a strong word to use, it is often because the patient has not given him-

or herself permission to recognize the affect and disposition as such, and to this extent kept it hidden, submerged, and dangerous.

The problem of destructiveness directed at an internalized object enters at this point. First elucidated by Abraham (1924) and Freud (1957), and given more sophisticated formulation in the self-psychology of Kohut (1978), it finds its anlage in the general tendency to direct negative feelings toward the self from earliest infancy. Winnicott's (1965) observations about the salutary influence of the mother who can tolerate overt aggression from the child have more forceful significance in this regard in that she not only presents the child with a model of bearing strong feelings but helps to deter the course of aggression from turning back onto the child itself. One must not be deceived by the vigorous expression of rage toward others as an indication that the patient is unlikely to turn it against the self. The first release may be transitory, and hate nursed toward others is ultimately hate nursed toward the self, if only in its implication that one cannot heal or surmount insult, but remains an injured party. The self-object is precisely self and object; hate directed at either side ultimately includes the other, and intolerance of some externally perceived qualities of other people too often entails intolerance to the same hidden within us. In some individuals, rage can be clearly seen as directed toward an internalized parent. More subtly, it finds direction toward aspects of the parent hidden in the superego, which, gaining force from the sadism of the superego, sets the stage for truly dangerous internal warfare.

Pathological guilt betrays its narcissistic origin in its grandiose assumption of blame, in its unrelenting punishment, in its unwillingness to be appeased by contrition, appropriate restitution, or undoing. It demands total and sadistic abasement of the self as all bad. This "self" may at times have significant characteristics of a disappointing parent; it may at the same time be an exaggerated image of the patient as a "selfish" child needing punishment. Alcohol is frequently the patient's drug of choice in attempting to relieve this burden. The internal pain already existing makes the patient entirely incapable of bearing fresh external disapproval or criticism; yet the tendency to externalize the conflict leads the patient to seek and find such negative attitudes everywhere and to assume they exist behind kinder words to the contrary. The only release may seem to be that of self-destruction. It is well to contrast this state of affairs with that of the integrated ego that can bear the affect of guilt, is less prone to good and bad judgments, and finds no need to blame or to moralize to maintain balance. The autonomous ego can assume appropriate responsibility, with fuller awareness of its own limitations and culpability. It treats the gulf between standards and reality with understanding. Too often patients feel their therapists are trying to seduce them away from good values, and miss the point that a lenient judge abides by the same laws as a hanging one: the sentence is what counts.

A less malignant form of the tendency to absorb hate can be found in those individuals who are so reminiscent of paintings of the martyred St. Sebastian, with varying quantities of arrows imbedded in his flesh. They are the "injured parties" who make up a large share of those manipulative individuals who threaten or make suicidal gestures. Nursing injury, they find it hard to love, and in themselves are not entirely lovable. They acquire thorns rather than beauty from the roses and never seem to be inclined to remove these thorns so that they might return to more productive pursuits. There is a curious aspect of these individuals, stranded between symbiosis and autonomy, that clearly betrays the self-object aspect of their relationships. They feel their pain always to be the responsibility of another, instead of recognizing that no matter how or where inflicted, it is now *their* pain, for them to process and work through. Blame, which is the inverse of envy, is always in conflict with autonomy.

The extreme of the masochistic position, of the reversal from hate directed toward others to the invitation of precisely the same toward the self, needs always to be kept in mind when treating suicidal individuals. This was well described by Asch (1980). It is the invitation to become the patient's executioner, to be the patient's accomplice in destruction. The need to bond with another seeks fulfillment in a mortal embrace. It is not uncommon in treating children with self-destructive tendencies to find parental behavior that clearly has this quality of collusion. Rosenn (1982) cited, for example, a 9-year-old who was given the board game "Hangman" a few months after he had tried to strangle himself, and the father of a premed college student who gave a copy of the *Physicians' Desk Reference* to his son after several nonlethal overdoses. The seduction of the therapist toward a similar pathological alliance may contain the wish to recreate such an earlier dynamic setting with a parent. This danger must certainly be kept in mind when supervising medication for potentially suicidal individuals. Similarly, manipulative threateners of suicide and stubbornly resistant depressed patients are likely to arouse the conscious, hateful wish that they go ahead and kill themselves. Those hungry for warmth may seek it out in the angry heat of those helpers they frustrate and offend.

Finally, one must give consideration to the defensive uses of hate, which become more amenable to interpretation when the directly responsive and the immediately self-satisfying aspects have been attenuated. The pleasure in hating must be given its full due before anyone nourishing it can consider giving it up. Hate blocks all true grief. It is antipathetic to the kindness and tenderness that are part of grief. It erases all memory of what lost good might be worth mourning, both in the other and in the self. Curiously, we are sad when our own goodness finds confirmation: a sense of worth both precedes and derives from grieving. Inability to bear and cope with grief is per se a variety of inferiority. Instead, too many patients experience sadness as a weakness to be ashamed of, rather than a strength signifying that reality has been accepted, digested, and integrated with one's experience. The hate of these patients may have an almost somatic quality, and they resist letting it go as they would resist feeling castrated, weakened, and undone. When true grief and sadness appear in the therapeutic process, the danger of suicide is significantly lessened.

In some psychotic individuals, many of these dynamic constellations of suicide can be discerned in the symbolic meaning of their irrational and deluded thinking. Menninger's (1938) emphasis on the symbolism of suicidal acts finds valuable application here. A young man who, over the course of a few years, had lost both parents, a brother, and a sister to cancer, heart disease, and accident heard voices telling him repeatedly to kill himself. Contact with others was painful, aggravating his feelings of estrangement and envious loneliness. He tried to deny all feelings—indeed, he was for the most part numb—and instead complained of the "toxins" that were building up inside of him. If he listened to the voices, he would simply take an overdose of medication and end his tormented existence. With a sardonic laugh, he would relish the thought of competitive triumph over the therapist that killing himself would mean and was deterred only by the reflection that he would not be around to savor it. His own theory of cure was that he needed to cut his arms to let the toxic blood out, and he practiced this repeatedly. In time, with a kind of distorted poetry, he came to a formulation that since his parents had made his heart bleed for them, by not caring for him and by leaving him, he would revenge himself on these "arms" that should have cradled and supported him by slicing up his own. As the affective meaning of his thinking and behavior was repeatedly translated for him, he began to show the first traces of tearfulness, and the threat of suicide palpably abated.

Many of these considerations concerning the breakdown in the integrity of the self have been succinctly described in a much earlier publication (Shakespeare's *Troilus and Cressida*):

> *Ulysses:* Take but degree away, untune that string,
>   And hark what discord follows! Each thing meets
>   In mere oppugnancy. The bounded waters
>   Should lift their bosoms higher than the shores
>   And make a sop of all this solid globe.

> Strength should be lord of imbecility,
> And the rude son should strike his father dead.
> Force should be right; or rather, right and wrong,
> Between whose endless jar justice resides,
> Should lose their names, and so should justice too.
> Then everything includes itself in power,
> Power into will, will into appetite;
> And appetite, an universal wolf,
> So doubly seconded with will and power,
> Must make perforce an universal prey,
> And last eat up himself. (I.iii)

Translate "degree" as the structure of normal social usages, and "bounded waters" as rage: self-destructive regression, with all its consequences, is perfectly described.

THE THERAPEUTIC ALLIANCE ACROSS THE LIFE CYCLE

Childhood

The concept of alliance is of special value in confronting the problem of suicide as it presents at different stages in the life cycle. It is readily apparent that any alliance with children can at best only be partial and that appropriate engagement of the family is essential. This is particularly the case insofar as almost all threats of suicide in childhood are found in the context of severe family pathology. Chaotic fighting, abuse of children and spouses, and/or threatened loss or collapse of the family as an entity are the common background for life-threatening behavior in children before adolescence. The parents need to be enlisted in the therapeutic process more than at any other time and clearly need ancillary help for their own troubles. Family as well as individual therapy for the child is almost always indicated.

Once assessed, it is particularly important to emphasize the real danger of suicide not only to the parents but to those immediately concerned with the child's welfare. Frequently, the tendency to idealize childhood persists to the extent that the danger is not sensed as real. Many laypersons cannot believe that all children have an intense curiosity about death and are well aware of its meaning from the age of 3 years on. The child may theorize that it is reversible, or wonder about the possibilities of an afterlife or rebirth, but the underlying concept of erasure and nothingness is always there. The child's longing for fusion finds satisfaction in ideas of reunion with loved ones after death and possible rebirth from this joining by coming alive again in new or happily altered form. But the ever-present oppositional side of narcissism gives strength to black-and-white divisions of good and bad selves, good and bad mothers. Too often the preservation of the good entails elimination of the bad. In this childish frame of reference, the wish to escape from intolerable conflict may find its way into a longing for the imagined peacefulness of death. The wish may be simply to die or may be coupled with the intent to preserve and protect the "good parent" by removing the "bad" self.

It is also common to find that suicide as a solution to problems is part of the family's world view, if not also part of its history. Manipulative suicidal threats by parents raise terror in the child. It can be perilous to assume that even healthy-appearing parents share the same attitudes toward suicide as the therapist, and exploration of this area must not be overlooked.

When the reliability of the parents is in question, and the child presents with a history of repeated near-fatal episodes, hospitalization is not only essential but may be the only means of conveying to both child and parent that they are being taken seriously and that there is real weight behind the words of the helpers. A crucial element of autonomy has bearing here. The use made of language develops alongside the growth of the ego. The first bondings made by the child are concurrent with language used as a manipulative tool. Words are stimuli that produce responses in important others. Only as separation and individuation progress does language come into its mature use, to convey what goes on inside one self to another, different self. Along the way, it may even be necessary to use language falsely, to lie, to be able to assure that one has secrets, to guarantee a sense of privacy. Individuals of envious, jealous, and rivalrous dispositions betray their immaturity in their readiness to use words for manipulative purposes; to enhance self-esteem by making others feel low, guilty, or needy; and to achieve a sense of power over others that diminishes their own sense of weakness. This is in contrast to the more give-and-take negotiating use of language that reflects a more mature ego. To the extent that parents are given to manipulative modes of communication, especially in their dealings with children, they may expect the same behavior toward themselves. These parents may be ready to discount warnings of danger to their children as simply attempts by the therapist to make them feel guilty, or to maneuver them contrary to their own inclinations. In some instances this is, of course, precisely the case. Better to call the situation with firmness and clarity than try to outmanipulate a manipulative parent.

Adolescence

The usage of language in establishing the rapport necessary for a working alliance is nowhere more crucial than in adolescence. Here the real personality of the therapist enters more significantly into the therapeutic equation. If the therapist cannot join with the adolescent in a mutuality of understanding, there is little hope of even a tenuous alliance. This does not mean speaking down to the patient or attempting to use adolescent jargon when it does not come naturally; it does mean avoiding didactic, pedantic, and moralizing postures. It means a lively awareness that the issues of envy, competition, jealousy, and rivalry are inflamed at this time of life, with all their associated confusion about identity, engagement, and withdrawal.

Intense envy, tinged by orality, can be mistaken by the self for evidence of homosexuality. Every fall, a parade of freshmen troop through college mental health centers to express their fears about their sexual identity. They need reassurance that theories about homosexuality deserve discussion, but have a different psychic structure than homosexuality itself.

One must always be alert to perverse twists of sexuality in the experimental adventurousness of adolescents. It is not uncommon for boys to flirt with partial asphyxiation by hanging themselves while masturbating to enhance their pleasure. Needless to say, the result is sometimes fatal.

Adolescents are also likely to form quite pathological "helping" alliances when in trouble. At a group meeting of relatives and friends of a young sophomore who had killed herself, convened to help clarify what had happened and to share grief, a roommate disclosed, with a sweet smile, that no one need feel really sorry for the dead girl. She was probably somewhere else, in a reborn state. The roommate had counseled her friend that suicide was a perfectly acceptable way out of her problems and would give her a fresh chance in life. The therapist had no inkling of these conversations, most probably because the girl had felt a need to protect the roommate. While not sufficient in themselves to have motivated suicide, the talks certainly contributed to the final outcome.

Adolescents are prone to gamble with fate, to take chances in Russian roulette, or wild driving, where they literally court disaster: as if an anthropomorphic Lady Luck must be challenged to either smile, or carry one out of existence. One triumphs in wresting hope from danger, or succumbs to nothingness.

Overt cruelty among peers, invidious comparisons, and mocking and ridicule are only some of the daily adversarial stresses adolescents endure. Seduction to drug and alcohol use, guilt-provoking delinquent behavior, and confusing sexual adventures distort the affiliative side of relationships. The therapist is often called on to be able to make fine discriminations in potentially dangerous situations. When does passionate defiance verge on suicidal heedlessness of reality? When is it a precursor of true independence, an overstated wish to attain autonomy? Some patients, adolescent or otherwise, may be drawn to dangerous situations in a counterphobic manner during the course of therapy. A young man who had always been troubled with separation anxiety decided to venture on skydiving as his confidence improved. While the possibility of suicidal intent might validly be explored, true alliance in this case meant recognition of the courageous aspects of the adventure, and a bit of therapeutic breath-holding. Similarly, it is important to recognize the different significance thoughts of death and dying have when they appear toward the conclusion of therapy, with patients of any age. Although occasionally of a threatening nature, they more often signal the wish to let go of an old part of the self, to say goodbye to the outworn hurt child inside, and an acceptance of limitation and mortality.

Adulthood

Among adults, special note must be taken of alcoholic patients, who have such striking representation among the diagnostic categories of completed suicides (see Flavin et al., Chapter 8, this volume). Alliance with an alcoholic patient is often tenuous, if not outright false. Just as some individuals do indeed present false selves to the world, some selves make false alliances. Lying and deception are common and not anticipated by those therapists whose work is principally with nonalcoholic populations. It would seem that for these people the only possible therapeutically significant alliance is that with a group whose members have a generally similar background, bound together by common experience and an explicit statement of conscious values to be shared. This is Alcoholics Anonymous (AA). Enlisting the aid of groups such as AA, or Narcotics Anonymous for addicted patients, is a sign of realistic good sense rather than defeat of the therapist.

On the other side of less than ideal dyadic alliances, it may be necessary to compromise strict confidentiality in the interests of containing suicidal danger. It may be important to have spouses or parents remove guns and potentially lethal medication from the environment of the patient. This is best accomplished by direct confrontation with the concerned individuals and firm insistence that no one in the patient's world is to facilitate or be an accomplice in disaster. Particular caution must be exercised with patients of high social or professional status, who may be accorded misguided respect for their privacy that allows them to jump from windows or to overdose.

Middle Age

Middle age is a unique time for both experiencing and delivering emotional hurt. Long dormant conflicts with parents are reawakened as mothers and fathers fall ill, become infirm, or pass away. Disappointments and dissatisfactions with spouses and children multiply and gather force. Because of the accumulation of defeats and failures in any middle-aged individual, their own feelings of relative worthlessness or inadequacy may blind them to the continuing emotional weight they carry with those close to them. Too often these primary relationships are betrayed or abandoned by those who convince themselves that there will be easily reparable emotional consequences. Other individuals, in a denial of feelings of weakness and mortality, or out of a confidence genuinely born of experience, are tempted to bolder actions, greater risks, and ultimately more serious injury to themselves or those near them. The result may be a resistant, guilt-ridden hangover that stirs thoughts of suicide as the only release. This is not to overlook the hurt and self-destructive responses of spouses and children caught up in such too-common family pathology, or the apathetic reactions of elderly parents, who too willingly welcome death in the face of abandonment by their children.

It is also precisely because of the disillusionment of middle age that establishing a therapeutic alliance depends more on the solid, commonsense understanding communicated to the patient than on the readiness to idealize one's helper or trust in the authority of the therapist, which might in other situations tide one over the initial stages of therapy. Perhaps more than at any other time of life, the means of self-destruction are easily available, and the sense of futility and hopelessness may be augmented by the conviction that real change or amelioration is no longer possible. It can be a time of great peril. The prospect of at least temporary relief from despair may be provided by the clinician's judicious use of pharmacotherapy, or electroconvulsive therapy; but unless a complementary helping alliance is established, the ultimate risk of suicide remains high.

Late Life/Incurable Illness

Persons of advanced age share an important aspect of alliance-making with those who suffer intractable illness: society readily accepts and tries to make available external supports and fosters appropriate dependency. At the same time, both groups are no less vulnerable to feelings of humiliation when such help is crudely offered or administered. A particular danger exists for those elderly individuals laboring under a depression that is mistaken for dementia. The importance of correct differential diagnosis here is not simply to distinguish those who may benefit from treatment from others with a more bleak prognosis. As at other times of life, the danger of suicide rises with depression and may be further aggravated by the many stresses suffered by those who are classified as irreversibly demented.

Similar alertness to suicidal potential must be observed for persons undergoing renal dialysis, for those with temporal lobe epilepsy, and for all individuals who, unlike the majority of us, have been given a clearer idea of when, and how, they will die of a fatal illness.

Finally, with the elderly or the incurably ill, the therapist's counteralliance meets a special stress. In these cases, suicide as a solution to human misery and suffering comes closest to being a rational choice. The therapist's own values, philosophy, and sensitivity to existential issues enter therapeutic deliberations with more conscious force. Insisting on the sanctity of life can at times take on the appearance of cruelty and unfeelingness. Dedication to the relief of pain may be in direct conflict with the value of preserving life. It is at these times that, in the hierarchy of values, understanding and respect for each individual's autonomy must take precedence. Certainly, all considerations must be explored and all consequences elaborated, but it is best to remember, with Job, that

He who wounds is He who soothes the sore,
And the hand that hurts is the hand that heals.

The temptation to play God is best avoided.

COUNTERTRANSFERENCE

While various considerations of countertransference have already been touched on, it may be of value to attempt a more general, unifying perspective of the therapist's less-than-rational responses to patients who challenge him or her with the threat of suicide. Human beings who have not been painfully hurt somewhere along life's way do not ordinarily appear in the consultation room. It is well to bear this in mind at those frequent times that the therapist feels attacked, devalued, overinflated in a hostile manner, threatened, manipulated, hopeless, and helpless in ministrations to the patient. Obnoxious behavior means underlying hurt. The therapist must on frequent occasion actively remind him- or herself of this more basic pain, than be seduced into too directly reflexive responses of withdrawal, disapproval, hostile criticism, or moralistic attack. Soma must be attended to as well as psyche: the simple physical presence of the patient in the consultation room is testimony to at least a rudimentary wish for help, no matter how camouflaged by a wall of words. As a corollary, missed appointments are ominous, notwithstanding ongoing benign verbal communications.

Insofar as the patient is in pain, the patient's first-order attempts at relief may be by either affiliative or oppositional means. In the former instance, the patient will be inclined to idealize the therapist. Anxiety roused by such elevation must be endured, even though it carries with it the implication of increased responsibility for the patient's welfare. While accepting such idealization, the therapist still maintains a clear sense of limitations. This is best contained, rather than too hastily communicated, in a move that relieves the therapist's distress but concomitantly leaves the patient stranded. Some therapists, particularly men, feel uncomfortable when they sense the patient wishes them to be an all-nurturant mother, ill at ease with this attribution of breasts rather than intellect. Others have difficulty with patients who search for a sturdy, powerful father, for fear that such strength may too quickly alter in perception to cruelty.

In general, such transferences must be allowed to develop and gradually to be interpreted. They should not be met with acted-out, complementary countertransference on the therapist's part, which always runs the risk of unnecessarily infantilizing the patient. Too much feeding, guidance, direction, and limit setting may be followed by too much rage when these interventions are withdrawn. It is not a good idea to try to prove that one can indeed be a better mother or father than the patient's parents. But neither is distance at all times in the interest of the patient. The concept of the counteralliance can be of value here, in permitting the therapist those direct interventions of appropriate giving and clarification of boundaries that are often necessary when working with people in great distress. The key is for the therapist to have a clear idea of what pain is in the background and what intervention will help the patient most appropriately deal with it. In many instances one must clarify that the pain is there and must be borne rather than evaded; in others, when it appears that the patient's (and not the therapist's) ego is being overwhelmed, medication must be offered or permission granted to resign gracefully from difficult circumstances, such as overtaxing work or school situations. For most suicidal patients, a position of professional passivity is more hazardous than overzealous intervention.

A special case of stress from affiliative repairs to narcissism occurs with those individuals who are more attracted to the institution that employs the therapist than to the actual therapist. This is not an infrequent situation in psychiatric emergency rooms. Those clinicians treating suicidal patients under these circumstances have both an extra measure of authority and expertise attributed to them as well as not too subtle pressure from invidious comparisons with others in the same working environment. It is best to see the resultant feelings of competitiveness evoked in the therapist as a complementary countertransference to the same sort of deeper issues in the patient. Idealization by the patient may also foster a resonating idealizing response by the therapist, in which the patient is seen as healthier than he or she is, and real danger mutually denied. In these circumstances, the therapist can often sense a current of underlying hostility that is being avoided: there is often a deeper negative transference on both sides, whose derivatives are feared.

Negative Countertransference

Adversarial engagement may similarly be hidden beneath apparent nonbinding by the patient. A therapist who feels erased, and of no consequence to the patient, will not often be wrong in assuming such a deeper dynamic. There may exist a parallel disguised, hidden erasure of the patient's own self-interest, so that only apathy and non-caring are manifest. For many disturbed individuals, or those in inferior or vulnerable circumstances, any binding at all is too close to bondage. It is fought off and opposed, by making the self passively uninteresting or actively distasteful. The therapist's first response to such people may be that of dislike or even repulsion. In these distanced engagements, it is of particular advantage to recall the prime parameter of transference strictly construed: history is being repeated. A lively awareness of this on the therapist's part is perhaps the best insurance against untoward, acted-out countertransference responses of reciprocal withdrawal, retaliatory rejection, or rationalized therapeutic pessimism. Obscure points in the patient's history and behavior should stimulate the curiosity that sustains many difficult therapeutic encounters.

The patient may be unconsciously driven to recreate an early environment of distanced or defective caring and rejection. Old identifications arise in disguised forms on the therapeutic stage, and roles are assigned accordingly. The therapist will be seen as both inadequate parent and unrewarding child, sexual antagonist and rivaled sibling. The drama may be played out through overt competition, threats, and challenges to rescue. Perhaps most difficult to bear are those instances when the piece requires a villain. The attribution of evil to the therapist, some of whose motivations may indeed be derived from reaction formation, is a special stress. With other patients, one must bear some degree of being manipulated. Helpless individuals feel less at a disadvantage if they feel they can have some impact on their therapists. The manipulations themselves have often a transference aspect of needing to wrest care and feeding from others rather than having trust in the processes of negotiation. Threats of suicide must similarly be endured and explored. They are a form of communication and evolve with repetition to disclose previously unsuspected dynamics.

Regression in the Counteralliance

The first sign of rising anger in the therapist may be a loss of patience, an edge of intolerance to the whole process of therapy that creeps into the hour. This impatience may be a harbinger of subsequent more overt anger, hostility, or direct hate. When contained and understood, this is part of all therapy. When instead of clearly seeing the picture, the therapist begins to blend into it, the therapeutic stance is compromised. The counteralliance may be conceived as an integration of several valuable sublimations of cruder urges. With frustration and attack, there is the danger that these sublimations will be undone, with the usual accompaniment of sadistic responses. Appropriate curiosity turns into hostile, intrusive questioning and cross-examination. Or, in apprehension of such a possibility, appropriate exploration is avoided. In the therapist's fearing to be a new hurter, old hurts—such as losses of parents by suicide, or circumstances of previous suicide attempts—are not examined. The therapist's regressive anger may be externalized so that the therapist becomes grossly mistrustful of the patient. The therapist may avoid questions about suicidal thoughts out of fear of making a suggestion or implanting an idea. At the same time, the clinician must recognize realistic fear in the counteralliance. This is a form of signal anxiety that there is indeed acute danger and not an indication of inner inadequacy that asks for denial. Hospitalization should not be avoided out of fear of looking frightened.

The therapist's regressive hostility may appear in the form of too stringent or harshly communicated limit setting. Communications become laced with a hurtful sarcasm where, somewhat like the Cheshire cat, the sneer remains long after the substance has vanished.

One may regard these departures from good technique as manifestations of regressions in the capacity to empathize. A much subtler example of the same is common with elderly and incurably ill patients, in whom there may be frequent conscious thoughts about how much easier things would be if they died. These may enhance the seduction to less than fully committed care. Similarly, the therapist may be tempted to agree subtly with some patients that their damaged egos are more worthy of elimination than repair.

On the more purely cognitive side, frustrations to the therapist's intuition may give rise to an increase in the use of intellectualization as a defense. Rigidity may supplant thoughtfulness. Some therapists lapse into a kind of sacramental psychotherapy, insisting on the external trappings of regular hours and compulsive disclosure by the patient of thoughts rather than truly sensitive responses to the problems at hand. Devotion to theory can blur clinical perceptiveness, just as zealous advocacy of any particular point of view may be at the cost of helping individuals who are suffering. This is a departure from the truly scientific inquiry, which relishes the "non-neat," the paradoxical, the departures from prediction. Indeed, relying too heavily on some comfortable metapsychology may make the therapist more vulnerable to panic when such structure and order is threatened by the unexplained.

Regression in the counteralliance may also take the form of the therapist turning hostility and anger on him- or herself. Therapists may devalue their own importance or the value of their efforts. In a particularly perverse manner, the therapist may give license to the patient that encourages the latter's hateful behavior toward the therapist or others, so that both ultimately feel more out of control and in danger.

Secondary Countertransferences

Significant figures in the patient's life also evoke strong and often irrational responses in the therapist. This holds for those figures who have been internalized as well as those who may actually be present on the scene. It is often difficult to appreciate just how hurtful the early parents may have been, and the therapist may be seduced into maintaining a blindspot in this area by his or her own and the patient's need to protect parental figures from damaging criticism. It may be hard to acknowledge where parents have neglected or dismissed their children, let alone where parents have clearly hated them, especially when they have a solid middle-class background where such things are not supposed to occur. The therapist's own history of hostility to younger or older siblings may also color his understanding and distort empathy with the patient's parallel relationships. Here, the therapist's own self-knowledge and the hopefully good results of the therapist's own therapy come in as a protective buffer. No protection is available, however, when the clinician is confronted directly with those parents, relatives, siblings, employers, teachers, and other witnesses who may hover in the wings when a suicidal patient is in therapy. These individuals may be truly caring, or they may be more interested in being judges or scapegoat-seekers. In either case, the task is to enlist them as potential allies, rather than take the bait of adversarial encounter that is frequently tendered. A similar situation exists with those colleagues, ward personnel, and consultants who are present to look over the therapist's shoulder with the hospitalized patient. Competitive stress is often present and best kept in place by focusing on the patient's distress. The temptation to develop a negative response to former therapists of the patient is also best scrutinized and not indulged.

There is one remaining significant area of countertransference response, and that is to the patient who has completed suicide. This is probably the greatest pain that a therapist must endure. Like a parent who has lost a child, the therapist is not easily, if at all, consoled. Unlike such a parent, the therapist often is tempted to bear the distress alone. It is wise at such a time to seek out some colleague or former therapist to help share this burden. All the usual manifestations of grief—anger, guilt, sadness—must be endured and worked through. It is not a process of a week or two, but many months. In this light, one can better comprehend the caution that it may be beyond the capacity of most therapists to have more than one or two acutely suicidal patients in therapy at any one time.

The workings of the counteralliance are also very important. The most constructive issue from the experience of a patient's completed suicide, when mourning has been eased, is the therapist's augmented ability to admit mistakes and limitations and then to reengage with patients, having transformed the pain of defeat and loss into new courage, wisdom, and integrity.

REFERENCES

Abraham K: A short study of the development of the libido, in Selected Papers on Psychoanalysis. Edited by Ernest Jones. London, The Hogarth Press, 1924

Asch SS: Suicide and the hidden executioner. International Review of Psychoanalysis 7:51–61, 1980

Browne T: Religio Medici and Other Writings of Thomas Browne, Part I. New York, EP Dutton (Everyman's Library), 1928

Durkheim E: Suicide: A Study in Sociology. Translated by Spaulding JA, Simpson G. New York, Free Press, 1897/1951

Freud S: Mourning and melancholia (1917), in The Standard Edition of the Complete Psychological Works of Sigmund Freud. Edited by Strachey J. London, The Hogarth Press, 1957

Gibbs JP, Martin WT: Status Integration and Suicide: A Sociological Study. Eugene, OR, University of Oregon Press, 1964

Glover E: The Techniques of Psychoanalysis. New York, International Universities Press, 1955

Henry A, Short JF: Suicide and Homicide: Some Economic, Sociological, and Psychological Aspects of Aggression. New York, Free Press, 1986

Horney K: Neurosis and Human Growth. New York, WW Norton, 1950

Kahn A: The moment of truth: psychotherapy with the suicidal patient, in Lifelines: Clinical Perspectives on Suicide. Edited by Bassuk EL, Schoonover SC, Gill AD. New York, Plenum, 1982a, pp 83–92

Kahn A: The stress of therapy, in Lifelines: Clinical Perspectives on Suicide. Edited by Bassuk EL, Schoonover, SC, Gill AD. New York, Plenum, 1982b, pp 93–100

Kahn A: The therapeutic stance, in Emergency Psychiatry. Edited by Bassuk EL, Birk AW. New York, Plenum, 1984, pp 75–80

Kernberg O: Severe Personality Disorders: Psychotherapeutic Strategies. New Haven, CT, Yale University Press, 1984

Klein M: Envy and Gratitude and Other Works. New York, Delacorte, 1975

Kohut H. The Search for the Self: Selected Writings of Heinz Kohut, 1950–1978. Edited by Orstein PH. New York, International Universities Press, 1978

Menninger KA: Man Against Himself. New York, Harcourt Brace, 1938

Modell AH: Affects and their non-communication. Int J Psychoanal 61:259–267, 1980

Peterson CV: John Davidson, Lammas (1896). New York, Twayne Publishing, 1972

Ranier J: Genetic factors in depression and suicide. Am J Psychother 38:329–340, 1984

Reece FD: School-age suicides: the educational parameters. Dissertation Abstracts International 27:2895–2896, 1967

Rosenn DW: Suicidal behavior in children and adolescents, in Lifelines: Clinical Perspectives in Suicide. Edited by Bassuk EL, Schoonover SC, Gill AD. New York, Plenum, 1982, pp 303–340

Seiden RH: Campus tragedy: a study of student suicide. J Abnorm Psychol 71:389–399, 1966

Shakespeare W: Troilus and Cressida, in the Arden Shakespeare. Edited by Palmer K. London, Methuen Press, 1982

Sullivan HS: Clinical Studies in Psychiatry. New York, WW Norton, 1956

van Praag HM, Plutchik R, Conte H: The serotonin hypothesis of (auto) aggression, in Psychobiology of Suicidal Behavior. Edited by Stanley M, Mann JJ. Ann NY Acad Sci 487:15–167, 1986

Winnicott DW: The Maturational Process and the Facilitating Environment. New York, International Universities Press, 1965

Chapter 17

Cognitive Approaches to Understanding and Treating Suicidal Behavior

Marjorie E. Weishaar, Ph.D.
Aaron T. Beck, M.D.

In THE PAST decade, increasing attention has been paid to cognitive factors that may contribute to suicidal behavior. The impetus for examining the role of cognitive processing in suicide has come largely from the paradigm shift in behavior therapy to the cognitive domain and, most notably, from research on cognitive aspects of depression and suicide dating from the early 1960s (Beck 1964, 1976, 1983, 1987; Beck and Young 1985; Beck et al. 1979b).

Current clinical research interest is focused on the cognitive deficits that impede active problem solving on the part of suicidal individuals and on models that describe the process of suicidality, from ideation to overt self-destructive behavior.

"Cognitive" pertains to how individuals perceive, interpret, and explain their environments. The process by which humans select stimuli to interpret, assign meanings to those stimuli, and respond affectively and behaviorally to them is often variable and is strongly influenced by prior learning and mental set. Thus cognitive processing is often accompanied by errors in perception and inference, which lead to faulty conclusions; narrow or inflexible thinking, which limits response repertoires; and deficits in conceptualizing the consequences of various courses of action.

Cognitive therapy, developed as a result of empirical investigations with depressed patients, has received attention because of its demonstrated efficacy in the treatment of unipolar depression. Research on the relationship between depression and suicide has identified hopelessness as an important mediating psychological variable. Cognitive therapy research has also yielded a taxonomy of suicidal behavior; scales for measuring suicidal ideation, suicidal intent, and hopelessness; and evidence that hopelessness is an important precursor of suicide (see Appendices III and IV).

In this chapter, we will review the contributions of cognitive approaches to our understanding of depression and suicidal behavior, present what is known about the contribution of cognitive factors to suicidal behavior, and describe the process of cognitive therapy with suicidal patients. To review the present status of cognitive approaches to suicide, the cognitive model of psychopathology, particularly depression, will be described, followed by other research developments concerning cognitive processes and suicide.

COGNITIVE MODEL OF PSYCHOPATHOLOGY

Cognitive therapy is based on an information-processing model: how people perceive, interpret, and assign meanings to events plays a primary role in their emotional and behavioral responses to those events (Beck 1967/1972, 1976).

Although people are bombarded with a plethora of stimuli, they integrate only a limited number of them. To the ones they attend to, they assign meaning. The meanings assigned to events and the selection of stimuli perceived are governed by each individual's "cognitive lens." In other words, the fundamental beliefs, attitudes, and assumptions we have about ourselves and the world form a template on which we impose our experience to explain it. The thoughts and images we have are called cognitions, and the basic assumptions forming the template or governing our interpretations of events are called basic beliefs. These basic beliefs are embedded in cognitive structures, labeled *schemas* (Beck 1967/1972).

Basic beliefs are derived from previous experience and are learned. They are messages usually acquired early in life from parents, teachers, peers, or the child's independent experience. They are often highly personal and idiosyncratic. Examples of basic beliefs are: "Life isn't fair," "I am unlovable," "I must be successful to be happy," "Nothing ever goes my way," "I cannot survive without depending on others," and "If I don't succeed at first, I never will." Basic beliefs may be expressed outright by the person or may not be in the person's immediate awareness. They are often attached to a person's value system and, therefore, may be fairly fixed. Negative beliefs established early in life are especially emotionally charged and emerge full-blown when triggered (Beck 1964). Depressogenic beliefs are negative, maladaptive, and idiosyncratic, as are those accompanying personality disorders. Some basic beliefs are very positive and promote self-confidence (e.g., "I can make it if I try"), but are not always borne out in particular situations (e.g., failure not due to the individual, but to some other cause). Because of their absoluteness and rigidity, basic beliefs can become problematic when they are applied universally to all situations.

Cognitive Distortions

Psychological disturbances frequently stem from specific, habitual errors in thinking (Beck 1967/1972). Errors are likely to occur when an individual perceives that his or her vital interests are at stake. At such times, a person is likely to make extreme, one-sided, absolutistic, and global judgments due to the activation of schemas specific to the syndrome manifested. For example, schemas focusing on danger or threat correspond to anxiety; those dealing with loss, deprivation, or defeat to depression. Normally, such judgments are then tested against reality, corrected, and refined. In psychopathology, however, corrective functions are impaired.

An individual is constantly classifying, evaluating, and assigning meaning to events. Thus one always has thoughts or pictorial images in one's mind. These "automatic thoughts" are spontaneous and involuntary. They are specific, discrete, and idiosyncratic to the individual. In cases of psychopathology, they share commonalities within the diagnosis. Automatic thoughts reflect the individual's underlying basic beliefs. By examining automatic thoughts across situations and over time, themes that reflect the person's basic beliefs emerge.

In cases of mild psychiatric disturbance, automatic thoughts are not always obvious to the individual, although they influence emotions and behavior (Beck 1976). As psychological disturbances intensify, there is a loss of volitional control over thinking and a reduced ability to "turn off" the intense schemas. Automatic thoughts become more salient, more extreme, and more believable to the individual.

Habitual errors in thinking are termed cognitive distortions (Beck 1967/1972). They include the following: 1) arbitrary inference, drawing a conclusion based on insufficient or even contradictory evidence; 2) selective abstraction, attending to only a portion of relevant information; 3) overgeneralization, abstracting a general rule from a single event and applying it to both related and unrelated events; 4) magnification and minimization, exaggerating or underestimating the magnitude and importance of events; 5) personalization, attributing causality to oneself when several factors contributed to an outcome; and 6) dichotomous thinking, categorizing people and events in absolutistic, black-and-white terms (e.g., good versus bad).

The Cognitive Model of Depression

The cognitive model of depression posits that there are a number of predisposing factors to depression, including hereditary predisposition, biochemical abnormalities, developmental traumas leading to specific vulnerabilities, inadequate personal experiences or identification to provide appropriate coping mechanisms, counterproductive cognitive patterns, unrealistic goals, unreasonable values and assumptions, and imperatives absorbed from significant others (Beck 1983). It is generally agreed that depressive illnesses have interactive biochemical, motivational, affective, behavioral, and cognitive components. The cognitive model of depression does not contradict the biochemical one. They are not competing theories, but rather reflect different levels of analysis of the same phenomenon (Beck 1983; Beck and Young 1985). A change in one level or component of the depressive system is likely to influence the other. Since cognitive phenomena are easily identifiable and readily investigated, they provide a logical entry point to the depressive constellation. Moreover, just as there may be a biological (genetic, neurochemical) vulnerability to depression, there is a cognitive one. Schemas based on negative views of the self, the world, and the future predispose individuals to depression.

According to the cognitive model of depression, a triggering event or series of events related to the individual's vulnerability activates a schema of defeat or deprivation. This generates negative expectations, self-blame, sadness, and apathy stemming from distorted thinking. As a consequence of pessimism, the individual is less active and avoids social contact. Reduced performance is taken as proof of the individual's worthlessness or failure, and this reinforces the negative schema.

Cognitive Triad

In depression, information processing is negatively biased so that the person views the self, the world, and the future in terms of defeat and/or deprivation. This is called the *cognitive triad* of depression (Beck 1967/1972). Depressed individuals view themselves as inadequate, deserted, and lacking the attributes or inherent qualities necessary for happiness. They blame themselves for negative events, even those beyond their control, and view themselves as bereft of the resources needed to cope with the simplest of life's demands. Low self-esteem, a low sense of self-efficacy, and little self-acceptance characterize the depressed individual. Automatic thoughts associated with the negative view of self reflect underestimates of resources and focus on personal qualities or the lack thereof as reasons for perceived loss or inability to cope.

Along with the negative view of the self is the individual's negative view of his or her personal world. Depressed persons tend to interpret events in a negative way. Interactions with others are viewed as defeats, trivial events appear as significant losses, and other people are seen as critical and better off. Depressed individuals perceive the world as making excessive and exorbitant demands on them, placing insurmountable barriers in their way, and offering punishments but no rewards. The depressed person's automatic thoughts reflect an overestimation of the demands on them. In the balance of power between the individual and the world, the world is winning.

The third element of the cognitive triad is the negative view of the future. Current difficulties are expected to persist unrelentingly, perhaps even get worse. There is no point in taking remedial action, for efforts are doomed to fail. Lack of action reinforces the person's self-image as ineffectual. In severe cases, depressed persons believe that they will continue to be worthless burdens and that those around them would be better off it they were dead. Automatic thoughts reflect hopelessness.

Given the negative view of the self as abandoned or defeated, incapable of dealing with problems in a world full of obstacles and demands yet empty of satisfactions and with a future that is an extension of the painful present, it is not surprising that depressed patients consider suicide as a way out of their gridlock, as a possible surcease for their suffering.

Other motivational and behavioral features of depression are also derived from this negative cognitive bias (Beck 1976). The paralysis of will or apathy, behavioral avoidance, and wishes to escape result from pessimism and hopelessness. Since depressed people have negative expectations, they will often not even try to achieve goals. This is also true of suicidal individuals. They may withdraw from activity and depend on others. Reduced performance is then taken as a sign of failure, which reinforces the schema of defeat or deprivation. This feedback loop can lead to the vegetative signs of depression. Pessimism leads to immobilization, fatigue, and low energy. Even eating becomes an effort. Decisions are avoided for fear of making the wrong one. Concentration difficulties increase as thinking becomes saturated with depressive themes and the dominant negative schemas interfere with reality testing and reasoning. The goal of the therapist is to reverse the negative spiral to suicide by first dealing directly with the person's hopelessness by correcting cognitive distortions and by problem solving.

Research on Risk and Prediction of Suicide

Cognitive therapy research on suicidal risk has entailed development of 1) a classification system of suicidal behaviors; 2) assessment scales that can be applied to prospective studies of suicide; 3) the exploration of hopelessness as a key psychological factor; 4) the elucidation of other cognitive features of suicidal behavior; and 5) the development of a model of suicidal behavior in which hopelessness is a critical mediating factor. These aspects of research will be discussed, and other cognitive factors related to suicidal behavior will be reviewed.

Classification

A critical element of suicide research is the appropriate use of a classification system to describe the suicidal behaviors under investigation. Cognitive therapy uses the tripartite classification of suicidal behavior formulated by a Task Force of the National Institute of Mental Health Center for Studies of Suicide Prevention: suicidal ideation, suicide attempt, and completed suicide (Beck et al. 1973a). Suicide intent, lethality of attempt, and method of suicide or attempted suicide are subdivisions of these categories. Intent and lethality are important distinctions because they are positively correlated only when the person has an accurate conception of the lethality of his or her chosen method of suicide (Beck et al. 1975a).

Assessment Scales

Assessment instruments have been developed and tested to assist the clinician's systematic evaluation and determination of the seriousness of an individual's suicidality and to serve as predictive tools.

Scale for Suicide Ideation. Suicide ideators think about suicide and may have a plan, but have not implemented this plan or overtly harmed themselves. The Scale for Suicide Ideation (SSI) (Beck et al. 1979a) was designed to assess the degree to which someone is presently suicidal (see Appendix III). The SSI assesses suicidal risk by investigating not only intention but other risk factors such as lethality of contemplated method, availability and opportunity of method, and presence of deterrents. It is used for both the initial assessment of a patient and throughout the course of treatment. Its semistructured format allows inserting relevant questions for that particular patient and guarantees that no vital question is forgotten. Thus it provides a means of eliciting critical information from a patient, often at a time of anxiety for both the patient and the clinician. The SSI is used during an initial assessment of the patient and throughout therapy as needed, for suicidal ideation may actually increase during therapy as a consequence of life events or due to confronting painful topics in therapy sessions. Items, such as the frequency and duration of suicidal thoughts, the patient's attitude toward the thoughts, the extent of the wish to die, subjective feelings of control against suicidal wishes, internal and external deterrents, history of previous attempts, desire to make an actual attempt, final acts including a suicide note, and reason for a contemplated attempt, were both empirically and clinically derived. The SSI is a 19-item scale. Each item has three alternative statements, which are graded in intensity from 0 to 2. The total score, computed by adding item scores, ranges from 0 to 38. The SSI is administered by the clinician during a semistructured interview with the patient. Studies of reliability, concurrent validity, and construct validity support the usefulness of the scale (Beck et al. 1979a).

The SSI asks the patient to compare the strength of the wish to live with the strength of the wish to die. Kovacs and Beck (1977) documented the clinical observation that suicide is the outcome of an internal struggle between the wish to live and the wish to die rather than the consequence of a single motivation. Fifty percent of their sample of 106 suicide attempters reported that, at the time of attempt, they both wanted to live and wanted to die. When the wish to die was stronger, it was reflected in a more serious suicide intent. These results underscore the importance of shifting the delicate balance between life and death in a positive direction.

Suicide Intent Scale. The Suicide Intent Scale (SIS) (Beck et al. 1974a) is used with patients who have attempted suicide (see Appendix IV). It evaluates the severity of the patient's psychological intent at the time of the attempt by examining all relevant aspects of the attempter's behavior before, during, and after his or her suicidal act. Intent, defined as "the seriousness or intensity of the wish of a patient to terminate his life" (Beck et al. 1974b, p. 45), is one component of suicidal risk or potential. Other risk factors include access to lethal methods, knowledge of how to use these methods, absence of protective individuals who could intervene, and sociodemographic factors (e.g., age, sex, social class). Thus the SIS examines the circumstances around the suicide attempt such as likelihood of being discovered, communications about intent, and final acts as well as purpose of the attempt, ambivalence about living, and the individual's understanding of the method's lethality.

The clinician scores the SIS during an interview with the patient.

The total score represents the summed scores for each item. The SIS has been validated as a measure of the seriousness of intent of suicide attempts (Beck et al. 1974a; Minkoff et al. 1973; Silver et al. 1971). Its ability to discriminate between attempted and completed suicides has also been demonstrated (Beck and Lester 1976; Beck et al. 1974a, 1974b, 1975b).

The SSI and SIS were developed as part of a larger project intended to provide systematic information regarding the determinants of suicide and depression. Two clinically significant factors linked to suicide are communication of intent and purpose of attempt. The verbalization of the wish to commit suicide is an indicator of suicidal risk. Some clinicians believe that those who "talk" about suicide are more intent, whereas others believe that those who "didn't talk" were at greater risk of suicide. Kovacs et al. (1976) found that "communicators" of suicidal ideas did not differ from "noncommunicators" in either severity of overall suicidal intent or the extent of their wish to die.

The clinical significance of this finding suggest that a patient's intent to die is not always volunteered. The therapist must ask about suicidal thoughts, plans, and actions repeatedly, particularly with more reticent patients.

> One very withdrawn young woman would not tell her therapist that she had suicidal thoughts, but would endorse the suicide item on the Beck Depression Inventory (Beck et al. 1961). The therapist and patient used this inventory at every session to monitor the patient's suicidality until the patient felt more comfortable discussing her thoughts with the therapist.

Determining and discussing the purpose of a suicide attempt also has importance as a guide to therapeutic interventions. Research on 200 suicide attempters (Kovacs et al. 1975b) found that 56% wanted to escape life or end their pain, 13% wanted to kill themselves to change others or something in their environments, and 13% reported a combination of escape and manipulation of their social environments. Patients who scored high on hopelessness—as measured by the Hopelessness Scale (Beck et al. 1974c)—and depression—as measured by the Beck Depression Inventory—were more likely to report that their suicide attempt was motivated by a wish to reduce suffering and escape from life. Lower hopelessness and depression scorers, in contrast, were more likely to report manipulation of others or the environment as reasons for their attempt (Kovacs et al. 1975b). Thus purpose of attempt is important as a reflection of hopelessness and as a guide for intervention. If the purpose of the attempt is to escape a seemingly hopeless situation, then therapy should focus on reducing cognitive distortions and increasing problem solving. If manipulation is the primary goal, then the suicidal behavior therapy would focus on the individual's need for revenge or expression of hostile feelings, maladaptive interpersonal techniques, and more effective strategies for obtaining love and affection.

The Hopelessness Scale. The Hopelessness Scale is a 20-item instrument to which the individual responds true or false to each item. A score of 20 is the maximum score. Hopelessness can be conceptualized as a state that occurs as the consequence of the activation of schemas and basic beliefs relating to negative expectations. Life events trigger schemas that affect the patient's beliefs about his or her future and well-being. Some individuals, regardless of diagnosis, are more prone to hopelessness than others. Each episode of depression or other form of psychiatric distress yields consistent levels of hopelessness. High hopelessness in one episode predicts high hopelessness in subsequent depressive episodes, sometimes ending in suicide (Beck et al. 1985). The Hopelessness Scale assesses the negative expectations a person might have about his or her ability to overcome an unpleasant life situation or to attain a goal. Items on the Hopelessness Scale include "I might as well give up because there's nothing I can do about making things better for myself," "I don't expect to get what I really want," and "My future seems dark to me." The Hopelessness Scale has been applied to diverse clinical populations and has been demonstrated to have a high degree of internal consistency (Beck et al. 1974c). It has a moderately high correlation with the Beck Depression Inventory (Minkoff et al. 1977) and with clinical ratings of hopelessness.

Hopelessness Research

Numerous studies have demonstrated that hopelessness is more strongly related to suicidal intent than is depression per se (Beck et al. 1975b, 1976; Bedrosian and Beck 1979; Dyer and Kreitman 1984; Goldney 1979; Minkoff et al. 1973; Petrie and Chamberlain 1983; Weissman et al. 1979; Wetzel 1976a; Wetzel et al. 1980). In a study of depressed and nondepressed schizophrenic patients, intent was more strongly correlated with hopelessness than with depression; even schizophrenic patients who showed little depression but who scored high in hopelessness had increased levels of suicidal intent (Minkoff et al. 1973). A further study of suicide attempters found hopelessness to account for 96% of the association between depression and intent (Beck et al. 1975b).

Factor analytic studies of the Beck Depression Inventory similarly link negative attitudes about the self and the future with suicide. Beck and Lester's (1973) study of the responses of suicide attempters found both cognitive (pessimism, sense of failure, self-hate) and affective (sad mood, crying spells) factors related to suicidal wishes. A further study by Lester and Beck (1977) replicated the previous finding with a sample of suicide ideators. As with attempted suicides, suicidal wishes in suicide ideators correlated most highly with cognitive factors such as pessimism and sense of failure and with items reflecting mood and feeling. Suicidal wishes had low correlations with somatic preoccupations, appetite disturbance, and sleep disturbance. Another study among depressed patients who had not attempted suicide found that negative attitude and anhedonia showed significantly greater association with suicidal wishes than did vegetative symptoms (Beck et al. 1973b).

One implication of these findings is that treatment directed at psychological factors may have a more immediate effect on suicidal wishes than pharmacotherapy directed at biological symptoms. Studies by Beck et al. (1979b) and by Rush et al. (1982) indicated that cognitive therapy yielded a greater reduction in hopelessness than pharmacotherapy combined with supportive contact.

Hopelessness has also been found to be a better indicator of intensity of current suicidal ideation among suicide attempters than is depression (Kovacs et al. 1975a). It has also been found to be a major source of variance in the relationship between alcoholism and suicide attempts (Beck et al. 1976) and a greater determinant of suicidal intent among abusers than drug use per se (Weissman et al. 1979).

The importance of hopelessness as a predictor of suicide in both inpatient and outpatient populations has been studied. Longitudinal research suggests than hopelessness is a predictor of eventual suicide among suicide ideators. A 10-year prospective study of patients hospitalized with suicidal ideation found that scores on the Hopelessness Scale were strong predictors of eventual suicide. Of 165 patients studied, 11 eventually committed suicide. Of those, 10 (90.9%) had Hopelessness Scale scores of 10 or above. Only one (9.1%) completer had a score of 9 or less (Beck et al. 1985).

Additionally, in examining 2,174 outpatient clinic records over a 10-year period, it was found that of the 10 who committed suicide, 90% had Hopelessness Scale scores of 10 or above. Only one patient who eventually committed suicide had a hopelessness score of less than 10%. A cutoff score of 17 identified a high-risk group among this outpatient sample in which the proportion of suicides was 15 times greater than the rest of the sample (Beck 1986). The role of hopelessness as a predictor of ultimate suicide has also been supported by studies by Fawcett et al. (1987) and Drake and Cotton (1986).

Other Cognitive Features of Suicidal Patients

In his review of the treatment of suicide, Ellis (1986, 1987) observed that most conventional therapies employ a crisis management approach, viewing each suicidal episode as an interruption of the normal course of therapy. The suicidal crisis is managed, with a subsequent return to other therapeutic issues for the patient. This perspective ignores the possibility of fundamental and critical differences between suicidal and nonsuicidal patients, which should be targeted in therapy. Specifically, the suicidal patient's cognitive distortions and problem-solving deficits may predispose the patient to another suicidal episode.

A number of studies have demonstrated cognitive differences between suicidal and nonsuicidal persons, even when level of depression or degree of pathology is controlled. Factors such as dysfunctional attitudes, dichotomous thinking, cognitive rigidity, and inability to generate or act on alternative solutions have been related to the general category of poor problem-solving ability. The cognitive matrix of negative expectancies creating hopelessness is likely to interact with other cognitive deficits, creating a mind-set in which suicide may seem like the only resolution to insoluble problems. Specific cognitive deficits related to suicidal behavior are examined below, including dysfunctional assumptions, dichotomous thinking, and problem-solving deficits.

Dysfunctional Assumptions. Ellis and Ratliff (1986) compared suicide attempters to equally depressed nonsuicidal psychiatric patients, using a battery of cognitive inventories. They found the suicidal patients to score higher in terms of irrational beliefs, depressogenic attitudes, and hopelessness than the nonsuicidal patients. Bonner and Rich (1987b) found dysfunctional assumptions to play a key role in predicting suicidal ideation among college students. Other factors operating in this college sample were emotional alienation and deficient adaptive resources (i.e., family cohesion and reasons for living). The role of reasons for living, a positive cognitive feature, is worth noting. Two studies indicated that those who think of and attempt suicide report fewer reasons to live than psychiatric and normal controls, when levels of stress are held constant (Bonner and Rich 1987b; Linehan et al. 1983). Thus the presence of dysfunctional assumptions and the absence of positive reasons for living are both considered cognitive variables or attitudes affecting suicidal behavior. Cognitive distortions may exacerbate stress while the lack of adaptive resources leaves the individual unprepared to cope (Bonner and Rich 1987b).

Dichotomous Thinking. Several types of cognitive distortions that relate to the cognitive triad of depression may contribute to suicidal behavior (Beck et al. 1979b). These include exaggerating one's problems, minimizing one's resources or ability to solve problems, and predicting the worst in the future. To date, there are no empirical data linking these specific distortions to suicide except as they relate to hopelessness. One cognitive distortion that has been systematically investigated is dichotomous thinking. Dichotomous or "all-or-nothing" thinking categorizes experiences into one of two extremes (e.g., either good or bad, a success or failure). It is a form of rigid thinking and is thus subsumed, in some research, under cognitive rigidity.

Early work by Neuringer (1961, 1967, 1968) found that suicidal persons rated certain concepts, such as life and death, more extremely than did nonsuicidal persons on semantic differential tests. Differential ratings were attributed to extremeness as a cognitive style. A later study (Neuringer and Lettieri 1971) supported the notion of extremeness as a style because this tendency persisted over time. However, Wetzel (1976b) interpreted differences on semantic differential ratings as reflecting attitudes toward specific concepts (e.g., life, death, self) rather than a generalized style of dichotomous thinking.

Problem-Solving Deficits. A number of studies have found rigid or dichotomous thinking to differentiate suicide ideators and/or attempters from both normal and psychiatric control groups. Cognitive rigidity was initially measured by tests of impersonal tasks such as arithmetic, map reading, and word associations. More recent research has investigated skills at interpersonal problem solving ("social cognition") (Arffa 1983; Schotte and Clum 1982). Of clinical relevance is the finding that suicide attempters report more difficulty with interpersonal problems than do suicide ideators, nonsuicidal psychiatric patients, and general population controls (Linehan et al. 1986).

Suicidal persons have been found to demonstrate a limited ability to find solutions to interpersonal problems. They are less able to consider alternatives (Cohen-Sandler and Berman 1982; Levenson 1974), and produce new ideas and think flexibly (Patsiokas et al. 1979), and may persist in ineffective problem solving even after a more effective strategy is presented (Levenson and Neuringer 1971). In terms of interpersonal problem solving, suicidal children appear less able to generate active cognitive coping strategies (e.g., self-comforting statements and instrumental problem solving) in the face of stressful life events than nonsuicidal children (Asarnow et al. 1987). These authors recommended teaching suicidal children coping skills to mediate their affective and behavioral responses to stress. Similarly, Linehan et al. (1987) found less active and greater passive interpersonal problem solving among suicide attempters than among suicide ideators and nonsuicidal medical patients. Further, higher levels of expectancy that suicide would effectively solve one's problems predicted greater suicidal intent. These researchers suggested that treatment of suicidal patients should combine interpersonal problem-solving training with assertiveness training.

Schotte and Clum (1987) found that psychiatric inpatients who had expressed suicidal ideation or made suicide attempts were deficient in both impersonal and interpersonal problem solving, as compared to nonsuicidal patients. They described the suicidal patients' deficits in terms of D'Zurilla and Goldfried's (1971) model of problem solving: suicidal individuals 1) lack an appropriate general orientation to problems; 2) have difficulty generating potential alternative solutions to problems once identified; 3) tend to focus on potential negative consequences of implementing the alternatives generated; and 4) have difficulty implementing viable alternatives.

Finally, McLeavey et al. (1987) compared patients who had overdosed with nonsuicidal patients and nonpatient controls using three measures of interpersonal problem solving. On all measures, the suicidal patients performed worse than the nonpatient controls, and this finding was even more striking on those measures with greater interpersonal content. The suicide attempters were less able to conceptualize the means to solve a problem, less capable of generating alternative solutions, less prepared to anticipate the consequences of various courses of action, and less able to deal with problems in their own lives than the nonsuicidal patients or normal controls. These researchers concluded that suicide attempters have less flexible social cognitions than other psychiatric patients or normal individuals, which helps explain multiple suicide attempts by these individuals.

Impulsivity and External Locus of Control. Two other cognitive factors, impulsivity and locus of control, have been investigated. There is little research evidence to support impulsivity (which has been clinically observed among suicide attempters) as a distinguishing feature of this group (Patsiokas et al. 1979). However, research on the biology of suicide has linked impulsivity to certain neurochemical abnormalities in violent suicide attempters (Winchel et al., Chapter 4, this volume). Studies of locus of control have found that suicide attempters were more likely than nonattempters to attribute problems to external events than to their interpretations of them (Ellis and Ratliff 1986). However, other researchers have found no difference in locus of control between suicide attempters and nonpatient controls (McLeavey et al. 1987) or have found external locus of control operating in only one age group of suicide attempters (Patsiokas et al. 1979).

As a distinguishing cognitive characteristic, locus of control is a vague concept because of theoretical disagreement about whether suicidal people are internally or externally oriented, or whether suicidal behavior is precipitated by a shift in locus of control from one end of the continuum to the other (Lester 1973). However, the locus of control research has implications for problem-solving abilities. The individual's general orientation toward problem solving may be more positive if the person believes a solution is within his or her control.

Models of Suicidal Behavior

Efforts have been made toward developing explanatory models of suicidal behavior, from suicidal ideation to suicide attempts. These models incorporate factors that have been found to correlate independently with suicidal behavior, including the cognitive factors discussed above.

Clum and colleagues (Clum et al. 1979; Schotte and Clum 1982) developed a model of suicidal behavior in which poor problem solving is a mediator between life stress and suicide attempts. Among a college student population, it was found that depression was the best predictor of suicide intent at low levels of suicidal ideation. At high levels of ideation, hopelessness was the best predictor of intent. The authors suggested that the combination of life stress and poor problem-solving ability led to hopelessness, which in turn discourages the individual from trying to solve problems. A later application of this model (Schotte and Clum 1987) with suicidal psychiatric patients found no relationship between hopelessness and levels of interpersonal problem-solving skill, thereby suggesting that hopelessness and problem-solving deficits are independent factors, both worthy of treatment.

Bonner and Rich (1987b) developed a model in which alienation, cognitive distortions, and deficient adaptive reasons for living predispose an individual to suicidal behavior while stress and increased hopelessness are more immediate precipitants to lethal suicidal behavior. A subsequent study (Bonner and Rich 1987a) validated the roles of these factors and included situational stress and cumulative life events as risk factors.

The Relationship of Hopelessness to Problem-Solving Skills

The relationship between hopelessness and other cognitive factors is not clear. Hopelessness has been conceptualized as the consequence of cognitive rigidity, dichotomous thinking, and deficient problem-solving skills (Ellis 1987; Patsiokas and Clum 1985). Patsiokas and

Clum (1985) found that problem-solving training lowered hopelessness among suicide attempters, lending support to the notion that hopelessness results from poor problem-solving skills.

Schotte and Clum (1987), however, found that hopelessness was not correlated with levels of interpersonal problem-solving skills. They argued that it is an independent variable reflecting a "maladaptive general orientation or set towards problems" (p. 53). Similarly, McLeavey et al. (1987) found that suicide attempters' performances on interpersonal problem-solving measures were not correlated with their hopelessness. Additional work (McLeavey et al. 1986) found no differences in hopelessness change scores between suicide attempters receiving problem-solving training and those receiving standard treatment. Thus there is evidence that interpersonal problem-solving deficits are not due to hopelessness, but rather reflect a more constant characteristic. Further support for the hypothesis that problem-solving deficits are traits of parasuicides and not state-dependent comes from the work of Linehan et al. (1987). They found that suicide attempters scored lower than ideators in interpersonal problem solving in general. However, first-time suicide attempters were more active in problem solving than ideators; repeat attempters were less able to solve problems than first-time attempters. Ideators with a history of parasuicide were also low in problem-solving skills. If poor problem-solving were an artifact of the stress of the current episode, then all current attempters, including first attempters, should have scored lower than ideators. However, this was not the case.

A longitudinal study of suicide ideators and suicide attempt "repeaters" (Beck 1987) shed some light on the distinctions between these groups in terms of problem-solving skills. The suicide ideators in this study were primarily patients hospitalized for depression. During their clinical depression, they were suicidal and hopeless, but these features resolved completely when the depression resolved. Additionally, when depressed, this group exhibited impaired problem solving but regained this ability when the depression was over. For this group, problem-solving deficits were state-dependent.

In contrast, the suicide attempt "repeaters" appeared much more trait-like in their problem-solving deficits. This group was comprised of individuals with personality disorders, those likely to have a history of alcoholism, and those with antisocial behavior problems. Although this group of repeaters distorted reality, their negative perceptions of themselves tended to be validated by society. When each suicidal crisis was over, these patients continued to view themselves in negative terms. While they may have experienced some depressive symptoms, their suicide attempts were usually related to a very recent precipitating life event. This group was also characterized by poor problem-solving ability, cognitive rigidity, and impulsivity that persisted after the suicidal crisis. Thus at the time of the suicide attempt, both groups exhibited elevated levels of hopelessness and problem-solving deficits, but they appear to stem from different "causes" (Figure 1).

COGNITIVE THERAPY FOR SUICIDAL BEHAVIOR

Features of Cognitive Therapy

Cognitive therapy is a very active, structured, problem-oriented form of therapy in which the therapist and patient collaborate in examining how the patient's attitudes and beliefs contribute to distress. It employs both verbal procedures and behavioral techniques to change maladaptive assumptions and the behaviors congruent or consistent with them. This type of therapy has been shown to be effective in the treatment of both depressed and suicidal patients. The following discussion will describe the critical elements of cognitive therapy and how it can be applied to the treatment of suicidal patients.

The three major features of cognitive therapy include collaborative empiricism, Socratic dialogue, and guided discovery. These elements are modified slightly when working with suicidal patients.

Collaborative empiricism is the process by which the therapist and patient work together to formulate the patient's beliefs as hypotheses to be tested rather than as "givens," and subsequently test them

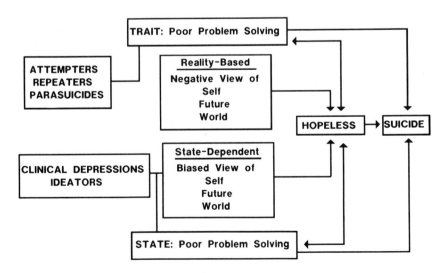

Figure 1. Progression of suicidality in ideators and attempters.

logically and empirically. Through Socratic dialogue, the therapist poses questions that reveal the patient's errors in logic. Guided discovery is the process by which the therapist uncovers the meanings of events with patients. Questioning leads the patient to examine the source, function, and utility of his or her beliefs. In working with suicidal patients, the therapist becomes even more active and directive, keeping the initial sessions focused on reducing risk. Collaboration at this stage means that the therapist focuses on the distortions that make the situation appear hopeless and on proposing solutions that the patient is unable to generate because of apathy, lack of information, rigid thinking, and decreased ability to concentrate, remember, or create.

Problem-solving deficits include cognitive rigidity, dichotomous thinking, failure to anticipate consequences or implement solutions, and viewing suicide as a desirable solution. These deficits become targets for intervention in the treatment of suicidal behavior. Along with poor problem-solving ability, hopelessness appears to be a related yet independent risk factor. It appears that problem-solving deficits are stable (Linehan et al. 1987; McLeavey et al. 1986, 1987), while hopelessness becomes more salient at higher levels of suicide intent (Bonner and Rich 1987b; Kovacs et al. 1975a; Schotte and Clum 1982).

Ellis (1987) distinguished among types of suicidal persons: 1) depressed/hopeless, 2) communication/control oriented, 3) psychotic, 4) alcoholic, 5) those with organic brain dysfunction, and 6) "rational" suicides. Cognitive interventions have generally focused on the depressed suicidal patient first to reduce the cognitive distortions that lead to hopelessness and second to increase problem solving. Cognitive therapy maintains that modifying the hopelessness underlying the depressed patient's suicidal wishes will reduce the risk of suicide, while problem solving will increase the patient's ability to cope with stressors.

Cognitive and Behavioral Techniques

As mentioned above, cognitive therapy is an active, collaborative effort aimed at modifying dysfunctional attitudes and behaviors. It employs both cognitive and behavioral techniques to promote therapeutic change. While behavioral techniques are efficacious in overcoming the inactivity of depression, cognitive techniques are most efficacious in treating hopelessness.

Cognitive techniques for the treatment of depressed, suicidal patients include the following: 1) identification of the relationships between negative thoughts and attitudes and affective and behavioral symptoms; 2) identification of the sequences between thoughts and motivation toward suicide; 3) exploration of depressive and suicidal thoughts and the meanings assigned to events; 4) examination, reality-testing, and revision of faulty cognitions using logic and empirical evidence; 5) consideration of alternative explanations for events; 6) generation of alternative ways of responding to psychological and environmental stressors; 7) identification, examination, and evaluation of underlying assumptions about self, others, world, and future; and 8) cognitive rehearsal, visualizing the steps necessary to carry out a plan.

Behavioral techniques used in the treatment of depressed, suicidal patients include 1) scheduling activities with the patient to combat inertia, structure the day, and build confidence; 2) graded task assignment, beginning with a simple assignment and increasing the complexity or duration of activities to give the patient a series of success experiences toward an identified goal; 3) mastery and pleasure therapy in which the patient rates daily activities both in terms of degree of satisfaction and amount of pleasure from doing the activity, which counteracts the tendency to minimize success and satisfaction; 4) role reversal in which the therapist plays the patient, helping the patient to view his or her problems with greater detachment; and 5) skills training, including assertiveness training, social skills training, and problem-solving training. Relaxation is also taught to enable the patient to tolerate the anxiety accompanying new behaviors.

Cognitive therapy for depressed, suicidal patients focuses on the following target areas (Ellis 1986, 1987): hopelessness, cognitive rigidity, dichotomous thinking and other cognitive distortions, ineffective problem solving, and the acceptance of suicide as a solution.

Hopelessness

Relieving the patient's hopelessness and shaking his or her rigid conclusions that things cannot improve are the immediate goals of treatment (Beck et al. 1979b). The patient may be overestimating the magnitude of problems or underestimating the resources available. The therapist must communicate to the patient that hopelessness is a consequence of negative expectations, not an accurate reflection of reality; other courses of action and alternative interpretations are possible; and they can work together to generate realistic alternatives.

Initially, the therapist may take a very active role in helping to generate solutions to problems. However, a thorough understanding of the patient's perspective is necessary first to prevent prejudgment or giving premature advice. If the patient views the therapist as overly optimistic or "Pollyannaish," collaboration is unlikely. The therapist's credibility begins with active and attentive listening from a neutral stance and grows as the therapist takes the position of co-investigator, examining how the patient's present ways of dealing with stress are dysfunctional. The therapist helps the patient to identify external and internal resources and supports (e.g., community resources, evidence from past experience that contradicts a present conclusion about the self) and tries to create some cognitive dissonance to shake the patient's maladaptive belief system.

To create disequilibrium in the patient's belief structure, the therapist introduces evidence that contradicts the patient's beliefs about the self, the situation, or suicide as a desirable solution. A chronic pain patient who said, "I can't stand this pain," was able to recall that a year ago she had tolerated even greater pain and her comfort had improved since then. Patients who overgeneralize by saying, "I know what I have to do, but I can't," benefit from such techniques as graded task assignment to feel less overwhelmed and by role playing to practice implementing an adaptive solution. For example, a patient who was isolating herself from social contact began by attending an office party for 15 minutes and eventually graduated to inviting an acquaintance to lunch. As the patient gains mastery over new behaviors, he or she challenges the belief of being ineffectual. The therapist works to have the patient suspend judgment before trying a new perspective or behavior. By beginning from the consensus that the patient's current strategies are not working and engaging the patient's interest in new strategies, the therapist decreases the likelihood that the patient will conclude, "Nothing works. It's no use." In addition to correcting cognitive distortions, the cognitive therapist teaches problem-solving skills, which contributes to reducing hopelessness in suicidal patients (Patsiokas and Clum 1985).

Cognitive Rigidity

Cognitive rigidity is challenged by framing the patient's beliefs as testable hypotheses and not fixed rules. The therapist and patient work together to generate other interpretations, to withhold harsh judgments that would eliminate other viewpoints, and to examine logically and test alternatives behaviorally.

Role playing with role reversal is a way to generate alternatives when the patient feels unable to assume another point of view. In this case, the therapist plays the patient, with the patient taking a more objective role and "assisting" the therapist in generating new solutions. Role reversal is also frequently used in training patients how to respond to powerful automatic thoughts. For example, the patient, playing his or her own critical voice, may heap abuse on the therapist, who is playing the patient. The therapist logically defends him- or herself. The roles are then reversed again, with the patient practicing adaptive responses to criticism.

Cognitive flexibility is enhanced through the use of visual imagery and cognitive rehearsal where the patient imagines a problematic scenario and its possible outcomes. Alternative solutions are generated by modifying the scenario ("If that happens then I could do this").

> A college student who had recurrent suicidal ideation whenever she was visiting her parents on holidays was able to picture and describe vividly a likely scenario of an upcoming visit. In the image, she portrayed herself as silent and passive while her parents criticized her for not being more attentive to their needs. She felt that if she countered their attacks, her parents would think she was insensitive. Rather than directly expressing her feelings, the patient would imagine suicide as a way out of her dilemma.

Visualizing and mentally rehearsing different responses to her parents helped the patient recognize other acceptable alternatives. Role playing helped her practice implementing these alternatives.

Visual imagery may be especially powerful in situations when patients have difficulty identifying their automatic thoughts. Guided imagery helps the patient describe details of an upsetting scene, often revealing the meaning of that event for the patient. For example, a businessman who had stolen from his company became depressed and suicidal. As he pictured a confrontation with his boss, he became tearful. The key feature of his image was not his shame at being discovered, but his sadness that his boss had never cared for him as a person.

Dichotomous Thinking

Dichotomous thinking is a particular kind of cognitive distortion in which experiences are categorized in one of two polar extremes. Patients who have a rapid escalation of affect are often thinking dichotomously. A suicidal thought revealing dichotomous thinking is, "I must have my job (marriage, money, reputation) restored or I'll kill myself." To challenge dichotomous thinking, a continuum between success and failure is designed, using specific criteria for assessment. Rating oneself on such a scale generally reveals that one is partly a success and partly a failure on any task.

> A woman had been suicidal for a year, ever since her boyfriend told her he would never marry her because she had less education and was of a different religion from him. The dichotomy of her thinking was, "If I can't have Larry, no one else is good enough. He was perfect."

The therapist worked to moderate her extreme thinking by reducing her idealization of Larry and by reframing the problem as an opportunity to find someone else who would treat her better, rather than as her last chance for happiness. The patient was able to list her criteria for a partner: kind, loving, respectful, understanding, and fun to be with. Then she rated Larry on these qualities. She found that although being with him allowed her to meet interesting people and go to exciting places, he had always criticized her lack of education and her background. In fact, there were a lot of things she didn't like about him. She was also able to use these criteria to evaluate other men she had dated. This allowed her to see that each man had positive qualities and that she needed to get to know some men better before she could evaluate them on some criteria.

The futility of dichotomous thinking can also be exposed by asking the patient for dichotomous value judgments on minor things, such as "Is the floor completely clean or totally dirty?" (Burns 1980), or by asking the patient to go through a day categorizing all their experiences in all-or-nothing terms.

Once patients know that they use dichotomous thinking to categorize experience, they may practice thinking and speaking in more conditional, less extreme terms (e.g., "I may not be the brightest guy in the world, but I'm not stupid.") and finding exceptions to extreme judgments ("My neighbor smiled and said 'Hello' to me. I'm not a total reject.").

Additionally, if the patient can learn to separate from his or her behavior, absolutistic judgments are less likely. For example, a person who thinks "I'm bad and should be punished" could be trained to separate "bad" or maladaptive behavior from his or her identity as a person. More realistic thinking would be along the lines of "I can change this behavior" rather than "I must punish myself," which helps reduce all-or-nothing perceptions.

Other Cognitive Distortions

In addition to dichotomous thinking, any of the cognitive distortions may be present in suicidal thinking. Selective abstraction is an error of perception in which the patient attends only to negative data, ignoring evidence that contradicts his or her negative conceptualization of things.

> A woman who had left several jobs because of social discomfort and problems with co-workers told her therapist that her day had been horrible because a co-worker had looked at her "funny." She concluded that he disliked her and might influence others to turn against her. She believed that she could not return to work. In reconstructing the day,

the patient recalled that this same co-worker had asked her opinion about something and had complimented her work. Additionally, there were other positive experiences that she had ignored. The patient was taught how to expand her view, incorporating all the available information before drawing conclusions.

Arbitrary inference is an interpretive error of jumping to a conclusion, even when that conclusion is contradicted by the facts.

A man became angry and despondent that a woman he had started to date broke up their relationship. "She found out what I'm really like. She saw my true self for the worthless person I am," stated the patient. Although the woman had told the patient that she felt they had nothing in common, the patient persisted in believing that she had only been trying to be nice to him, that she really thought he was worthless. In discussing their brief relationship, the patient discovered how little he knew about this woman. The therapist pointed out that the same might be true about her knowledge of him. It was unlikely that, after a couple of dates, she was rejecting him for anything but superficial reasons.

In cases of arbitrary inference, patients are asked to present evidence in support of their conclusions and then gather evidence in support of other, more realistic interpretations.

Overgeneralization can be undone by finding evidence that contradicts the patient's conclusion or by logically finding an exception to the stated rule. Evidence that contradicts the patient's conclusion is generated by examining the patient's past and present experiences.

A patient who labeled himself "a lazy bum" and stated he was "always that way" remembered that he made an effort in school when teachers demonstrated an interest in him. Moreover, when tasks were broken into manageable steps, he found them easier to approach and accomplish.

Magnification or exaggeration of events, personal flaws, or barriers facing the patient can be approached in several ways. One is to use a standard of comparison based on consensus to gain perspective. For example, is the patient's "horrible" behavior as heinous as a criminal's? Another technique is to provide education or information.

A young woman who learned she had to wear a hearing aid became suicidal, thinking she was destined to live in a group home and would never marry. She was educated about her hearing loss and what she might expect. She was also told of several celebrities who wore hearing aids, including a glamorous television actress who is entirely deaf in one ear and partially deaf in the other.

Another technique to deal with magnification is to use "what if" questions (e.g., "What if your family discovered that you fathered an illegitimate child?"). This type of question allows the patient to test reality (e.g., "After a while, they would acknowledge it and maybe accept it," the patient decided), engage in problem solving (e.g., the patient developed ways of responding to his family), and discover the meaning of the situation for the patient (e.g., "It would be a public embarrassment," the patient stated).

Personalization is an error in attribution in which the patient either assumes too much or too little responsibility for an event. A therapeutic goal is to have the patient recognize the influence of other factors operating in the situation as well as accept responsibility for his or her own contribution.

> A reclusive, suicidal woman concluded she was being "victimized" by the community because her car was stolen. As she went over the details of the car theft, she recalled that she hadn't locked the car, making it easy to steal. In addition, the police told her that cars are frequently stolen from her neighborhood.

Another type of faulty attribution is believing that one's problems are due to external events rather than to one's interpretations of events (Ellis and Ratliff 1986). The possibility that a person has control over their own thoughts, emotions, and behavior may be a novel idea to the patient, but can be demonstrated by eliciting thoughts about being in therapy and then tying those thoughts to affect and behavior. Further demonstration of the patient's control over his or her reactions is to have the patient consider alternative ways of viewing a recent, yet nonthreatening, life situation. Finally, patients often assume responsibility for persons or events outside their control. Helping them to distinguish factors under their control from factors beyond their control clarifies the problem, sets realistic limits on their expectations and behaviors, and allows them to see that they are neither the passive victims of external events nor the sole determinant of most outcomes.

The most effective way for a patient to begin to correct cognitive distortions is to write down his or her negative, automatic thoughts between sessions. Negative thoughts may be written in one column, with more adaptive responses written next to them in another column. The Daily Record of Dysfunctional Thoughts (Beck et al. 1979b) is a form used for the recording of negative automatic thoughts and adaptive responses to them. Writing automatic thoughts requires that the patient recognize specific thoughts and not dismiss them or ignore them. If thoughts are ignored or remain unchallenged, they will persist. In responding to negative automatic thoughts, the aim is to correct the distortion with a realistic interpretation, less extreme language, or a more objective evaluation. Initially, the therapist and patient work together to develop responses, with the patient assuming more responsibility for this task as he or she learns to identify distortions, gather evidence, and generate alternative interpretations.

Ineffective Problem Solving

Nezu's (1987) review of social problem-solving deficits of depressed persons elaborates on the cognitive factors operating in this population. According to D'Zurilla and Nezu's (1982) model, the components of the problem-solving process are problem orientation, problem definition, generation of alternatives, decision making, and solution implementation and verification.

Problem orientation requires an accurate recognition of a problematic situation, acceptance of problems as a normal and inevitable part of life, and belief that one is capable of solving problems. Cognitive distortions about the self and the situation ("I can't handle this. Life is unfair.") maximize difficulties and minimize resources.

Problem definition includes obtaining information in clear and specific terms, differentiating fact from inference, identifying what makes the situation a problem, and setting a realistic goal. Cognitive distortions such as arbitrary inference, emotional reasoning (equating feelings with facts), selective abstraction, overgeneralization, magnification, and minimization skew a person's perceptions of the problem, thus leading to ineffective solutions.

Generating alternatives requires eliciting as many solutions as possible from the patient. It also requires that the patient defer judgment about a possible solution before a fair evaluation of it. Suicidal patients often give up when their standard solutions fail.

Decision making entails evaluating alternatives with regard to their consequences for self and others, immediately and in the long run. Both the value and the probability of various consequences are examined. When suicide is viewed as a solution to a problem, many consequences of that act are ignored or minimized by the patient.

Implementing a solution and evaluating its effectiveness can be hampered by overgeneralization ("I can't") and not making one's standard of evaluation clear and explicit. For example, a patient may report that the chosen solution worked terribly because of anxiety while following through with the task, even though the goal was actually achieved. In addition, patients may not implement a solution correctly or give it a fair trial. Therapy may be directed at increasing the patient's tolerance for frustration, anxiety, or discomfort as solutions are tested, given that it often takes time to resolve certain problems. Beck et al. (1979b) recommended cognitive rehearsal for future problems combined with a stress inoculation technique to distract the patient from interfering suicidal thoughts while problem solving is being undertaken.

Problem solving has much promise as a treatment for depressed and suicidal patients, including children and adolescents. Researchers have found that suicidal children were more able to generate solutions and plans to deal with difficult situations following problem-solving training (Cohen-Sandler and Berman 1982). Beck et al. (1979b) described a case of problem solving done by a suicidal 12-year-old boy. Additionally, problem solving has been found to reduce depression (Nezu 1986, 1987) and hopelessness (Patsiokas and Clum 1985).

View of Suicide as a "Desirable Solution"

Suicidal people have a unique "cognitive deficit" in solving highly charged interpersonal problems: when their usual way of dealing with problematic situations fails, they become paralyzed, viewing suicide as a way out. These individuals have a low tolerance for uncertainty and may prematurely abandon problem solving. Suicide is thus a kind of "opiate," a relief and escape from problems (Beck et al. 1979b).

The clinician must challenge the patient's assumptions that suicide will achieve a desired goal without causing further complications. For example, the goal of punishing someone by the suicide might not be achieved because the intended person may not blame him- or herself for the patient's death. Suicidal patients often want to relieve loved ones of the burden of their suicidality. The therapist can point out that getting better will relieve that "burden." Thus, in reviewing the patient's reasons for wanting to die, cognitive distortions become apparent. *At no time* are the patient's reasons dismissed or minimized, but rather are challenged logically. This helps the patient to increase his or her objectivity, consider both the short- and long-term consequences of suicide, and identify other solutions.

The balance between reasons for living and reasons for dying is delicate. The balance may be shifted in favor of living by having the patient list past and present reasons for staying alive. The therapist may prompt the patient if it is apparent that the patient has forgotten, ignored, or negated positive factors in his or her life. Therapists' familiarity with the Reasons for Living Inventory (Linehan et al. 1983) may be especially helpful in adding to a list of reasons to live.

A list of cognitive techniques for the treatment of suicidal behavior appears in Table 1.

CONCLUSION

Research in the past decade has revealed common cognitive characteristics of suicidal individuals, including dichotomous thinking, cog-

Table 1. Cognitive techniques for the treatment of suicidal behavior

Cognitive characteristic	Intervention
Dichotomous thinking	Build a continuum between extreme points of view. Specify criteria used to categorize things in all-or-nothing terms. Find "shades of gray" in judgments. Use conditional, or less absolute, language.
Problem-solving deficits	Apply problem-solving training, including accepting problems as a normal part of life, precisely defining the problem, generating alternatives, and implementing solutions. Minimize cognitive distortions that interfere with this process.
Cognitive rigidity	Employ collaborative empiricism: test the patient's assumptions logically and empirically. Role play with role reversal to generate alternatives. Look for evidence in support of alternative interpretations.
Hopelessness	View hopelessness as a symptom and not as an accurate reflection of the situation. List all of the problems making the patient feel hopeless. Reduce cognitive distortions to define problems clearly. Share optimism with the patient about finding solutions. Use problem-solving training. Use skills training to aid implementation of solutions (e.g., assertiveness).
View of suicide as desirable	Elicit reasons for dying and reasons for living. Describe advantages and disadvantages of suicide relative to other solutions. Correct cognitive distortions about advantages of dying.

nitive rigidity, problem-solving deficits, hopelessness, and the acceptance of suicide as a desirable solution. Cognitive therapy targets these features to foster more fundamental changes in the patient, thereby decreasing the chance of future suicidality.

The elements of cognitive therapy with suicidal patients are similar to those of standard cognitive therapy: 1) establishing a collaborative relationship between therapist and patient; 2) using questioning as a means of assisting the patient to reach his or her own conclusions; and 3) testing the validity of the patient's assumptions. However, in working with suicidal patients, the therapist is much more active and directive. Collaboration does not mean that the therapist, at any time, agrees that suicide is an acceptable alternative. Rather, patient and therapist work together to generate other perspectives, interpretations, and solutions to presenting problems. As in standard cognitive therapy, the ultimate goal is to modify the patient's maladaptive assumptions, which in this case predispose the patient to self-destruction.

REFERENCES

Asarnow JR, Carlson GA, Guthrie D: Coping strategies, self-perceptions, hopelessness, and perceived family environments in depressed and suicidal children. J Consult Clin Psychol 55:361–366, 1987

Arffa S: Cognition and suicide: a methodological review. Suicide Life Threat Behav 13:109–122, 1983

Beck AT: Thinking and depression. 1: Idiosyncratic content and cognitive distortions. Arch Gen Psychiatry 9:324–333, 1964

Beck AT: Depression: Clinical, Experimental, and Theoretical Aspects. New York, Harper & Row, 1967; republished as Depression: Causes and Treatment. Philadelphia, PA, University of Pennsylvania Press, 1972

Beck AT: Cognitive Therapy and the Emotional Disorders. New York, New American Library, 1976

Beck AT: Cognitive therapy of depression: new perspectives, in Treatment of Depression: Old Controversies and New Approaches. Edited by Clayton PJ, Barrett JE. New York, Raven Press, 1983, pp 265–290

Beck AT: Hopelessness as a predictor of eventual suicide, in Psychobiology of Suicidal Behavior. Edited by Mann JJ, Stanley M. Ann NY Acad Sci, Vol 487, 1986

Beck AT: Cognitive approaches to hopelessness and suicide. Paper presented at the annual meeting of the Association for the Advancement of Behavior Therapy, Boston, MA, 1987

Beck AT, Lester D: Components of depression in attempted suicides. J Psychol 85:257–260, 1973

Beck AT, Lester D: Components of suicidal intent in completed and attempted suicides. J Psychol 92:35–38, 1976

Beck AT, Young JE: Cognitive therapy of depression, in Behavioral Treatment of Adult Disorders. Edited by Barlow D. New York, Guilford, 1985, pp 206–244

Beck AT, Ward CH, Mendelson M, et al: An inventory for measuring depression. Arch Gen Psychiatry 4:561–571, 1961

Beck AT, Davis JH, Frederick CJ, et al: Classification and nomenclature, in Suicide Prevention in the Seventies (DHEW Publ No HSM-72-9054). Edited by Resnick HCP, Hawthorne BC. Washington, DC, U.S. Govenment Printing Office, 1973a, pp 7–12

Beck AT, Lester D, Albert N: Suicidal wishes and symptoms of depression. Psychol Rep 33:770, 1973b

Beck RW, Morris JB, Beck AT: Cross-validation of the Suicide Intent Scale. Psychol Rep 34:445–446, 1974a

Beck AT, Schuyler D, Herman I: Development of suicidal intent scales, in The Prediction of Suicide. Edited by Beck AT, Resnick HCP, Lettieri D. Bowie, MD, Charles Press, 1974b, pp 45–56

Beck AT, Weissman A, Lester D, et al: The measurement of pessimism: the Hopelessness Scale. J Consult Clin Psychol 42:861–865, 1974c

Beck AT, Beck R, Kovacs M: Classification of suicidal behaviors. I: Quantifying intent and medical lethality. Am J Psychiatry 132:285–287, 1975a

Beck AT, Kovacs M, Weissman A: Hopelessness and suicidal behavior: an overview. JAMA 234:1146–1149, 1975b

Beck AT, Weissman A, Kovacs M: Alcoholism, hopelessness and suicidal behavior. J Stud Alcohol 37:66–77, 1976

Beck AT, Kovacs M, Weissman A: Assessment of suicidal intention: the Scale for Suicide Ideation. J Consult Clin Psychol 47:343–352, 1979a

Beck AT, Rush AJ, Shaw B, et al: Cognitive Therapy of Depression. New York, Guilford, 1979b

Beck AT, Steer RA, Kovacs M, et al: Hopelessness and eventual suicide: a ten-year prospective study of patients hospitalized with suicidal ideation. Am J Psychiatry 142:559–563, 1985

Bedrosian RC, Beck AT: Cognitive aspects of suicidal behavior. Suicide Life Threat Behav 9:87–96, 1979

Bonner RL, Rich AR: A prospective investigation of suicide ideation: a test of a model. Paper presented at the annual meeting of the American Psychological Association, New York, 1987a

Bonner RL, Rich AR: Toward a predictive model of suicidal ideation and behavior: some preliminary data in college students. Suicide Life Threat Behav 17:50–63, 1987b

Burns D: Feeling Good: The New Mood Therapy. New York, William Morrow, 1980

Clum GA, Patsiokas AT, Luscomb RL: Empirically based comprehensive treatment program for parasuicide. J Consult Clin Psychol 47:937–945, 1979

Cohen-Sandler R, Berman AL: Training suicidal children to problem-solve in nonsuicidal ways. Paper presented at the annual meeting of the American Association of Suicidology, New York, April 1982

Drake RE, Cotton PG: Depression, hopelessness, and suicide in chronic schizophrenia. Br J Psychiatry 148:554–559, 1986

Dyer JAT, Kreitman N: Hopelessness, depression and suicidal intent in parasuicide. Br J Psychiatry 144:127–133, 1984

D'Zurilla TJ, Goldfried MR: Problem-solving and behavior modification. J Abnorm Psychol 78:107–126, 1971

D'Zurilla TJ, Nezu A: Social problem-solving in adults, in Advances in Cognitive-Behavioral Research and Therapy, Vol 1. Edited by Kendall PC. New York, Academic, 1982, pp 201–274

Ellis TE: Toward a cognitive therapy for suicidal individuals. Professional Psychology: Research & Practice 17:125–130, 1986

Ellis TE: A cognitive approach to treating the suicidal client, in Innovations in Clinical Practice: A Source Book. Edited by Keller PA, Ritt LG. Sarasota, FL, Professional Resource Exchange, 1987, pp 93–107

Ellis TE, Ratliff KG: Cognitive characteristics of suicidal and nonsuicidal psychiatric patients. Cognitive Therapy and Research 10:625–634, 1986

Fawcett J, Schefter W, Clark D, et al: Clinical predictors of suicide in patients with major affective disorder: a controlled prospective study. Am J Psychiatry 144:35–40, 1987

Goldney RD: Attempted suicide: correlates of lethality. Unpublished doctoral dissertation, University of Adelaide, Australia, 1979

Kovacs M, Beck AT: The wish to die and the wish to live in attempted suicides. J Clin Psychol 33:361–365, 1977

Kovacs M, Beck AT, Weissman A: Hopelessness: an indicator of suicidal risk. Suicide 5:98–103, 1975a

Kovacs M, Beck AT, Weissman A: The use of suicidal motives in the psychotherapy of attempted suicides. Am J Psychother 29:363–368, 1975b

Kovacs M, Beck AT, Weissman A: The communication of suicidal intent: a reexaminaton. Arch Gen Psychiatry 33:198–201, 1976

Lester D: Suicide and internal-external orientation. Psychology 10:35–39, 1973

Lester D, Beck AT: Suicidal wishes and depression in suicidal ideators: a comparison with attempted suicides. J Clin Psychol 33:92–94, 1977

Levenson M: Cognitive characteristics of suicide risk, in Psychological Assessment of Suicide Risk. Edited by Neuringer C. Springfield, IL, Charles C Thomas, 1974, pp 150–163

Levenson M, Neuringer C: Problem-solving behavior in suicidal adolescents. J Consult Clin Psychol 37:433–436, 1971

Linehan MM, Goodstein JL, Nielsen SL, et al: Reasons for staying alive when you are thinking of killing yourself: the Reasons for Living Inventory. J Consult Clin Psychol 51:276–286, 1983

Linehan MM, Chiles JA, Egan KJ, et al: Presenting problems of parasuicides versus suicide ideators and nonsuicidal psychiatric patients. J Consult Clin Psychol 54:880–881, 1986

Linehan MM, Camper P, Chiles J, et al: Interpersonal problem-solving and parasuicide. Cognitive Therapy and Research 11:1–12, 1987

McLeavey BC, Daly RJ, Murra CM: Evaluation of an interpersonal problem-solving training programme for self-poisoning patients (abstract). Psychological Abstracts 1986

McLeavey BC, Daly RJ, Murray CM, et al: Interpersonal problem-solving deficits in self-poisoning patients. Suicide Life Threat Behav 17:33–49, 1987

Minkoff K, Bergman E, Beck AT, et al: Hopelessness, depression, and attempted suicide. Am J Psychiatry 130:455–459, 1973

Neuringer C: Dichotomous evaluations in suicidal individuals. J Consult Psychol 25:445–449, 1961

Neuringer C: The cognitive organization of meaning in suicidal individuals. J Gen Psychol 76:91–100, 1967

Neuringer C: Divergencies between attitudes towards life and death among suicidal, psychosomatic, and normal hospitalized patients. J Consult Clin Psychol 32:59–63, 1968

Neuringer C, Lettieri DJ: Cognition, attitude, and affect in suicidal individuals. Life Threatening Behavior 1:106–124, 1971

Nezu AM: Efficacy of a social problem-solving therapy approach for unipolar depression. J Consult Clin Psychol 54:196–202, 1986

Nezu AM: A problem-solving formulation of depression: a literature review and proposal of a pluralistic model. Clinical Psychology Review 7:121–144, 1987

Patsiokas AT, Clum GA: Effects of psychotherapeutic strategies in the treatment of suicide attempters. Psychotherapy 22:281–290, 1985

Patsiokas AT, Clum GA, Luscomb RL: Cognitive characteristics of suicide attempters. J Consult Clin Psychol 47:478–484, 1979

Petrie K, Chamberlain K: Hopelessness and social desirability as moderator variables in predicting suicidal behavior. J Consult Clin Psychol 51:485–487, 1983

Rush A, Beck AT, Kovacs M, et al: Comparison of the differential effects of cognitive therapy and pharmacotherapy on hopelessness and self-concept. Am J Psychiatry 139:862–866, 1982

Schotte DE, Clum GA: Suicide ideation in a college population: a test of a model. J Consult Clin Psychol 50:690–696, 1982

Schotte DE, Clum GA: Problem-solving skills in suicidal psychiatric patients. J Consult Clin Psychol 55:49–54, 1987

Silver MA, Bohnert M, Beck AT, et al: Relation of depression of attempted suicide and seriousness of intent. Arch Gen Psychiatry 25:573–576, 1971

Weissman A, Beck AT, Kovacs M: Drug abuse, hopelessness, and suicidal behavior. Int J Addict 14:451–464, 1979

Wetzel RD: Hopelessness, depression and suicide intent. Arch Gen Psychiatry 33:1069–1073, 1976a

Wetzel RD: Semantic differential ratings of concepts and suicide intent. J Clin Psychol 32:4–13, 1976b

Wetzel RD, Margulies T, Davis R, et al: Hopelessness, depression, and suicide intent. J Clin Psychol 41:159–160, 1980

Chapter 18

Community Strategies for Suicide Prevention and Intervention

Patrick W. O'Carroll, M.D., M.P.H.

IN RECENT YEARS, suicide has been explicitly identified as an important public health problem. The United States Surgeon General has included a specific health objective related to suicide as part of the national public health agenda (U.S. Department of Health and Human Services 1980). Suicide ranks eighth as a cause of death in the United States. Among persons aged 15 to 34 years, it is now the second leading cause of death (Centers for Disease Control 1986a). Unlike many diseases, suicide rates are substantial among both young and old people. As a result, suicide is the fourth leading cause of premature death, as defined by years of potential life lost before age 65 years (Centers for Disease Control 1987). Moreover, the problem of suicide has been worsening among our nation's youth. The rate of suicide among persons 15 to 24 years of age has tripled since 1950 (Centers for Disease Control 1986b).

Identifying suicide as a public health problem has important implications for our approach to this issue. The main focus of public health practice is the primary prevention of disease. Because primary prevention frequently cannot be accomplished solely in the clinical setting, public health interventions have necessarily been multidisciplinary (Mercy and O'Carroll 1988). Providing a clean water supply, pasteurizing milk, investigating potentially infected contacts of persons with tuberculosis or sexually transmitted diseases, legislating building safety codes, and implementing the Special Supplemental Food Program for Women, Infants and Children (WIC program) are all public health interventions that have required expertise and action from a number of different disciplines in addition to contributions from clinical practice.

The prevention of suicide will likewise require a multidisciplinary effort. That no single discipline or profession has all the necessary resources to address the problem of suicide adequately has been vividly demonstrated in communities that have experienced so-called suicide clusters. These suicide clusters have frequently involved teenagers and young adults and have almost invariably resulted in the rapid development of a crisis atmosphere in the affected communities. In most cases, the intense concern of parents, students, teachers, and others led to enormous pressure on community leaders to address the crisis and prevent the cluster from spreading. Yet in almost every community, the early days of the crisis were marked by confusion over who was responsible for addressing the problem. Various community sectors had a tendency to alternate between claiming jurisdiction over the problem and blaming some other community sector for failing to address it. Underlying this confusion was the failure to recognize that persons in a number of different community sectors— including mental health, medicine, education, public health, and municipal government—can and should play important roles in suicide prevention.

CRISIS RESPONSE RECOMMENDATIONS AS A MODEL FOR GENERAL SUICIDE PREVENTION

Of course, a number of disciplines and societal sectors already contribute to suicide prevention. What has been lacking in most communities is a recognition that these efforts must be coordinated as part of a community plan for suicide prevention. A useful model for a community strategy for suicide prevention has developed out of the experiences of communities that have faced suicide clusters (see Gould, Chapter 19, this volume). Following an episode of multiple suicides in New Jersey, the New Jersey Department of Health and the Centers for Disease Control (CDC) jointly sponsored a workshop to develop recommendations for controlling suicide clusters. Participants at that workshop included persons who had played key roles in community responses to nine different suicide clusters, as well as representatives from the American Association of Suicidology, the Association of State and Territorial Health Officials, the Indian Health Service, and the National Institute of Mental Health. Table 1 summarizes the 10 recommendations developed at that workshop; they have

Table 1. The Centers for Disease Control recommendations for a community plan for the prevention and containment of suicide clusters

1. A community should review these recommendations and develop its own response plan before the onset of a suicide cluster.

2. The response to the crisis should involve all concerned sectors of the community and should be coordinated by:

   A. Coordinating committee, which manages the day-to-day response to the crisis

   B. Host agency, whose responsibilities would include "housing" the plan, monitoring the incidence of suicide, and calling meetings of the coordinating committee when necessary

3. The relevant community resources should be identified.

4. The response plan should be implemented under either of the following two conditions:

   A. When a suicide cluster occurs in the community

   B. When one or more deaths from trauma occur in the community, especially among adolescents or young adults, which may potentially influence others to attempt or complete suicide.

5. If the response plan is to be implemented, the first step should be to contact and prepare those groups who will play key roles in the first days of the response.

6. The response should be conducted in a manner that avoids glorification of the suicide victims and minimizes sensationalism.

7. Persons who may be at high risk of suicide should be identified and have at least one screening interview with a trained counselor; these persons should be referred for further counseling or other services as needed.

8. A timely flow of accurate, appropriate information should be provided to the media.

9. Elements in the environment that might increase the likelihood of further suicides or suicide attempts should be identified and changed.

10. Long-term issues suggested by the nature of the suicide cluster should be addressed.

been recently published and widely disseminated (Centers for Disease Control 1988).[1]

Although these recommendations were developed to assist communities to develop a plan for response to suicide clusters, they are largely applicable to and consistent with general community suicide prevention efforts. In this chapter, the recommendations for responding to a suicide cluster will be reviewed point by point to illustrate how these recommendations may be used to develop a number of major components of a coordinated community suicide prevention plan. In doing so, the important roles that can be played by physicians and mental heatlh professionals in promoting, coordinating, and assisting in this response will be underscored.

It should be remembered, however, that these recommendations were developed for the specific purpose of responding to a crisis situation. A general community plan for suicide prevention would include several measures not addressed by these crisis response recommendations. Some of these measures will be reviewed in the final part of this chapter.

1. A community should review these recommendations and develop its own response before the onset of a suicide cluster. As noted previously, in the context of an evolving suicide cluster, there is typically a great deal of confusion and little initial coordination of community effort to contain the cluster. For this reason, it is important that communities develop a plan for community response in advance. Of course, communities are highly motivated toward some sort of preventive action when faced with a suicide cluster—this motivation is not so easily generated in the absence of a crisis. Yet the actions suggested in the following recommendations for suicide cluster control will inevitably be hindered if communities wait until there is a crisis to adapt the plan to their own resources. This places a challenging responsibility on those interested in preventing and containing suicide clusters to provide the impetus for action in the absence of any crisis by persuading appropriate community leaders of the importance of this preparatory step.

[1]I would like to acknowledge Eugene Aronowitz, Ph.D.; Ines Assafi, M.S.W.; Dennis Blomquist; Ronald G. Burmood, Ph.D.; Betsey S. Comstock, M.D.; Karen Dunne-Maxim, R.N., M.S.; John W. Farrell, M.S.W.; Louis C. Goetting IV; Madelyn S. Gould, Ph.D.; Myra Herbert, M.S.W.; Karen Hymbaugh; Elizabeth N. Jones, Ed.S.; Alan J. Krumholz, M.D.; James A. Mercy, Ph.D.; William Parkin, D.V.M., Dr.P.H.; Michael Petrone, M.D.; Julie Rayburn-Miller, M.S.W.; Jon Shaw, M.D.; Carol E. Steele, R.N., M.S.; and John A. Steward, M.P.H., all of whom actively participated in the development of the CDC Recommendations for a Community Plan for the Prevention and Containment of Suicide Clusters. I would also like to acknowledge Mark L. Rosenberg, M.D., who contributed substantially to the original conceptualization of those recommendations.

This responsibility is even more challenging when it comes to the general prevention of suicide. In this case, the evocative image of a community in crisis is not available to help convince community leaders of the importance of developing a coordinated, multidisciplinary suicide prevention plan. Yet such a plan would potentially address a much larger segment of the suicide problem than one focused solely on suicide clusters. It is estimated that only 1% to 4% of all suicides occur in clusters (Gould et al. 1987). Thus, even if every community were to develop a plan for suicide cluster control and even if these plans were uniformly, completely effective, 96% to 99% of the suicides in this country would still occur.

Health professionals can play at least two important roles in providing the impetus for developing a community suicide prevention plan. First, they might provide a leadership role by becoming personally involved in developing the community plan, as described later. Second, they can provide an effective advocacy role by contacting persons who may be in a better position to lead and coordinate community suicide prevention efforts, and convincing them of the need for community-wide suicide prevention efforts. Such persons may be found, for example, in municipal government, public health or mental health agencies, and state or local mental health associations.

2. The response to the crisis should involve all concerned sectors of the community and should be coordinated by a committee of individuals from various community agencies, and a "host agency." The concept of a coordinating committee—individuals from education, public health, mental health, local government, suicide crisis centers, and other concerned agencies—was developed so that the response to a suicide cluster would truly be a community endeavor. The coordinating committee would be responsible for incorporating the CDC's recommendations into a suicide cluster response plan that reflects the needs and resources of their particular community, deciding when the plan should be implemented and coordinating its implementation. The individual representing the "host agency" would be responsible for enlisting members of the coordinating committee, calling the initial meeting of the committee to develop the suicide cluster control plan, establishing a mechanism by which the agency would be notified of a potentially evolving suicide cluster, and convening a meeting of the coordinating committee when it is suspected that a suicide cluster is occurring or might be about to occur.

The advantages inherent in this approach apply to preventing suicide in general, as well as to controlling suicide clusters. In both cases, no single agency has all the necessary resources for a comprehensive response. Cooperation and coordination among the various community sectors that might contribute to suicide prevention are thus necessary. Furthermore, an existing coordinating committee should eliminate some of the "turf" issues that sometimes arise in suicide prevention. Each agency represented on the committee could contribute to the suicide prevention effort according to its particular expertise. Having one agency serve as the host for the community plan would allow for a necessary locus of responsibility, but should allow the committee to avoid identifying any one agency as the "lead." Finally, local input during the plan's development allows for the best possible use of a community's resources.

3. The relevant community resources should be identified. Clearly, identifying resources is as applicable to suicide prevention in general as it is to the control of suicide clusters. It may seem to be an intuitive and straightforward step, but most communities that have faced suicide clusters have found that enumerating, contacting, and developing a working relationship with a variety of agencies and community organizations in the space of a few days is an exceedingly difficult task. Assembling the coordinating committee alone should help with this step, but many other potential resources need to be considered when constructing a community suicide prevention plan, including hospitals, emergency medical services systems, high school and college health clinics, local physicians, parents' groups, students, clergy, survivor groups, police, and the local news media.

The role of each group included in the plan should be clearly identified and should be agreed on and reviewed by persons representing each group. Most of those involved in the community plan will already be familiar with their likely roles in a community suicide prevention effort, but in some cases training for the staff of the involved groups may be necessary (Dunne et al. 1987).

It is particularly important that members of the local news media be included in the plan's development. In the context of suicide clusters, the media has often been accused of being part of the problem; but for both preventing suicide in general and controlling suicide clusters, the news media can be part of the solution. For example, the local media might be instrumental in announcing and publishing the location of various community resources and agencies that offer treatment and support services.

4. The response plan should be implemented when a suicide cluster occurs, or when one or more deaths from trauma occur (especially among adolescents or young adults), which members of the coordinating committee think may potentially influence others in the commu-

nity to attempt or complete suicide. At first glance, this recommendation for conditional implementation of the suicide cluster control plan would seem conceptually to separate this plan from an ongoing community suicide prevention effort. As the first three recommendations indicate, however, the cluster response plan is not something that is meant to be kept on the shelf until a cluster occurs. Rather, the plan requires ongoing notification of the host agency when suicides occur in the community; frequent examination of the numbers and patterns of suicides in the community; and occasional meetings of the coordinating committee to decide whether the response plan should be implemented in the face of an unusual pattern or number of suicides in the community. Even when the response plan is implemented, it is not an all-or-nothing decision. Implementation of the plan can be quite subtle and limited (as might be the case, for example, if it were feared that a suicide cluster were about to start) or highly visible and extensive. Finally, even in the absence of unusual numbers or patterns of suicides, the coordinating committee would need to meet regularly to maintain and revise the plan.

Thus, the suicide cluster response plan might fit very neatly into the ongoing operations of a general community suicide prevention plan.

5. If the response plan is to be implemented, the first step should be to contact and prepare the various groups identified above. This point primarily applies to crisis-response situations. In several past school-based suicide clusters, persons who might otherwise have been instrumental in helping identify high-risk students during the early days of the crisis were not contacted and prepared. These people were therefore unaware of the various resources for referral and of the potential role they might play as gatekeepers to those resources.

This point is best illustrated with an example. In one community in which two high school students committed suicide over a weekend, both the teachers and the students learned of the deaths at the same time on the following Monday, when the suicides were announced over the school loudspeaker. The teachers were entirely unprepared to deal with the emotional response of the students and did not know what to say to them or where to refer those who were most upset. It would have been far preferable to have called a meeting with the teachers before the start of the school day to outline the problem, discuss the appropriate roles of the teachers, and announce the various resources that were available (Dunne et al. 1987).

A number of benefits might have accrued from this approach. First, the teachers could have provided input concerning the manner in which the deaths were announced to the students. They might, for example, have suggested that the students be in a small, supervised setting, such as a homeroom class, when the deaths were announced and that the announcement be made by individual teachers rather than over the loudspeaker. Second, the teachers would have been in a very good position to identify students who seemed particularly affected by the news, to ensure that these students were properly referred for counseling, and to see that others were made aware of counseling resources. Finally, the teachers would have had time to react to the news and prepare themselves to provide support to the students later on.

6. The crisis response should be conducted in a manner that avoids glorifying the suicide victims and minimizes sensationalism. This recommendation is certainly relevant to a suicide cluster response, since sensationalism and glorification of suicide victims have been conspicuous elements in several past suicide clusters. A number of investigators have hypothesized that suicide clusters may occur due to "contagion," a process by which one's risk of suicide is increased by exposure to the suicides of others (Davidson and Gould 1989; Robbins and Conroy 1983). Sensationalizing suicide may augment the effect of contagion. In addition, glorifying victims of suicide may unintentionally increase the likelihood that someone who identifies with the decedents or who is having suicidal thoughts will also attempt suicide, so as to be similarly glorified or to receive similar positive attention (Rosenberg et al. 1987).

This recommendation is equally applicable to general suicide prevention efforts. If exposure to another person's suicide increases one's own risk of suicide, there is no reason to suppose that it only has this effect in the context of a suicide cluster. Although a large number of people may be exposed in any given suicide cluster, these clusters appear to be quite rare compared to the number of noncluster suicides that occur. Overall, more people may be exposed to noncluster than cluster suicides. Although the contagion hypothesis has yet to be formally tested, it would seem prudent in the meantime to avoid sensationalizing suicide or glorifying suicide victims, regardless of whether the suicides were committed in the context of a suicide cluster.

7. Persons who may be at high risk of suicide should be identified and have at least one screening interview with a trained counselor; these persons should be referred for further counseling or other services as needed. In response to a suicide cluster, all of the preceding steps may be considered preparatory to this step. Because the central goal of a suicide cluster response is to prevent any further suicides or suicide attempts from occurring, the response should be focused on those who are considered most likely to become part of the cluster. In addition, identifying high-risk persons allows for efficient and effective use of community resources for suicide prevention. Those who were emotionally close to the suicide victims (e.g., relatives, girlfriends/boyfriends, close friends, fellow employees) should be identified and screened, if possible. In addition, persons who were exposed to the suicides (e.g., students in the same school as a suicide victim) who have other known risk factors for suicide (e.g., depression, history of suicide attempt, recent loss) should be identified and provided with an opportunity to express their feelings about and reactions to the suicide deaths.

This recommendation is also entirely applicable to the general prevention of suicide. Physicians have long been aware that patients with depression and certain other mental illnesses are at increased risk of suicide (Hagnell et al. 1981), and doctors are usually very careful both to screen such patients for suicidal ideation and to avoid dispensing potentially lethal quantities of medications to them (Blumenthal 1988). Physicians may not be as sensitized, however, to the increased suicide risk of persons who have been recently widowed or divorced (MacMahon and Pugh 1965; Smith et al. 1988), who have lost other close family members (Bunch et al. 1971), who are alcoholic (Miles 1977; Roy and Linnoila 1986), who have recently lost their jobs (Platt 1985), or who have recently had their normal social supports disrupted (South 1987). Again, although the contagion hypothesis has not yet been formally tested at the individual level, the anecdotal and ecological evidence to date is sufficiently compelling that physicians should consider the possibility of suicide for any patient who has been recently exposed to another person's suicide. This is particularly true if the patient has other risk factors for suicide, such as a past history of attempted suicide (Paerregaard 1975) or one of the risk factors mentioned above.

Unfortunately, an approach based entirely on physician identification of suicidal patients is not sufficient. Thirty-five years ago, most suicide victims were older men, and the chief risk factor for suicide in this group was clinical depression (Rosenberg et al. 1987). Teaching physicians to diagnose and treat depression in this group was, therefore, a very reasonable and theoretically comprehensive means of preventing suicide. Indeed, the suicide rates in this age-sex group have declined during the past several decades (Centers for Disease Control 1985) and some of that decline may be due to better recognition and treatment of depression. Now, however, suicide rates are also high among adolescents and young adults, and research suggests that a much smaller proportion of suicide victims in this age group satisfy clinical criteria for depression (Shaffer et al. 1986). In the younger age groups, suicides are frequently impulsive acts, and there may be risk factors for youth suicide (such as contagion) that are not risk factors for suicide among older persons (Gould et al. 1987). More importantly, risk factors such as impulsiveness and exposure to another's suicide are not such as to require contact with a physician.

This is one of the main reasons that a community-wide suicide prevention effort is necessary. Persons who are at high risk of suicide do not uniformly come to the attention of a single category of professionals, such as physicians or mental health practitioners. Instead, teachers, relatives, fellow workers, police, and others may sometimes be in the best position to identify suicidal persons. Unfortunately, there has usually been no well-publicized, coordinated community plan of action for people who are worried about the possibility of suicide by someone they know.

Actively identifying and providing potentially suicidal persons with a screening interview with a counselor will not prevent all suicides. But this active approach should at least be more effective than a solely passive approach based on self-referral. Whether passive measures such as suicide hotlines or walk-in suicide crisis centers actually reduce the suicide rate is still an open question; the evidence is mixed, at best (Miller et al. 1984). Absence of evidence is not evidence of absence, of course, and it is difficult to believe that no suicide has ever been prevented because of the presence of hotlines or walk-in centers. The coordinating committee must weigh the costs and potential benefits of various mixes of active and passive efforts to identify suicidal persons in the community.

8. A timely flow of accurate, appropriate information should be provided to the media. The controversy regarding the media's role in reporting suicides has escalated during the past few years because of the intense media coverage of suicide clusters. Leaders in several communities that faced suicide clusters reported that news media demands for information during the crisis were overwhelming. In addition to disrupting the crisis response, the intense news coverage is believed by several community leaders to have been at least partly to blame for some of the subsequent suicides through a sensationalism that fostered a preoccupation with suicide—that is, through promoting contagion.

For this reason, it is especially important that communities learn how to satisfy the legitimate needs of the news media in the context of a suicide cluster in a way that avoids sensationalism and minimizes disruption of the community response to the crisis. The CDC recommends that "media spokespersons" be appointed to represent the various community sectors involved in the response and that a single "information coordinator" be appointed to ensure that the various media spokespersons have complete and current information, to refer inquiries to the appropriate spokespersons, and to schedule and hold press conferences, if necessary. Perhaps the most effective single step that can be taken is to develop a working relationship with local media representatives before any crisis occurs.

Even in the absence of a suicide cluster, communities must work with the news media to ensure that suicides are reported appropriately so that the risk of imitative suicides is not unwittingly increased. For example, it is accurate to state that a person committed suicide by carbon monoxide poisoning, but it is not necessary—and is potentially very dangerous—to explain that the decedent acquired a hose from a hardware store, hooked it up to the tail pipe of a car, and then sat in the car with its engine running in a closed garage at a particular address. Such details practically constitute a recipe for imitative suicide and can only make such suicides more likely.

In the context of a general community suicide prevention plan, an information coordinator and various media spokespersons could work with the local news media to try to avoid such needlessly detailed and lurid accounts. The American Association of Suicidology has developed guidelines for reporting suicide[1] that may also be helpful. The coordinating committee should review these guidelines with local media representatives and use them as a starting point for agreement on what is and is not appropriate news coverage of suicide.

9. Elements in the environment that might increase the likelihood of further suicides or suicide attempts should be modified and changed. Passive environmental modifications, such as fences around swimming pools, household fuses, collapsing automobile steering wheels, and childproof closures on containers with toxic substances, have proven highly effective in preventing a variety of unintentional injuries (National Research Council 1985; O'Carroll et al. 1988). In the case of suicide, the fact that the injury is intended adds another dimension to the issue, a dimension that provides us with another avenue for intervention. For example, persons who are considering suicide may reveal this intention to physicians, counselors, or friends, and these individuals may then intervene to prevent the suicidal act. This opportunity for intervention, however, should not blind us to the potential power of environmental modifications as a tool for suicide prevention.

---

[1]A copy of these guidelines may be obtained by writing to the American Association of Suicidology, 2459 South Ash, Denver, CO 80222.

There are a number of examples where environmental modification has been used as part of a community's effort to control a suicide cluster. In one community where four adolescents committed suicide together by carbon monoxide poisoning in a garage, the coordinating committee arranged to have the garage door locked and instituted police surveillance of the area. By all accounts, this police surveillance was responsible for saving the lives of two other adolescents who broke into the locked garage and also attempted suicide by carbon monoxide poisoning. After this incident, the garage door was removed—a more definitive environmental intervention. In another suicide cluster among Native Americans, many of the victims committed suicide by hanging in their jail cell on the morning following an arrest. Efforts were stepped up to remove articles of clothing or other elements that might be used to commit suicide, and surveillance of the jail cells was increased.

Environmental modification may contribute to the general prevention of suicide, as well as to the control of suicide clusters. Reducing the carbon monoxide content in domestic gas apparently led to a sustained decrease in the suicide rate in England (Kreitman 1976). In Australia, a change in the prescribing practices of physicians also apparently led to a decrease in the rate of suicide by overdose (Goldney and Katsikitis 1983). Unfortunately, modifications of the environment are not always so successful (Pan American Health Organization 1986), and certain methods of suicide do not readily lend themselves to comprehensive environmental solutions. For example, suicide by jumping cannot be completely prevented by environmental modification because it is impractical to erect barriers on every tall building, bridge, parking garage, and cliff. Similarly, firearm suicides could presumably be completely eliminated if potential victims did not have access to such lethal weapons. Restricting access to firearms is a highly contentious social and political issue, however, and it is therefore unlikely that we will greatly reduce the availability of firearms in the near future. In any case, some investigators argue that even if certain means of suicide are restricted, persons who are truly suicidal will simply substitute some alternative means of suicide (Rushforth et al. 1984).

Despite these caveats, environmental modifications should be considered even when they are not likely to be totally effective. For example, although barriers will not prevent every suicide by jumping, they should nevertheless be erected if possible at any site where more than one suicide has occurred. Such sites have sometimes become "suicide magnets" (Seiden 1988), where potential suicide victims would come to join the growing—and well-publicized—list of preceding victims. Anecdotal evidence suggests that if these potential victims cannot attempt suicide from the site in question, they do not all simply go elsewhere to attempt suicide from some other high place. Similarly, although the coordinating committee cannot eliminate access to all firearms, they can recommend that parents reduce their children's risk of suicide by keeping any firearms locked up and separate from the ammunition. Even if some suicidal adolescents substitute an alternate method of suicide when their access to firearms is restricted, this substitution may increase their chances for survival. Most methods of suicide are not as immediately lethal as firearms. Nonfirearm suicide attempts thus present a greater opportunity for lifesaving medical or surgical intervention.

10. Long-term issues suggested by the nature of the suicide cluster should be addressed. In retrospect, common characteristics among the victims in certain suicide clusters have suggested that various community issues need to be addressed. For example, many of the victims in one cluster were troubled adolescents who, by dropping out of school, had become excluded from the life of an otherwise closely knit community. In this instance, community leaders felt that greater efforts might be made to bring such persons back into the mainstream of community life. In another case, many of the victims had not been identified before their suicides as being depressed or otherwise troubled about anything. Resources for help in this community might be developed or made more accessible so that persons who were troubled could receive help in the future before they reached the stage of overt suicidal behavior.

But for both suicide cluster control and for suicide prevention in general, the one long-term issue that most communities face is the need to develop a community plan for preventing and responding to suicide. Community problems that appear to contribute to suicide should certainly be addressed, but this should be conducted in the larger context of the community suicide prevention plan described above.

LIMITATIONS INHERENT IN THIS APPROACH

Although these recommendations for responding to a suicide cluster might be used as a model for major components of a general community suicide prevention effort, the model is not comprehensive. These recommendations are limited because they were developed with a specific need in mind: the response to a rapidly evolving crisis situation. This need is reflected both in the inclusion of numerous examples of crisis control measures and in the relative dearth of suggestions for primary prevention of suicide.

The Report of the Secretary's Task Force on Youth Suicide presents a comprehensive list of suggestions for preventing suicide (Alcohol, Drug Abuse, and Mental Health Administration 1989). Some of these suggestions, such as those relating to improving the quality of national suicide data, are not immediately relevant to community suicide prevention. Other suggestions, such as those relating to media coverage of suicide, have been mentioned previously. But there are numerous other recommendations in the report that communities should carefully consider when formulating a general suicide prevention plan. These include developing a local suicide attempt surveillance system; creating specific intervention programs for identified suicide attempters; teaching gatekeepers (e.g., school personnel, counselors, coaches, family members, friends, youth group leaders) how to identify those at high risk of suicide; restricting lethal means of suicide, especially for newly incarcerated prisoners and potentially suicidal adolescents; increasing access to suicide prevention services; and integrating suicide prevention into programs focused on preventing antecedent risk factors for suicide, such as depression, substance abuse, and delinquency.

CONCLUSION

Although suicide is by no means a new problem, the recent delineation of suicide as a public health problem provides the context for a renewed, more cooperative approach to prevention. The suicide cluster control recommendations prepared by the CDC provide a useful (although not comprehensive) outline for the general prevention of suicide at the community level. At a minimum, they highlight the need to establish a locus of responsibility for suicide prevention that involves all concerned sectors of the community and the need to develop a community plan for suicide prevention that makes the best use of existing local resources. This is best accomplished before any crisis occurs.

Physicians and mental health professionals can play a number of important roles in this process, ranging from minimal involvement as clinicians during actual implementation of the crisis response plan to active leadership in forming a coordinating committee and in developing the community plan. As health practitioners who have seen the tragedy of suicide at close hand, physicians and mental health professionals are well-suited to be effective advocates for developing a community-wide suicide prevention effort. This advocacy might be all that is needed to galvanize certain communities into a concerted effort to prevent suicide.

REFERENCES

Alcohol, Drug Abuse, and Mental Health Administration: Report of the Secretary's Task Force on Youth Suicide (DHHS Publ No ADM-89-1621). Washington, DC, U.S. Government Printing Office, 1989

Blumenthal SJ: A guide to risk factors, assessment and treatment of suicidal patients. Med Clin North Am 72:937–971, 1988

Bunch J, Barraclough B, Nelson B, et al: Suicide following bereavement of parents. Soc Psychiatry 6:193–199, 1971

Centers for Disease Control: Suicide surveillance: summary 1970–80. Atlanta, GA, U.S. Department of Health and Human Services, Public Health Service, 1985

Centers for Disease Control: Homicide surveillance: high-risk racial and ethnic groups: blacks and Hispanics, 1970 to 1983. Atlanta, GA, Centers for Disease Control, 1986a

Centers for Disease Control: Youth suicide in the United States, 1970–80. Atlanta, GA, U.S. Department of Health and Human Services, Public Health Service, 1986b

Centers for Disease Control: Premature mortality due to suicide and homicide: United States, 1984. MMWR 36:531–534, 1987

Centers for Disease Control: CDC recommendations for a community plan for the prevention and containment of suicide clusters. MMWR 37(suppl S-6):1–12, 1988

Davidson L, Gould MS: Contagion as a risk factor for youth suicide, in Alcohol, Drug Abuse, and Mental Health Administration: Report of the Secretary's Task Force on Youth Suicide, Vol 2, Risk Factors for Youth Suicide (DHHS Publ No ADM-89-1622). Washington, DC, U.S. Government Printing Office, 1989, pp 88–109

Dunne EJ, McIntosh JL, Dunne-Maxim K (eds): Suicide and Its Aftermath: Understanding and Counseling the Survivors. New York, WW Norton, 1987

Goldney RD, Katsikitis M: Cohort analysis of suicide rates in Australia. Arch Gen Psychiatry 40:71–74, 1983

Gould MS, Wallenstein S, Kleinman M: A study of time-space clustering of suicide: final report (Contract RFP 200-85-0834). Atlanta, GA, Centers for Disease Control, 1987

Hagnell O, Lanke J, Rorsman B: Suicide rates in the Lundby study: mental illness as a risk factor for suicide. Neuropsychobiology 7:248–253, 1981

Kreitman N: The coal gas story: United Kingdom suicide rates, 1960–71. British Journal of Preventative and Social Medicine 30:86–93, 1976

MacMahon B, Pugh TF: Suicide in the widowed. Am J Epidemiol 81:23–31, 1965

Mercy JA, O'Carroll PW: New directions in violence prediction: the public health arena. Violence and Victims 3:285–301, 1988

Miles CP: Conditions predisposing to suicide: a review. J Nerv Ment Dis 164:231–246, 1977

Miller HL, Coombs DW, Leeper JD, et al: An analysis of the effects of suicide prevention facilities on suicide rates in the United States. Am J Public Health 74:340–343, 1984

National Research Council, Committee on Trauma Research: Injury in America: a continuing public health problem. Washington, DC, National Academy Press, 1985

O'Carroll PW, Alkon E, Weiss B: Drowning mortality in Los Angeles County, 1976 to 1984. JAMA 260:380–383, 1988

Paerregaard G: Suicide among attempted suicides: a 10-year follow-up. Suicide 5:140–144, 1975

Pan American Health Organization: Paraquat poisoning in two Caribbean countries. Caribbean Epidemiology Centre (CAREC) Surveillance Report 12:1–9, 1986

Platt S: Unemployment and suicidal behavior: a review of the literature. Soc Sci Med 19:93–115, 1984

Robbins D, Conroy R: A cluster of adolescent suicide attempts: is suicide contagious? J Adolesc Health Care 3:253–255, 1983

Rosenberg ML, Smith JC, Davidson LE, et al: The emergence of youth suicide: an epidemiologic analysis and public health perspective. Annu Rev Public Health 8:417–440, 1987

Roy A, Linnoila M: Alcoholism and suicide. Suicide Life Threat Behav 16:244–273, 1986

Rushforth NB, Ford AB, Sudak HS, et al: Increasing suicide rates in adolescents and young adults in an urban community (1958–1982): tests of hypotheses from national data, in Suicide in the Young. Edited by Sudak HS, Ford AB, Rushforth NB. Boston, MA, J Wright, 1984, pp 45–67

Seiden R: Suicide prevention in public places. Paper presented at the 21st annual meeting of the American Association of Suicidology, Washington, DC, April 1988

Shaffer D, Gould MS, Phillips D, et al: Developments in teen suicide research. Paper presented at the 33rd annual meeting of the American Academy of Child Psychiatry, Los Angeles, October 1986

Smith JC, Mercy JA, Conn JM: Marital status and the risk of suicide. Am J Public Health 78:78–80, 1988

South SJ: Metropolitan migration and social problems. Social Science Quarterly 68:3–18, 1987

U.S. Department of Health and Human Services, Public Health Service: Promoting health/preventing disease: objectives for the nation. Washington, DC, U.S. Government Printing Office, 1980

Section 3

Special Issues

Chapter 19

Suicide Clusters and Media Exposure

Madelyn S. Gould, Ph.D., M.P.H.

INCREASING CONCERN ABOUT the role of imitation and contagion as risk factors for suicide has been associated with a number of highly publicized suicide outbreaks in teenagers and young adults and with evidence that an increased number of suicides appear to be associated with suicide stories in the mass media. A review of the research and literature on suicide clusters and the impact of suicide stories in the mass media is the focus of this chapter.

The interchangeable usage of the terms *clusters, contagion,* and *imitation* in the literature leads to difficulties in communication and understanding of the contribution of these factors to suicide (Biblarz 1988). A suicide *cluster* refers to an excessive number of suicides occurring in close temporal and/or geographic proximity. Suicide *contagion* is the process by which one suicide facilitates the occurrence

This work was partially supported by Faculty Scholars Award 84-0954-84 from the W.T. Grant Foundation, Grant R01 MH38198 from the NIMH and Contract #200-85-0834 from the Centers for Disease Control.

Portions of this material were adapted from Gould MS, Davidson L: Suicide contagion among adolescents, in *Advances in Adolescent Mental Health, Volume III: Depression and Suicide.* Edited by Stiffman AR, Feldman RA. Greenwich, CT, JAI Press, 1988; and from Davidson L, Gould MS: Contagion as a risk factor for youth suicide, in *Alcohol, Drug Abuse and Mental Health Administration: Report of the Secretary's Task Force on Youth Suicide, Volume 2: Risk Factors for Youth Suicide* (DHHS Publ No ADM-89-1622). Washington, DC, U.S. Government Printing Office, 1989.

of a subsequent suicide. Contagion assumes either direct or indirect awareness of the prior suicide. *Imitation*, the process by which one suicide becomes a compelling model for successive suicides, is one underlying theory to explain the occurrence of contagion.

Although suicide is not a disease per se, the application of an infectious disease model highlights factors that may influence the process of suicide contagion and emphasizes the multiple causation of disease. An infectious disease model focuses on the forces within the individual, as well as the environment that influences the individual's state of health. The components of an infectious disease model relevant to suicide contagion include host susceptibility, modes of transmission, degree of virulence, dose dependency, and a spectrum of disease (Davidson and Gould 1989).

Host susceptibility involves the individual's own capacity to shape the manifestations of disease (Susser 1973). An individual's resistance or immunity to a disease can prevent the occurrence of illness even if the individual is exposed to an outbreak of the disease. There are multiple host factors that affect susceptibility to disease, including inherited or genetic attributes as well as acquired characteristics. In the case of suicide, a genetic predisposition to depression may increase the probability of engaging in suicidal behavior. Good baseline emotional health may be analogous to an affective immune system in being capable of warding off challenges. The cognitive and affective ability to identify and speak about feelings may make an individual less susceptible to suicide (Davidson and Gould 1989).

A central aspect of the spread of infectious disease is the transmission of infection (Mausner and Kramer 1985). Transmission may be direct (person-to-person) or indirect. An outbreak of suicides among friends within the same social network implies direct, person-to-person transmission. The suicide of a celebrity may be an indirect exposure to suicide for millions of people. Thus various suicide contagion pathways may exist: direct contact or friendship with a victim, word-of-mouth knowledge, and indirect transmission through the media.

Virulence refers to the ability of an infective agent to produce serious illness. The degree of virulence varies for different infective agents. For suicide, the characteristics of the individual whose death was the first in a potential cluster may yield different degrees of virulence or influence. For example, the suicide of a highly esteemed role model may function as a more virulent agent than the suicide of a loner who was considered to be odd or disturbed.

The likelihood of an infection is dose dependent (Davidson and Gould 1989). For youth suicide, the risk to an individual for suicide may increase as the number of suicides increases in the individual's peer group or community or as the number of suicide reports or publicity increases in the media. The spectrum of disease is characterized by a wide variety of manifestations, ranging from inapparent infection to severe clinical illness or death. The consequences of suicide contagion may be inapparent, either because the "illness" was arrested before the appearance of effects or because the apparent effect was unobserved, ignored, misclassified, or unreported (an actual suicide recorded on the death certificate as an accident). Inapparent infections are not available for study, and their absence may result in an underestimate of the significance of contagion as a risk factor for youth suicide (Davidson and Gould 1989).

EVIDENCE OF SUICIDE CLUSTER OUTBREAKS

Contagion is presumed to play a role in suicide epidemics or clusters, referring to unusually high numbers of suicides occurring in a small area within a limited time period (Blonston 1985; Coleman 1987; Doan 1985; Fox et al. 1984; Gelman and Gangelhoff 1983; McCain 1984; Robbins and Conroy 1983; Taylor 1984; Ward and Fox 1977). Evidence of epidemic suicides has been reported in accounts from ancient times through the 20th century (Bakwin 1957; Popow 1911). Davidson and Gould (1989) reported that, in England in the year 665, "distraught persons," preferring a speedy death to the lingering torture from the plague, crowded to the seaside cliffs and threw themselves over. In 1190 in York, more than 500 Jews committed suicide to avoid religious persecution. In 1928, an epidemic of 150 suicidal drownings in the Danube occurred during 2 months. A "suicidal flotilla," a boat squadron to patrol the river, was established to control the epidemic. Between May 1908 and October 1910, 70 children in one school district in Moscow killed themselves.

The reports of epidemics of suicides (detailed in Davidson and Gould 1989; Gould and Davidson 1988) can be examined for characteristics suggesting that suicide contagion may be part of the etiology. The anecdotal reports of cluster suicides have addressed diverse populations, including psychiatric inpatients (Anonymous 1977; Crawford and Willis 1966; Kahne 1968; Kobler and Stotland 1964; Sacks and Eth 1981), high school and college students (Robbins and Conroy 1983; Seiden 1968), community samples (Ashton and Donnan 1981; Nalin 1973; Rubinstein 1983; Walton 1978), Native Americans (Ward and Fox 1977), marine troops (Hankoff 1961), prison inmates (Niemi 1978), and religious sects (Rovinsky 1898).

A number of studies highlight the choice of identical methods among suicides in a cluster (Ashton and Donnan 1981; Crawford and

Willis 1966; Hankoff 1961; Nalin 1973; Rovinsky 1898; Seiden 1968; Walton 1978). A clear imitation of method was seen in Seiden's (1968) report of five cases of suicide by jumping that occurred within a month on a college campus. Identical methods, however, may not always reflect direct imitation of another decedent in the cluster. Cultural factors may also predominate in the choice of method.

More recent clusters indicate that it is not necessary for the decedents to have had direct contact with each other (Davidson and Gould 1988). Indirect knowledge of the suicides appears to have been obtained through the news media in some cluster situations. Other clusters have a mixture of members from one social network plus individuals unknown to each other directly. Among those who knew another decedent, the degree of acquaintance varied from closest friends to those in the same school or church who knew of each other but had little direct personal contact. The extent to which direct and indirect exposure is associated with cluster suicides is currently controversial (Davidson et al. 1989).

Nineteenth-century writers (Winslow 1895) as well as contemporary researchers (Ashton and Donnan 1981; Niemi 1978; Robbins and Conroy 1983; Walton 1978; Ward and Fox 1977) have considered the impact of poor baseline emotional functioning on increasing susceptibility to suicide in a cluster. Winslow (1895) observed that "all human actions are under the influence and power of example more than precept." He attributed the outbreak of suicides to "the force of imitation being so great and acting prejudicially on weak-minded persons or on those predisposed to mental disorders." Another 19th-century writer, in considering the role of the potential suicide's intrinsic vulnerability and the impact of outside events, said that "it is difficult to determine how much was due to the psychopathic tendencies of the actors . . . and how much to the external circumstances which probably served only as the spark applied to the inflammable material" (Rovinsky 1898, pp. 238–239). Emotional well-being, then, could be viewed as a determinant of host susceptibility. However, the proportion of noncluster suicides with psychiatric problems (Robins 1981) may not differ from proportions reported in case series of cluster suicides.

The anecdotal reports of outbreaks are difficult to interpret. There is no systematic surveillance or reporting system of suicide clusters. Therefore, these case series have selection biases that affect their representativeness. As descriptive studies, comparison groups or statistical analyses have rarely been included. Without reference to a comparison group, descriptions of the demographic and psychological characteristics of suicides that occur within the context of a cluster are speculative. What may appear to be a ubiquitous characteristic of cluster suicides may not differentiate them from sporadic, noncluster suicides and, therefore, may be of limited value in preventing this particular type of death. Moreover, even if suicides occurred essentially at random, some clustering would be bound to arise by chance alone, and if enough people are looking for it, some are bound to find it. What is necessary to determine is whether or not outbreaks are occurring to an extent greater than would be expected by chance variation. Until recently there has been no systematic research on the extent to which cluster outbreaks occur.

A project by the author (Gould et al., in press, a, b) developed and adapted epidemiologic techniques to detect the occurrence and to assess the significance of time-space clusters. These methods establish clustering by demonstrating an excess frequency of suicide in certain times and places or a significant relationship between the time and space distances between pairs of suicides. The epidemiologic techniques to detect clusters were applied to U.S. mortality data on suicides obtained from the National Center for Health Statistics Mortality Detail Files for 1978 through 1984. The analyses indicated that suicide clusters occur predominantly among teenagers and young adults; a cluster situation does not appear to accelerate suicidal behavior in individuals who would have killed themselves anyway, as indicated by the lack of a "vacuities" in the number of suicides following the clusters. Rather, the cluster represents a significant excess of suicides, and cluster suicides account for approximately 1% to 5% of all teenage suicides. The estimates do not reflect all clusters that occur because there appears to be variability in temporal and geographic patterns among clusters; yet, the time-space cluster analytic methods require a predefined set of time and space units to characterize a cluster (e.g., suicides occurring within a county). Moreover, these estimates do not include clusters of attempted suicides. It is not possible to enumerate suicide attempts adequately because no registry of attempts exists. Therefore, the estimates of clustering represent a lower bound due to the set definitions of a cluster and the sole employment of mortality data.

Summary of Suicide Outbreaks

Anecdotal accounts and epidemiologic research of epidemic suicides indicate that significant clustering of suicides does occur. Cluster suicides appear to be multidetermined, as are noncluster suicides, but imitation and identification are factors hypothesized to increase the likelihood of cluster suicides. Among susceptible individuals, the route of exposure to the model may be direct or indirect. Examples of direct exposures include close friendship with a suicide or observing a suicidal act. Indirect exposures include watching television news coverage of a prominent person's suicide or hearing about a suicide by word of mouth.

Nonfictional Suicide Stories

Research on the impact of suicide stories has largely focused on the reporting of nonfictional suicides in the mass media (Baron and Reiss 1985; Barraclough et al. 1977; Blumenthal and Bergner 1973; Bollen and Phillips 1981, 1982; Littman 1985; Motto 1967, 1970; Phillips 1974, 1979, 1980; Phillips and Carstensen 1986; Stack 1984; Wasserman 1984). Consistent findings in support of an imitation hypothesis have been reported by the majority of studies despite their variation in method, location, and type of variables. A number of studies examined an excess of deaths following the appearance of suicide stories (Barraclough et al. 1977; Bollen and Phillips 1981, 1982; Phillips 1974, 1979; Wasserman 1984). Other studies examined the decrease in deaths during the cessation of newspaper stories (Blumenthal and Bergner 1973; Motto 1970). Different types of "control" periods have been employed—varying from control periods immediately prior to the suicide story (Bollen and Phillips 1981), control periods in different years (Motto 1970; Phillips 1979), and indirect control periods used in time-series analyses (Wasserman 1984). Both quasi-experimental designs (e.g., Phillips 1974) and regression analytic strategies (e.g., Bollen and Phillips 1981) have been employed.

There is general consensus from the majority of research of studies that prominent newspaper coverage of a suicide has the effect of increasing suicide behavior within the readership area of the newspaper. The magnitude of the increase is related to the "attractiveness" of the individual whose death is being reported and the amount of publicity given to the story (Bollen and Phillips 1981, 1982; Phillips 1974, 1979, 1980; Phillips and Carstensen 1986). This finding has been replicated with American (Bollen and Phillips 1982) and Dutch data (Ganzeboom and de Haan 1982). Despite the substantial support for the association of nonfictional suicide stories and an increase in subsequent suicides, there are a few studies that have been contradictory (Baron and Reiss 1985; Littman 1985; Stack 1984). Some of the inconsistencies that exist among studies could have arisen as a result of significant methodological differences between them (Gould and Davidson 1988).

Fictional Suicide Stories

Little research has been carried out on the impact of fictional stories; the few studies prove to be controversial, with findings of significant imitative effects (Gould and Shaffer 1986; Holding 1974, 1975; Schmidtke and Hafner 1986), no imitative effects (Berman 1986, 1988; Phillips and Paight 1987), and sex- and age-specific imitative effects (Platt 1987).

Previous research by the author suggested that an increase in teenage suicides in the greater New York area followed fictional films featuring suicidal behavior that were broadcast on television in the fall and winter of 1984–1985 (Gould and Shaffer 1986). The examination of the variation in youth suicide was extended to the metropolitan regions of Cleveland, Dallas, and Los Angeles. The results indicated a significant interaction by location (Gould et al. 1988).

Phillips and Paight (1987) published results that indicated that there was no significant effect of the same movies in the states of California and Pennsylvania. These results might be explained by an interaction between the locations where the films were shown and the effect of the films. Berman's (1988) data also suggest variability in the impact of fictional stories by geographical locale. This interaction is not an unreasonable supposition because the way the suicide broadcasts were presented varied according to location. The affiliates were encouraged to develop local education programs to go along with the film, and these varied in intensity. Phillips and Paight hypothesized that there is a dose-response effect between suicide and the media. More exposure produces more effect. If this is true, it might explain regional variation. However, the extent of affiliate coverage in the areas studied has not been documented.

Methodological Considerations

The major limitation of the studies examining the impact of media coverage of suicides is that all have employed aggregate data (Davidson and Gould 1989; Gould and Davidson 1988). A major constraint of this design is that it cannot demonstrate whether the suicide victims were actually exposed to the media events. Therefore, there is always the danger of an "ecological fallacy," which involves making spurious individual-level inferences from aggregate relationships.

There are a number of other methodological factors that may underlie the controversial findings. These include low statistical power, different sources of data, variability in broadcast reception, and differing baseline/comparison periods (Gould et al. 1988). Given the small number of completed suicides and a small number of stimuli (i.e., broadcasts), the statistical power to detect a significant effect, even when it exists, is low. For example, the power to detect a significant effect on completed suicides in the author's original report (Gould and Shaffer 1986) was less than .15. In other words, a media effect would be able to be significantly detected in only 15 of 100 examinations, even when an effect really existed. One of the advantages of the author's original study was that the number of examined cases was increased by extending the study to suicide attempts. The fact that identical trends were found in both completions and attempts and that the effect was repeated after three of four movies offers good internal replication as well as increasing the power of the analysis.

Variability in the completeness of case identification among different sources of data could impact on the likelihood of finding a significant effect. For example, an examination of data from the national and state vital statistics and local medical examiner's office in the New York metropolitan area highlighted a discrepancy in that cases identified in the local data did not appear in the state or national data. It appears that pending cases may obtain a verdict after the deadline for submitting data to the state vital statistics, and thus these cases are also never submitted for entry into the national mortality tapes (Gould et al. 1988). Since the incidence of suicide is low, the deletion of even a few cases could preclude the detection of a significant effect. The extent to which this inconsistency in data exists in other geographic areas has implications for the adequacy of the data sources and needs to be examined further.

Variability in broadcast reception can pose a problem in examining statewide data (e.g., Phillips and Paight 1987). Television coverage for the major networks varies across different nonurban locations, but is generally quite uniform in urban areas. Therefore, the use of statewide data can introduce "noise" and diminish the ability of the study to examine the impact of the media adequately.

Estimates of stable baseline expectations of suicides are necessary to compare with the "experimental" period(s) under study. It is not sufficient to limit the examination to weeks before and after the broadcast. Because each control period precedes the experimental period, the possibility exists that a significant increase (or decrease) in suicides after the broadcasts may merely reflect a tendency for suicides to increase (or decrease) over time. The examination of one alternative year as the comparison period may also be misleading because circumstances unbeknownst to the investigator may have yielded a high (or low) incident comparison year. The employment of several comparison years is preferable in establishing a stable estimate of the expected number of suicides.

Summary of Media Influences

Growing evidence forcefully supports the existence of imitative suicides following media coverage of nonfictional suicides. While there is evidence that fictional suicide stories can have a negative impact (Gould and Shaffer 1986; Holding 1974, 1975; Schmidtke and Hafner 1986), there is clearly a need to engage in further careful research in this area to resolve the issue.

The evidence from continuing research efforts will have to be evaluated. In this light, it is useful to present criteria that assist judgments about the causal significance of associations (Susser 1973) and the extent to which existing evidence from research on the impact of the media fulfills the following criteria. First is the time sequence of variables. The increase in mortality occurred only after the media events. Several studies on the impact of media coverage of nonfictional suicides (Bollen and Phillips 1981, 1982; Phillips 1974, 1979; Wasserman 1984) have established the time sequence of the variables. The suicide stories did not occur during a "suicide wave," but before it. The second criterion is consistency of association on replication. Consistent findings in support of a contagion hypothesis have been described earlier in the chapter. The third criterion is strength of association. The stronger the association, the more likely it is to be causal. The strength of the association is indicated by the reports that suicide stories had larger effects on suicide rates than did day of the week, month, or holidays, variables known to affect the suicide rate (Bollen and Phillips 1982), and by the fact that the reports of celebrities' suicides resulted in an increase of approximately 134 suicides (Wasserman 1984). The fourth criterion is coherent explanation; the association supports preexisting knowledge and is coherent with other known facts about the outcome and the causal factor. The association of media coverage of suicides with an increase in subsequent suicides as well as the findings that the increase is a function of the amount of publicity and is restricted to the area in which the stories are publicized is coherent with the consensus of laboratory findings that mass media violence can elicit aggression (Comstock 1975). The association is also coherent with a number of mechanisms of contagion, such as imitation and familiarity with the idea of suicide. These mechanisms will be discussed in the next section.

MECHANISMS OF SUICIDE CONTAGION

Behavioral contagion has been described as the situation in which some mood or behavior spreads quickly and spontaneously through a group and is defined as a composite of four factors: 1) motivation to perform a particular behavior, 2) knowledge of how to perform the behavior, 3) observation of a model performing the behavior, and 4) performance of the behavior after observing the model (Wheeler 1966). Individual susceptibility (e.g., preexisting mental health problems, family history of suicidal behavior) is probably a major influence of the individual's motivation. The occurrence of suicides in the community or in the media may also impact on the individual's motivation by providing a model that serves to reduce the observer's internal restraints against performing the behavior (Wheeler 1966). The occurrence of a suicide or report in the media can also increase the knowledge of how to perform the behavior.

Social learning theory also provides a foundation on which many aspects of suicide contagion may build. According to this, most human behavior is learned observationally through modeling (Bandura 1977). Imitative learning is influenced by a number of factors, including the characteristics of the model and the consequences or rewards associated with the observed behavior (Bandura 1977). Models who possess engaging qualities or who have high status are more likely to be imitated. Behaviors depicted as resulting in gains, including notoriety, are more effective in prompting imitation.

Consistent with these principles, Phillips and his colleagues have reported that the magnitude of the increase in suicide behavior after prominent newspaper coverage is related to the amount of publicity given to the story (Phillips 1974, 1979). Wasserman (1984) found that a significant rise in the national suicide rate occurred only after celebrity suicides were covered on the front page of *The New York Times.*

People cannot learn much by observation unless they attend to the modeled behavior (Bandura 1977). A number of factors, some involving the observers' characteristics, regulate the amount of attention to an observed behavior. To date, the host characteristics that may yield a greater susceptibility to suicide imitation have not been studied. One host characteristic proposed by Sacks and Eth (1981) is a history of similar past experiences that lead to "pathological identification" with the victim.

In addition to imitative effects, the occurrence of suicides in the community or in the media may produce a familiarity and acceptance of the *idea* of suicide. This mechanism was postulated by Rubinstein (1983) in his study of a suicide epidemic among Micronesian adolescents. Familiarity with suicide may eliminate the "taboo" of suicide, lower the threshold at which point the behavior is manifested, and introduce suicide as an acceptable alternative response or option to life stresses.

RECOMMENDATIONS

Cluster Outbreaks

A detailed examination of a representative sample of cluster suicides is a recommended research strategy to identify mechanisms of initiation and persistence of clusters. Although suicide clusters are thought to occur through a process of contagion, the mechanisms have not been systematically examined. For example, the time-space cluster analytic research, previously described, is not designed to indicate whether clusters were due to the influence of an initial suicide, acting as a model, or whether the presumed model merely happened to be the first individual who committed suicide in response to conditions that then led others to kill themselves. Field studies are better suited to identify the mechanisms of the clusters.

Guidelines for community responses to a cluster of suicides have been developed by the Centers for Disease Control. A suicide cluster creates a crisis atmosphere in the communities in which they occur, and there is usually a great deal of confusion and little coordination in what should be done in the early stages of a cluster. An effort by professionals and community leaders to implement and evaluate these guidelines is recommended (see O'Carroll, Chapter 18, this volume). The guidelines include the following:

1. A community should develop a response plan before the onset of a suicide cluster.
2. The response to the crisis should involve all concerned sectors of the community (e.g., education, public health, mental health, local government, suicide crisis centers) designated to serve on a coordinating committee.
3. The response plan should be implemented when a cluster of suicides or attempts occurs in the community or when one or more traumatic deaths occur in the community. The occurrence of traumatic deaths has been implicated as a precipitating factor in anecdotal reports of a few clusters (O'Carroll 1988).
4. The response to the crisis should be conducted so as to avoid glorification of the suicide victims and to minimize sensationalism.
5. An accurate, appropriate flow of information to the media should be provided.
6. Individuals who may be at high risk (e.g., relatives, boyfriends/girlfriends, close friends, past and present suicide attempters) should be identified for follow-up referrals and counseling.

7. The availability of existing hotlines or suicide crisis centers should be announced.
8. Counselors should be provided at a particular site (e.g., school).
9. The local media should be enlisted to publish sources of help.
10. Elements of the environment may need to be modified (e.g., barriers erected on a bridge, a garage door removed).

The psychiatrist and other mental health professionals in the community can facilitate the implementation of the response plan. The mental health professional is a necessary member of a coordinating committee and will be a source of information on the identification and treatment of high-risk individuals. If the mental health professional is unaware of the existence of a response plan or crisis committee in his or her community, then the Centers for Disease Control, Division of Injury Epidemiology and Control, can be consulted.

Media Presentations

Highlighting potential problems in media presentations will focus the presentation of recommendations for the type and extent of media coverage. There are several characteristics of media stories of suicide that may encourage "copycat" suicides:

1. Detailed depictions of methods are often presented, yielding potential demonstrations on "how to" commit suicide.
2. Physical consequences of an attempt (e.g., paralysis, brain damage) are minimized or not presented.
3. There is minimal or no presentation of mental health problems in the victim. For example, captions of the "All-American" have been noted in newspaper headlines. There is usually an emphasis on stressors, whereas most suicide victims have chronic mental health problems (Shaffer and Gould 1988).
4. Precipitants or triggers to a suicide act are trivialized (e.g., low grade on the Scholastic Aptitude Test) and simplistic psychological processes, such as "pressure," are often endorsed.
5. Victims possess engaging qualities, attractiveness, or high status— characteristics that may encourage modeling.
6. Rewards associated with suicide (e.g., "getting even," gaining notoriety) are presented.
7. No models of effective treatment are presented. Rather, simplistic and inappropriate strategies are endorsed, such as, "reaching out and touching."

Moreover, the excessive responsibility put on significant others may foster undue guilt in the surviving family members and friends. This delineation of media characteristics is based on informal reviews of six suicide dramatizations and approximately 50 newsclippings. Systematic content analyses of media stories are required to determine the validity of these impressions.

Voluntary media guidelines need to be developed to avoid the problems noted previously. These include such recommendations as 1) the method should not be depicted in the story; 2) hotline or other service agency numbers should accompany newspaper articles and television coverage of suicide stories; 3) "massive" or repeated doses of media coverage should be discouraged; and 4) ongoing dialogues between local mental health agencies and media representatives (e.g., editors, journalists, schools of journalism) should be encouraged.

These recommendations should be kept in mind by the mental health professional when asked to comment on a particular case of suicide or the topic in general so as to avoid the pitfalls of previous media presentations.

CONCLUSIONS

There appears to be increasing support for the role of contagion and imitation as a mechanism in suicidal behavior. However, emphasizing these factors exclusively, as in the term "copycat" suicides, trivializes the many other factors contributing to suicide. Suicides are multi-determined events even when they occur in clusters or are influenced by media displays. Evidence of imitation should not negate the importance of the contribution of individual susceptibility and stresses in each suicidal act.

REFERENCES

Anonymous: A suicide epidemic in a psychiatric hospital. Diseases of the Nervous System 38:327–331, 1977

Ashton VR, Donnan S: Suicide by burning as an epidemic phenomenon: an analysis of 82 deaths and inquests in England and Wales in 1978–79. Psychol Med 11:735–739, 1981

Bakwin H: Suicide in children and adolescents. J Pediatr 50:749–769, 1957

Bandura A: Social Learning Theory. Englewood Cliffs, NJ, Prentice-Hall, 1977

Baron JN, Reiss PC: Reply to Phillips and Bollen. American Sociological Review 50:372–376, 1985

Barraclough B, Shepherd D, Jennings C: Do newspaper reports of coroners' inquests incite people to commit suicide? Br J Psychiatry 131:528–532, 1977

Berman AL: Mass media and youth suicide prevention. Paper prepared for the National Conference on Prevention and Interventions in Youth Suicide,

Department of Health and Human Services' Task Force on Youth Suicide, Oakland, CA, 1986

Berman AL: Fictional depiction of suicide in television films and imitation effects. Am J Psychiatry 145:982–986, 1988

Biblarz A: Minimizing the contagion phenomenon. Panel at the 21st annual conference of the American Association of Suicidology, Washington, DC, 1988

Blonston G: Suicides among Arapahoe youths tied to "cultural identity crisis." Hartford Courant, October 1985

Blumenthal S, Bergner L: Suicide and newspaper: a replicated study. Am J Psychiatry 130:468–471, 1973

Bollen KA, Phillips DP: Suicidal motor vehicle fatalities in Detroit: a replication. American Journal of Sociology 87:404–412, 1981

Bollen KA, Phillips DP: Imitative suicides: a national study of the effects of television news stories. American Sociological Review 47:802–809, 1982

Coleman L: Suicide Clusters. Boston, MA, Faber & Faber, 1987

Comstock B: Television and Human Behavior: The Key Studies. Santa Monica, CA, Rand, 1975

Crawford JP, Willis JH: Double suicide in psychiatric hospital patients. Br J Psychiatry 112:1231–1235, 1966

Davidson L, Gould MS: Contagion as a risk factor for youth suicide, in Alcohol, Drug Abuse and Mental Health Administration: Report of the Secretary's Task Force on Youth Suicide, Vol 2: Risk Factors for Youth Suicide (DHHS Publ No ADM-89-1622). Washington, DC, U.S. Government Printing Office, 1989

Doan M: As "cluster suicides" take toll of teenagers. U.S. News and World Report 97:49, 1985

Fox J, Manitowabi D, Ward JA: An Indian community with a high suicide rate—5 years after. Can J Psychiatry 29:425–427, 1984

Ganzebom HBG, de Haan D: Gepubliceerde zelfmoorden en verhoging van sterfte door zelfmoord en ongelukken in Nederland 1972–1980. Mens en Maatschapij 57:55–69, 1982

Gelman D, Gangelhoff BK: Teen-age suicide in the sunbelt. Newsweek 15:70–74, 1983

Gould MS, Davidson L: Suicide contagion among adolescents, in Advances in Adolescent Mental Health, Vol 2: Depression and Suicide. Edited by Stiffman AR, Felman RA. Greenwich, CT, JAI Press, 1988, pp 29–59

Gould MS, Shaffer D: The impact of suicide in television movies: evidence of imitation. N Engl J Med 315:690–694, 1986

Gould MS, Shaffer D, Kleinman M: The impact of suicide in television movies: replication and commentary. Suicide Life Threat Behav 18:90–99, 1988

Gould MS, Wallenstein S, Kleinman M: Time-space clustering of teenage suicide. Am J Epidemiol (in press, a)

Gould MS, Wallenstein S, Kleinman M: Suicide clusters: an examination of age-specific effects. Am J Public Health (in press, b)

Hankoff LD: An epidemic of attempted suicide. Compr Psychiatry 2:29A-8, 1961

Holding TA: The B.B.C. "Befrienders" series and its effects. Br J Psychiatry 124:470–472, 1974

Holding TA: Suicide and "The Befrienders." Br Med J 3:751–753, 1975

Kahne MJ: Suicide among patients in mental hospitals. Psychiatry 1:32–43, 1968

Kobler ALL, Stotland E: The end of hope: a social-clinical study of suicide. London, Free Press of Glencoe, 1964

Littman SK: Suicide epidemics and newspaper reporting. Suicide Life Threat Behav 15:43–50, 1985

Mausner JS, Kramer S: Mausner and Bahn Epidemiology: An Introductory Text. Philadelphia, PA, WB Saunders, 1985

McCain M: Suicides at an early age. Boston Globe, March 25, 1984, A12

Motto JA: Suicide and suggestibility: the role of the press. Am J Psychiatry 124:252–256, 1967

Motto JA: Newspaper influence on suicide. Arch Gen Psychiatry 23:143–148, 1970

Nalin DR: Epidemic of suicide by malathion poisoning in Guyana. Trop Geogr Med 25:8–14, 1973

Niemi T: The time-space distances of suicides committed in the lock-up in Finland in 1963–1967. Israel Annals of Psychiatry and Related Disciplines 16:39–45, 1978

O'Carroll P: A plan for preventing and containing suicide clusters. Paper presented at the 21st annual conference of the American Association of Suicidology, Washington, DC, 1988

Phillips D: The influence of suggestion on suicide: substantive and theoretical implication of the Werther effect. American Sociological Review 39:340–354, 1974

Phillips DP: Suicide, motor vehicle fatalities, and the mass media: evidence toward a theory of suggestions. American Journal of Sociology 84:1150–1174, 1979

Phillips DP: Airplane accidents, murder, and the mass media: towards a theory of imitation and suggestion. Social Forces 58:1001–1004, 1980

Phillips DP, Carstensen LL: Clustering of teenage suicides after television news stories about suicide. N Engl J Med 315:685–689, 1986

Phillips DP, Paight DJ: The impact of televised movies about suicide: a replicative study. N Engl J Med 317:809–811, 1987

Platt S: The aftermath of Angie's overdose: is soap (opera) damaging to your health? Br Med J 294:954–957, 1987

Popow NM: The present epidemic of school suicides in Russia. Nevrol Nestnik (Kazan) 18:312–355, 592–646, 1911

Robbins D, Conroy RC: A cluster of adolescent suicide attempts: is suicide contagious? J Adolesc Health Care 3:253–255, 1983

Robins E: The Final Months. New York, Oxford University Press, 1981

Rovinsky A: Epidemic suicides. Boston Medical and Surgical Journal 138:238–239, 1898

Rubinstein DH: Epidemic suicide among Micronesian adolescents. Soc Sci Med 17:657–665, 1983

Sacks M, Eth S: Pathological identification as a cause of suicide on an inpatient unit. Hosp Community Psychiatry 32:36–40, 1981

Schmidtke A, Hafner H: Die vermittlung von selbstmordmotivation und selbstmordhandlung durch fiktive modelle. Nervenarzt 57:502–510, 1986

Seiden RH: Suicidal behavior contagion on a college campus, in Proceedings of the Fourth International Conference for Suicide Prevention. Edited by Farberow NL. Los Angeles, CA, Suicide Prevention Center, 1968, pp 360–365

Shaffer D, Gould MS: Study of completed and attempted suicides in adolescents: progress report (NIMH grant MH-38198). Washington, DC, National Institute of Mental Health, 1988

Stack S: The effect of suggestion on suicide: a reassessment. Paper presented at the annual meeting of the American Sociological Association, San Antonio, TX, 1984

Susser M: Causal Thinking in the Health Sciences: Concepts and Strategies in Epidemiology. New York, Oxford University Press, 1973

Taylor P: Cluster phenomenon of young suicides raises contagion theory. Washington Post, March 15–16, 1984

Walton EW: An epidemic of antifreeze poisoning. Med Sci Law 18:231–237, 1978

Ward JA, Fox J: A suicide epidemic on an Indian reserve. Canadian Psychiatric Association Journal 22:423–426, 1977

Wasserman IM: Imitation and suicide: a reexamination of the Werther effect. American Sociological Review 49:427–436, 1984

Wheeler L: Toward a theory of behavioral contagion. Psychol Rev 73:179–192, 1966

Winslow F: Suicide considered as a mental epidemic. Bulletin of the Medico-Legal Congress, 1895, pp 334–351

Chapter 20

An International Perspective on the Epidemiology and Prevention of Suicide

Rene F. W. Diekstra, Ph.D.

SUICIDE IS A paradoxical phenomenon. On the one hand, it appears to be the most personal action an individual can take. On the other hand, it has occurred throughout human history in all corners of the world, and often under circumstances that show such a striking similarity that one must conclude that social factors play an important, if not a decisive, role in its causation. For example, for centuries, loss of a love relationship and death of a spouse have been reported to be precipitants of suicide in regions as diverse as Southeast Asia, Africa, and Central Europe. The same can be said of loss of face or defeat in battle, which has been reported as a reason for suicide by warriors in the Roman empire as well as in medieval Japan.

It was long believed by laypersons as well as scientists that suicidal behavior was a by-product and dubious prerogative of Western industrialized societies while other parts of the world, particularly more "primitive" societies, were free of it. Over the past 80 years, the study of the distribution of suicide across populations and countries over the world has clearly established that this thesis is not defensible.

This chapter is reprinted, with permission, from the article "Suicide and Attempted Suicide: An International Perspective." *Acta Psychiatrica Scandinavica*. 80 (suppl. 354):1–24, 1989. Copyright 1989, Munksgaard International Publishers, Ltd., Copenhagen, Denmark.

In fact, suicide occurs in almost all cultures and societies across different phases of the life cycle.

This life-cycle phenomenon has been demonstrated by Wisse (1933), who showed that, among the Inuit (Eskimos) of northern America as well as the Mongols of Asia, suicide and suicide attempts are behaviors frequently found among both the disabled elderly and the healthy but unhappy young. The Greek historian Plutarch reported suicides across the life cycle in classical Greece during the fourth and third centuries B.C., indicating that even among early adolescents, suicidal behavior, both in its fatal and nonfatal forms, was not uncommon.

It seems that the frequency of suicidal behavior not only fluctuates over the life cycle of an individual, depending on psychological, social, and cultural conditions, but also correlates with the life cycle of cultures or societies themselves. In his milestone work on the history of moral attitudes toward suicide, Bayet (1922) pointed out that cultures at the zenith of their power and development or just beyond it show more permissive attitudes toward suicide as well as a considerable increase in frequency of this behavior. Conversely, cultures in the early states of growth and development have a more restrictive attitude toward suicide, with a concomitant lower frequency of the phenomenon. Therefore, differences in the frequency of suicide between cultures and societies may not only be related to differences in values, socioeconomic structure, and related conditions, but also to their stage of development.

In this chapter, differences in the frequency of suicidal behavior in different countries in the world will be analyzed. Although the term *suicidal behavior* comprises several categories of action (i.e., completed suicide, attempted suicide or parasuicide, and suicidal threats and communications), the data presented here are mainly on completed suicide. International comparisons with regard to suicide attempts and communications are generally not possible because there are no countries that record national statistics on these behaviors.

Insofar as data are available, international comparisons with regard to differences in suicide rates across gender and age groups will be presented. An attempt will be made to explain differences observed between countries and regions in the world. As will be shown, there are substantial international differences with regard to the changes in suicide rates over the last 25 years. For a number of European countries, an attempt has been made, on the basis of a number of social indicators, to explain these differences. The main results of that study will be summarized and discussed. Finally, public policy implications based on the presented data will be reviewed, and conclusions for prevention, intervention, and treatment will be drawn.

INTERNATIONAL VARIATION IN SUICIDE RATES

There are large international variations in death rates from suicide among the countries in the world (Table 1). (For reasons of convenience, the term *country* [or *state*] in this chapter is to mean any territory with mortality statistics reported to WHO Headquarters, Geneva.) Of the countries that report to the World Health Organization (WHO) and whose suicide rates are published in the 1987 WHO Health Statistics Annual (WHO 1987) or are available in the WHO data bank for at least one year after 1979, the range in suicide rates spans from approximately zero (where there are no deaths from suicide) in countries including Malta and Egypt to the remarkably high rate of nearly 1,000 per million on the Falkland Islands. In 1987, the highest rate of suicide (5,000 suicides per million population) was for 20- to 24-year-old males on the Falkland Islands.

An inspection of Table 1 shows a pattern in the suicide rates. Arabic countries have relatively low rates of suicide. The Latin American countries also tend to have lower suicide rates. European nations and countries mainly populated by people of European descent (such as Australia, the United States, and Canada) tend to have relatively high rates. There is also a discernible pattern among the European countries. Southern European countries have relatively low suicide rates, whereas northern and middle European countries usually have higher rates. The Asians have rates more evenly distributed across the range. It would, however, be unjustified to consider Table 1 as a totally accurate or complete reflection of the international mortality by suicide. First of all, only 71 countries of the 166 member states of WHO are reported here (some of them not being nations in the legal sense of the word). Notable exceptions to the reporting states are the People's Republic of China, the Union of Soviet Socialist Republics (U.S.S.R.), and most African nations. Second, the validity of the figures reported is questionable for a number of reasons (which will be discussed in the conclusion section of this chapter).

Of particular note is that the rate of suicide for males is considerably higher than that for females in every country. However, in his analysis of WHO annual statistics over the period 1973–1985, Barraclough (1988), found equal or higher rates for 15- to 24-year-old women in four Asian countries (i.e., Thailand, Hong Kong, Philippines, and Singapore). As will be shown later in this chapter, this reversal of the classic sex distribution in suicide appears to be limited to the 15- to 24-year-old age group.

INTERNATIONAL CHANGES IN SUICIDE RATES 1960–1980/86

For a number of the industrialized countries in the Western Hemi-

Table 1. Suicide rates in countries reporting to WHO (per million of population)

Country	Males	Females	Country	Males	Females
Falkland/Maldives	1000	—	Trinidad and Tobago	121	50
Hungary	661	259	Italy	110	43
Suriname	436	128	Chile	107	18
Finland	430	113	Argentina	105	34
Austria	421	158	Ireland	92	39
Sri Lanka	377	197	Venezuela	76	20
Denmark	351	206	Israel	75	35
France	331	127	Costa Rica	74	15
Switzerland	330	132	Thailand	69	62
Belgium	326	153	Spain	68	23
Czechoslovakia	292	92	Greece	57	25
Japan	278	149	Ecuador	55	36
Federal Republic of Germany	266	12	Cape Verde	44	6
Sweden	250	115	Martinique	44	13
Bulgaria	232	94	Bahrain	40	6
Yugoslavia	228	97	Mauritius	40	16
Poland	220	44	Paraguay	33	15
Norway	208	74	Dominica	28	—

Country			Country		
Luxemburg	207	74	Mexico	25	7
Iceland	206	58	Barbados	25	15
Canada	205	54	Panama	22	5
United States	197	54	Saint Vincent	20	0
Australia	182	51	Grenadine	17	—
Puerto Rico	176	23	Santa Lucia	17	0
Scotland	166	60	Iran	16	4
Uruguay	159	—	Belize	13	—
New Zealand	157	50	Kuwait	12	5
El Salvador	148	61	Bahamas	10	—
Singapore	147	107	Guatemala	9	1
Netherlands	146	81	Philippines	5	4
Korea	139	49	Syria	2	—
Hong Kong	137	107	Papua New Guinea	1	2
Portugal	136	51	Egypt	0	0
Northern Ireland	131	39	Malta	*	6
England and Wales	121	57	German Democratic Republic	*	—
			Cuba	*	—

*No figures reported.
Source. Figures taken from World Health Statistics Annual (World Health Organization 1987), latest year of reporting.

sphere, an increase in suicide rates has been reported over the past several decades (Diekstra 1985). Tables 2 and 3 illustrate how common this trend is at a global level. Suicide rates are presented for the 62 countries that reported to WHO both in 1960 and for at least one of the years 1980 to 1986.

A comparison of the rates for 1960 and 1985 indicates that the rank order of countries over the past 25 years has changed somewhat, but is not all that different from today's ranking. This is true despite the often substantial changes in suicide rates (Table 4). It appears that more countries have witnessed an increase (42) than a decrease (20) in suicide rates over the past 20 to 25 years. The average percentage of change is about 37%, with a range of −82% to 437%. The logical conclusion to draw from these data is that suicide mortality on a global level has apparently increased over the last quarter of a century. However, closer inspection of Table 4 in conjunction with Tables 2 and 3 shows a remarkable pattern.

Relatively large increases are observed in most countries in northwest and central Europe. Countries populated in the majority by people of European descent show a similar trend, although generally less sizeable. A striking fact is that Latin countries, both around the Mediterranean as well as on the American continent, have witnessed decreasing suicide rates. For Asian countries, the picture is mixed, with relatively large increases for the southeastern Asia (Sri Lanka, Thailand, and Singapore) and no changes or decreases for the Far East (Hong Kong, Japan, and the Philippines).

This strikingly consistent geographic distribution of changes in suicide rates around the world suggests that they are probably not simply a reflection of changes in classification procedures, but rather a consequence of sociocultural developments, the nature of which still remains unclear.

The Relationship of Age and Sex With Suicides Rates

As was mentioned earlier in the chapter, the total suicide rates for males are higher than those for females in every country reported in the 1987 WHO Health Statistics Annual (World Health Organization 1987). This picture remains the same if one examines different age groups. Tables 5 and 6 compare the rates by gender for 19 countries across three different age groups (15–29, 30–59, and 60 and over) in 1970 and for the latest year of reporting (1985 or 1986).

It appears that in only one of the 57 possible comparisons, the female suicide rate exceeds the rate for males (Singapore, 1970, age group 15–29). (In contrast to Barraclough's findings (1988), Thailand, Hong Kong, and the Philippines do not appear in this list, which is

Table 2. Suicide rates (per 100,000 of population) in 62 countries: 1960

Country	Rate	Country	Rate
1. Federal Republic of Germany	37.0	32. Chile	7.5
2. Hungary	25.0	33. Argentina	7.4
3. Austria	23.1	34. Martinique	6.8
4. Czechoslovakia	22.3	35. Netherlands	6.6
5. Japan	21.6	36. Suriname	6.5
6. Finland	20.5	37. Norway	6.4
7. Denmark	20.3	38. Venezuela	6.1
8. Switzerland	19.2	39. Italy	6.1
9. German Democratic Republic	18.6	40. Spain	5.5
10. Sweden	17.4	41. Panama	4.1
11. France	15.8	42. Northern Ireland	4.4
12. Belgium	14.6	43. Greece	4.3
13. Yugoslavia	13.9	44. Guadeloupe	3.9
14. Luxemburg	13.4	45. Thailand	3.5
15. Uruguay	12.7	46. Mauritius	3.5
16. El Salvador	12.1	47. Trinidad and Tobago	3.2
17. England and Wales	11.2	48. Ireland	3.0
18. Hong Kong	11.1	49. Colombia	2.7
19. Cuba	11.1	50. Guatemala	2.7
20. United States	10.6	51. Costa Rica	2.5
21. Australia	10.6	52. Jamaica	2.0
22. Iceland	10.6	53. Mexico	1.9
23. Puerto Rico	10.3	54. Antigua and Barbuda	1.8
24. Sri Lanka	9.9	55. Peru	1.5
25. New Zealand	9.7	56. Malta	0.9
26. Bulgaria	8.7	57. Equador	0.8
27. Portugal	8.7	58. Dominican Republic	0.8
28. Singapore	8.6	59. Philippines	0.7
29. Poland	8.0	60. Nicaragua	0.4
30. Scotland	7.9	61. Egypt	0.1
31. Canada	7.6	62. Papua New Guinea	0.1

Source. WHO data bank latest year of reporting as per July 1, 1988.

Table 3. Suicide rates (per 100,000 of population) in 62 countries: 1980/86

Country	Rate	Country	Rate
1. Hungary	45.3	32. Uruguay	9.6
2. Federal Republic of Germany	43.1	33. Northern Ireland	9.3
3. Sri Lanka	29.0	34. Portugal	9.2
4. Austria	28.3	35. England and Wales	8.9
5. Denmark	27.8	36. Trinidad and Tobago	8.6
6. Finland	26.6	37. Guadeloupe	7.9
7. Belgium	23.8	38. Ireland	7.8
8. Switzerland	22.8	39. Italy	7.6
9. France	22.7	40. Thailand	6.6
10. Suriname	21.6	41. Argentina	6.3
11. Japan	21.2	42. Chile	6.2
12. German Democratic Republic	19.0	43. Spain	4.9
13. Czechoslovakia	18.9	44. Venezuela	4.8
14. Sweden	18.5	45. Costa Rica	4.5
15. Cuba	17.7	46. Ecuador	4.3
16. Bulgaria	16.3	47. Greece	4.1
17. Yugoslavia	16.1	48. Martinique	3.7
18. Norway	14.1	49. Colombia	2.9
19. Luxemburg	13.9	50. Mauritius	2.8
20. Iceland	13.3	51. Dominican Republic	2.4
21. Poland	13.0	52. Mexico	1.6
22. Canada	12.9	53. Panama	1.4
23. Singapore	12.7	54. Peru	1.4
24. United States	12.3	55. Philippines	0.5
25. Hong Kong	12.2	56. Guatemala	0.5
26. Australia	11.6	57. Malta	0.3
27. Scotland	11.6	58. Nicaragua	0.2
28. Netherlands	11.0	59. Papua New Guinea	0.2
29. El Salvador	10.8	60. Jamaica	0.1
30. New Zealand	10.3	61. Egypt	0.1
31. Puerto Rico	9.8	62. Antigua and Barbuda	—

Source. WHO data bank latest year of reporting as per July 1, 1988.

Table 4. Percentage of change in mortality by suicide in 62 countries between 1960 and 1986

Country	%	Country	%
1. Hungary	81	32. Uruguay	−24
2. Federal Republic of Germany	21	33. Northern Ireland	111
3. Sri Lanka	193	34. Portugal	6
4. Austria	25.5	35. England and Wales	21
5. Denmark	37	36. Trinidad and Tobago	169
6. Finland	30	37. Guadeloupe	102
7. Belgium	63	38. Ireland	160
8. Switzerland	19	39. Italy	25
9. France	44	40. Thailand	89
10. Suriname	232	41. Argentina	−15
11. Japan	−2	42. Chile	−17
12. German Democratic Republic	2	43. Spain	−11
13. Czechoslovakia	−15	44. Venezuela	−21
14. Sweden	6	45. Costa Rica	80
15. Cuba	59	46. Ecuador	437
16. Bulgaria	87	47. Greece	−5
17. Yugoslavia	16	48. Martinique	−46
18. Norway	120	49. Colombia	7
19. Luxemburg	4	50. Mauritius	−20
20. Iceland	25	51. Dominican Republic	200
21. Poland	62	52. Mexico	−16
22. Canada	70	53. Panama	−66
23. Singapore	48	54. Peru	−7
24. United States	16	55. Philippines	−29
25. Hong Kong	1	56. Guatemala	−82
26. Australia	9	57. Malta	−67
27. Scotland	41	58. Nicaragua	−50
28. Netherlands	67	59. Papua New Guinea	100
29. El Salvador	−15	60. Jamaica	−50
30. New Zealand	6	61. Egypt	0
31. Puerto Rico	−6	62. Antigua and Barbuda	—

Source. WHO data bank.

Table 5. Suicide in females: comparison of rates for 1970 and 1985/6 (per 100,000)

	1970			1985/6		
Country	15–29	30–59	60+	15–29	30–59	60+
1. Australia	6.2	12.4	12.3	5.3	6.9	8.4
2. Belgium	3.4	15.1	25.7	6.5	21.3	26.2
3. Bulgaria	5.0	8.5	27.7	5.7	8.0	31.3
4. Canada	5.9	10.3	6.9	4.6	8.3	6.3
5. Czechoslovakia	11.5	15.4	35.5	4.8	10.3	27.0
6. Denmark	6.4	25.4	23.3	9.9	30.4	29.5
7. England and Wales	2.9	8.9	11.9	10.5	7.6	17.7
8. France	5.4	10.3	18.2	6.3	16.2	26.2
9. Federal Republic of Germany	8.1	20.7	26.6	6.6	12.6	23.1
10. Hungary	9.6	20.8	59.3	11.3	29.7	65.7
11. Ireland	0.3	1.1	1.1	1.2	6.3	5.1
12. Japan	12.8	13.4	53.0	9.5	10.3	45.5
13. Mexico	1.0	0.7	0.3	1.4	0.9	0.7
14. Netherlands	3.3	9.3	15.3	5.4	11.9	12.5
15. New Zealand	4.1	10.9	14.9	6.0	7.0	6.1
16. Scotland	2.5	11.2	6.1	3.4	7.0	10.4
17. Singapore	10.9	7.9	56.3	8.0	12.7	69.4
18. United States	6.0	11.7	8.3	4.7	7.6	6.5
19. Venezuela	9.0	4.1	5.2	10.9	2.7	2.7

Source. WHO data bank.

Table 6. Suicide in males: comparison of rates for 1970 and 1985/6 (per 100,000)

Country	1970			1985/6		
	15–29	30–59	60+	15–29	30–59	60+
1. Australia	15.3	29.1	33.2	26.1	22.3	28.6
2. Belgium	8.8	27.0	76.0	22.7	38.6	85.8
3. Bulgaria	9.8	16.2	82.5	14.0	22.8	102.5
4. Canada	17.1	27.1	23.9	25.6	26.2	28.2
5. Czechoslovakia	32.5	52.3	87.9	18.1	43.4	79.7
6. Denmark	15.3	44.7	50.0	24.3	47.1	72.5
7. England and Wales	6.7	13.0	21.4	10.5	16.7	19.9
8. France	11.3	32.2	68.5	22.7	41.5	93.7
9. Federal Republic of Germany	22.8	39.5	67.7	19.7	32.3	59.2
10. Hungary	33.2	70.6	131.3	33.5	98.3	156.9
11. Ireland	2.8	5.0	4.2	15.9	15.9	16.1
12. Japan	16.5	20.8	70.2	18.4	40.3	64.7
13. Mexico	3.1	3.4	5.8	4.3	4.1	9.6
14. Netherlands	6.0	14.1	35.1	10.0	17.7	37.7
15. New Zealand	11.1	21.2	26.8	19.6	18.5	33.1
16. Scotland	6.7	14.9	20.8	15.8	23.4	21.1
17. Singapore	10.4	20.3	98.4	12.7	18.1	99.4
18. United States	16.2	25.4	39.3	22.6	23.6	43.4
19. Venezuela	14.6	17.4	19.1	10.9	13.4	23.4

Source. WHO data bank.

due to the fact that he used the 15–24 age range.) For many countries, the gender gap appeared to have widened over the period 1970 to 1985/86. In the age range 15–29, the rates for males increased in 16 countries, with only Czechoslovakia and Venezuela showing a decrease and Hungary showing no change. For females in this age group, seven countries showed decreasing rates. The differences in trends between the sexes are less striking for the other two age groups, although here the number of countries and the magnitude of the increase are both greater for males.

Generally speaking, for both sexes the increase in suicide rates over the period (1970–1985/86) is not dramatic except for the 15- to 29-year-olds. However, there are some exceptions to this rule that are noteworthy. For example, in Japan the total suicide rate showed a decline that is reflected in all age and sex subgroups, with the exception of males between 30 to 59 years of age. The total suicide rate in this latter age group almost doubled in a relatively short period of about 15 years. Something similar, although at a less dramatic level, is found for Hungarian males, who had a stable rate of suicide for the 15–29 age group but a considerable increase in the rate for 30- to 59-year-olds. For females this same pattern is found in Singapore.

The data in Tables 5 and 6 confirm the general observation that suicide rates increase with advancing age. The countries where this regularity is violated include two Latin American countries, Venezuela and Mexico, where in both 1970 and 1985 young females aged 15 to 29 had the highest rates. Remarkable also is the fact that in 1986 males aged 15 to 29 in Australia and New Zealand had higher rates than males aged 30 to 59. This was a consequence of a strong increase in the suicide rate for the first group and a decrease for the latter age group. In other countries, including Canada, the United States, and Ireland, a somewhat similar development can be observed in that the rates of male suicides for ages 15 to 29 are approximately the same as the rates for 30 to 59 year olds. For females, the same trend can be observed in England and Wales, Australia, and New Zealand. It is of interest to note that all of these countries are predominantly Anglo-Saxon. This suggests that there may be common contributory factors operating in these countries.

Czechoslovakia particularly stands out because it is the only country that shows declining suicide rates over the period 1970–1985 for all age and sex groups. One explanation for this phenomenon might be that in 1968 this country was invaded and occupied by armies of the Warsaw Pact countries, evoking desperate emotional reactions, especially by young people (e.g., the self-burning in 1968 by Jan Palach at the Wenceslas Square shortly after the invasion). By 1985 there was a new generation of adolescents and young adults who had not experienced the aftermath of this traumatic event. The fact that the greatest drop in suicide rate is among 15- to 29-year-olds appears to lend some support to this hypothesis.

THE IMPORTANCE OF SUICIDE AS A CAUSE OF DEATH

Tables 7 and 8 show a breakdown of the percentage of all deaths caused by suicide in three age groups for a selected number of countries. The age groups have been chosen to represent the two groups with the highest and the one group with the lowest percentage of suicidal mortality. Two facts emerge very clearly. First of all, the 25–34 age group has the highest relative mortality risk from suicide. In some countries, such as Japan and Denmark, approximately one of every three males and one of every four females who die in that age group does so by suicide. Second, two Asian countries, Singapore and Japan, are the only countries in the world in which the relative mortality by suicide is higher for females than for males among 15- to 24-year-olds. In Singapore this is also true for the 25–34 age group. This distinct difference from other countries in the world, especially Europe and North America, might well reflect cultural differences regarding the status and role of women in these societies (Barraclough 1988; Headley 1983).

Table 7. Suicide in males across the life cycle as a percentage of all causes of death

Country	Age (years)			
	15–24	25–34	65–74	All ages
Australia	17.7	20.3	0.5	2.2
Bulgaria	10.8	9.6	1.1	1.7
Czechoslovakia	13.0	20.0	1.0	2.3
Canada	20.7	20.6	0.8	2.6
Denmark	18.6	28.2	1.4	2.9
England and Wales	10.9	18.1	0.4	1.0
France	13.9	21.7	1.7	3.1
Hungary	18.8	27.8	2.0	4.4
Ireland	9.0	14.3	0.4	0.9
Japan	19.5	29.6	1.6	4.1
Netherlands	15.2	21.5	0.7	1.6
New Zealand	12.8	14.4	0.9	1.8
Scotland	16.6	17.4	0.5	1.3
Singapore	12.6	13.6	1.2	2.6
United States	14.5	14.3	0.9	2.1

Source. WHO data bank.

Table 8. Suicide in females across the life cycle as a percentage of all causes of death

Country	Age (years)			All ages
	15–24	25–34	65–74	
Australia	10.3	8.5	0.1	0.7
Bulgaria	9.9	7.9	0.8	0.9
Czechoslovakia	10.4	13.5	0.7	0.8
Canada	9.6	12.5	0.4	0.9
Denmark	23.3	25.0	1.5	1.9
England and Wales	6.2	9.5	0.5	0.5
France	10.1	16.2	1.7	1.4
Hungary	18.8	18.6	1.6	2.0
Ireland	8.5	7.0	0.2	0.5
Japan	28.0	24.9	2.3	2.7
Netherlands	11.2	10.5	0.9	1.0
New Zealand	9.0	7.3	0.4	0.6
Scotland	9.4	11.1	0.5	0.5
Singapore	15.0	17.6	0.6	2.5
United States	8.6	8.9	0.3	0.7

Source. WHO data bank.

Factors Influencing Contemporary Trends in Suicide Rates

One obvious conclusion from this analysis of international suicide rates is that there is much unexplained variation between countries in the incidence of suicide. A second conclusion is that many countries show a considerable to very strong increase in the frequency of suicide in the 15–29 age group over the past two decades. This tendency is especially strong in European states, but is also clearly present in North America, Asia, Oceania, and in certain Latin American countries. It is stronger for males than females.

The fact that the rise in total rates of suicide in several countries is mainly due to the increased rates in younger age groups and that even countries with a stable or decreasing rate often still show an increase in rates among young adults raises the question of what makes young people more vulnerable to suicide. Since the rise in youth suicide occurred in many Western countries around 1965, some authors suggested that there may be a cohort effect (e.g., Häfner and Schmidtke 1987). Around this time, the children of the post–World-War-II baby boom were coming of age. The numbers of youth were so large that the law of the critical mass demography came into effect. Increased numbers of young people became a factor in political destabilization, expressing itself among other things in the "student revolts" in France and other continental European countries as well as on many college campuses in the United States. The size of the youth population also increased intrageneration competition and stresses related to finding jobs and establishing careers. It has been shown (Holinger et al. 1988) that there is a positive relationship between the rate of youth suicide and the percentage of young people in the total population. The relationship is stronger for males than for females, which might partially be attributed to women less frequently seeking jobs outside of the home than men, a difference that was still rather strong in the post–World-War-II baby-boom generation.

However, the continuing rise over the period 1970–1985/86 in suicide rates among young males (15–19 and 20–24), who are certainly not a part of the baby-boom generation, suggests that other important contributory variables are needed to explain the contemporary trends in suicide.

In epidemiology, the search for causative factors is often facilitated if "an explosion of cases" occurs at points in time that are quite separate, enabling a hypothesis generated for one period to be re-tested using data from the other period. For certain countries that have kept national suicide statistics for the whole of this century or even beyond, an examination of trends in their suicide rates over the last 85 years reveals that the present peak in young suicides has an historical precedent. The United States has had two peak periods in youth suicides in this century: one in the 1980s and another in the beginning of the century, around 1910 (Figure 1). Additionally, several other European countries such as the Netherlands also experienced this 1910 peak.

Interestingly, the first scientific meeting on suicide took place in Vienna in 1910. This meeting of the Viennese Psychoanalytic Society was chaired by Alfred Adler. Sigmund Freud was one of the conference discussants, and, most significantly, suicide among students was the theme of the meeting. The increased rates in youth suicide in Austria and other middle European countries and several "school epidemics" were the stimulus for the meeting. Unfortunately, no studies have been carried out to explain the 1910 peak in youth suicide. It is safe to assume, however, that the peak was closely related to a number of pervasive social changes that took place in many European and other Western countries at that time, changes that led to intense political and cultural destabilization and finally to dramatic international and national conflicts, such as World War I in 1914 and the Russian Revolution in 1917. Of importance may have been the rapid development toward urbane societies under the influence of industrialization; the introduction of (prolonged) obligatory education in many countries, which was a major factor in creating

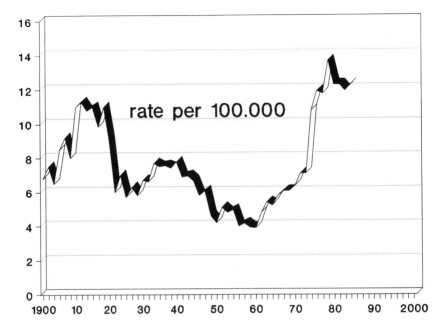

Figure 1. Suicide rates in the United States for 15- to 24-year-olds.

adolescence as we know it today; changes in the status of women, such as the right to vote or to be elected to political office; and separation of church and state and concomitant secularization. The latter expressed itself, among other ways, in large masses of people turning away from traditional religion toward socialism. Furthermore, it was a period of very rapid population growth, which was fostered in part by the effects of the public health and sanitation movement, including decreased infant mortality and increased life expectancy at the end of the 19th century. Finally, it was a period in which the production and consumption of alcoholic beverages in many countries reached an all-time high.

Despite the absence of analytical epidemiologic research to test the possible influence of such factors on the suicide rates at the beginning of this century, these trends can inform important directions for explanatory research regarding the current trends in youth suicide. However, before examining the results of the few available studies in this area, the trends in youth suicide in a number of countries in the world for the period 1970–1985/86 will be examined. Separate analyses of suicide rates for the age groups 15–19, 20–24, and 25–29 in 13 selected countries (Figures 2–4) demonstrate the following.

For the 15- to 19-year-olds, nine countries show a moderate to

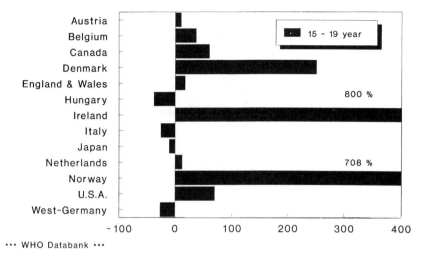

Figure 2. Percentage of increase in suicide mortality for 15- to 19-year-olds: 1970–1985.

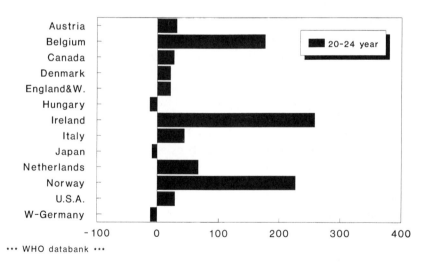

Figure 3. Percentage of increase in suicide mortality for 20- to 24-year-olds: 1970–1985.

very dramatic increase in suicide rates. This is especially the case for Ireland, Norway, and Denmark. Four countries show small to moderate decreases. Of interest is that three of these are countries with traditionally high suicide rates: Hungary, Japan, and the Federal Republic of Germany. For the 20–24 age group, the picture is quite

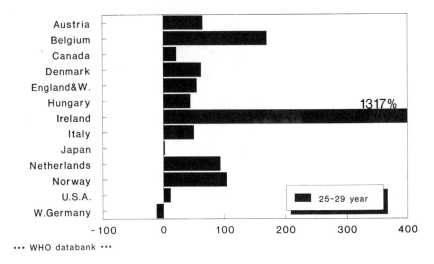

••• WHO databank •••

Figure 4. Percentage of increase in suicide mortality for 25- to 29-year-olds: 1970–1985.

similar. Most countries have had a moderate to strong rate increase, but again Hungary, Japan, and the Federal Republic of Germany show a small decrease. However, the picture for the 25- to 29-year-olds is somewhat different. Most countries show a considerable increase in suicide rates, with Ireland experiencing an enormous rise. The Federal Republic of Germany is now the only country with a small decrease, and Japan shows a very small increase in rate.

While for each age category the countries that show an increase do so both for males and to a somewhat lesser extent for females, the situation is different wherever countries show decreasing rates. Both Hungary and Japan show a small increase for males in the 15–19 and 20–24 age groups, but a considerable decrease for females. Taken together, the combined rate is decreasing. On the other hand, the Federal Republic of Germany shows decreasing rates for both females and males.

What is the explanation for why some countries have had a widespread increase in youth suicide, while other nations have witnessed decreasing rates of suicide in young females? Are these trends the result of social forces such as the ones suggested above for the 1910 peak? If so, how do these developments translate themselves into a particular individual's self-destructive behavior?

One obvious approach to answer these questions would be to look at the nation most at risk, which is Ireland, and see whether some pertinent clues can be found there. In a study carried out by Kelleher and Daly (1988), evidence suggesting a relationship between certain indicators of social change (e.g., anomie) and suicide was found.

The Irish suicide rate rose during the same period as increases occurred in the illegitimate birth rate, the crime rate, and the rate of referrals for treatment of alcohol dependency. That period was also characterized by a decrease in marriages. The study does not provide information on the relationship between changes in suicide rate and unemployment rate, but studies in England and Wales and in Scotland strongly suggest that such a relationship exists (Figure 5; Platt 1988).

Since the effects of social factors, as the ones mentioned here for Ireland and Great Britain, are not expected to be independent of one another, nor are they the only social forces related to changes in suicide rates, the question arises concerning what constellation of social factors might help explain the prevailing trends in suicide rates among adolescents and young adults.

Sainsbury et al. (World Health Organization 1982), in cooperation with the WHO, investigated for 18 European countries the relationship between changes in social conditions and changes in their suicide rate after 1960. The social characteristics of countries in 1961–1963 that predicted a subsequent increase in their rates of suicide were 1) a high divorce rate, which may be interpreted as an indicator of the level of alienation prevailing in a society; 2) a low percentage of the population under the age of 15 years, which may be interpreted as an

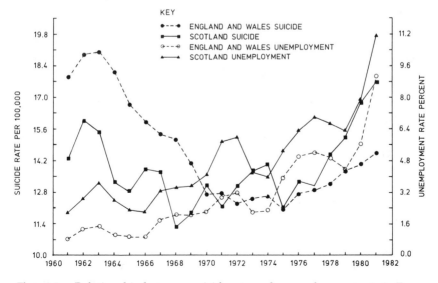

Figure 5. Relationship between suicide rate and unemployment rate in England and Wales and in Scotland for males age 15+.

indicator of the extent to which people are not living in family groups; 3) a high unemployment rate; and 4) a high homicide rate. These last two factors can be interpreted as indicators of "anomie"—the state of normlessness and lack of social regulation in a society that Durkheim (1951) suggested would lead to more suicides. Additionally, Sainsbury et al. found a high proportion of employed women in these countries, which may reflect the change in status for women and the stresses on them in a society. Taken together, the first three predictors can also be considered as indicative of pervasive changes in the structure of the family in a society.

Sainsbury et al. (World Health Organization 1982) also carried out an analysis in which changes in social conditions after 1960 were related to changes in national suicide rates. The results indicated similar but not identical factors to be associated with suicide trends. Increased suicide rates were associated with 1) a reduction in the population of those aged 15 and under; 2) an increase in the percentage of the population aged 65 and over, that is, the age group with the relatively highest suicide rate in European countries; and 3) an increase in "females' tertiary education"—possibly another indicator of the changing status of women and of the family structure.

Since Sainsbury et al.'s study examined only the relationship between social factors and changes in total suicide rates, it did not provide information on changes in rates among adolescents and young adults specifically. Diekstra et al., within the framework of the WHO Project on Preventive Strategies for Suicide (World Health Organization 1988), carried out a similar analysis of the 15–29 age group. Changes in the suicide rates for this age group for the same European countries over the period 1960–1961 and 1984–1985 were related to changes in social conditions. The extent to which seven of these conditions (listed in Table 9) accurately predict changes in national suicide rates is depicted in Figure 6.

Five of these factors are either identical or quite similar to the variables shown by Sainsbury et al.'s (World Health Organization 1982) study to be associated with changes in national suicide rates. Unlike Sainsbury et al.'s findings, however, Diekstra et al.'s study showed a negative relationship between the percentage of young people in the population and an increase in suicide rate. This may, however, be a consequence of the fact that the latter study used the percentage of persons younger than 30 years of age as a predictor, as well as the suicide rate in that same age group as a dependent variable.

Two other variables related to the change in youth suicide rates were the change in use of alcohol and the percentage of change in church membership (nine countries only), an indicator of seculariza-

Table 9. Suicide rates in Europe: factors of change—1960–1980

Percentage of unemployed (+)

Percentage of population under 15 (−)

Percentage of women employed (+)

Divorce rate (+)

Homicide rate (+)

Percentage of change in alcohol use (+)

Percentage of change in church affiliation (+)

tion. These factors are interesting for several reasons. First of all, the percentage of change in alcohol use has the highest single correlation (.71) with changes in the suicide rate. This factor seems to point to the increasing emergence of a pattern of behavior involving the use of psychoactive substances to cope with life's problems. Many suicides and particularly many "attempted" suicides or parasuicides are just that.

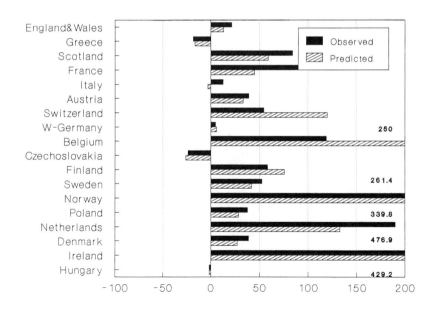

Figure 6. Percentage of change in suicide rate between 1960–1961 and 1984–1985.

The association between the percentage of change in church membership and the suicide rate suggests the influence of changing moral values and attitudes toward suicide impacting on the frequency of its occurrence. It might also be an indicator of decreasing social integration, given that churches have for centuries functioned as social "havens."

In conclusion, the results from these two studies indicate that societies, communities, or social groups that are increasingly subject to conditions like economic instability or deprivation (unemployment), breakdown of traditional primary or family group structure, interpersonal violence, increases in criminal behavior, secularization, and increasing substance use/abuse are at high risk for an increase in suicides in youth. Therefore, it is expected that the developing world will show a sharp increase in suicides among the young in the coming decades. Many of the developing countries, as a consequence of a dramatic growth of urban areas, are witnessing a disruption of traditional family structure, values, and ways of life as well as a demographic explosion of young people who are often unemployed and vulnerable to the seductions of substance abuse (see Diekstra 1988). A striking trend is that patterns of mortality in large urban areas in the developing world are beginning to resemble more and more the patterns of mortality in the industrialized world (Mahler 1987).

NONFATAL SUICIDE ACTS

In numerous clinical studies (e.g., van Egmond and Diekstra 1989), previous suicidal behavior in the form of one or more nonfatal suicide attempts has emerged as the most powerful predictor of suicide. Many suicides (estimates range from about 40% to 65%) are the last in a series of suicide attempts for an individual. Follow-up studies show that between 10% and 14% of those who made a nonfatal attempt will eventually die as a result of a subsequent attempt. Since no countries in the world keep national statistics on attempted suicides, it is not possible to relate trends in completed suicide to trends in attempted suicides on a national or international scale. However, it would seem safe to assume that both trends are intimately related. Data from centers in well-defined catchment areas collected in several countries over a number of years (Diekstra 1985; World Health Organization 1982) indicate that hospital admission rates for attempted suicides for adolescents and young adults rose sharply during the same period (1965–1980/81) when the national suicide rates were also increasing. In Great Britain and the Netherlands, data on attempted suicides from hospital inpatient registers revealed the same pattern.

For a number of reasons, the term *suicide attempt* is misleading, because the majority of such acts are not intended to be fatal. The wish to die is just one among the many motives for an "attempt" (Table 10). Three different types of motivations can be delineated: 1) cessation, to die, to stop conscious experience now and forever; 2) interruption, to interrupt conscious experience for a while, to sleep; and 3) appeal, to mobilize or change others. Most "attempts" are motivated by a combination of interruption and appeal (Diekstra 1987). Such acts can be viewed as coping behaviors that may or may not be appropriate under the circumstances. For these reasons, a nonfatal suicide attempt would more appropriately be called "deliberate self-harm," as it has been termed in the draft of the 10th International Classification of Diseases. (For reasons of consistency, however, the term *suicide attempt* will still be used in the remainder of this chapter.)

How common is deliberate self-harm in the world today? One indication can be found from a study carried out in 1979 of the nine countries that formed the European Economic Community (EEC) (Diekstra 1982). Based on data provided by medical centers with well-defined catchment areas, it was extrapolated that for the year 1976 in the whole of the EEC (comprising about 200 million persons at that time), approximately 430,000 acts of deliberate self-harm were treated in either inpatient or outpatient facilities (Table 11).

Table 10.   Reason for taking overdoses: self-report

To make others feel sorry, give them a sense of guilt, to shock or pay them back

To make it clear to others how desperate you are

To influence someone else, make him/her change mind

To escape from an unbearable state of mind

To seek help

To find out whether someone really loves you

To escape temporarily from an unbearable situation

To show how much you love someone else, to make things easy for other

To die

Source.   Adapted from Bancroft and Marsack (1977) and Diekstra (1987).

Table 11. Attempted suicides in the EEC: hospital and general physician contacts—1976

Country	Rate/100,000		Absolute number	
	Men	Women	Men	Women
Denmark	179	282	3,468	5,681
France	133	247	26,012	51,796
Ireland	127	227	1,382	2,498
Italy	26	82	5,383	18,260
Netherlands	94	147	4,834	7,779
Great Britain	353	527	73,413	118,968
Federal Republic of Germany	151	231	34,352	60,159
Belgium and Luxemburg	—	—	6,260	929
EEC Total	**162**	**265**	**155,104**	**266,070**

Note. EEC = European Economic Community.
Source. Adapted from Diekstra (1982).

This amounts to an average of 215 cases (i.e., episodes) for the EEC per 100,000 persons, aged 15 years and older. Actually, between countries, a wide variation in rates occurred, which can be explained in part by the differences in referral and data recording procedures (Diekstra 1982). Given how common the "tip-of-the-iceberg" phenomenon is in the area of mental illness, there is good reason to suspect that the figures reported in Table 11 represent only a small part of the overall problem. This hypothesis is supported by a number of survey studies in samples of the general population (see Table 12) indicating that the lifetime prevalence of deliberate self-harm ranges from 1% to 5% of persons 15 years and older. Suicide attempts were fairly uncommon in the 1950s but increased with dramatic rapidity in the 1960s and 1970s in a number of EEC countries (Diekstra 1982). Additionally, because the majority (60%) of these acts are carried out by persons below the age of 30, the lifetime prevalence figures strongly suggest that the rates reported in Table 12 significantly underestimate the "true" attempt rates in most countries. One survey study (Diekstra 1982) that examined the possibility of a tip-of-the-iceberg phenomenon discovered that three of four cases of deliberate self-harm did not lead to contact with health services (Figure 7).

The reasons for this low rate of health care system interventions include the following: 1) the act was not considered medically serious; 2) there was deliberate negligence; and 3) the act was no longer effective in mobilizing others because of many preceding attempts. The estimated yearly figure of 700 to 800 suicide attempts per 100,000

Table 12. Percentage of suicide attempters in the population: lifetime and 1-year prevalence

Study	Lifetime	1975
Diekstra and van de Loo (1978)	4.04	0.55 0.70 (events)
Diekstra and Kerkhof (1981)	5.01	
Hallström (1977)	4.50	
Mintz (1970)	3.90	
Paykel et al. (1974)	1.10	0.60 (persons)

Source. Adapted from Diekstra (1982).

of population for people aged 15 years and over clearly indicates that attempted suicide in certain European countries is not (in contrast to suicide) a rare phenomenon. In certain population groups, it is very common behavior and appears to be a habitual coping response to recurring life stresses (Kreitman 1976).

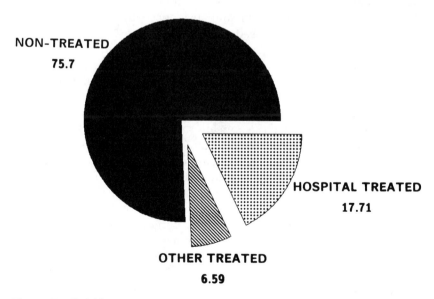

Figure 7. Suicide attempts: treated and nontreated. From Diekstra (1982).

Suicide Attempts and Suicide: Overlapping Phenomena

If the population of persons engaging in suicide attempts comprises a pool from which many future suicides are recruited, two key questions for the prevention of suicide arise. What causes nonfatal attempts? What factors are responsible for repeated attempts that ultimately lead to death?

State-of-the-art knowledge concerning both issues is quite limited. In a recent meta-analysis of the literature on the predictability of suicidal behavior, van Egmond and Diekstra (1989) reviewed 81 published studies from a number of countries comprising 106 comparisons between clinical and nonclinical suicidal and nonsuicidal groups.

Results from 17 studies concerning the characteristics of suicide attempters as compared to people who never engaged in suicidal behavior revealed the following profile of the attempters. They are more often unmarried or divorced and suffer more often from depressive disturbances and interpersonal conflicts. Depressive symptomatology includes agitation, hostility, and feelings of hopelessness and helplessness. Cognitive distortions that are associated with a depressive disturbance (e.g., a negative view of oneself, a negative view of others and of the future) were found more often among the suicide attempters. Their interpersonal conflicts were not limited to problems with partners, but extended to the majority of persons in their social networks. They also had poorer employment records as well as more alcohol and drug abuse. In addition to their own history of suicidal behavior, there was much greater incidence of a family history of suicide or deliberate acts of self-destruction.

A review of 12 studies comparing characteristics of first-ever attempters with those of repeaters (persons who have made two or more nonfatal attempts) found that persons who make recurrent attempts are more often diagnosed as sociopathic personalities than are first-time attempters (van Egmond and Diekstra 1989). The differences also indicate that the repeaters more often had an unstable life-style as compared to the first-time attempters as evidenced by frequent change of residence, unemployment, poor work histories, substance abuse, a criminal record, and chaotic family environments. Repeat suicide attempters are more likely to have been in psychiatric treatment, often as a consequence of earlier suicidal behavior, which sometimes led to an intensive, lengthy period of inpatient or outpatient treatment. Many of the attempts made by repeaters were not very serious. A review of the studies comparing differential characteristics of completed suicides and individuals who engaged in nonfatal attempts suggests the following profile: suicides are more likely to be older men who are unmarried, divorced, or widowed; who live alone;

and who are unemployed or retired. In their early attempts, they often use a more lethal method and leave suicide notes.

Other differences between the two groups include the following. Suicides have a higher prevalence of long-term use of prescribed psychotropic drugs and a higher prevalence of the psychiatric diagnoses of schizophrenia and depression. Furthermore, among the completed suicide group, there are more persons with a criminal record, repeated antisocial behavior, long-term alcohol and (nonprescribed or illicit) drug abuse, a history of psychiatric treatment, and contacts with medical services in the period just before their fatal attempt.

Additionally, there is accumulating evidence that social factors influencing the rates and trends in completed suicide are similar to those affecting the rates of attempted suicide. Platt (1986), for example, demonstrated that in Scotland there is a relationship between unemployment and both the rates of suicide and of attempted suicide. Other studies indicate that most social factors related to changes in the suicide rate (see Table 9) are also related to rates of attempted suicide (Diekstra and Hawton 1987).

COMPLEXITY OF CAUSE AND CURE

The data presented in this chapter clearly indicate, and this is confirmed by the general literature in suicidology, that both suicide and suicide attempt are very complex phenomena. The search for one single responsible agent, a "suicidococcus," has proven to be unfruitful. Every act of suicidal behavior has notable causes and grows out of an array of individual and societal factors.

Blumenthal (Chapter 26, this volume) underscores the complex causation of suicidal behavior, emphasizing the need for parallel complex solutions. The call for multifaceted, multidisciplinary solutions has occurred in the past for a number of other public health problems (e.g., the reduction of violence). However, it has seldom been heard before in the area of suicidology, presumably because most of the work on intervention and prevention of suicidal behavior has been in clinical settings. Although in more recent years a number of authors have proposed to approach the problem of the prevention of suicidal behavior from a broader community perspective (e.g., Diekstra and Hawton 1987), most of these intervention activities have usually taken the form of rather isolated projects, such as school curricula for suicide education. Apart from the danger that such activities might be counter productive because they might not only provide explicit information on suicide but also provide models for that behavior, they also have the disadvantage of not being directed toward those population groups that carry the highest risk for suicidal behavior, especially for completed suicide (Pardes and Blumenthal, Chapter 25, this volume). Additionally, while these interventions might be useful in certain developed nations, they might not have applicability in other countries, especially in the developing world. The generalizability of such programs may be further limited by the fact that cultures differ widely with regard to their attitudes toward suicidal behavior and therewith to the acceptability of programs that speak openly and frankly about it. Therefore, from an international and a WHO perspective, successful programs to prevent and reduce self-destructive behavior must be oriented at the entire system: the individual, family, school, workplace, other organizations, as well as to the larger community context. Furthermore, an optimal complex prevention program designed to reduce suicide rates should seek to accomplish this goal through a variety of channels. It may be that one reason why intervention and prevention programs tried over the past few decades in a number of countries have not been able to withstand empirical tests of their efficacy is that they have not been based on the "complex-cause–complex-cure" approach (World Health Organization 1982). Simply put, complex problems require complex solutions.

The growing awareness of that effect has recently led to the establishment of national task forces on suicide in several countries (the United States, Canada, the Netherlands), which have been charged with developing comprehensive national programs for the prevention of suicidal behavior. The recommendations of these task forces (Alcohol, Drug Abuse, and Mental Health Administration 1989; Diekstra 1986; Simmons 1987; Syer-Solursh, personal communication, 1986) generally agree with the recommendations made by the WHO (World Health Organization 1982). The main categories of public policy recommendations that emerged from these national and international strategies are described by Pardes and Blumenthal (Chapter 25, this volume).

TOWARD A COMPREHENSIVE STRATEGY FOR THE PREVENTION OF SUICIDAL BEHAVIOR

Both from international and national perspectives, prevention of suicidal behavior depends on the degree to which the following four conditions are met: 1) the assembly of scientifically sound information and research on the causation of suicidal behavior, on the efficacy of intervention and prevention schemes, and on effective methodologies for implementing such strategies in a variety of cultural and socioeconomic settings; 2) the improvement of services dealing with suicidal persons or persons at high risk for suicidal behavior; 3) the effective provision of information and training to relevant organizations and the general public; and 4) the provision of special services to high-risk groups.

Research

There is an urgent need for more and better information concerning the causes of suicidal behavior, methods for preventing suicide, and the reasons why there are international differences in rates. Compared with other health problems, the amount of knowledge available in this field is extremely limited. Effective intervention and prevention programs must be based on results from carefully designed and implemented national and international research programs. Essential components of such research programs should include the following:

1. The collection of national and international data on the incidence of suicide and suicide attempts and the characteristics of individuals who make suicide attempts and commit suicide. To accomplish this goal it is necessary that:

   (a) the classification or certification of suicidal behavior be improved through the international adoption of uniform definitions and operational criteria for suicide and suicide attempts, preferably in systems like the International Classification of Diseases (World Health Organization 1978);

   (b) measures are taken to ensure that the authorities or persons whose responsibility it is to establish suicide as the cause of death do, in fact, apply the criteria referred to above;

   (c) data collection at the national and international level be developed in such a way that the information can be used for analytic-epidemiologic studies of the characteristics of high-risk groups and the changes in those characteristics that take place over time;

   (d) data collection be conducted so that the effects of local and regional prevention or intervention programs can be tested;

   (e) general hospitals and other medical and social services that treat suicide attempters be encouraged to maintain records of these cases that would be regularly reviewed by a regional or local body.

2. The funding of carefully designed multidisciplinary international research programs in which a range of relevant risk factors for suicidal behavior are investigated. These programs must be planned and directed in such a way that existing research projects and available knowledge are made use of and that they

provide the information necessary for effective prevention or intervention programs. They should also study, among other things, the interaction between multiple risk factors, such as emotional disturbance and alcohol and drug abuse as well as the question of possible causal relationships between biological, environmental, and cultural factors and suicidal behavior.

3. The carrying out of well-planned research studies using control groups that examine methods for treating suicide attempters and of prevention programs for high-risk groups (e.g., relatives and close friends of people who have committed suicide).

4. The conducting of studies to determine the most effective and safe way of informing the public about suicide, examining the positive and negative effects the media can produce in this context.

Improving Services

It is of great importance that available services designed to help those with a high risk of suicidal behavior be expanded and improved. This should occur within the public mental health system, the welfare and social services, *and* the judicial and law enforcement agencies. Pending the results of research into the effectiveness of methods of prevention and intervention, improvements can be made in a number of areas.

Increased competence of professionals in the health and mental health system who identify and treat suicidal and depressed persons must be achieved. Training for physicians, psychiatrists, clinical and health psychologists, psychotherapists, social workers, and general and social/psychiatric nurses must include the following obligatory components: 1) information on the epidemiology of suicide and attempted suicide and the risk factors for suicidal behavior; 2) information on and training in the skills necessary to identify those with a high risk of suicidal behavior; 3) training in interview techniques, treatment, and aftercare of suicidal individuals, the relatives of those who have committed suicide, and the families or friends of those who have made a suicide attempt; and 4) training in the appropriate referral of suicidal individuals to appropriate health care professionals and agencies.

Models or scenarios should be developed to assist institutions and staff within the health and mental health system to give more specific and better coordinated assistance or aftercare to suicidal individuals and their relatives. One way to achieve this goal is to make community mental health systems on the primary health care level responsible for the coordination of care and treatment of suicidal persons and for developing models that will ensure that the following tasks are fulfilled: 1) the provision of direct and specific assistance and intervention in crisis situations; 2) making thorough assessments of suicide risk and appropriate plans for treatment; 3) referral and transfer of suicidal individuals to other services and the provision of appropriate help and aftercare by various agencies; 4) the provision of mental health consultations to primary health care professions, their suicidal patients, and their relatives; and 5) maintaining records to monitor the extent of the problem and to evaluate the care provided.

The implications of the above recommendations are that the primary health care system will assume a coordinated role in ensuring that appropriate expertise and sufficient access to services are available within each community. Primary health care workers or agencies will have to establish contact with other relevant services available in the community (e.g., police, general practitioners, emergency telephone services, social health services, ambulance services) and ensure collaboration with inpatient health care institutions (general hospitals, psychiatric units in general hospitals, psychiatric hospitals, and university psychiatric clinics). Every effort must be made to ensure that the designated agency's address and telephone number in a community becomes so well known and so accessible that it can operate as the central point from where immediate assistance in case of emergencies can be obtained.

Measures should also be taken to ensure that in every hospital providing medical (emergency) treatment for attempted suicides, a formal policy be established with regard to psychiatric assessment, treatment, and referral of suicide attempters and their relatives. The help given to suicide attempters in hospitals should be organized to incorporate clinical psychiatric and psychological knowledge, skills, and expertise in crisis intervention. Facilities should be established for prolonged observation of suicidal persons in hospitals, even when medical treatment has ended. Formal arrangements should be made between the primary health care facilities and inpatient psychiatric institutions for the referral and aftercare of suicide attempters and their relatives. To improve the care provided to suicide attempters in general psychiatric hospitals, research must be carried out on the short-term and long-term factors that have contributed to the rise in suicide rates in such hospitals. Greater emphasis should be placed on training people to work with suicidal patients in psychiatric hospitals. More attention should be devoted to health care workers' own attitudes toward suicide. In this regard, research into effective treatment methods for patients who repeatedly attempt suicide is of great importance.

Training and Information Regarding the Problem of Suicide

The provision of appropriate information and training to relevant organizations and groups and the general public is essential if the suicide rate is to be substantially reduced and to mitigate effects on survivors. The following points are worthy of particular consideration.

Curricula of primary and secondary school teachers and counselors should include information and training on assessing depression, the risk of suicide, and appropriate referral of suicidal pupils. The same holds true for the curricula of workers dealing with out-of-schoolers or school dropouts. Relevant curricula models must include 1) information concerning the acute and chronic risk factors associated with suicidal behavior; 2) information on the characteristic symptoms of depression and other psychological disturbances as they may manifest within the school context; 3) information on criteria and methods for referral of students who are clearly at risk and identification of referral institutions; 4) training in interpersonal and communication skills necessary to approach and establish an understanding relationship with such pupils; and 5) information on how linkages between mental health services and the schools can best deal with and respond to suicide or attempted suicide by pupils.

With regard to the role of the police, the following recommendations are made. Senior police officials should ensure that in the event of a suicide or an attempted suicide, police duties be carried out, whenever possible, by officers who have the necessary skills and appropriate attitudes. Policies and guidelines should be established based on police experience that can be followed in cases of suicide and attempted suicide. These might include the wearing of civilian clothes, providing support to surviving relatives until other helpers arrive, and contacting the family physician. Arrangements must be made to ensure that items seized at the time of a suicide, such as suicide notes, diaries, and other evidence of a personal nature, be returned to the family as soon as investigations have been completed.

To assess the role of emergency telephone services and their potential in suicide prevention, research should be undertaken to investigate how the role of these services can be optimally used to prevent suicide. The focus should be on such aspects as the training of volunteer workers, the telephone services' relationship with agencies providing assistance, and the linkages to mental health professionals. Research should also be undertaken to study the long-term follow-up of suicidal persons who have contacted emergency telephone services. The information obtained should help clarify the role of these services in suicide prevention and determine whether they should receive more governmental support than currently is the case. With regard to the general public, efforts are needed to increase awareness of the symptoms of depression and other warning signs of suicide. In addition, more publicity should be given to organizations that can offer confidential and professional advice and/or assistance to suicidal persons and their families.

The media can be very helpful in accomplishing the above-mentioned objectives, but may also play a role in provoking or encouraging suicidal behavior. It is recommended that in the interests of suicide prevention, the media should exercise great prudence and restraint in publishing news items and articles or broadcasting fictional programs concerning suicide. It is suggested that efforts be made to discuss such material and the method of presentation with professional experts in suicide before it is made public.

Special Groups

It is suggested that the following provisions be made for special high-risk groups. Provisions for identifying and preventing suicidal behavior among adolescents should be clearly organized. In the case of school-attending adolescents, collaboration between schools and the primary mental health services within each community should be established. Where possible, parents should be involved. Furthermore, arranging for a psychiatrist or psychologist to consult at the school on certain days with pupils who have psychological problems would be advisable. In the case of youngsters not attending school, special community outreach activities should be established.

Care of potentially suicidal elderly persons should include an active outreach policy directed at elderly people living alone, and in particular those who have recently experienced the death of their partner. These programs must be set up as part of primary health care services. Efforts must be made to make regular checks on the physical condition of the widow or widower (which can often deteriorate rapidly after the death of the partner) and to encourage socialization. Such an approach is of particular importance with childless elderly couples and should be continued for at least a year after the death of the partner. The various agencies involved must (under coordination of primary health care agencies) establish clear policies at regional levels regarding such activities. It is further recommended that regional geriatric services provide better information about depressive disorders and their treatment to health care professionals and to the elderly.

More research is needed on suicidal behavior in correctional institutions and prisons, particularly on methods of preventing such behavior. Training of prison staff to identify and to intervene with suicidal inmates is needed.

It is recommended that health care professionals who care for the chronically ill (including AIDS patients) be trained to identify and to discuss suicidal thoughts and plans with patients, to assess the risk of suicidal behavior, and to evaluate the degree to which suicidal wishes are related to acceptance of illness or disability and the extent to which an acceptable quality of life, given the disability, is possible. They must also be trained in counseling such patients or, where this is not part of their job, in appropriately referring them.

Agencies and individuals involved in treating alcoholics and substance abusers should be alert to the risk of suicide among their patients/clients and should be trained to identify and deal with an increased risk of suicidal behavior. To enhance suicide prevention efforts, it is important that national measures be taken to combat alcohol and drug abuse.

Relatives of people who have committed suicide should be considered at high risk for suicide and, therefore, an important target group for preventive measures. Given that they do not often ask for help themselves, an active approach must be used to contact and assist them. It is an important responsibility of the primary mental health services to get in touch with relatives of people who have committed suicide as soon as possible thereafter to offer help and to repeat this offer in subsequent contacts. These support interventions should continue for at least a year after the suicide.

Assistance should include both individual counseling and support for the surviving family members as a group. Primary health care agencies should organize grief support groups for survivors of those who have committed suicide to facilitate their working through their bereavement and grief. Additionally, information (e.g., brochures) should be immediately made available to survivors, describing in simple terms the process of coming to terms with complex feelings of grief, loss, and guilt; social consequences and ways of dealing with them; and ways of seeking help from others.

An assessment of community organization provisions for dealing with suicidal persons should be made. Where services are lacking, it is recommended that the federal or state governments request these organizations to make such provisions.

Conclusion

Suicide is an international problem affecting virtually every country in the world. Suicide and attempted suicide can be prevented, but the development, implementation, and evaluation of effective large-scale prevention programs is still in its infancy. The organizational structures required for well-coordinated programs of research and practice in the area of suicide prevention are only beginning to be built. Adequate training of health care professionals and other relevant groups in the assessment and management of suicide risk is lacking. These deficiencies in current programs across the world have promoted the establishment of national task forces on suicide prevention in the United States, Canada, and the Netherlands, as well as a WHO strategy on suicide prevention. These groups have formulated comprehensive strategies for the prevention of suicide. The main components of these programs are 1) the design and implementation of national research programs; 2) the improvement of services; 3) the provision of information and training on suicide prevention to relevant professional groups, organizations, and the general public; and 4) formulation of strategies and techniques to deal with special risk groups.

In this chapter, the scope of suicide and attempted suicide from an international perspective has been reviewed. Sociodemographic trends have been analyzed and explanatory theories for international differences proposed. Public policy recommendations for the prevention of suicide, both nationally and internationally, have been proposed. Three national task forces on suicide and an international strategy have been discussed and their recommendations presented. These efforts are seen as important steps in translating comprehensive national plans to prevent suicide into clinical, research, and community programs that can effectively prevent these tragedies around the world.

REFERENCES

Alcohol, Drug Abuse, and Mental Health Administration: Report of the Secretary's Task Force on Youth Suicide, Vol 1–4 (DHHS Publ No ADM-89-1623). Washington, DC, U.S. Government Printing Office, 1989

Bancroft J, Marsack P: The repetitiveness of self-poisoning and self-injury. Br J Psychiatry 131:394–399, 1977

Barraclough B: International variation in the suicide rate of 15-24 year olds. Soc Psychiatry 23:75–84, 1988

Bayet A: Le Suicide et la Morale. Paris, Alcon, 1922

Diekstra RFW: Epidemiology of attempted suicide in the EEC, in New Trends in Suicide Prevention. Edited by Wilmott J, Mendlewicz J. Basel, S Karger, Bibliotheca Psychiatrica, 1982, pp 1–16

Diekstra RFW: Suicide and suicide attempts in the European economic community: an analysis of trends with special emphasis among the young. Suicide Life Threat Behav 15:402–421, 1985

Diekstra RFW: Health Council of the Netherlands. Rapport inzake suicide (report on suicide). The Hague, The Netherlands, Health Council of the Netherlands, December 1986

Diekstra RFW: The complex psychodynamics of suicide, in Suicide in Adolescence. Edited by Diekstra RFW, Hawton K. Dordrecht/Boston, Martinus Nijhoff, 1987, pp 30–55

Diekstra RFW: City lifestyles. World Health, June 1988, WHO Geneva, pp 18–19

Diekstra RFW, Hawton K (eds): Suicide in Adolescence. Dordrecht/Boston, Martinus Nijhoff, 1987

Diekstra RFW, Kerkhof A: Suicide-pogingen in de bevolking. Vakgroep Klinische Psychologie, RU Leiden, 1981

Diekstra RFW, van de Loo KJM: Attitudes towards suicide and incidence of suicidal behaviour in a general population, in Aspects of Suicide in Modern Civilization. Jerusalem, Academic, 1978

Durkheim E: Suicide. New York, Free Press, 1951

Häfner H, Schmidtke A: Suizid und Suizidversuche-epidemiologie und aetologie. Nervenheilkunde 6:49–63, 1987

Hallström T: Life-weariness, suicidal thoughts and suicidal attempts among women in Gothenburg, Sweden. Acta Psychiatr Scand 56:15–20, 1977

Headley LA: Suicide in Asia and the Near East. Los Angeles, CA, University of California Press, 1983

Holinger PC, Offer D, Zola MA: A prediction model of suicide among youth. J Nerv Ment Dis 176:275–279, 1988

Kelleher MJ, Daly M: Suicide in Cork and Ireland. Paper presented at the second European Conference on Suicide Research, Edinburgh, 1988

Kreitman N: Age and parasuicide ("attempted suicide"). Psychol Med 6: 113–121, 1976

Kreitman NS: Parasuicide. Chichester, John Wiley, 1977

Mahler H: Epidemiology, Health Promotion and Health for All by the Year 2000. Paper presented at the 11th Scientific Meeting in Epidemiology, Helsinki, 1987

Mintz RS: Prevalence of persons in the city of Los Angeles who have attempted suicide. Bulletin of Suicidology 7:9, 1970

Paykel ES, Myers JJ, Lindenthal AO: Suicidal feelings in the general population: a prevalence study. Br J Psychiatry 124:460–469, 1974

Platt S: Parasuicide and unemployment. Br J Psychiatry 149:401–405, 1986

Platt S: Data from Royal Infirmary, Edinburgh, 1988

Simmons K: Task Force to make recommendations for adolescents in terms of suicide risk. JAMA 257:3330–3332, 1987

van Egmond M, Diekstra RFW: The predictability of suicidal behavior: the results of a meta-analysis of published studies, in Suicide Prevention: The Role of Attitude and Imitation. Edited by Diekstra RFW, Maris RA, Platt S, et al. New York, Leiden, Canberra, Brill Publishers, 1989, pp 37–61

Wisse J: Selbstmord und Todesfurcht bei den Naturvolkern. Zutphen, Thieme, 1933

World Health Organization: International Classification of Diseases (ICD-9). Geneva, World Health Organization, 1978

World Health Organization: Changing patterns in suicide behaviour. Copenhagen, WHO/EURO Reports and Studies, 74, 1982

World Health Organization: World Health Statistics Annual. Geneva, World Health Organization, 1987

World Health Organization: Correlates of Youth Suicide, Division of Mental Health. Geneva, World Health Organization, 1988

Chapter 21

Suicide in Minority Groups: Epidemiologic and Cultural Perspectives

Felton Earls, M.D.
Javier I. Escobar, M.D.
Spero M. Manson, Ph.D.

THE TOPIC OF suicide in minorities is important for at least four very practical reasons. First, it is a leading cause of premature death among minority groups. Second, the social, economic, and political disadvantages associated with minority status have inevitably resulted in poorer living conditions for members of these groups compared to those in the majority. To the extent that poorer material conditions are translated into greater psychosocial stress, it might be expected that the frequency of suicide would be higher in minority groups. Third, the economic disadvantage of minorities in American society also results in inferior health care. This means that they are less likely to receive treatment for health problems, such as mental disorders, chronic physical illnesses, and substance abuse, any one of which could elevate the risk of suicide. Fourth, cultural beliefs and attitudes may serve to either heighten or reduce the risk of suicide. Each of these functional concerns is important to understand in the planning and provision of mental health services, since they may not only influence the actual or perceived need for care but dictate particular ways in which the treatment should be given. This chapter will review the problem of suicide in minority populations. General popu-

Supported by MacArthur Network III on Risk and Protective Factors in Major Mental Disorders and NIMH Grant Number MH-31302.

lation characteristics will be discussed and the prevalence of suicide, risk factors for suicide, and intervention strategies will be reviewed.

Beyond these instrumental motives, there are other reasons to study suicide in minorities. Both majority and minority groups live within permeable barriers in American society. For all groups, specific cultural attitudes and practices are accepted, but the integrity of a group is challenged as these barriers are transversed as they must be in our open society. The effects of such adjustments go in both directions, from majority to minority group and from minority to majority. What this means for the study of suicide is that what were originally culturally specific risk or protective factors for an ethnic minority group may evolve over time to become characteristic of the more prevailing cultural characteristics established by the majority. Therefore, to reach a full understanding of this phenomenon in relation to suicide, it is necessary to place each group's experience within a changing historical context.

Another important reason to study suicide in culturally different groups is that an uncertain relationship exists between suicide attempters and those people who complete suicide. The two demographic correlates that have traditionally demarcated attempted or unsuccessful suicide from completed suicide are age and sex. Younger age groups and females predominate among attempters; older age groups and males are overrepresented among suicide completers. In this chapter we will add cultural factors to this exploration, since they may help illuminate what accounts for contrasts and similarities in suicide in the total American population.

For each of the three minority groups chosen (American blacks, Hispanics, and American Indians and Alaska Natives), population-based estimates on the prevalence of suicide will be given; their demographic and psychological correlates examined, and culturally distinctive approaches to prevention and treatment of persons who are at high risk for suicide explored. Space limitations prevented the inclusion of a section on Asian-Americans in this chapter. This topic has been discussed in some detail by Liu and Yu (1985).

SUICIDE IN AMERICAN BLACKS

Population Characteristics

With a population of 26.5 million, making up 11.5% of the total United States population, blacks constitute the largest minority group. Children are overrepresented and the elderly are underrepresented among blacks relative to the larger population. In both males and females, life expectancy is reduced in blacks by 5 to 7 years compared to whites. Most of this difference is accounted for by higher rates of infant mortality and cardiovascular diseases and a dramatically higher rate of homicide in blacks. In fact, while homicide accounts for far fewer deaths than cardiovascular disease (the most frequent cause of death in the United States), it rivals all other causes in accounting for premature death or, using the Centers for Disease Control's index, years of potential life lost. Thus when considering the topic of suicide in blacks, a parallel concern with homicide is required. This issue is particularly salient given the category of "intentional violence," which combines homicide and suicide into reportable causes of death.

Poverty, unemployment, and single-parent family composition are believed to be related to reduced life expectancy. Each of these demographic indicators is significantly more common in blacks than in whites. The disease-specific mechanisms through which these social and economic conditions work to increase mortality, however, are poorly understood and may not share much in common.

Just as the experience of several hundred years of economic exploitation and racial oppression has created maladaptive behaviors, which may be reflected, for example, in such forms as intraracial violence, the fact that blacks have survived underscores an important role for adaptive strategies. Such adaptive strategies involve the cultivation of resilience in the face of adversity, the maintenance of strong family ties, and the use of religion to promote personal and community harmony. As efforts to explain and eliminate various causes of premature death among blacks are pursued, it is important to keep in mind that these adaptive strategies are also at work and that they may serve as protective factors in some selective ways, one of which may relate to death by suicide.

A final point needs to be made in regard to race and culture. Racial identity has historically operated to create the appearance of a monolithic black culture. But, in fact, considerable variation exists and is defined by place of birth and regional differences.

Prevalence of Completed Suicide

The prevalence of suicide in black males (10.5 per 100,000) is several times higher than it is in black females (2.2 per 100,000) (U.S. Department of Health and Human Services 1985). This sex difference is similar to that found in whites, although the rates are appreciably lower for black males and females. As shown in Figure 1, the age distribution in black males demonstrates that peak rates occur in the 20- to 34-year-old age group. This is distinctly different from the age distribution for white males, which peaks toward the end of the life cycle. Differences between black and white females contrast much less

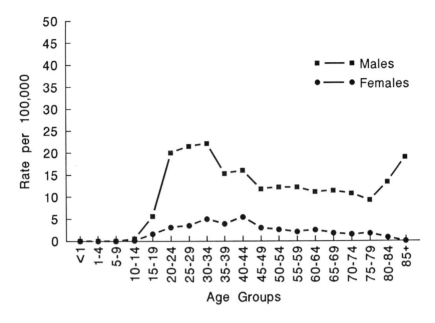

Figure 1. Death rates for suicide by 5-year age groups in black males and females, 1980.

sharply than the difference between black and white males.

The profile presented in Figure 1 could be made more dynamic by the addition of two features: geographical differences and secular changes. Geographic differences relate to urban-rural contrasts, the population size and density of urban areas, time since migration from the rural South to industrialized cities of the Midwest and Northeast, proportion of blacks in a given area, and degree of segregated versus integrated housing. Data of this sort will remain difficult to amass because of the rarity of suicide, but they are, nevertheless, important strategies to consider in studying suicide in blacks.

Secular changes could also provide important clues regarding the causes of suicide. Over the past few decades the most striking secular change has occurred in young white males, for whom the rate of suicide has tripled. The frequency in young black males has also increased, although not as strikingly as in white males. Efforts are being made to explain this secular change as either a cohort effect or a period effect. These different explanations carry special significance for black males. For example, if the increased incidence of suicide is caused by the induction of new socialization experiences in a birth cohort, then the current trend for young black males to die at higher rates will continue as this and subsequent cohorts age. As premature death increases in black males, the gap in life expectancy between white and black males will widen. Period effects, on the other hand, suggest that as an environmental condition linked to suicide changes, so will the suicide rates. Thus if the availability of drugs decreased or if employment opportunities for young black males increased, the rate of suicide (and homicide) should decrease.

It is important to contrast differences in the frequency of suicide with figures for homicide. Figure 2 shows the age and sex distribution for homicidal deaths in blacks. The death rate for homicide in males is approximately seven times the rate for homicide in females. The figure shows how decisively the rate of homicide peaks in early adulthood among males: in the same age range as the peak rate of suicide. The relationship between homicide and suicide in whites is different than it is for blacks; suicide is nearly twice as common as homicide for both sexes and at all ages (U.S. Department of Health and Human Services 1985).

Analysis of the demographic profile for suicide raises a number of concerns. First, differential reporting of rates for suicide in blacks and whites could contribute to some of the disparity between homicide and suicide rates. Specifically, underreporting of suicide and overreporting of homicide in blacks could account for some of the difference, but probably not enough to make up for the huge difference of death

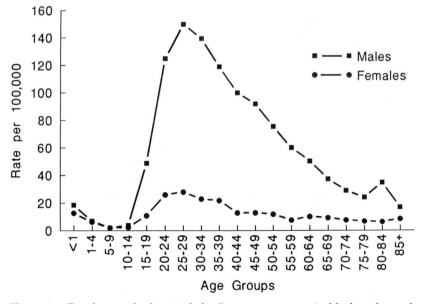

Figure 2. Death rates for homicide by 5-year age groups in black males and females, 1980.

rates for homicide. Second, it is possible that early death by homicide may be removing individuals at risk for suicide. This explanation is plausible if the risk factors for homicide and suicide are either the same or closely related. Third, the strikingly low rate of suicide among black females is in need of close examination. A recent attempt to examine stress-buffering or protective factors in black teenage females failed to produce practical results (Brown et al. 1989). Most of the females with high levels of psychosocial stress also had some form of psychopathology. In this study of adolescent medical patients, a very low rate of alcohol and drug use was found among black females. This may be a clue to explaining the low suicide rate, but more investigation is needed.

As a final step in examining differential suicide rates, information on the methods used in suicide were examined. Existing data show that the use of firearms is the primary method among both black and white males. However, black males are more likely to die by hanging, as the second most common method of suicide, whereas white males are more likely to use carbon monoxide poisoning.

Risk Factors for Completed and Attempted Suicide

Efforts to estimate numbers of potential suicides in the population have typically been based on the prevalence of suicide attempters in treated samples. Until fairly recently, there has not been a large representative population from which accurate estimates of suicidal behavior could be derived. The Epidemiologic Catchment Area (ECA) study of the National Institute of Mental Health has provided the sample needed to make such estimates and to explore the types of psychiatric symptoms and psychosocial factors that correlate with suicide (Regier et al. 1984).

Based on findings from the ECA study, Robins et al. (1989) constructed an index of suicidality that combines measures of suicidal ideation and suicidal behavior. The questions used in this study to elicit information about suicidality were: "Have you ever felt so low you thought of committing suicide?" and "Have you ever attempted suicide?" The frequency of suicidality in blacks is shown in Table 1. While female rates are higher in both age groups shown in the table, the differences are not nearly as striking as they are for completed suicide. The sex differences would have been greater if only the rates for suicide attempters had been considered. But since males are more likely to die from suicidal acts (and, therefore, not survive to report it), an estimate of their potential for suicide may include ideators as well as attempters. The extent to which ideators and attempters represent distinct groups as opposed to different levels of risk for completed

Table 1. Percentage of suicidality in 4,058 black adults by age and sex

Age	Males	Females
<45	7	9
≥45	4	5

suicide requires more research, particularly in regard to age and sex differences.

In the same analysis, risk factors associated with suicidality were examined. These included measures of psychiatric symptoms, such as depression, alcohol and drug abuse or dependence, childhood conduct disorder, and adult antisocial behavior, as well as a number of psychosocial characteristics. These variables were separately examined for black males and females. In both cases, the strongest correlations were for psychiatric symptoms. In ranking these variables, depressive symptoms (particularly hopelessness), daily drug use, multiple childhood conduct problems, and multiple somatic symptoms were more strongly correlated with suicidality in males than were having an unstable marriage, being unemployed, earning wages below the poverty level, or having less than a high school education. A very similar rank ordering of these characteristics was obtained for females.

In this same study we extended this analysis to include other violent behaviors such as fist fighting, using a weapon in fighting, and child abuse (Robins et al. 1989). A strong association with suicidality was found for each of these problems. There was also a strong association between being victimized in a violent incident and suicidality. Thus it appears that suicidality may be part of a violent repertoire of behavior and life circumstances.

The extent to which suicidality is a risk for completed suicide in blacks and whites is another important area in which the available evidence is inconclusive. It may be possible that the presence of suicidal ideation and behavior is less of a risk factor for blacks than whites and that this accounts for the lower death rate. One of the few studies to examine this question was completed almost 20 years ago (Pedersen et al. 1973). Given the secular changes that have occurred since then, these results may not accurately reflect the contemporary situation. Another limitation of that study is that it is based on the experience of the emergency service of a single hospital in Rochester, New York. Nevertheless, two conclusions from that work may have relevance. First, fewer blacks than whites received treatment following their suicide attempt. Second, despite higher rates of suicide attempts in blacks than whites in this sample, all of the deaths due to suicide occurring over a short follow-up interval were in whites. This may have been due to the small proportion of blacks in the sample. On the other hand, most of the deaths occurring in the sample were due to causes other than suicide. The investigators did not report these other causes, but one wonders if those deaths of blacks may have been due to accidents or homicide.

Intervention Strategies

The ECA study was also used to investigate the proportion of individuals with various types of psychiatric disorders who received treatment (Sussman et al. 1987). Since questions pertaining to suicide are a subset of the inventory of questions on depression, the extent of treatment for depression may provide a useful estimate of intervention for suicidal behavior. On comparing blacks and whites who had experienced a recent depressive episode, whites were more likely to seek mental health care than blacks. However, when the severity of depressive illness was considered, blacks were just as likely to seek help as whites. Thus it was only for milder forms of depression (fewer symptoms, shorter durations, fewer lifetime episodes) that blacks were less likely to seek help. Among the reasons given were the fear of treatment and hospitalization. Evidence was also obtained, however, indicating that blacks perceive themselves as being able to better tolerate mild to moderate levels of depression than do whites. In another study of adolescent medical patients, only about a quarter of patients with suicidal ideation and behavior informed their doctors about this problem (Earls 1989). So, even among those suicidal youth who are seeking care for some other reasons (most commonly for prenatal care), considerable effort will be required to detect the majority of youths at risk for suicide. Thus, while access to health services remains an issue, training in detecting and treating suicide is also important.

To provide effective treatment and quality care to black patients at risk for suicidal death, the training of psychiatrists and other mental health professionals must expose them to experiences that foster an appreciation of and sensitivity toward cultural differences. These training experiences should provide supervised management of black patients that takes account of how behavioral, linguistic, and attitudinal factors influence the therapeutic process. They should also assist the trainee in overcoming the propensity to stereotype behavior. Only through such experiences can a professional help a black patient overcome fears and hostility related to stigmatization of being a psychiatric patient, the use of medication or other biologic therapies, and hospitalization. These types of experiences need to be required for both white and black professionals. Being black does not, in itself, guarantee that a therapist's approach to a black patient will be more finely tuned to cultural nuances than a therapist of different ethnic origin. These same issues of training are just as applicable to other minority groups as they are to blacks, since all minority groups are subject to be viewed from the perspective of the norms and values established by the majority.

Beyond issues directly related to treatment, there is the need to gain a perspective on how black culture influences the quality of care received. This involves the use of language, the role of religion, and ways in which blacks have learned to cope with racism and powerlessness. Intellectual and cultural efforts have been made to legitimize styles of English used among blacks. When such styles and patterns of usage are regularly encountered by professionals who are unfamiliar with them, an effort should be made to study them.

Religion has occupied a dominant place in the black community for centuries. Religious expressions in music and art reflect an ethos of fortitude, endurance, and resiliency in the face of adversity. The extent to which this orientation toward life contributes to mental health is unknown. It is likely, however, that it has helped blacks maintain a sense of dignity and remain creative in American society. The professional working with black patients should be knowledgable about the role that religion plays in a patient's life. The failure to do so may cause the patient to feel that a therapist disrespects or trivializes an important aspect of the patient's life (Mendes 1982).

The attitudes fostered by the black church have not been uniformly incorporated into a life-style orientation by all blacks. The segment of the black population least influenced by this perspective may be young black men. Without the religiously oriented cultural supports to endure despite adversity, they, more than any other group, may have adopted violent and self-destructive behaviors. This is a major problem facing blacks.

New approaches are needed to encourage help-seeking behavior among black males. Young black females are much more likely to seek health care than young males, primarily for advice and treatment for contraceptive use and for prenatal care. For females, the issue is how to improve rates of early detection and treatment of suicidal behavior for those already in a health service. The problem for males is how to motivate them to see a doctor or counselor. One approach that has not been exploited involves linkage between mental health and criminal justice systems. This is of particular importance because of the association between antisocial behavior and suicide (Earls and Jemison 1986). The problems that led blacks to be grossly overrepresented in the jails and prisons are closely associated (if not the same) problems that place them at risk of early death. It makes sense to think that every black male entering the criminal justice system should be screened for suicidality and given preventive counseling or treatment, if it is needed. To accomplish this, more research is needed. But just as importantly, political and social interventions are needed to address intentional violence (i.e., homicide and suicide) as a most serious public health problem in the United States (Earls 1977).

Suicide In Hispanics

Population Characteristics

Hispanic from Hispania (Iberian peninsula, Spain) is the term applied to the 20 million United States residents who trace their roots to a Latin American country. (The 1980 Census [U.S. Bureau of Census, 1984] counted approximately 15 million Hispanics, and conservative estimates place the number of undocumented Hispanics at about 5 million.) In official statistics, the term *Hispanic* is used to separate those of Mexican origin from the rest of Texans. Although surrounded by controversy, the term is now firmly entrenched in American tradition following imprimatur by the Office of Management and Budget in the 1970s. Demographers predict that Hispanics will number 35 million in the early portion of the 21st century, thus becoming the largest single United States ethnic group, surpassing blacks and any other single nationality. Mexican Americans constitute the largest Hispanic subgroup (60% of the total), followed by Puerto Ricans (15%) and Cubans (6%). The remaining 19% includes at least 20 other nationalities. Hispanics are young (mean age, 23 years), congregate in households (more than one-half of Hispanic households report having more than four members compared to about one-fourth of the general United States population), and inhabit predominantly urban areas (90% live in cities or suburban towns). Geographically, Mexican-Americans tend to be localized in the Southwest, Puerto Ricans in the Northeast, and Cubans in the Southeast. These geographic distributions are important in a number of ways. The proximity of Mexican-Americans to the Mexican border, for example, allows for a frequent back and forth flow and ongoing contact with the Mexican culture, thus facilitating retention of traditional values despite generational shifts.

Major common features of United States Hispanics include 1) using Spanish as a first or second language (as many as 40% of Hispanics in the United States exclusively or predominantly speak Spanish); 2) living in a traditional close-knit family unit with hierarchies; and 3) having "traits" relating to the original colonial culture (Spain) and the prevailing religion (Catholic). These characteristics may impact on the form and course of mental disorders in this population and affect their observed prevalence. In fact, many of these traits may have a "protective" effect on the development of psychiatric disorders. It must be emphasized, however, that United States Hispanics are a very heterogenous group—racially (White, Black, Indian elements, and their complex assortments constitute the Hispanic "race"), educationally, economically, nationally (national origins can be traced to at least 20 different countries), historically (e.g., countries like Mexico have enjoyed long periods of autonomy while others have always been under some form of colonialism), and politically (awareness and use of the relative "power" conveyed by a minority status differs for many Hispanic subgroups).

Even for regionally distinct subgroups such as Mexican-Americans in the Southwest, the degree of incorporation of American culture or retention of traditional values differs widely. The concept of acculturation refers to the psychosocial changes that occur when individuals from one culture come into contact with a host culture. When the individual maintains most of the original culture's mores and motivations, that person is said to have low levels of acculturation, whereas high acculturation implies a thorough assimilation of the host culture's values. Acculturative "stress" and low levels of acculturation have been traditionally believed to increase the risk for mental illness. The "stress" of migration may also have important consequences on the prevalence of mental disorders and their complications.

Prevalence of Completed Suicide

Statistical information on Hispanics in the United States has lagged behind that for other United States groups. In 1984, the United States vital statistics included for the first time specific information on mortality of Hispanic groups based on data from only 15 states accounting for about 45% of the United States Hispanic population (Vital Statistics of the United States 1984). According to these reports, less than 5% of all suicide deaths in the 15 states considered were identified as "Hispanic." This proportion is lower than the proportion of Hispanics in the total United States population (6.5%), thus suggesting that United States Hispanics have lower mortality rates due to suicide than the rest of the United States population. The largest number of Hispanic deaths due to suicide was reported for the 15- to 24-year-old age group, whereas for the general population deaths due to suicide peaked in the 25- to 34-year-old age group. Vital statistics in Puerto

Rico (Gonzalez-Manrique and Rodriguez-Llauger 1986) have shown an annual prevalence of completed suicide among Puerto Ricans of 9.2 per 100,000, a rate that has remained stable for the last 25 years.

Smith et al. (1985) reviewed suicide deaths reported for Hispanics and non-Hispanic whites (Anglo) in five southwestern states (Arizona, California, Colorado, New Mexico, and Texas) for the years 1975–1980. Overall, the suicide rate for non-Hispanic whites was approximately twice as high as that for Hispanics (19.2 versus 9 per 100,000 population). The ratio of male to female suicides was greater for Hispanics than for non-Hispanic whites (4 to 1 versus 2.3 to 1). Hispanic suicides were particularly frequent among younger groups (e.g., those individuals below the age of 25 years).

Hoppe and Martin (1986) reported on suicide trends in San Antonio, Texas (Bexar County), for Mexican-Americans and non-Hispanic whites during three different time periods (1959–1961, 1969–1971, and 1979–1981). Mexican-Americans of both sexes had substantially lower suicide rates than non-Hispanic whites during the three periods. Rates for Mexican-Americans were on the average more than four times lower than corresponding rates for non-Hispanic whites (range, 1.3–3.4 for Mexican-Americans; 6.2–14.3 for non-Hispanic whites). Although suicide for both groups increased from 1960 to 1980, the percentage of increase was much higher for non-Hispanic whites (males, 66%; females, 74%) than for Mexican-Americans (males, 14%; females, 38%).

The above data on suicide rates suggest that Hispanics are less likely to die from suicidal intent than non-Hispanics. Obviously, these rates may be affected by the underreporting of suicidal deaths or by the misclassification of suicide deaths as due to "undetermined causes." The impact that the high number of undocumented deaths among Hispanics might have on vital statistics is unknown. It seems reasonable to assume that misclassification and underreporting should affect Hispanic and non-Hispanic suicide statistics about equally, suggesting that "protective" factors are operating in Hispanic populations.

Risk Factors for Completed and Attempted Suicide

Information on suicide ideation and behavior in Mexican-American and Puerto Rican community populations has become available through the Los Angeles ECA (Karno et al. 1987) and a similar survey in Puerto Rico (Canino et al. 1987). The information in both cases was obtained from the section of the Diagnostic Interview Schedule (DIS) on depressive symptoms. Four questions specifically inquire whether for a period of 2 weeks or longer the respondent felt so despondent that he or she thought about death, wanted to die, thought of committing suicide, or actually attempted suicide. In Los Angeles, fewer Hispanics than non-Hispanic whites reported both suicide ideation (9% versus 19%) and suicide attempts (3% versus 5%). In Puerto Rico, the lifetime rate of suicide ideation and suicide attempt was 14% and 6%, respectively. Interestingly, these proportions exceed those reported for Hispanic samples in the United States (a majority of whom were Mexican-American).

The Los Angeles-ECA survey collected extensive information on psychopathology, acculturation, social support, and use of available services, which allowed for secondary analyses on the relationship of such variables to suicide ideation and attempts. These analyses showed that the prevalence of suicide attempts among Hispanics and non-Hispanic whites remained stable across different educational levels. However, suicide ideation was lowest among those with low levels of education and highest for the most educated (8% for those who had less than a high school diploma versus 24% for those with college degrees). As expected, females had higher prevalences of suicide ideation and attempts than males, and both males and females who were married had lower prevalences of ideation and attempts than the single, separated, or divorced (Sorenson and Golding 1989). Respondents who met criteria for a lifetime psychiatric diagnosis were more likely to think of or attempt suicide. Individuals with bipolar affective disorder had the highest prevalence of suicide ideation (72%), followed by those with obsessive-compulsive (63%), panic (59%), and schizophrenic (57%) disorders. Regarding suicide attempts, the prevalence was highest for respondents who met criteria for dysthymia or major depression (23% in each case), followed by those with bipolar (20%), obsessive-compulsive (18%), and antisocial personality (17%) disorders. Finally, respondents who had been recently victimized were at greater risk for depression (15%) or suicide ideation or attempts (6%) than those not reporting any recent criminal victimization (10% and 2%, respectively).

Although Mexican-Americans with low levels of acculturation had lower rates of suicide ideation or attempts than the highly acculturated, these differences disappeared when controlling for country of birth (Sorenson and Golding 1989). Mexican-Americans born in Mexico reported a lower prevalence of suicide ideation (4.5%) or suicide attempts (2%) than Mexican-Americans born in the United States, 13% of whom reported suicide ideation and 5% suicide attempts. When religious affiliation is considered, the data show that, regardless of ethnicity, those who described themselves as Catholic were less likely to attempt suicide than non-Catholics (Sorenson and Golding 1989).

Intervention Strategies

Although detailed studies on the treatment of suicidal Hispanic patients are not available, there are five characteristics that should be considered in planning treatment and selecting high-risk samples for further study: religion, social supports, place of birth, acculturation, and somatization.

Mortality statistics indicate that suicide deaths are low in those European countries with a prevailing Catholic influence, such as Spain, Northern Ireland, or Italy (Sainsbury 1986). Since a majority of United States Hispanics maintain a Catholic affiliation, this might be an important deterrent for suicidal intent. Interestingly, according to the ECA data, United States Catholics are also less likely to report having ever thought about suicide compared to non-Hispanic whites.

A close-knit family system with hierarchies remains as a central feature of many United States Hispanic groups. These highly supportive systems may provide protection against suicidal behaviors by "buffering" the impact of environmental stressors and by providing assistance in times of need. Randolph and Escobar (1983) reported that Mexican-American psychiatric patients are more likely than non-Hispanic white patients to have intact families that provide unrelenting support. These family support systems seem to have a high tolerance for psychopathology and may be responsible at least in part for the lower hospitalization rates reported in the case of United States Hispanics with mental disorders.

In the case of Mexican-Americans, being born in Mexico instead of the United States seems to augur a healthier psychiatric outlook. This low risk for mental disorder for those born in Mexico may be related to a selection process; for example, those who migrate from Mexico may be particularly resilient and less likely to succumb to the ravages of social stress. The reverse seems to apply to Mexican-Americans born in the United States, possibly due to frustrated expectations in regard to achievement and social status (Burnam et al. 1987).

Those Mexican-Americans who identify strongly with the Mexican culture (the less acculturated) report less suicide ideation or intent than those who show more affinity for the North American culture. It is not yet known whether low acculturation status within the mainstream culture of the United States protects individuals from death by suicide, but this is a plausible issue for future research. As the acculturation status of Mexican-Americans increases, it might be expected that suicide rates will increase proportionately. If such a direct relationship can be shown to exist, it would present an important opportunity to examine social, behavioral, and cognitive mechanisms that could explain this association.

The presence of somatic symptoms suggestive of physical disorder but for which physical and laboratory assessments provide no clues has been found to be a rather common phenomenon among Hispanic populations (Escobar 1987; Escobar et al. 1987a, 1987b). Although some degree of somatization traditionally accompanies depression, this is particularly pronounced in the case of depressed Mexican-Americans and Puerto Ricans. Somatization may be highly disabling and leads to preferential use of medical over psychiatric services (Escobar et al. 1989). However, somatization may work as a coping mechanism (Nichter 1981), which may yield potentially beneficial results such as lower levels of guilt (Kleinman 1982) and might also lower the risk for suicide ideation or intent. The clinician should be alert to use of this mechanism in Hispanic patients and be particularly vigilant in questioning about emotional issues as part of the diagnostic workup.

SUICIDE IN AMERICAN INDIANS AND ALASKA NATIVES

Population Characteristics

According to the 1980 census (U.S. Bureau of Census 1984a), slightly less than 1.5 million American Indians and Alaska Natives reside in the United States, comprising 0.6% of the population. More than 300 different tribes are recognized by the federal government, distributed across 278 reservations and 209 Native villages. More than half of their members, however, now live in urban settings. The average income for Indian/Native families ($13,678) is considerably lower than the national average ($19,917); twice as many Indians/Natives (27.5%) are below the poverty line (U.S. Bureau of Census 1984a, 1984b). The unemployment rate for American Indians and Alaska Natives is two times greater than that of the nation as a whole and reaches over 80% in some communities. The Indian/Native population is generally younger (median age, 22.9 years) than the general United States population (median age, 30.0 years), due in large part to its higher fertility rate over the last three decades. The degree of educational attainment by Indians/Natives is far below that of their white and nonwhite counterparts (Brod and McQuiston 1983). The poorer health status and concomitant shorter life expectancy of American Indians and Alaska Natives in comparison to whites and even other ethnic minorities have been amply documented (Office of Technology Assessment 1986; U.S. Department of Health and Human Services 1986). Of particular note is the major contribution of alcohol abuse to 5 of the 10 leading causes of death among most tribes. One of these causes of death, suicide, constitutes a particularly grave concern, especially for adolescents (May 1987a).

Prevalence of Completed Suicide

The average suicide rate for American Indians and Alaska Natives from 1980–1982 was 19.4 per 100,000, which is 1.7 times the rate for the nation as a whole. Suicide rates for Indians and Natives ages 10–14, 15–19, and 20–24 were considerably higher than the national averages, specifically 2.8, 2.4, and 2.3 times greater, respectively (May 1987a). In contrast to the general trends for the general United States population, Indian suicide occurs predominantly among the young as opposed to the elderly (McIntosh and Santos 1981).

Several general patterns of suicide among Indians and Natives can be discerned from the approximately 116 studies that have been published on the subject since 1960 (for an annotated bibliographic review, see May 1987b). In this special population, suicides are most likely to be male, to have occurred in association with heavy alcohol consumption, and to have been carried out by highly lethal means (i.e., guns and hanging). These individuals more typically belong to tribes with loose social integration, which emphasize a high degree of individuality, that are undergoing rapid socioeconomic change. However, despite this fairly common pattern, actual rates vary dramatically, ranging from well below the national average in some southwestern communities to well above the national average in intermountain tribes of the Rockies (Shore 1974, 1975).

In addition to the high rates of suicide among Indian/Native adolescents, there appears to be an increasing tendency for these to occur in clusters, defined as any series of three or more suicides closely related in time and space (Coleman 1986). Several articles have recently appeared in the literature specific to this population (Bechtold 1988; Davis and Hardy 1986; Long 1986). Unfortunately, little is known about this phenomenon among adolescents in general, much less Indian/Native youth. Conventional wisdom holds that clustering occurs more frequently among females than males, despite the latter's higher rates (Phillips and Carstensen 1986). Moreover, serial suicides seem to be linked by imitative behavior. Subsequent suicides may be stimulated by personal knowledge of the victim and of the circumstances surrounding the death, and by the interpersonal proximity of a relatively closed community. Extensive media coverage may also contribute to the increased probability of serial suicides by dramatizing the death and focusing widespread attention on the victim (Gould and Shaffer 1986). Reports of cluster suicides among Indian/Native youth differ slightly in that the victims are predominantly males, although many attempts by females occur, usually by less lethal means, at similar points in time. Clearly, serial suicides by Indian/Native adolescents are fueled by the same interpersonal and social dynamics as those that underpin this phenomenon in the population at large, as indicated in Bechtold's (1988) penetrating analysis.

Risk Factors for Completed and Attempted Suicide

A wide range of individual risk factors has been considered in regard to Indian/Native suicide (Shore and Manson 1983). Frequent interpersonal conflict (Biernoff, unpublished manuscript, 1969; May 1973; Maynard and Twiss 1970; Miller and Schoenfeld 1971; Ross and Davis 1986); prolonged, unresolved grief (Devereux 1961; Jilek-All et al. 1978); chronic familial instability (Dizmang et al. 1974; May and Dizmang 1974; Resnik and Dizmang 1971; Swanson et al. 1971); depression (National Task Force on Suicide in Canada 1987; Termansen and Peters 1979); alcohol abuse or dependence (Westermeyer and Brantner 1972); and unemployment (Spaulding 1985–86; Travis 1983, 1984; Trott et al. 1981) have been shown to be major correlates of this phenomenon. In addition, a family history of psychiatric disorder— particularly alcoholism, depression, and suicide—often has been noted (Shore et al. 1972).

The suicide rate also is higher among Indian/Native adolescents who have been seen for psychiatric problems, those with physical illnesses, those who have previously attempted suicide, those with frequent criminal justice encounters, and those who have experienced multiple home placements (Berlin 1986; Dizmang et al. 1974; Fox and Ward 1977). Social disintegration and acculturation also have captured a great deal of attention as possible causes of suicide in this segment of the population (Kraus and Buffler 1979; Levy 1965; Levy and Kunitz 1971, 1987; Van Winkle and May 1986; Westermeyer 1971, 1979). Culture conflict and concomitant problems in identity formation are believed to produce a chronic dysphoria and anomie, which render Indian youth vulnerable to suicidal behavior during periods of acute stress (Hochkirchen and Jilek 1985).

Even more unique cultural dynamics appear to be at work in determining risk for suicide among Indian adolescents. For example, Levy and Kunitz (1987) illustrated that among the Hopi, suicide rates are not only high in "progressive villages" and off-reservation bordertowns, but along certain lines in traditional villages as well. Specifically, Hopis at special risk for suicide include the children of parents who entered into traditionally disapproved marriages (e.g., across tribes, mesas, and even clans of disparate social status). The labeling of parents as "deviant" in this regard stigmatizes their children, thereby engendering a distinct series of stressors. In an earlier example, Levy (1965) suggested that suicide among Navajo males may indicate their relative lack of integration into a changing, matrilineal society. Moreover, he described how these individuals seem to employ suicide to withdraw from intolerable situations, and yet, by virtue of its social, cultural, and spiritual affront to the survivors, accomplish a final act of aggression. Lastly, tribes that emphasize a high degree of individuality generally exhibit higher rates of suicide than those that emphasize conformity. Classic comparisons include the Apache, Navajo, and Pueblo communities, with the former representing "looser" social integration and the latter two representing "tighter" integration (Levy 1965; May 1987a; Van Winkle and May 1986).

Intervention Strategies

A literature review by Manson et al. (1987a) revealed published accounts of more than 45 different preventive interventions targeted to suicide and related risk factors among American Indians and Alaska Natives. Using Caplan's (1964) nosology, the authors characterized the programmatic foci of these efforts in terms of promotional, primary, and secondary types of intervention. Specific activities included counseling/psychotherapy, education/training, recreation, unique sociocultural institutions, consultation, legal regulation, registers, and provision of special facilities.

Nearly three-quarters of these interventions were promotional in nature, seeking to ensure the continued well-being of Indian/Native people by enhancing their psychosocial strengths and coping resources. Education, training, recreation, and unique sociocultural activities predominated. Project DARE, a culture-specific curriculum launched by the Ute Mountain Ute Tribe, emphasized decision-making abilities, assertiveness, self-respect, and self-esteem among local school-age youth (Beiser and Manson 1987). The Toyei Model Dormitory project increased the ratio of Navajo houseparents to students and provided special training to dorm aides in techniques for encouraging and reinforcing positive behaviors among residents (Goldstein 1974). The Chemawa Indian Boarding School Recreational Program employed the planning and implementation of outdoor adventures (ballooning, white-water rafting, mountain climbing) to increase a sense of mastery, self-efficacy, and interpersonal competence among the student participants (Beiser and Manson 1987). The Tiospaye Project on the Rosebud Sioux Reservation revolved around a traditional Lakota way of life that depends on extended family and shared responsibility. The Tiospaye organized a range of community activities that promoted group cohesion, cooperation, and collective identity (Mohatt and Blue 1982). Similarly, the Wido-Ako-Da-De-Win Project, named after the Chippewa word for "networking," encouraged ethnic identity, communication skills, self-analysis, and parenting skills among inner-city Indian adolescents by establishing social support groups and fictive kin networks (Red Horse 1982).

An equal number of interventions have entailed primary prevention programming, focusing on Indians and Natives known to be at high risk for suicide and related disorders. The delivery mechanisms included targeted counseling, program consultation, and the provision of special facilities. The Developmental Task Framework Project strengthened care-giver–toddler relationships, increased cultural identification, enhanced self-image, and facilitated child development through teaching isolated, rural Navajo families culture-specific interactional activities (Dinges 1982; Dinges et al. 1974). The suicide prevention center at the Fort Hall reservation established a medical holding facility for Shoshone/Bannock adolescents and young adults who had been arrested by local police for disruptive behavior, thereby dramatically reducing the likelihood of their suicide in an off-reservation jail (Dizmang et al. 1974; Shore et al. 1972). A similar detention facility was instituted on the Manitoulin Island Indian Reserve (Ward 1984). Yet another effort targeted a series of individual and group counseling sessions to fourth-, fifth-, and sixth-grade Indian children of dysfunctional, alcoholic families (Berlin 1985). The Whipper Man Project incorporated the culturally salient concept of tribal disciplinarian into the development of a group home for displaced, antisocial children and adolescents (Shore and Keepers 1982; Shore and Nicholls 1975). Numerous examples can be found of program consultation with courts, jails, schools, and primary-care clinics (Kinzie et al. 1972; Robbins 1982; Schottstaedt and Bjork 1977).

Far fewer of the programs described in the literature represent secondary preventive interventions. The most common types of activities were suicide registers, crisis hotlines, and psychotherapy with individuals who had attempted suicide. Confidential suicide registers have been used for surveillance as well as case management through local mental health programs and Indian Health Service regional offices (Dizmang et al. 1974; Shore 1975). Suicide centers have operated 24-hour crisis hotlines on the Fort Hall and Blackfeet reservations (Shore et al. 1972). Suicidal adolescents on the Manitoulin Island Indian Reserve were placed in a special residential facility and trained to perform specific community services (Fox et al. 1984; Ward 1984). Tribal elders have conducted group sessions about leadership for adolescent suicide attempters in a boarding high school. These bright and capable students appeared to suffer inordinate stress because they stood out as achievers.

Considerable debate has emerged among providers, within health care organizations such as the Indian Health Service, and across Indian/Native communities, about the relative emphasis that should be placed on these intervention modalities (Neligh 1988). By and large, communities press for essentially promotional approaches, which hold considerable appeal because of their nonstigmatizing aspects and emphasis on the collectivity. Interventions of this nature, however, may not be the most cost-effective in regard to suicide. They clearly require long periods of time before one can expect to observe outcomes. Health care organizations, on the other hand, which are subject to greater accountability, prefer primary and secondary forms of preventive intervention. They are more easily staged and delivered within institutional settings, appear to relate more directly to patient needs, and can be readily credited to an agency. The answer lies somewhere in between and is beginning to be modeled by innovative, comprehensive programs such as the Blue Bay Healing Center on the Flathead Indian Reservation in western Montana and the Jack Brown Center among the Cherokee Nation in northeastern Oklahoma—examples that, hopefully, will soon find their place in the literature.

CONCLUDING REMARKS

The inclusion of three cultural groups in a single chapter on suicide provides the opportunity to examine similarities across different strata of American society. The similarities begin with their shared status as minority groups in American society and extend to certain demographic and health indicators. Each of the three minority groups is overrepresented by youths and underrepresented by the elderly compared to the majority. They also have in common reduced life expectancy stemming from higher rates of infant deaths and violent deaths in adolescents and young adults. Despite these similarities, the differences between them are prominent. Each group has had a very different historical experience in the United States. Language, religion, and customs are also different. These characteristics justify their designation as unique cultural or ethnic groups, just as their relative size in the total population and their political influence warrant the status of being a minority.

Given this background, there is an important perspective to be gained in studying suicidal behavior in minorities. In all three groups, peak rates of suicide occur in young males. Although young black and Hispanic males have lower rates than white males of comparable ages, the gap is narrowing. Among American Indians and Alaska Natives, the gap is already closed. Predicting secular trends in suicide is complicated given our lack of understanding about cohort versus period effects; but one possible scenario is that the age-adjusted rates of suicide in minority-group males will eventually resemble the bimodal distribution that currently exists for white males. This makes for an unsettling state of affairs since it anticipates a trade-off between increasing life expectancy derived from improved health care and living circumstances, and a higher rate of suicide among males in the advancing years.

Just as in the white population, all three minorities demonstrate higher rates of suicide ideation and attempts in females than in males. Indeed, this has become a robust finding for which we do not have convincing explanations. Is the marked difference in sex ratio between completed and attempted suicide simply a reflection of more lethal methods used by males, or are there more substantive differences in their mental and physiologic states or help-seeking behavior that bring about suicidal thinking and behavior?

In examining the efforts to document risk factors across the three groups, most attention has been given to the presence of suicide ideation, depressive symptoms, and a past history of suicidal behavior. While we have explored the relationship between suicidality and other forms of violent behavior in blacks, this type of analysis should also be conducted in other minority groups (Earls and Jemison 1986; Robins et al. 1989). It is also the case that sufficient efforts to document the role of alcohol and drugs in suicidal behavior do not appear to have been made. This is essential since both suicide and alcohol and drug use have increased in young people over the same time period in the last 20 to 30 years. While alcohol and drug use tend to be less common among blacks and Hispanics than among whites, alcohol use among American Indians and Alaska Natives (Manson et al. 1987b) constitutes one of the most prevalent and serious health threats. It is important to ask if the differential experience with alcohol and drugs among minorities is linked to differential rates of suicide. Because imitation, based on either direct or vicarious experiences, may also lead to suicide, specifically in young people, it is important to continue efforts to document the clustering of suicides not only in American Indians and Alaska Natives but in other minorities as well.

Studies of suicide in minorities have not yet matured to the point of considering the interaction of both biological and psychosocial risk factors. While the contribution of a positive family history for completed suicide or affective disorder leaves open the question of how genetic and environmental factors are transmitted, studies of suicide in minorities can make an important contribution to our understanding. Cultural factors and psychosocial stressors may operate more powerfully than genetic factors in minorities to bring about changes in the expression of suicidal behavior because of the adaptations required to adjust to historical changes.

We have emphasized the importance of several putative protective factors along with the discussion of risk factors for suicide. To the extent that a protective factor is found to exist in a minority group, it is most likely to be detected in females. The question will then become the extent to which characteristics such as low acculturation, religious affiliation, and somatization constitute conditions that mental health agents will want to influence.

There is a persistent concern that our current estimates of suicide are underestimated because the degrees of misclassification and nonreporting are virtually unknown. Whether this "bias" operates uniformly across age, race, sex, and ethnic groups is also unknown. Yet, its significance for minorities is obvious since the combination of accidental death, homicide, and suicide represent major causes of premature death.

Although the accurate documentation of suicide as a cause of death remains suspect, methods available to measure psychiatric symptoms and disorders have improved considerably. The feasibility of conducting cross-cultural studies has been considerably advanced by the introduction of measures of known reliability and validity, such as the DIS, the Center for Epidemiologic Studies Depression Scale, and several other checklists and diagnostic interviews. With more accurate methods to document risk and protective factors that could become incorporated into preventive interventions, the need to adopt accurate methods of recording death rates for suicide is made all the more imperative.

Our final and most pressing concern is with the development of specific and culturally sensitive strategies for treatment and prevention. Current evidence indicates that blacks must experience more severe symptoms before telling a health professional about depressive symptoms (Sussman et al. 1987). This hesitation to reveal aspects of poor mental health functioning may constitute more of a barrier to improved care than the actual location or accessibility of services. This means that continued emphasis on the training of physicians and therapists in treating minorities is needed. Once the risks for suicide have been adequately addressed, treatment strategies useful with minorities should not be so different than they are for any other group (Blumenthal and Kupfer 1988). The areas in which unique strategies are necessary relate to the role of family, cultural considerations, and community supports. As pointed out earlier in this chapter, it is necessary that training programs view it as their responsibility to expose students and trainees to supervised experience in the management of minority patients. For some, this exposure will provide an enriching experience, serving to correct stereotypes and increase awareness of cultural diversity both within and between minority groups.

In terms of prevention, we have emphasized the need to target educational and high-risk strategies, particularly toward young males in all three groups examined. Indeed, we have pointed to an acute need for further research in this area because the age- and class-related changes that are occurring in minorities constitute a foreboding sign for an increased rate of suicidal death in future generations.

REFERENCES

Bechtold DW: Cluster suicide in American Indian adolescents. American Indian and Alaska Native Mental Health Research 1:36–45, 1988

Beiser M, Manson SM: Prevention of emotional disorders in Native North American Children. Journal of Preventive Psychiatry 3:225–240, 1987

Berlin IN: Prevention of adolescent suicide among some native American tribes, in Adolescent Psychiatry: Developmental and Clinical Studies. Edited by Feinstein SC. Chicago, IL, University of Chicago Press, 1985, pp 77–93

Berlin IN: Psychopathology and its antecedents among American Indian adolescents. Advances in Clinical Child Psychology 9:125–152, 1986

Blumenthal SJ, Kupfer DJ: Generalizable treatment strategies for suicidal behavior. Ann NY Acad Sci 487:327–340, 1988

Brod RL, McQuiston JM: American Indian adult education and literacy: the First National Survey. Journal of American Indian Education 1:1–16, 1983

Brown LJ, Powell J, Earls F: Stressful life events and psychiatric symptoms in black females. Journal of Adolescent Research 4:140–151, 1989

Burnam MA, Hough RL, Karno M, et al: Acculturation and lifetime prevalence of psychiatric disorders among Mexican-Americans in Los Angeles. J Health Soc Behav 28:89–102, 1987

Canino GJ, Bird HR, Shrout PE, et al: The prevalence of specific psychiatric disorders in Puerto Rico. Arch Gen Psychiatry 44:727–735, 1987

Caplan G: Principles of Preventive Psychiatry. New York, Basic Books, 1964

Coleman L: Teen suicide clusters and the Werther effect. The Network News 3:1–6, 1986

Davis BR, Hardy RJ: A suicide epidemic model. Soc Biol 33:291–300, 1986

Devereux G: Mohave ethnopsychiatry: psychic knowledge disturbances of an Indian tribe (Smithsonian Institution Bureau of American Ethnology Bulletin 175, Part 7, Suicide). Washington, DC, U.S. Government Printing Office, 1961, pp 286–484.

Dinges N: Mental health promotion with Navajo families, in New Directions in Prevention Among American Indian and Alaska Native Communities. Edited by Manson SM. Portland, OR, Oregon Health Sciences University, 1982, pp 119–143

Dinges N, Yazzie M, Tollefson GD: Developmental intervention for Navajo family mental health. Personnel and Guidance Journal 52:390–395, 1974

Dizmang LH, Watson J, May P, et al: Adolescent suicide at an Indian reservation. Am J Orthopsychiatry 44:43–49, 1974

Earls F: A failure of constituency. J Natl Med Assoc 69:803–805, 1977

Earls F: Studying adolescent suicidal ideation and behavior in primary care settings. Suicide Life Threat Behav 19:99–107, 1989

Earls F, Jemison A: Suicidal behavior in American Blacks, in Youth in Despair: Preventive Aspects of Suicide and Depression Among Adolescents and Young Adults. Edited by Klerman GL. Washington, DC, American Psychiatric Press, 1986, pp 131–145

Escobar JI: Cross-cultural aspects of the somatization trait. Hosp Community Psychiatry 38:174–180, 1987

Escobar, JI, Burnam MA, Karno M, et al: Somatization in the community. Arch Gen Psychiatry 44:713–718, 1987a

Escobar JI, Golding J. Hough RH, et al: Somatization in the community: relationship to disability and use of services. Am J Public Health 77:837–840, 1987b

Escobar JI, Rubio M, Canino G, et al: Somatic Symptom Index (SSI): a new and abridged somatization construct: prevalence and epidemiological correlates in two large community samples. J Nerv Ment Dis 177:140–147, 1989

Fox J, Ward JA: Indian suicide in northern Ontario. Paper presented at annual meeting of the Canadian Psychiatric Association, Saskatoon, Saskatchewan, 1977

Goldstein G: The model dormitory project. Psychiatric Annals 4:85–92, 1974

Gonzalez-Manrique MA, Rodriguez-Llauger A: Epidemiological trends of suicide in Puerto Rico: 1931–1985. Paper read at the 22nd annual convention of the Puerto Rico Medical Association, Psychiatry, Neurology and Neurosurgery section, San Juan, Puerto Rico, September 1986

Gould M, Shaffer D: The impact of suicide in television movies: evidence for imitation. N Engl J Med 315:690–694, 1986

Hochkirchen B, Jilek W: Psychosocial dimensions of suicide and parasuicide in Amerindians of the Pacific Northwest. Journal of Operational Psychiatry 16:24–28, 1985

Hoppe SK, Martin HW: Patterns of suicide among Mexican Americans and Anglos, 1960–1980. Soc Psychiatry 21:83–88, 1986

Jilek-All L, Jilek W, Flynn F: Sex role, culture and psychopathology: a comparative study of three ethnic groups in western Canada. Journal of Psychological Anthropology 1:473–488, 1978

Karno M, Hough RL, Burnam MA, et al: Lifetime prevalence of specific psychiatric disorders among Mexican Americans and non-Hispanic whites in Los Angeles. Arch Gen Psychiatry 44:695–701, 1987

Kinzie JD, Shore JH, Pattison EM: Anatomy of psychiatric consultation to rural Indians. Community Ment Health J 8:196–207, 1972

Kleinman A: Neurasthenia and depression: a study of somatization and culture in China. Cult Med Psychiatry 6:117–190, 1982

Kraus RF, Buffler PA: Sociocultural stress and the American native in Alaska:

an analysis of changing patterns of psychiatric illness and alcohol abuse among Alaska natives. Cult Med Psychiatry 3:111–151, 1979

Levy JE: Navajo suicide. Human Organization 24:308–318, 1965

Levy JE, Kinitz SJ: Indian reservations, anomie, and social pathologies. Southwestern Journal of Anthropology 27:97–128, 1971

Levy JE, Kunitz SJ: A suicide prevention program for Hopi youth. Soc Sci Med 25:931–940, 1987

Liu W, Yu E: Ethnicity and mental health, in Urban Ethnicity in the United States: New Immigrants and Old Minorities. Edited by Maldonaldo L, Moore J. Beverly Hills, CA, Sage Publications, 1985.

Long KA: Suicide intervention and prevention with Indian adolescent population. Issues on Mental Health Nursing 8:247–253, 1986

Manson SM, Shore JH, Bloom JD, et al: Alcohol abuse and major affective disorders: advances in epidemiologic research among American Indians, in The Epidemiology of Alcohol Use and Abuse Among U.S. Ethnic Minority Groups (National Institute on Alcohol Abuse and Alcoholism Monograph Series). Edited by Spiegler D. Washington, DC, U.S. Government Printing Office, 1987a

Manson SM, Walker RD, Kivlahan DR: Psychiatric assessment and treatment of American Indians and Alaska Natives. Hosp Community Psychiatry 38:165–173, 1987b

May PA: Suicide and Suicide Attempts at the Pine Ridge Reservation. Pine Ridge, SD, P.H.S. Community Mental Health Program, 1973

May PA: Suicide and self-destruction among American Indian youths. American Indian and Alaska Native Mental Health Research 1:52–69, 1987a

May PA: Suicide and Suicide Attempts Among American Indians and Alaska Natives: An Annotated Bibliography. Albuquerque, NM, Office of Mental Health Programs, Indian Health Service, 1987b

May PA, Dizmang LH: Suicide and the American Indian. Psychiatr Ann 4:22–28, 1974

Maynard E, Twiss G: Suicide attempts, in That These People May Live: Conditions Among the Oglala Sioux of the Pine Ridge Reservation (Hechel Lena Oyate Kin Nipi Kte) (DHEW Publ No HSM-72-508). Washington, DC, U.S. Government Printing Office, 1970, pp 147–148

McIntosh JL, Santos JF: Suicide among minority elderly: a preliminary investigation. Suicide Life Threat Behav 11:151–166, 1981

Mendes H: The role of religion in psychotherapy, in The Afro-American Family: Assessment, Treatment, and Research Issues. Edited by Bass BA, Wyatt GE, Powell GJ. New York, Grune & Stratton, 1982, pp 203–210

Miller SI, Schoenfeld LS: Suicide attempt patterns among the Navajo Indians. Int J Soc Psychiatry 17:189–193, 1971

Mohatt GV, Blue AW: Primary prevention as it relates to traditionality and empirical measures of social deviance, in New Directions in Prevention Among American Indian and Alaska Native Communities. Edited by Manson SM. Portland, OR, Oregon Health Sciences University, 1982, pp 91–118

National Task Force on Suicide in Canada: Suicide in Canada. Ottawa, Ontario, Health and Welfare Canada, 1987

Neligh G: Secondary and tertiary prevention strategies applied to suicide among American Indians. American Indian and Alaska Native Mental Health Research 1:4–18, 1988

Nichter M: Idioms of distress: alternatives in the expression of psychosocial distress: a case study from South India. Cult Med Psychiatry 5:379–408, 1981

Office of Technology Assessment: Indian Health Care. Washington, DC, U.S. Government Printing Office, 1986

Pedersen AM, Awad GA, Kindler AR: Epidemiological differences between white and nonwhite suicide attempters. Am J Psychiatry 130:1071–1076, 1973

Phillips DP, Carstensen LL: Clustering of teenage suicides after television news stories about suicide. N Engl J Med 315:685–689, 1986

Randolph ET, Escobar JI: Ethnicity, social networks and schizophrenia. Paper read at the annual meeting of the American Psychiatric Association, New York, May 1983

Red Horse Y: A cultural network model: perspectives for adolescent services and paraprofessional training, in New Directions in Prevention Among American Indian and Alaska Native Communities. Edited by Manson SM. Portland, OR, Oregon Health Sciences University, 1982, pp 173–188

Regier D, Myers JK, Robins LN, et al: The NIMH Epidemiologic Catchment Area Program: historical context, major objectives, and study population characteristics. Arch Gen Psychiatry 41:934–941, 1984

Resnik HLP, Dizmang LH: Observations on suicidal behavior among American Indians. Am J Psychiatry 127:882–887, 1971

Robbins M: Project Nak-nu-we-sha: a preventive intervention in child abuse and neglect among a Pacific Northwest Indian community, in New Directions in Prevention Among American Indian and Alaska Native Communities. Edited by Manson SM. Portland, OR, Oregon Health Sciences University, 1982, pp 233–251

Robins LN, Carlson V, Bucholz K, et al: Violence as a black health problem. Paper for the National Research Council study on the status of Black Americans, 1989

Ross CA, Davis B: Suicide and parasuicide in a northern Canadian native community. Can J Psychiatry 31:331–334, 1986

Sainsbury P: The epidemiology of suicide, in Suicide. Edited by Roy A. Baltimore, MD, Williams & Wilkins, 1986

Schottstaedt MF, Bjork JW: Inhalant abuse in an Indian boarding school. Am J Psychiatry 134:1290–1293, 1977

Shore JH: Psychiatric epidemiology among American Indians. Psychiatr Ann 4:56–66, 1974

Shore JH: American Indian suicide: fact and fantasy. Psychiatry 38:86–91, 1975

Shore JH, Keepers G: Examples of evaluation research in delivering preventive mental health services to Indian youth, in New Directions in Prevention Among American Indian and Alaska Native Communities. Edited by Manson SM. Portland, OR, Oregon Health Sciences University, 1982, pp 325–340

Shore JH, Manson SM: American Indian psychiatric and social problems. Transcultural Psychiatric Research Review 20:159–180, 1983

Shore JH, Nicholls WM: Indian children and tribal group homes: new interpretation of the whipper man. Am J Psychiatry 132:454–456, 1975

Shore JH, Bopp JF, Waller TR, et al: A suicide prevention center on an Indian reservation. Am J Psychiatry 128:1086–1091, 1972

Smith JC, Mercy JA, Warren CW: Comparison of suicides among Anglos and Hispanics in five Southwestern states. Suicide Life Threat Behav 15:14–26, 1985

Sorenson SB, Golding JM: Suicide ideation and attempts in a community sample of Hispanics and non-Hispanic whites: demographic and psychiatric disorder issues. Suicide Life Threat Behav 18:322–333, 1989

Spaulding JM: Recent suicide rates among ten Ojibwa Indian bands in northwestern Ontario. Omega 16:347–354, 1985–86

Sussman LK, Robins LN, Earls F: Treatment-seeking for depression by black and white Americans. Soc Sci Med 24:187–196, 1987

Swanson DM, Bratrude AP, Brown EM: Alcohol abuse in a population of Indian children. Diseases of the Nervous System 32:835–842, 1971

Termansen PE, Peters RW: Suicide and attempted suicide among status Indians in British Columbia. Paper presented at the World Federation for Mental Health Congress, Salzburg, Austria, 1979 (Available from: P.E. Termansen, 1415 Bellevue Avenue, West Vancouver, British Columbia, V7T 1C3 Canada)

Travis R: Suicide in northwest Alaska. White Cloud Journal 3:23–30, 1983

Travis R: Suicide and economic development among the Inupiat Eskimo. White Cloud Journal 3:14–21, 1984

Trott L, Barnes G, Dumoff R: Ethnicity and other demographic characteristics as predictors of sudden drug-related deaths. J Stud Alcohol 42:564–578, 1981

U.S. Bureau of Census: American Indian Areas and Alaska Native Villages, 1980 (Suppl Rep PC80-51-13). Washington, DC, U.S. Government Printing Office, 1984a

U.S. Bureau of Census: A Statistical Profile of the American Indian Population: 1980 Census. Washington, DC, U.S. Government Printing Office, 1984b

U.S Department of Health and Human Services: Report of the Secretary's Task Force on Black and Minority Health, Vol 1: Executive Summary. Washington, DC, U.S. Government Printing Office, 1985, pp 81–84

U.S. Department of Health and Human Services: Bridging the Gap: Report on the Task Force on Parity of Indian Health Services. Washington, DC, U.S. Government Printing Office, 1986

Van Winkle NW, May PA: Native American suicide in New Mexico, 1957–1979: a comparative study. Human Organization 45:296–309, 1986

Vital Statistics of the United States: General Mortality, Section 1, 1984, pp 358–359

Ward JA: Preventive implications of a native Indian mental health program: focus on suicide and violent death. Journal of Preventive Psychiatry 2:371–385, 1984

Westermeyer J: Disorganization: its role in Indian suicide rates. Am J Psychiatry 128:123, 1971

Westermeyer J: Ethnic identity problems among ten Indian psychiatric patients. Int J Soc Psychiatry 25:188–197, 1979

Westermeyer J, Brantner J: Violent death and alcohol use among the Chippewa in Minnesota. Minn Med 55:749–752, 1972

Chapter 22

Suicide Among Physicians

Valerie F. Holmes, M.D.
Charles L. Rich, M.D.

SUICIDE ACCOUNTS FOR 3% of all male physician and 6.5% of all female physician deaths in the United States (American Medical Association Council on Scientific Affairs 1986a). Additionally, it is responsible for 35% of the premature deaths among all physicians (Thomas 1976). Despite the annual death rate for physicians decreasing by almost 60% from 1949 to 1981 (AMA Council on Scientific Affairs 1986b), more than 100 physicians commit suicide annually (Rich and Pitts 1979). No human life can be considered more valuable than another; however, the premature and untimely death of a physician represents a loss of society's investment in his or her education and potential professional contributions as well as the personal loss to the family, friends, and patients.

What do we know about physicians who commit suicide? Are the reports of a higher incidence of suicide correct? Do they resemble and differ from other people who commit suicide? In this chapter, these questions will be explored in more detail.

The studies discussed in this chapter deal almost exclusively with those who have obtained the "M.D." degree. Therefore, the terms *physician* and *doctor* will be used synonymously with "M.D." We recognize the legitimacy of these terms being applied to those with other medical degrees. However, we are not aware of similarly detailed suicide statistics being reported for them. It would be inappropriate, therefore, to include them in any conclusions reached about M.D. physicians using such data. Finally, in this discussion, data about medical students will not be automatically included because it is not possible to predict how many students who commit suicide would have graduated from medical school. Also, many physicians in the United States are not graduates of United States medical schools. It should also be noted that conclusions about United States medical students may not be applicable to graduates of foreign medical schools.

Facts About the Rates

Over the past 100 years, despite the variability reported from individual states (Blachly et al. 1963; Rose and Rosow 1973; Revicki and May 1985), the national rate per 100,000 for physician suicide has averaged between 35 and 40 (Rose and Rosow 1973). While this is about three times the rate for the general population in the United States, it is equivalent to that for white males over age 25 (Craig and Pitts 1968), the group that until recently comprised the vast majority of physicians in the United States. It is with the rates for this age group that physician suicide rates must be compared, not to the general population rates. This comparison reveals that, in general, physicians in this country have not been at greater risk for suicide than the general population.

Data on physicians in postgraduate training are harder to interpret because of the even smaller sample size and the low number of deaths in that age range. One report suggests that the suicide rate for house officers is also not higher than age-, race-, and sex-matched controls in the general population (Craig and Pitts 1968). The same authors reached a similar conclusion about medical students. This finding was supported by a later survey of students at United States medical schools (Pepitone-Arreola-Rockwell et al. 1981). Other researchers have argued that these are tenuous conclusions because of the small sample size. However, no satisfactory contradictory data have yet been established.

Some investigators from other countries have reported higher than expected suicide rates among physicians in their countries. Richings et al. (1986) found high standardized mortality ratios for suicide in England and Wales among both male and female physicians under the age of 40. In this study, young women doctors significantly surpassed their male counterparts. Arnetz et al. (1987) found that male physicians in Sweden suicided at a rate comparable to the general population. Female Swedish physicians, however, had elevated suicide rates when compared to the general population. Rimpela et al. (1987) compared age-adjusted suicide rates in Finnish physicians and found that the rate for males was 1.3 times higher than that for the general population. In this study, rates could not be calculated for female physicians. Simon (1986) reviewed the German-language literature and concluded that the suicide rate for male physicians in Bavaria was 1.5 times that for the general male population over age 25. The rate for female physicians was 3 times higher than the comparable group in the general population. Some variations in methodology make generalization of these studies to United States statistics difficult. However, these European data do point to one issue that has been consistently reported as well in the American literature: the much higher than expected rate of suicide among women physicians.

The annual suicide rate for women physicians in the United States has been calculated at around 40 per 100,000 (Craig and Pitts 1968; Pitts et al. 1979), which is about four times the rate for white women over age 25 in the general population. Some researchers have argued that the small number of women physicians precludes any significant conclusion about their rate of suicide (Carlson and Miller 1981). No contradictory data have been offered, however, and, as mentioned above, the European data support a conclusion that this difference is real. It seems, then, that the possibility of a much higher than expected rate of suicide for women doctors must be addressed in any consideration of the physician suicide.

Differences in suicide rates have also been reported among various medical specialties. Three studies have found that psychiatrists have a twofold higher rate among physician suicides in the United States (Craig and Pitts 1968; DeSole et al. 1969; Rich and Pitts 1980). Ophthalmologists, otolaryngologists, and anesthesiologists also may have higher rates, but these incidents may not have been reported as consistently or to the same degree. Small sample sizes limit the power of conclusions about suicide rates among the medical specialties. The replication of the high suicide rate among psychiatrists indicates that this specialty should be examined with greater scrutiny as a potential high-risk group.

It is very difficult to draw any conclusions about sex differences among the medical specialties. Suicides among female specialists are usually included with those for males because of the small numbers of female physicians who suicide in a given study period. Given the growing number of women doctors, as the balance in the United States between male and female physicians equalizes, any gender differences that may exist in this country should emerge.

To summarize, the rate of physician suicide in the United States seems to have remained stable for the last century. For male doctors, the rate is comparable to the rate for white males over the age of 25 in the general population. The female physician suicide rate is essentially the same rate as for male doctors, but is significantly greater than that for white females over age 25 in the general population. There may also be several medical specialties that have higher than expected suicide rates. Psychiatry repeatedly stands out in this regard. Certainly, as we explore the other factors related to physician suicide, special attention must be paid to the questions of gender and specialty. It must be remembered, however, that, in general, physicians do not appear to have a higher rate than does the general population. Therefore, risk factors for the general population probably apply equally to physicians.

DEMOGRAPHIC VARIABLES

General population suicide rates for the United States have consistently shown that whites have approximately twice the suicide rate of nonwhites for both men and women (Centers for Disease Control 1985). Revicki and May (1985) found that 18% of the doctors in their study were nonwhite, but the authors did not present suicide data on that group. No other study has reported the ethnic breakdown of the sample. As more balance is achieved in the ethnic distribution of physicians in the United States, it may be possible to determine whether any differences exist between white and nonwhite physician suicide rates as they do in the general population.

Overall, physician suicide primarily occurs during the most professionally productive years. The average age of the male doctor who takes his own life is reported to be around 50 years (Rich and Pitts 1979); for female physicians it is a few years younger (Pitts et al. 1979). These average ages are perhaps slightly higher than the general population mean suicide ages, but physicians generally do not include persons under age 25. Considering male suicides in the general population, the mean age tells us very little, since suicide rates increase steadily over the life span. This steady increase with age is true for male doctors as well.

Married physicians tend to have the lowest rates of suicide. Divorced and widowed doctors have higher rates when compared to married colleagues (Revicki and May 1985; Rose and Rosow 1973). This has been found repeatedly in general population suicides as well.

In summary, the demographic characteristics of physician suicides do not greatly differ from those of the general population. However, until better gender and ethnic balance is achieved in the profession, this conclusion about physician suicide applies mostly to white male doctors.

GENETIC AND BIOLOGICAL FACTORS

A number of investigators have reported on genetic and biological factors contributing to suicide. These include, of course, factors that may relate to specific psychiatric disorders associated with suicide as well as to the isolated act of suicide. These factors have been reviewed in depth elsewhere in this volume. As far as we can tell, there is no reason to suspect that any of these factors relates uniquely to physicians. However, it should be reiterated that a family history of suicide or the presence of biological factors related to suicidal behavior should be considered as seriously with a physician as with another person.

PSYCHIATRIC DISORDERS AMONG PHYSICIAN SUICIDES

Systematic interview studies of unselected consecutive suicides have uniformly reported the presence of psychiatric disorders in more than 90% of the cases (Barraclough et al. 1974; Chynoweth et al. 1980; Dorpat and Ripley 1960; Rich et al. 1986; Robins et al. 1959). There have been no similar systematic interview studies of unselected consecutive physician suicides. It seems reasonable to conclude, however, that psychiatric illness is as necessary a condition for physician suicide as it is for anyone else.

Certain differences in the pattern of illness might be expected. For example, because of the usually early age of onset of schizophrenia (which has a nearly 15% lifetime suicide rate) and its devastating effects on vocational performance, it seems unlikely that many people with schizophrenia would enter or actually complete medical school. Consequently, we would expect, perhaps, to see more of the other two most common disorders associated with suicide—substance abuse and depression—and less schizophrenia among physician suicides. A report by the American Medical Association and the American Psychiatric Association (AMA Council on Scientific Affairs 1986a) cited a higher rate of substance use problems (34%) and psychiatric hospitalization (33%) among the physician suicides than the controls. The report states that "chronic mental disorders were especially prominent among physicians who took their own lives" (p. 314). No other diagnostic details were given despite the fact that the systematic structured interviews with informants were done by psychiatrists. It is also unfortunate that the study did not examine the issues of gender and specialty differences, which, as mentioned above, had been identified prior to the study. Finally, it was not a randomly or consecutively collected sample.

An earlier study reported a 40% to 60% rate of substance abuse among 80 physician suicides (Blachly and Roduner 1968). However, it was not clear if the 40% with alcoholism overlapped with the 20% with drug abuse. Again, no further diagnostic specificity was reported, and the issues of gender and specialty were not addressed. The sample represented only a 41% return of questionnaires mailed to relatives.

In summary, we still do not know what the distribution of psychiatric disorders is among physicians who commit suicide. Clearly, a large study of consecutive unselected physician suicides systematically examining the issue of psychiatric diagnoses is warranted. Attention should also be given to significantly large unselected groups of women physicians and high-risk specialists.

PSYCHIATRIC DISORDERS AMONG PHYSICIANS

Another way of examining the relationship between physician suicide and the presence of a psychiatric disorder would be to see how often the three major psychiatric illnesses associated with suicide occur among physicians. If these disorders occur in physicians with similar frequency to their occurrence in nonphysician controls, it would add further support to the conclusion that doctors who suicide are similar to general population suicides. As mentioned above, one might expect to find depression and/or substance abuse more commonly among physicians than in the general population, and schizophrenia less commonly. Again, unfortunately, there are no studies of unselected physicians to determine their base rates of psychiatric disorders.

A study that sampled virtually all the women physicians in St. Louis reported that from 39% (Clayton et al. 1980) to 51% (Welner et al. 1979) (depending on the definition of the syndrome) had a history of primary affective disorder. This is considerably less than the speculated rate for affective disorder in women doctors of over 60% suggested by Pitts et al. (1979), but is considerably more than the depression rate for women in the general population (Robins et al. 1984). It should be recognized, however, that all the subjects in Clayton et al.'s study had not yet passed through the age of greatest risk for affective disorder (25 to 45 years of age) (Carlson and Miller 1981). Clayton et al. found very little alcoholism and other drug abuse in the sample, so this would seem to support Pitts et al.'s (1979) speculation that depression may be responsible for the entire difference in suicide rates between women physicians and women in the general population. However, as will be discussed in a following section, other data suggest a greater frequency of substance abuse among women physicians than was reflected in the Clayton et al. study.

In a mail survey study of interns, residents, and fellows in

Canada, women house officers reported more depression than men, but the data collection was uncontrolled and the sample was unselected (Hsu and Marshall 1987). It would be tenuous to consider this supporting evidence for Clayton et al.'s (1980) study, but its findings do point in the same direction.

Unfortunately, there are no similar studies of psychiatric illness among unselected physicians from various specialties, particularly the ones that have been identified as possibly high risk. Surveys of selected postgraduate medical trainees have targeted psychiatric residents (Russell et al. 1975) as having a high frequency of psychiatric disorders and anesthesiology residents (Ward et al. 1983) as having increased substance abuse problems. No controls were offered to demonstrate that these problems occurred more than in other specialty training programs. A Swiss study (Willi 1983) found an increased rate of psychiatric disorder in 19-year-old conscriptees who later selected psychiatry as a specialty as compared to medicine and surgery (prior to even obtaining their medical degrees). Willi concluded that the nature of the impairment determined the choice of medical specialty rather than the specialty training determining the disorder. Rich and Pitts (1979) speculated that the high suicide rate in psychiatrists might be completely due to the presence of affective disorder in this group. This study suggested that the rate of depression among psychiatrists was two to three times greater than in the general population. Since there is no study of psychiatrists comparable to the Clayton et al. (1980) study of women physicians, this question remains unanswered.

In summary, except for the one excellent study of women physicians, there is little known about the incidence and prevalence frequencies of psychiatric disorders associated with high suicide risk among doctors. The study of women physicians is particularly important, however, because it is consistent with one possible explanation of their apparently high suicide rates. Similar studies should be done of high-risk specialties to see if the findings are consistent with those found for women physicians.

PSYCHIATRIC DISORDERS AMONG PHYSICIAN PSYCHIATRIC PATIENTS

One other way, albeit even less scientifically powerful, to address the relationship of psychiatric illness to physician suicide is to examine the frequency of various psychiatric disorders among identified physician psychiatric patients. A number of reports have been published describing groups of doctors who are psychiatric patients, but there are only five that include controls (A'Brook et al. 1967; Franklin 1977; Jones 1977; Murray 1977; Small et al. 1969). These studies, summarized in Table 1, consisted primarily of inpatients, and only two studies were from the United States. Since a variety of diagnostic frameworks were used in these investigations, only broad comparisons among them are possible. All used nonphysician patient controls from the same setting, but the first three studies (see Table 1) also were controlled for higher socioeconomic class. Several observations are apparent. First, both depression and substance abuse occur more frequently among physicians than among the controls across all five studies. Substance abuse appears to be the most prominent diagnosis, with an average difference of 9% compared to 4% for depression. Second, if the Indiana study is excluded as an outlier, the physicians had on the average 7% fewer schizophrenic patients than controls. The difference is more striking if the two studies that used upper-class controls (mean difference 1%) are compared to the two studies that did not control for socioeconomic class (mean difference 14%). Since none of the five studies cited above examined the diagnostic data by gender or specialty, they cannot shed light on these questions. Although not conclusive, these studies do consistently support the hypothesis that substance abuse and affective disorder are major contributors to suicide in physicians, whereas schizophrenia has only a minimal role.

Of particular concern is the greater preponderance of substance abuse among physician patients. Substance abuse is frequently mentioned in reviews of physician suicide. However, it is not known whether the rate of substance abuse is higher among doctors than in the general population, and estimates vary widely. For example, one survey of physicians found a rate of only 7% probable alcoholism, which was comparable to a group of medical patient controls (Niven et al. 1984). This contrasts rather strikingly with the general population estimate of 24% definite alcoholism for males (Robins et al. 1984) using more rigorous criteria. The high rate of substance abuse among physician patients as indicated in Table 1 could possibly reflect a greater tendency for doctors to receive treatment. On the other hand, a considerable anecdotal literature on and clinical experience in dealing with impaired physicians suggest that, in fact, doctors may be considerably less inclined than others to enter treatment (Keeve 1984). Nevertheless, it seems reasonable to conclude that the 7% estimate cited above is low and can be attributed to sampling problems. The true rate of substance abuse among physicians or physician patients remains unclear.

Also complicating the determination of the rate of substance abuse is the growing frequency of polysubstance use. McAuliffe et al. (1986) surveyed more than 700 medical students and physicians and found that, respectively, 77.2% and 59% reported using a psychoactive drug at some time for self-treatment, recreational use, or "instrumental" use (to stay awake, to facilitate work, or for sports). This is done regularly by 16% of medical students and 9.5% of physicians. More than 5% of the students and more than 3% of the physicians admitted to drug dependence. A significant association between drug abuse and suicide has been described among young people (Fowler et al. 1986; Shafii et al. 1985). It may be expected that the growing use of drugs among young physicians may change the pattern from alcoholism to polysubstance abuse among physician suicides.

In contrast to the study of women physicians by Clayton et al. (1980), Bissell and Skorina (1987) reported on a sample of 100 alcoholic women doctors. Despite being a selected sample gathered by personal contacts, some interesting observations emerged. First, only 40% of women physicians in the study were addicted to alcohol alone. Second, they found that often (number not given) the substance abuse problem was not discovered until after a serious suicide attempt, if then. In some instances, the suicide attempt was ascribed to depression, and no investigation was made into possible drug or alcohol abuse. This anecdotal evidence suggests the possibility that Clayton et al. could have missed some degree of substance abuse among the women physicians in their study since it focused on affective disorder. A report by Rich et al. (1988b) also suggests that the major contributor to the greater rate of suicide by men than women in the general population in the United States may be due to the greater rate of alcoholism among men. These data suggest that a partial explanation for the comparable suicide rate for men and women physicians could be due to undetected substance abuse.

In another uncontrolled but interesting survey of 98 (97 male) sober alcoholic doctors, Bissell and Jones (1976) analyzed the sample by specialty. They found that 17% of the sample were psychiatrists, which contrasted to the American Medical Association's estimate of 6% of all United States physicians being psychiatrists. In the survey described above, Bissell and Jones found that 22% of the alcoholic women physicians were psychiatrists compared to 9.5% of the women doctors. This, again, can be considered only anecdotal evidence and not representative of physicians in general. However, it does suggest that substance abuse may play a larger than previously recognized role in the high rate of suicide by psychiatrists as well as by women physicians.

In summary, the data concerning the incidence of psychiatric disorders among physician patients add further weight to the conclusion that substance abuse and depression are major contributing factors to physician suicide. It also seems likely that substance abuse substantially contributes more to the disproportionate numbers of

Table 1. Controlled studies of physician psychiatric patients

| | | | Number | | \multicolumn{8}{c}{Percentage with psychiatric illness} |
| | | | | | Depression | | Drug abuse/ alcoholism | | Schizophrenia | |
Study	Location	Patient source	MDs	Controls	MDs	Controls	MDs	Controls	MDs	Controls
A'Brook et al. (1967)[a]	England	Inpatient & outpatient	192	197	42	41	29	15	9	9
Small et al. (1969)[a]	Indiana	Inpatient	40	47	15	13	33	19	52	36
Murray (1977)[a]	Scotland	Inpatient	110	379	31	30	43	34	5	7
Franklin (1977)[b]	England	Inpatient	100	100	40	30	30	27	2	14
Jones (1977)[b]	Pennsylvania	Inpatient	100	9567	24	16	12	5	6	21

[a]Controlled for socioeconomic class.
[b]Not controlled for socioeconomic class.

women physician and psychiatrist suicides than previously suspected. The diagnosis of schizophrenia occurs less frequently than among general population suicides, but it is occasionally associated with physician suicide.

ROLE STRAIN

It has been repeatedly demonstrated that virtually everyone who commits suicide has some active psychosocial stressor (Rich et al. 1988a). The problem in assessing the importance of stressors in the etiology of suicide is that good population controls do not exist. Not only is it an incredibly difficult task to gather such data, but also no agreement exists on the methods of measuring the relative value of various stressors. It seems reasonable to conclude that physicians are as vulnerable to the common stressors and precipitants associated with suicide (e.g., disruption of interpersonal relationships, financial difficulties, physical illness) as anyone else.

The question remains as to whether there are unique stressors associated with medical training and practice that, if alleviated, would decrease the physician suicide rate. Again, much has been written on the subject, but little controlled data have been generated (DeSole et al. 1969; Ellard 1974; Krakowski 1982; Mawardi 1979; McCue 1982). Three general categories of physician stress have been described: 1) inordinate time and work demands; 2) responsibility for human life and death; and 3) inadequate psychosocial supports. Clearly, these conditions exist, but the degree of their contribution to physician suicide has not yet been determined. It must be remembered that, except for certain subgroups of doctors (see above), the suicide rate for physicians is not higher than that for the general population. This makes it difficult to conclude that the stress of being a physician plays a unique role in their suicides.

There is evidence, in fact, that even the stress and role strain associated exclusively with being a doctor may be important only within the context of a preexisting vulnerability to psychiatric disorder. Several findings support this conclusion. First, only a proportion of doctors (who all presumably experience similar professional pressures) develop psychiatric illness (Vaillant et al. 1972). Second, long hours, demanding patients, and ready access to narcotics were not problematic for physicians who appeared psychologically intact by the time they reached college (Vaillant et al. 1972). Third, substance abuse among physicians seems to be due to individual vulnerability rather than to the stresses of medical training (Hurwitz et al. 1987). Finally, there is strong evidence that psychiatric illness in physicians is correlated with family histories of psychiatric disturbance and the presence of symptomatology prior to medical school (Garfinkel and Waring 1981; Hunter et al. 1961; Vaillant et al. 1972).

The two major physician subgroups with high suicide rates do bear further discussion in regard to stressors. First, we have seen that the rate for women doctors is higher than population rates for women but the same as for male physicians (Pitts et al. 1979). This might lead to the conclusion that whatever protects women in general from suicide (as compared to men) does not operate for women doctors. Assuming that similar numbers of men and women physicians have a high-risk psychiatric disorder, it may be that the stress of being a doctor equalizes their suicide rates. We have shown above, however, that there is evidence to suggest that women physicians do have a higher than expected rate of depression (Clayton et al. 1980). In fact, Clayton et al. found that many of the women physicians in their study had a first episode of depression prior to medical school. This information seems to indicate that the presence of depression in women physicians is often independent of (rather than secondary to) the stresses of medicine and that whatever legitimately unique stressors women face from the practice of medicine may have little to do with the reason their suicide rate is as high as (but not higher than) male physicians. While prejudice and discriminatory practices, lack of female role models, and lack of family and institutional supports have been cited as unique stressors for women in medicine (Lloyd and Gartrell 1981), no factual information exists to substantiate whether these factors influence the incidence of psychopathology and/or suicide among female physicians.

There has also been much speculation in the literature about the relative degree of professional stress associated with the various medical specialties. There has been little logic associated with these predictions. It might be argued that because psychiatrists commit suicide at twice the rate of general surgeons (Rich and Pitts 1980), the practice of psychiatry is twice as stressful as surgery. As mentioned above, agreement about the quantification of stressors has not been reached. Certainly, there are obvious differences in the types of stressors between the practice of psychiatry and surgery. However, without quantifiable measures, the debate over who has the "tougher" job would be endless.

One survey of practicing physicians (Mawardi 1979) reported similar degrees of satisfaction with choice of profession between surgeons and psychiatrists. The author pointed out that no correlation emerged between practice satisfaction and suicide rate by specialty. Although this finding is highly anecdotal, it does make the point that if the relative stresses of different specialties are important in the suicide formula, they may not be apparent to the practitioners who face them.

In summary, the problem of assessing the role of stressors in physician suicide is similar to the assessment problems for the population. It has not been demonstrated that either general stressors or physician-specific stressors (including those that may apply uniquely to a particular gender or specialty) occur more frequently in physician suicides than in other doctors or in the population at large. Given the nature of human existence, it is not hard to imagine that most (if not all) people, including physicians, experience stressors throughout their life cycle. On the other hand, far from a majority of people, including physicians, ever have a diagnosable psychiatric disorder. It is reasonable to conclude that if stressors play a role in physician suicide, it is most likely (as it is in the general population) they do so by increasing the vulnerability of those people who have a preexisting high-risk psychiatric disorder.

IDENTIFICATION AND MANAGEMENT OF SUICIDAL BEHAVIOR IN PHYSICIANS

As with any person, correct identification of potentially suicidal physicians is the first step to prevention. As stated above, it is reasonable to assume that the vast majority of doctors who suicide, like others in the general population, have an identifiable psychiatric disorder. There is no reason to believe that affective disorders, substance abuse, or other psychiatric disorders are more difficult to identify in doctors than in anyone else. It has been alleged by many authors, however, that physicians and their families, colleagues, and even treating physicians are less inclined to recognize these high-risk conditions among doctors for a variety of personal and professional reasons. Although this contention makes sense, there are no controlled data to verify that it is any truer for physicians than for appropriately matched population controls. On the other hand, the possibility that such difficulties may exist should not be discounted in educational efforts relating to physician suicide. It must be underscored that doctors are not protected from suicide risk factors by virtue of their "physician-hood." When risk factors for suicide are present, doctors must be considered serious suicide risks. Family, friends, and colleagues must not assume that a physician should know when and how to take care of him- or herself. There should be no reluctance or hesitation in encouraging the suicidal physician to obtain psychiatric treatment under such circumstances. In the case of substance abuse in particular, this might even involve enforced participation in monitoring and treatment programs.

Much has been written suggesting that doctors cooperate poorly with psychiatric treatment. As far as we can tell, however, there are no data to support the contention that physicians are different in this respect from other persons with similar disorders. For example, A'Brook et al. (1967) reported that 33% of physician substance abusers discontinued treatment early, and 25% of physician inpatients signed out against medical advice. Comparisons are not given, however, for nonphysician patients. Many characteristics have been ascribed to physician patients to explain why they are particularly difficult to manage in the hospital. These relate mainly to staff perceptions about the manipulativeness of the physician patient. Again, these observations are not controlled, making it difficult to conclude whether doctors are, in fact, more difficult to treat than other patients or whether they are just perceived that way by others. However, it is safe to say that physician patients should be managed with just as much caution as any other suicidal person. The physician patient has rights *equal* to those of any other patient to be protected from his or her own suicidal impulses.

Another hazard that has been suggested in treating suicidal physicians is that the treating psychiatrist will underestimate the severity of the physician patient's condition, potentially leading to inadequate treatment and an ultimately tragic outcome. Many possible reasons for this have been suggested but, as discussed above, there are no data to suggest that this really occurs any more frequently for physician patients than for others. Treatment of the suicidal physician is no different from that of other patients with similar problems or psychiatric disorders. Physician patients are often relieved when they are not expected to be experts in their own care. They deserve the same considerations regarding involvement in planning their care as anyone else. Regardless of the physician patient's apparent familiarity with his or her diagnosis and proposed treatment plan, the treating psychiatrist must provide adequate information, allow time for discussion, and answer any questions.

We know of no data that indicate any particular differences in identification or treatment of psychiatric disorders based on physician gender or specialty. It is important to remember that higher-risk subgroups (e.g., women and psychiatrists) exist, but this should not lead to complacency when dealing with other suicidal physicians.

In summary, there is considerably strong opinion that doctors are more difficult to deal with as psychiatric patients than other people. It has not been demonstrated that this is the case. If it is true, it is not clear whether it is the physician patient or the potential caretakers who may contribute more to the problem. In either case, it is reasonable to conclude that doctors deserve the same aggressive, concerned care and treatment as anyone else when suicide is a risk.

SUICIDE PREVENTION FOR PHYSICIANS

Two other approaches to prevention should be mentioned. First, it is conceivable that limiting the entry of high-risk individuals into the medical profession might decrease the physician suicides. There are two major drawbacks to this strategy. First, screening out susceptible candidates (were that possible) may spare the medical profession, but it is of little value to the individual. While the practice of medicine may be quite stressful, there is no evidence to support the hypothesis that an eventual suicide can be averted by changing the occupation of potentially suicidal individuals. This applies as well to the concept of specialty choice. Second, while there may be a multitude of factors that are frequently associated with suicide, the false positive rate for them is quite high (Pokorny 1983). That is, a large number of people with these risk factors will never commit suicide. Great contributions to medicine would undoubtedly be lost if preventing entry to medical school or particular specialties were based on these risk factors with low specificity for predicting which individual will eventually die by suicide.

A second approach might be to attempt to intervene with at-risk populations of physicians before overt psychiatric disorder develops. There are three major limitations to this concept. First, even in the highest-risk subgroup, psychiatrists, only a very small number actually die by suicide. It would be hard to justify imposing prophylactic measures that would result in such an overall small payoff (in numbers) without data indicating that such interventions would indeed be effective. Second, aside from the problem of deciding who should receive these prophylactic efforts, there is little evidence that such measures have a demonstrated prophylactic effect on suicide, much less on psychiatric illness. Assuming that drug and alcohol abuse might be directly responsible for suicidal behavior, it is conceivable that enforced abstinence for all doctors could protect against physician suicide. This seems unrealistic given the human experience with attempts at prohibition. Third, it would be impossible to know which treatment of the many available should be chosen for any individual prior to the development of overt symptomatology.

In summary, the prospects of excluding potentially high-suicidal-risk individuals or enforcing presumably prophylactic measures as an approach to prevention of physician suicide seem unrealistic at best. At worst, such actions might be construed as unjustifiably prejudicial and also may deny medicine many significant contributions from productive individuals.

Probably the most rational and clinically useful approach to reducing the suicide rate among physicians would be to couple early detection of those who are at risk with education of both the physician and the physician's family. In addition, identification and strengthening of personal and community supports may provide significant contributions to intervention and treatment.

THE AFTERMATH

In the same way that physicians who commit suicide are similar to others in the general population who kill themselves, there is little reason to believe that survivors of physician suicide are much different from other suicide survivors. Consequently, it is important to remember that they will need the same degree of support in their period of grieving. It should not be assumed that they will have any easier or harder time coping with the tragedy because of their close association with the medical profession.

CONCLUSIONS

Despite intense interest in the topic of physician suicide by numerous authors, scientifically solid research in the area is in short supply. Several of the best studies have been conducted outside the United States and, therefore, may have limited applicability in this country. Nonetheless, there are some threads that can be woven together to draw some general conclusions.

It would appear that doctors are more alike than different from the general population with regard to suicide. Overall, the rate of suicide among physicians in the United States is probably not different from the population at large. In general, the demographic risk factors are similar. The major difference, of course, is that the rate for women physicians is equivalent to the rate for male physicians rather than two-thirds lower as it is in the general population. The debate over whether this is an artifact of the low numbers of women physicians or a true finding will not be settled until a sufficient balance in the numbers of men and women physicians has been achieved. However, it should be noted that gender difference in rates has been observed in other countries as well.

Debate rages as to what contributes to the high rate of suicide among women physicians. As yet there are no clear conclusions. The only systematic psychiatric study of unselected women doctors (or any doctors, for that matter) substantiated the speculation that a high rate of depression exists among them. There is some suggestion that this depression might mask substance abuse in this population. This hypothesis deserves future study. While the question of role strain among women physicians may be important from a variety of standpoints, it has not been clearly implicated in their risk for suicide. The other identified major high-risk group for physician suicide are psychiatrists. It seems likely that depression and/or substance abuse are important contributing factors. However, other evidence supports the conclusion that high-risk individuals may choose psychiatry as a specialty. This conclusion deserves further debate and further systematic study. The psychiatric community should not ignore this potential problem out of concern for their professional image. For example, radiologists are wearing lead aprons now because they were willing to admit that more of them were dying of leukemia than should have been.

Furthermore, changing patterns of medical specialty susceptibility should be monitored. The growing problem of substance abuse and suicide among young people suggests that there may be a carry-over to future generations of doctors. Reports of increasing problems with substance abuse among anesthesiologists, for example, should be kept in mind.

Issues of practice stress should also be evaluated and dealt with as part of the treatment of physicians with psychiatric illness. Poor practice performance can certainly lead to many of the stressors associated with suicide, such as loss of income, self-esteem, and interpersonal support. The answer to the question about the relationship between psychiatric illness and stressful life events awaits further study.

The identification and management of a potentially suicidal physician may be more difficult than with other patients. Regardless of where the difficulty lies, it is incumbent on the care givers to be as aggressive as necessary in ensuring that the physician patient receives appropriate treatment as would any other suicidal patient.

Finally, there is much debate about the subject of suicide among physicians generating many opinions based on anecdotal clinical experience. Certainly, the management of an individual suicidal physician is a matter for a responsible and competent clinician. However, the facts about physician suicide require scientific scrutiny and must be based on systematically collected controlled data. Only in this way can we expect to make headway in solving this puzzle about whether there are unique characteristics of suicide among physicians.

REFERENCES

A'Brook MF, Hailstone JD, McLauchlan IE: Psychiatric illness in the medical profession. Br J Psychiatry 113:1013–1023, 1967

American Medical Association, Council on Scientific Affairs: Physician mortality and suicide: results and implications of the AMA-APA physician mortality project: Stage II. Chicago, American Medical Association, 1986a

American Medical Association, Council on Scientific Affairs: Physician mortality and suicide: results and implications of the AMA-APA pilot study. Conn Med 50:37–43, 1986b

Arnetz BB, Horte LG, Hedberg A, et al: Suicide patterns among physicians related to other academics as well as to the general population. Acta Psychiatr Scand 75:139–143, 1987

Barraclough B, Bunch J, Nelson B, et al: A hundred cases of suicide: clinical aspects. Br J Psychiatry 125:355–373, 1974

Bissell L, Jones RW: The alcoholic physician: a survey. Am J Psychiatry 133:1142–1146, 1976

Bissell L, Skorina JK: One hundred alcoholic women in medicine: an interview study. JAMA 257:2939–2944, 1987

Blachly PH, Roduner G: Suicide by physicians. Bulletin of Suicide, 1968, pp 1–18

Blachly PH, Osterud HT, Josslin R: Suicide in professional groups. N Engl J Med 268:1278–1282, 1963

Carlson GA, Miller DC: Suicide, affective disorder, and women physicians. Am J Psychiatry 138:1330–1335, 1981

Centers for Disease Control: Suicide Surveillance, 1970–1980. Atlanta, GA, U.S. Department of Health and Human Services, Public Health Service, March 1985

Chynoweth R, Tonge JI, Armstrong J: Suicide in Brisbane: a retrospective psychosocial study. Aust N Z J Psychiatry 14:37–45, 1980

Clayton PJ, Marten S, Davis MA, et al: Mood disorder in women professionals. J Affective Disord 2:37–46, 1980

Craig AG, Pitts FN: Suicide by physician. Diseases of the Nervous System 29:763–772, 1968

DeSole DE, Singer P, Aronson S: Suicide and role strain among physicians. Int J Soc Psychiatry 15:294–301, 1969

Dorpat TL, Ripley HS: A study of suicide in the Seattle area. Compr Psychiatry 1:349–359, 1960

Ellard J: The disease of being a doctor. Med J Aust 2:318–322, 1974

Fowler RC, Rich CL, Young D: San Diego suicide study. II: Substance abuse in young cases. Arch Gen Psychiatry 43:962–965, 1986

Franklin RA: One hundred doctors at The Retreat: a contribution to the subject of mental disorder in the medical profession. Br J Psychiatry 131:11–14, 1977

Garfinkel PE, Waring EM: Personality, interests, and emotional disturbance in psychiatric residents. Am J Psychiatry 138:51–55, 1981

Hsu K, Marshall V: Prevalence of depression and distress in a large sample of Canadian residents, interns, and fellows. Am J Psychiatry 144:1561–1566, 1987

Hunter RCA, Prince RH, Schwartzman AE: Comments on emotional disturbances in a medical undergraduate population. Can Med Assoc 85:989–992, 1961

Hurwitz TA, Beiser M, Nichol H, et al: Impaired interns and residents. Can J Psychiatry 32:165–169, 1987

Jones RE: A study of 100 physician psychiatric inpatients. Am J Psychiatry 134:1119–1123, 1977

Keeve JP: Physicians at risk: some epidemiological considerations of alcoholism, drug abuse, and suicide. J Occup Med 26:503–508, 1984

Krakowski AJ: Stress and the practice of medicine. II: Stressors, stresses, and strains. Psychother Psychosom 38:11–23, 1982

Lloyd C, Gartrell NK: Sex differences in medical student mental health. Am J Psychiatry 138:1346–1351, 1981

Mawardi BH: Satisfactions, dissatisfactions, and causes of stress in medical practice. JAMA 241:1483–1486, 1979

McAuliffe WE, Rohman M, Santangelo S, et al: Psychoactive drug use among practicing physicians and medical students. N Engl J Med 315:805–810, 1986

McCue JD: The effects of stress on physicians and their medical practice. N Engl J Med 306:458–463, 1982

Murray RM: Psychiatric illness in male doctors and controls: an analysis of Scottish hospitals in-patient data. Br J Psychiatry 131:1–10, 1977

Niven RG, Hurt RD, Morse RM, et al: Alcoholism in physicians. Mayo Clin Proc 59:12–16, 1984

Pepitone-Arreola-Rockwell F, Rockwell D, Core N: Fifty-two medical student suicides. Am J Psychiatry 138:198–201, 1981

Pitts FN, Schuller AB, Rich CL, et al: Suicide among U.S. women physicians, 1967–1972. Am J Psychiatry 136:694–696, 1979

Pokorny AD: Prediction of suicide in psychiatric patients: report of a prospective study. Arch Gen Psychiatry 40:249–257, 1983

Revicki DA, May HJ: Physician suicide in North Carolina. South Med J 78:1205–1207, 1985

Rich CL, Pitts FN: Suicide by male physicians during a five-year period. Am J Psychiatry 136:1089–1090, 1979

Rich CL, Pitts FN: Suicide by psychiatrists: a study of medical specialists among 18,730 consecutive physician deaths during a five-year period, 1967–1972. J Clin Psychiatry 41:261–263, 1980

Rich CL, Young D, Fowler RC: San Diego suicide study. I: Young vs old subjects. Arch Gen Psychiatry 43:577–582, 1986

Rich CL, Ricketts JE, Fowler RC, et al: Differences between men and women who suicide. Am J Psychiatry 145:718–722, 1988a

Rich CL, Fowler RC, Fogarty LA, et al: San Diego suicide study. III: Relationships between diagnoses and stressors. Arch Gen Psychiatry 45:589–592, 1988b

Richings JC, Khara GS, McDowell M: Suicide in young doctors. Br J Psychiatry 149:475–478, 1986

Rimpela AH, Nurminen MM, Pulkkinen PO, et al: Mortality of doctors: do doctors benefit from their medical knowledge? Lancet 1:84–86, 1987

Robins E, Murphy GE, Wilkinson RH, et al: Some clinical considerations in the prevention of suicide based on a study of 134 successful suicides. Am J Public Health 49:888–899, 1959

Robins LN, Helzer JE, Weissman MM, et al: Lifetime prevalence of specific psychiatric disorders in three sites. Arch Gen Psychiatry 41:949–958, 1984

Rose KD, Rosow I: Physicians who kill themselves. Arch Gen Psychiatry 29:800–805, 1973

Russell AT, Pasnau RO, Taintor ZC: Emotional problems of residents in psychiatry. Am J Psychiatry 132:263–267, 1975

Shafii M, Carrigan S, Whittinghill JR, et al: Psychological autopsy of completed suicide in children and adolescents. Am J Psychiatry 142:1061–1064, 1985

Simon W: Suicide among physicians: prevention and postvention. Crisis 7:1–13, 1986

Small IF, Small JG, Assue CM, et al: The fate of the mentally ill physician. Am J Psychiatry 125:1333–1342, 1969

Thomas CB: What becomes of medical students: the dark side. Johns Hopkins Medical Journal 138:185–195, 1976

Vaillant GE, Sobowale NC, McArthur C: Some psychologic vulnerabilities of physicians. N Engl J Med 287:372–375, 1972

Ward CF, Ward GC, Saidman LJ: Drug abuse in anesthesia training programs: a survey: 1970 through 1980. JAMA 250:922–925, 1983

Welner A, Marten S, Wochnick E, et al: Psychiatric disorders among professional women. Arch Gen Psychiatry 36:169–173, 1979

Willi J: Higher incidence of physical and mental ailments in future psychiatrists as compared with future surgeons and internal medical specialists at military conscription. Soc Psychiatry 18:69–72, 1983

Chapter 23

Surviving a Suicide in Your Practice

Harvey L. Ruben, M.D., M.P.H.

WHEN YOUR PATIENT COMMITS SUICIDE

One of the most difficult and upsetting experiences for a mental health professional is the suicide of a patient. This event occurs in the professional lives of many clinicians; yet, it is not widely written about in the literature or discussed very often as a topic of case conferences or meetings (Chemtob et al. 1988). A review of the literature on the subject over the past two decades has revealed only a small number of articles concerning the effects of a patient's suicide on the therapist (Brown 1987; Carter 1971; Chemtob et al. 1988; Goldstein and Buongiorno 1984; Gorkin 1985; Kolodny et al. 1979; Litman 1965; Marshall 1980; Sanders 1984). Most of these reports have focused on the personal reactions of the therapist. Clearly, the suicide of a patient is an event that is disturbing and disruptive to the life of any therapist; yet, it is an event that has received only minimal professional attention.

Until 1988, the most extensive study of the effects of a patient's suicide on a therapist was conducted in the early 1960s by Litman (1965). He interviewed more than 200 psychotherapists shortly after the death of a patient by suicide and concluded that therapists have two basic types of reactions. The first is related to the experience of loss. Like other people who are mourning the loss of a valued person, the clinician experiences guilt, anger, denial, and repression. However, the clinician also responds as a therapist who has lost a patient. As a result, the clinician may experience feelings of self-blame, personal inadequacy, and a sense of responsibility for the death. Initially, the therapist may be in a state of shock or disbelief, as is anyone undergoing a grief reaction: "It can't be true; this hasn't really happened." This response usually gives way to a sense of anger: "Why did the patient do this? How could the patient have done this to me?" This emotion is often accompanied by feelings of guilt: "What did I do wrong? What could I have done differently? How could I have prevented this from happening?"

These initial feelings of grief, which are part of the therapist's human reaction, are intensified by the need to maintain professional balance. Clinicians often find themselves in the position of having to respond to questions about the patient's death from family members, colleagues, hospital administrators, and others. At a time when the therapist is feeling most upset and distressed by this catastrophic event, he or she is forced to continue to respond and often to minister to the needs of others. Since many therapists will experience shame or self-doubt during this early phase, it makes it even more difficult to respond appropriately.

An extensive national survey of psychiatrists completed in the mid-1980s found that more than half of the 259 respondents had patients who committed suicide (Chemtob 1988). Of these, 50% reported symptoms and reactions similar to those described above. Gorkin (1985) discussed specific symptoms of pathologic mourning that might be experienced at the time of a patient's suicide. He pointed out the depressive manifestations of the reaction, which included exaggerated feelings of guilt, expectations of severe judgment and recrimination from colleagues, and pervasive ruminations about one's worth as a therapist and the value of therapy. He also pointed out that some therapists might use narcissistic defenses, such as denying guilt and feelings of failure or feeling indifferent and blaming others for the patient's death. He reported that some therapists who have experienced a patient's suicide become overly anxious and cautious when confronted with suicidal ideation in other patients.

As a result, therapists must be very sensitive to their own feelings during this time; they must be aware that they are experiencing a grief reaction like any other human being. They should also expect some unavoidable negative impact on their professional functioning for a short period of time. Keeping this in mind, clinicians must be particularly careful to ensure that any negative effects do not cause harm to other patients or to themselves.

Goldstein and Buongiorno (1984) interviewed 20 therapists who had a patient commit suicide. At some point after the event, all of the therapists realized that the effects were much greater than they had initially thought. As in other studies, these therapists documented an initial phase of guilt, anger, disbelief, and shock, which gave way to a second phase of grief, shame, and a loss of self-esteem and self-confidence. The therapists interviewed in this study managed the initial flooding of feelings through the use of some denial, which facilitated reestablishment of their sense of equilibrium. The investigators found that the therapists had to experience the feelings and attempt to deal with them before they were able to share their emotions with anyone else. This may cause problems for the treating therapist because, invariably following a patient's suicide, the clinician must respond to questions about the event and yet may not be prepared to do so psychologically. One clinician reported that after his patient suicided, he needed help from his supervisors and friends (Carter 1971). He especially felt the need for reliable information from neutral sources; he pointed out that very often, what the therapist learns about the patient's death is initially inaccurate or tainted by the assumptions or interpretations of others.

Therefore, in the early phase of learning about the death of a patient, it is critically important for the therapist to gather all of the pertinent information about the suicide before reaching conclusions or making statements to others about the patient or his or her own role or responsibility relating to the patient's death. An example of this is drawn from a negligence case where a psychiatrist whose patient had eloped from an inpatient unit told the family that there was no way of knowing that the patient had been suicidal and that there had been no warning signs. However, had the psychiatrist spoken to the hospital staff, he would have learned that the patient had made comments to several staff members that he felt life was no longer worth living. In addition, the staff had been sufficiently concerned to call the psychiatrist at the time that the patient was leaving the unit. The psychiatrist's premature comments to the family without having adequate information put him in a difficult situation, and this ultimately had a negative effect on the outcome of the malpractice action.

Kolodny et al. (1979), all of whom were trainees when their patients committed suicide, discussed how lonely and isolated they felt following the event. In addition to feelings of shame, embarrassment, and inadequacy, each of these young therapists felt a sense of desolation and lack of support from their peers. Even though many of their colleagues attempted to make supportive statements, no one initially took the time to sit down and discuss the situation with them extensively. Each felt a great need for an in-depth discussion with their supervisors, harboring the fantasy that this session might allow them to feel exonerated. The authors emphasized the need for intensive discussion of the event with supervisors or peers before discussing the suicide in a case conference or staff meeting format.

Brown (1987) studied 55 graduates of the Cambridge Hospital's Psychiatric Residency Program and found that one-third of them had a patient who committed suicide during training. He reported that this event occurred far more frequently than has been generally recognized and suggested that training programs should take specific steps to help their students deal with this issue. The tragedy can be an opportunity for growth if it is dealt with correctly. It can also have a very negative impact on the trainees, sometimes precipitating their leaving psychiatry for another field. Brown contends that young therapists will have great difficulties dealing with the suicide of a patient until their professional development is complete, and yet the completion of that development may only occur from the working through of a patient's death by suicide. Thus, training programs must ensure that trainees receive adequate support and appropriate interventions to facilitate successful coping with such an overwhelming event.

While it is critical for therapists to grieve, bereavement following the aftermath of a suicide is extremely difficult (Sanders 1984). The family struggles to deal both with its grief and its anger in a society that still scorns suicide and gives little support to the survivors. However, the grieving professional may be in a worse predicament. The family often displaces its anger and guilt onto the care givers, intensifying the clinician's burden and guilt. The fact that many malpractice suits occur following a suicide suggests that the family may use this vehicle as an attempt to expiate some of its own guilt. Therefore, the therapist's grieving process may be complicated by the possibility of being blamed by others. This only exacerbates feelings of self-doubt and guilt. Given the complexity and severity of reactions to patient suicides, Marshall (1980) suggested that every mental health treatment facility should have an established procedure for dealing with patient suicides to provide therapists with the kind of support and input they need following this event. Marshall also pointed out that therapists may become suicidal following the death of a patient, just as do family members, and unless other colleagues and supervisors are aware of this possibility and intervene, the outcome may be fatal.

In summary, when a patient commits suicide, therapists should be prepared to have the same kind of reaction as any other bereaved person. A typical grief reaction occurs with feelings of shock and disbelief, followed by anger and denial. Most clinicians will experience a sense of guilt as they examine their behavior and question how they might have prevented the tragedy. Therapists will blame themselves, and many experience feelings of inadequacy to work with other patients. Following the suicide of a patient, it is critical that the clinician gather as much information as possible from neutral, reliable sources to enhance the probability of accurately reconstructing the events that contributed to the patient's suicide. Clinicians should refrain from making statements to others concerning their role and responsibility for the patient's death. Most therapists will talk with family members, colleagues, and/or administrative personnel concerning the suicide. This should be done with care and caution. It is not inappropriate in such a situation for the clinician to temporize, by suggesting to those who are inquiring that he or she will get back to them when more information about what has happened is available. The clinician should thoroughly review the case with a trusted colleague or supervisor to facilitate increased understanding of the event before commenting on it in a public forum such as a staff meeting or a case conference. It is not uncommon for the therapist to experience disturbed sleep or nightmares under these circumstances. Depending on the degree of symptoms, the clinician should consider seeking the professional help of a colleague. Therapists should be strongly advised not to attempt to treat their own reactions by self-medication.

INTERVENING WITH THE PATIENT'S FAMILY

Concurrent with experiencing and working through his or her own grief for the patient's death, the clinician must often interact with the patient's family. This work has been termed *postvention*. Its goal is to help family members cope with their anguish, guilt, shame, anger, and perplexity. Very often, it is the treating professional who has the responsibility of informing the family of a patient's death. This should be undertaken with extreme sensitivity and skill. In contrast to the death of a patient by a heart attack, where the professional does not usually feel personally responsible, a patient suicide often engenders feelings of guilt and self-blame for the tragedy. Therefore, the task is that much harder. If the patient was hospitalized, it is advisable to ask the family to come to the hospital, telling them that a problem has occurred, rather than attempting to inform them of the patient's death over the telephone. When the family has been told of the patient's death by someone else, such as the police or a hospital authority, it is useful for the therapist to call the family and ask to meet with them at the hospital or office as soon as possible to discuss the situation and to help them cope with the loss.

Resnik (1969) has written extensively about "psychological resynthesis," an approach that helps the survivors of a suicide to cope. The first step in the resynthesis is "resuscitation." This means visiting the family and talking with them about the patient's death within 24 hours of the suicide. This includes a discussion of what the suicide means, what motivated it, and what the consequences might be. In some respects, this intervention can be viewed as psychological first-aid. As mentioned earlier, caution should be exercised about discussing the circumstances surrounding the patient's suicide until the clinician has adequate knowledge of the event. The clinician may need to postpone answering certain questions from the family with the understanding that responses will be forthcoming when more information is available.

The second phase of the resynthesis process is called "psychological rehabilitation" (Resnik 1969). The aim is to help the survivors work through their mourning to cope with the loss. This phase may take several months; over this period, it is quite appropriate for the therapist to meet with the family several times to facilitate this process. The third phase of resynthesis is termed "psychological renewal" (Resnik 1969). This is the period following the active grieving process when the family ceases its mourning and moves on with life. According to Resnik, the therapist should be available to the family throughout the entire process to help survivors understand and cope with the loss.

The initial phase (immediately following the suicide) is perhaps the most critical period for determining how family members will deal with their anger toward the therapist. If the therapist is available as a helpful supportive person, then the likelihood of the family displacing their anger onto the clinician is greatly reduced. In addition to the clinician meeting with the family immediately after the event, attending the wake or the funeral is appropriate and may also help the family deal with their anger and distress.

One of the greatest mistakes a therapist can make is to avoid the family, should the family seek the therapist out. Cases have been reported of therapists who did not return the family's call or who made flippant comments to family members that they were not responsible for the patient's death at the same time when the family was reaching out to the clinician for help. Needless to say, these actions serve only to mobilize the family's anger against the therapist.

Even if the clinician had minimal contact with the family prior to the patient's death, it should be recognized that the family will now need care and assistance. If the clinician strongly feels that such family interventions are inappropriate for him or her to administer, then the clinician should arrange for a colleague to consult with the family. However, even if the clinician does not choose to become involved with the postventive work, the clinician should at least meet with the family to discuss the patient's death and to help the survivors initiate their "working-through" process. At this time, the therapist can suggest to the family that it would be better if a colleague were to meet with them. It should be underscored that not talking or meeting with the family under these circumstances is a most foolhardy course of action; it has the greatest potential for inciting family members to initiate legal actions against the therapist.

DEALING WITH COLLEAGUES AND STAFF

Since the suicide of a patient usually becomes a visible event in the community (even if the patient is being treated in a solo private practice), one's professional colleagues and peers are often aware of the occurrence. Additionally, patients frequently suicide during or just following hospitalization or a clinic visit. Consequently, various staff members may have been involved with the patient's care. Therefore, it is important to consider how to intervene with these colleagues after the death of a patient by suicide.

Let us first address the issue of colleagues who have not been involved in the patient's treatment. Colleagues usually will attempt to reach out and be helpful when they learn that another clinician's patient has committed suicide. Sometimes, colleagues' seemingly well-meaning comments may not feel that way, given the stress of the grieving process. Kolodny et al. (1979) pointed out that some colleagues may wish to share with the clinician their experiences with a patient suicide. In this regard, they may make offhand comments intended to be helpful that have the result of being very upsetting to the clinician. They may even directly inquire about the clinician's responsibility for the suicide or ask about why certain actions were not undertaken that may have prevented the death. Such inquiries may feed directly into the therapist's own feelings of self-doubt and guilt. Similar to the intervention with the family, it is important to avoid lengthy discussions with colleagues concerning the suicide until the therapist has had a chance to explore it, to understand it, and to work it through. Certainly, it is important for the clinician to find one or two colleagues with whom an in-depth discussion and review of the case can occur to help work through the process. However, the clinician should be cautious in informally discussing with a colleague possible mistakes that may have been made because, should there be a malpractice action, such discussions might be discoverable in court. It often makes sense for the clinician to schedule a professional consultation with a trusted colleague or mental health professional so that an exploration of feelings about the patient's death can occur in a setting that is protected by the confidentiality of the physician-patient relationship or the psychotherapist-patient relationship.

If the patient was being treated in the hospital or in an outpatient clinic setting, it is very important for the primary therapist to help other staff members deal with their feelings about the patient's death. Similar to the reactions discussed for the primary therapist, other staff members who have been involved with the patient's care will also experience a range of feelings in response to the patient's death. Neill et al. (1974) pointed out that a suicide on an inpatient unit may adversely affect the staff's ability to work together and with other patients. Following a suicide on an inpatient unit, the anxiety of being held responsible by one's co-workers, the questioning of one's skill, and the threat to one's feelings of professional competence may impede effective functioning. The authors suggested that performing a psychological autopsy may help the staff to work through feelings and concerns following such an event. Failing to deal with these staff feelings openly on a unit can have a very destructive effect on both staff and patients (Neill et al. 1974). In addition, ignoring the impact of a suicide or attempting to suppress reactions to it may make the staff more vulnerable to misinterpreting future suicidal behavior by other patients. Conversely, gaining a better understanding of each staff member's role with the patient and how this may have affected the ultimate suicide can be useful in working through staff feelings about the occurrence.

The method of a psychological autopsy has two phases. The first is a process of information gathering; the second is a meeting of all staff members who were involved in the patient's care. Initially, the psychological autopsy team, comprised of staff members who were not directly involved in the patient's care, reviews all records to obtain a complete understanding of the patient's medical and psychiatric history and the course of treatment and hospitalization. After reviewing the records, the team interviews the involved staff members and as many of the patient's family members and/or friends as possible. Once the information is gathered, a staff meeting is convened where the findings are presented and thoroughly discussed to gain understanding and insight into the patient's suicide.

While this procedure can be very helpful and therapeutic, several caveats must be observed. Goldstein and Buongiorno (1984) pointed out that while 8 of the 20 therapists they interviewed found the psychological autopsy beneficial, 12 experienced it as threatening, contributing to their increased self-doubt and distress. Kolodny et al. (1979) suggested that the psychological autopsy is most helpful for the primary therapists if carried out after the clinician has thoroughly explored his or her own feelings and role in the suicide with a supervisor or colleague as discussed above. Thus it should be emphasized that a premature staff meeting may, in fact, have harmful effects for those involved.

The therapist should also carefully consider the possible legal consequences of such a staff meeting since it is *not* a privileged forum. Although it is crucial for mental health professionals to explore and understand their role in a patient's suicide, especially to determine if there were errors in the management and treatment plan so that corrective actions can be taken in the future, it should be remembered that this information may be discoverable in a malpractice action and used against the therapist. For example, in one malpractice action a general staff meeting was held by the hospital's chairman of psychiatry shortly after the suicide. A psychological autopsy was performed, the patient's records were reviewed with the entire staff present, and it was determined that the patient had told different staff members of her wishes to die. Although the staff had noted the patient's suicidal ideation in the record, it was not communicated directly to the treating psychiatrist. As a result of this meeting, the staff agreed that, in the future, in addition to recording notes about a patient's suicidality in the chart, the psychiatrist would also be phoned immediately. Unfortunately, this information became known to the plaintiff's counsel and was used during the malpractice proceedings to ascribe blame to the hospital staff who had failed to take appropriate action.

Fortunately, there is a way to convene such a staff meeting so that the discussion will not become discoverable in most jurisdictions. Peer review proceedings are considered privileged communications in order that colleagues may examine each other's behavior and treatment of patients for the purposes of improving and monitoring the course of treatment. As a result, had the case conference or staff meeting in the above example been constituted as a peer review meeting by the hospital peer review committee, then this particular meeting could have been considered privileged and possibly could not have been used in the malpractice proceeding.

Thus, while it is of utmost importance to help staff explore and work through their feelings in relation to the suicide of a patient to understand their role and to improve future care of suicidal patients, it is also important to consider involving the hospital attorney or risk management department so that the conference can be conducted in a manner that will not be prejudicial to any of the professionals involved. Morever, should such an event occur in a setting such as an outpatient clinic or a group practice, it is advised that the clinician discuss management of the situation with colleagues and co-workers with a personal attorney present to avoid legal ramifications.

Another case illustrates the importance of legal consultation. In this example, a patient who subsequently committed suicide was being treated by two clinicians in an outpatient group practice setting. Her primary therapist was a psychologist who was treating her in weekly psychotherapy, with the managing psychiatrist evaluating the patient monthly to prescribe antidepressant medications. Unfortunately, after the suicide, the psychiatrist and the psychologist discussed their roles and what each had known about the patient's suicidal ideation. These discussions were discovered during the pretrial depositions and were used by the plaintiff's counsel to demonstrate that each of the professionals thought that the other was responsible for mismanagement of the patient. As a result, even though there had been no negligence and neither of the professionals had been the proximate cause of the patient's death, both of their insurance companies decided to settle, rather than to defend the case. So while it is important to discuss these issues with colleagues and co-workers, it must be done in such a way as to avoid legal jeopardy.

Since the treatment of potentially suicidal patients is a common occurrence in most inpatient and outpatient settings, it is recommended that ongoing in-service training procedures be instituted for staff that focus on staff feelings about suicidal behavior and death (Marshall 1980). These meetings should occur on an ongoing basis and be followed up with a staff conference whenever a patient evidences suicidal behavior. These in-service training sessions should include a discussion of the personal philosophy of each staff member concerning the morality or the rationality of suicide, clarifying for each person his or her own sense of responsibility for patients as well as determining realistic limits for health care professionals on that responsibility. The sessions should also provide information on the agency's guidelines for treating suicidal patients and clarify procedures to be followed in the event of a patient's suicide. Following this training program, the primary focus of the staff meeting in the event of a patient suicide is neither identification of responsibility nor determination of the cause for the patient's death. Rather, the primary goals of the meeting are to examine staff members' feelings and attitudes about the patient's death and to identify carefully factors that may have contributed to the suicide. Marshall found that this process helped staff members to resolve their grief and guilt without ascribing blame or responsibility in ways that could be used in legal proceedings.

In summary, appropriate interactions with staff and colleagues after a patient commits suicide are essential both in terms of personal resolution of feelings about the suicide and also to prevent legal actions.

THE CLINICIAN'S LEGAL RESPONSIBILITIES

When a patient commits suicide, the treating professional has a number of legal responsibilities that must be fulfilled. In addition to the general discussion of these responsibilities that follows, it is advisable that the clinician consult the hospital attorney or lawyer in the community to discuss the particular requirements and state laws. This helps to ensure that the clinician will fulfill these responsibilities in the event of a patient suicide. Failure to be aware of the requirements of such laws may result in legal jeopardy for the clinician. Victoroff (1983a) described at length the obligations of a physician following a patient suicide. The first obligation of the treating professional is to be available to the survivors of the suicide victim. As previously discussed, family members and close friends will need explanations, assurances, sympathy, and expressions of human concern. They almost always need professional intervention. The absence of prompt and appropriate consultation may lead to symptoms of pathologic grief. In some cases, other family members may become suicidal. A failure on the part of the therapist to respond to family members under these circumstances may result in adverse consequences if legal actions are taken; it might contribute to inciting the family to legal action as their anger becomes mobilized against the therapist. Although there is no specific legal requirement to be available to the family, it should be considered sound medical practice.

The clinician's first *legal* obligation following a patient's suicide is to notify the coroner or medical examiner. If the physician files a medical certificate that contains false information, or fails to cite the cause of death, the physician is guilty of a misdemeanor in virtually all jurisdictions. The death certificate is a legal document, and the physician who completes it attests to the correctness of the information. Falsifying or distorting the data, in addition to being unethical, is a significant breach of the law. In addition, if (because the clinician does not properly fill out a death certificate) the burial is delayed, this may mobilize the family's anger toward the physician.

Another legal issue pertains to the therapist's notes and records. As with all medical records, states have statutes that require physicians to maintain records in confidence for a period of years following the death of a patient. This is 7 years in many states; however, clinicians should be certain of the requirements of the laws in their own state. Even though the patient has committed suicide, a factor that may be known publicly, the confidentiality of the physician-patient or psychotherapist-patient relationship (which is protected by state law) still pertains to all information that the therapist possesses about the patient. The right to divulge such information, however, now belongs to the legal representative of the deceased. Therefore, if the therapist receives requests from the police who are investigating the patient's death for information about the course of the patient's treatment, the clinician must receive a release of information from the patient's administrator or estate executor in order to comply. Should you be contacted by a representative of the press or the media who is seeking information to report on the suicide, confidentiality prevents the therapist from making any comment. The clinician should not even acknowledge being the treating professional, but rather explain that state laws of confidentiality prevent any comments about any patient or suicide.

Another critically important area pertains to what information the clinician records in the patient's chart immediately following the suicide. When a patient commits suicide, the clinician should immediately write a comprehensive note in the patient's record of all the information remembered about interactions with the patient from the time of the last recorded note in the chart until the time of the patient's death. This should include notes about any phone calls from the patient or the patient's family, any discussions about the patient with colleagues or with hospital or clinic staff members, any changes in medication that might not have been noted in the record since the last visit, any impressions or anything else that might have pertinence. Of the utmost importance is that the clinician notes the *exact date* and *time* at which this information was recorded to acknowledge that it was written after the patient's death to ensure accurate memory of all relevant events should the need arise for discussion of them in the future. The necessity of this procedure should be clear. If a legal action occurs, the clinician's ability to have accurate recall of the events will be greatly enhanced by having made such a record.

A word of extreme caution: Under no circumstances should the clinician in any way alter the record or make additions to notes previously recorded in the chart. The only way that additional information can be added is by putting an addendum to the record such as previously discussed, clearly stating the date and the time of the note and acknowledging that it was written after the patient's death. Several lawsuits have been brought against professionals where an addition to the record was made after the patient's death that did not contain acknowledgement that it had been made after the suicide. These omissions led to the insurance companies' settling the suits when, in fact, there had been no negligent care. In one unfortunate situation, a psychiatric resident had forgotten to chart that his patient had no suicidal ideation, although he had asked the question several hours before the patient committed suicide. In the midst of a discussion with the attending psychiatrist, the resident was instructed to write a note in the chart to this effect. Rather than making a separate note as an addendum, the resident added the statement to his preexisting note. He then decided that it did not look right and, therefore, proceeded to recopy the entire page of his notes, including the statement of no suicide intent, as though he had written it at the time he had asked the question. In the ensuing legal action, it came out during pretrial deposition that this event had in fact occurred. The insurance company believed that it was so detrimental to the defense of the case that they decided to settle.

The final area that merits discussion is of a slightly different nature. What do you do about your bill? Although the physician's bill is not a legal responsibility, every responsible professional bills for his or her services. However, after the suicide of a patient, it may be difficult for the clinician to do this. Considering what we have discussed about the professional's feelings following a patient suicide, including his or her own grief and the frequent sense of responsibility and self-blame, it is not unusual that the clinician may consider not billing for his or her services. Unfortunately, although this may seem to have humanitarian merit, it is rarely a wise thing to do tactically. Given that the clinician has been billing the patient for services throughout the course of treatment, the fact that an invoice is not sent for all services rendered since the last bill until the time of the patient's death might be construed as an admission of the therapist's guilt or responsibility for the death of the patient. There have been cases where the plaintiff's attorney used this fact as a weapon against the treating professional, implying that the clinician had decided not to bill because of guilt and a sense of responsibility for the patient's death. This does not go unnoticed by the jury. Therefore, a bill sent to the patient's family in the same manner as any other bill would be sent to the patient or to his or her family throughout the course of the treatment is most appropriate. Certainly, if the therapist has been involved with the family in the postventive efforts that we have discussed above, they will not be surprised to receive such a bill. Moreover, this is the practice of all other medical specialists when a patient dies. Therefore, failure to follow this procedure may have negative consequences for the clinician.

MALPRACTICE ISSUES

While psychiatric malpractice is an uncommon occurrence, suicide is the most threatening of malpractice risks for the psychiatrist. Perr (1979) pointed out:

What is unusual about suicide litigation is that the behavior that caused the death is not that of the defendant but of the deceased. A psychologic salve is involved in attributing blame for that behavior to others, and that process is compounded by the vast monetary rewards sometimes made in such litigation. The dead person is absolved—more or less in a fashion comparable to the exculpation for criminal responsibility. (p. 95)

The threat of being sued increases the stress and burden for the professional following a patient's suicide. Unlike other medical specialties, it is only in psychiatry that the physicians are asked to be responsible for the behavior of their patients (Rachlin 1984). In one California study, 2% of psychiatrists had been sued. Of those, more than one-quarter of the cases involved suicide, making it the most frequent event for which a legal action was instituted (Rachlin 1984). In a study of malpractice actions in New York, half of the suits against psychiatrists involved suicide. Consequently, the clinician's concerns about being sued after the suicide of a patient are not unrealistic, especially considering the increased numbers of malpractice actions that have occurred over the past decade.

Lawsuits against professionals or hospitals often take the form of wrongful death actions. Professional liability exists in every state for any wrongful act, neglect, or default that causes the death of a patient. The damages in these suits are based on assessment of the pain and suffering of the deceased, medical expenses incurred, trauma and loss to survivors, and the loss of prospective earnings over the victim's projected life. Victoroff (1983b) pointed out that these malpractice suits do not arise from an intentional act by the clinician, but rather occur through negligence or the failure to act by the defendant. This professional negligence is commonly called malpractice, and it is defined as the bad, wrong, or injudicious treatment of a patient, which becomes the proximate or immediate cause of an injury to or the death of the patient. In order for malpractice to exist, not only must there be harm to a patient and an action or a lack of action by the professional that has caused that harm, but there also must be a deviation from nationally recognized standards for the management of the patient's illness. In other words, the professional cannot be sued merely for a bad result or a bad outcome. Therefore, should there be an unfortunate outcome, such as a patient committing suicide, as long as the professional has performed his or her duty reasonably and according to well-accepted standards of practice, the professional will not be held responsible in most cases. Since legal actions often occur months to years after the death of a patient, the need for keeping accurate and adequate contemporaneous records of the course of the patient's treatment and all interactions with the patient is critical to the clinician's defense. The issue of proximate cause is exceedingly important, because even if it can be demonstrated that the professional performed in a negligent manner, if it can be shown that the action was not the direct cause of the patient's death, then the professional cannot be held accountable in a negligence action. In one particular malpractice suit, the court accepted all of the allegations of negligence attested to by the plaintiff's expert witness after a schizophrenic patient made a suicide attempt by hurling himself into a plate-glass window. But the court found the defendant not to be responsible because, in the court's opinion, it was not possible to predict when or if a schizophrenic patient might make a suicide attempt.

In addition to making appropriate and specific notes in the record and detailing exactly when the notes were written, it should be underscored that the clinician should exercise great caution in discussing the patient's suicide with colleagues or staff members. Despite the fact that the clinician may initially feel responsible for the patient's death, a statement to this effect should never be made and no effort to assess fault or blame should be attempted other than in the context of a professional consultation protected by physician-patient confidentiality or in a privileged, peer review conference. The clinician should not issue any statements about the patient or the suicide without complete command of all relevant information pertaining to the patient's death. Furthermore, as previously discussed, the clinician's interactions with the family will have an important bearing on whether the family chooses to blame the therapist for the death and institute a malpractice action. Clinical outreach to the survivors is both humane and the best prevention against legal actions. In one malpractice action, a patient had chosen to change psychiatrists and was in the midst of switching from one doctor to another at the time that she committed suicide. She actually had seen the new psychiatrist but was scheduled for an appointment with her former psychiatrist on the day that she killed herself. When the family called and spoke to the original psychiatrist about the patient's death, he told them that he no longer had medical responsibility for the patient since she had transferred her treatment to a colleague. He had, in fact, been treating the woman for several months, and the family considered him to be her doctor. In addition, during his deposition he stated that he did not understand why he was being sued nor did he feel concerned about the situation because she had transferred to another doctor. Even though he had not behaved negligently, nor were any of his actions the proximate cause of the patient's death, the insurance company was so concerned about his attitude and appearance as a witness that they settled the case against him out of court.

The essential message should be quite clear. No matter how

appropriate the clinician's treatment has been, when a patient commits suicide, the therapist is at greater risk for a malpractice action than at any other time in the course of his or her professional career. Consequently, the clinician's behavior at this time is critically important to the outcome. Therapists must be as thoughtful, sensitive, and cautious about what they say and how they behave with colleagues and family members as they would be with any patient in a therapy session. The clinician should keep in mind that most malpractice suits do not lead to judgments against psychiatrists. In many instances, when suits are settled by the professional's insurance company, it is not because the clinician has rendered negligent treatment, but rather for many of the other reasons discussed above. Thus the clinician's humane and caring attitude and appropriate professional manner is the best defense against legal action following the suicide of a patient.

PICKING UP THE PIECES

The discussion so far has focused on the clinician's immediate reaction to the death of a patient, how to work with the family, strategies for staff and colleague interaction, and legal responsibilities and considerations. (See Table 1 for a summary of these points.) This last section will focus specifically on how the clinician picks up the pieces after a patient suicides. Earlier in this chapter, the normal human reactions of therapists to the death of a patient were discussed. In this regard, most therapists will feel guilt, shame, and a sense of inadequacy at having been unable to prevent the death of their patient. It is these feelings that are the most detrimental to the clinician's future functioning and that must be resolved to continue productive professional activities. Several authors documented therapists' suicidal ideation and attempts following the death of a patient (Carter 1971; Litman 1965; Marshall 1980). Given the frequency of these feelings, it is incumbent on us as clinicians to be aware that they may occur and to be certain that appropriate actions are taken for our colleagues in distress. Just as impaired physician committees have been established in local medical societies to help colleagues who are suffering from disabling illnesses or alcohol or drug abuse, so would it be helpful for local mental health professional societies to have committees that would assist their members to deal with the suicide of a patient. In larger urban areas where there might be several professionals who have had a patient commit suicide, a self-help group under the auspices of the professional society would be very appropriate. Kolodny et al. (1979) described how such a group for trainees facilitated their ability to work through the loss of patients by suicide. Such a technique would also be very helpful for fully trained professionals working in the community.

Table 1. When a patient commits suicide

Personal responsibilities

Reach out to the family.

Reach out to other staff and colleagues.

Do not discuss and assess fault or blame.

Obtain a professional consultation with a colleague to help work through your own feelings.

Legal responsibilities

Know the laws of your own state.

Consult a personal and/or hospital attorney and the hospital risk management team.

Record in chart all your recollections about the case and the events preceding the suicide with *accurate* dates and times.

Never alter medical records!

Notify medical examiner as required by law.

Avoid discussions of case in nonprivileged settings, such as a case conference or with colleagues.

Maintain confidentiality of the patient's psychiatric records, including the course of treatment.

Earlier in this chapter, the technique of psychological resynthesis was described as a method that professionals can use to help the surviving family of the suicide victim (Resnik 1969). This process has also been suggested to be of value for professionals following the suicide of a patient. The phases of psychological resuscitation, rehabilitation, and renewal would be worked through in individual treatment or in a group setting for several professionals who have had a patient suicide under the auspices of the local psychiatric society.

It should be underscored that the trauma experienced when a patient commits suicide is unavoidable. Every attempt should be made to acknowledge this pain in a suffering colleague. Whenever a professional loses a patient by suicide, at the very least there should be an individual response from a caring and sensitive colleague and, where possible, an organizational response from the professional society. If we, as health care professionals, notice that a colleague is suffering and do not reach out or suggest that a professional consultation with another colleague might be helpful, we are failing to fulfill our moral and ethical responsibility to our peers. If we do not support an organized response on the part of our professional society, we are also failing to fulfill our responsibilities. These are difficult issues to confront, and it is never easy to approach a colleague and suggest that he or she may be in emotional pain. The odds are extremely high that any active mental health practitioner will have one or more patients commit suicide throughout the course of his or her career. We must acknowledge that the risk of patient suicide is inherent in our practice. We must establish institutional and organizational responses to deal with the sequelae of such an event. In that clinicians may be the "professional victims" in these unfortunate situations, we must acknowledge our own humanity and vulnerability and turn to our colleagues in appropriate ways to obtain the help that is needed to pick up the pieces so that we can continue with our professional lives.

References

Brown HN: The impact of suicide on therapists in training. Compr Psychiatry 28:101–112, 1987

Carter RE: Some effects of client suicide on the therapist. Psychotherapy: Theory, Research and Practice 8:287–289, 1971

Chemtob CM, Hamada RS, Baver G, et al: Patient's suicide: frequency and impact on psychiatrists. Am J Psychiatry 145:224–228, 1988

Goldstein LS, Buongiorno PA: Psychotherapists as suicide survivors. Am J Psychother 38:392–398, 1984

Gorkin M: On the suicide of one's patient. Bull Menninger Clin 49:1–9, 1985

Kolodny S, Binder RL, Bronstein AA, et al: The working through of patients' suicides by four therapists. Suicide Life Threat Behav 9:33–46, 1979

Litman RE: When patients commit suicide. Am J Psychother 19:570–576, 1965

Marshall KA: When a patient commits suicide. Suicide Life Threat Behav 10:29–40, 1980

Neill K, Benensohn HS, Farber AN, et al: The psychological autopsy: a technique for investigating a hospital suicide. Hosp Community Psychiatry 25:33–36, 1974

Perr IN: Legal aspects of suicide, in Suicide: Theory and Clinical Aspects. Edited by Hankoff LD, Einsidler B. Littleton, MA, PSG Publishing, 1979, pp 91–101

Rachlin S. Double jeopardy: suicide and malpractice. Gen Hosp Psychiatry 6:302–307, 1984

Resnik HLP: Psychological resynthesis: a clinical approach to the survivors of a death by suicide, in Aspects of Depression. Edited by Schneidman ES, Ortega MJ. Boston, MA, Little, Brown, 1969, pp 213–224

Sanders CM: Therapists too need to grieve. Deaf Education (Suppl) 8:27–35, 1984

Victoroff VM: Obligations and liabilities of the physician, in The Suicidal Patient: Recognition, Intervention, Management. Oradell, NJ, Medical Economics Books, 1983a, pp 194–199

Victoroff VM: Suicide and the law, in The Suicidal Patient: Recognition, Intervention, Management. Oradell, NJ, Medical Economics Books, 1983b, pp 173–193

Chapter 24

Suicide, Ethics, and the Law

Jess Amchin, M.D.
Robert M. Wettstein, M.D.
Loren H. Roth, M.D., M.P.H.

ASSESSMENT AND TREATMENT decisions for suicidal patients ideally reflect the clinician's experienced clinical judgment. Many mental health professionals, however, find their clinical judgment compromised by conflicting ethical principles, the threat of litigation, or other restrictions imposed by the legal system.

Underlying both ethical and legal aspects of suicide is a basic conceptual struggle. While society seeks to promote individual freedom and autonomy, it also seeks to protect a person from self-injury. When does the threat of self-destructive behavior justify protective intervention by mental health professionals, even though the intervention may compromise an individual's autonomy and civil rights? This tension between promoting individual freedom and protecting people from self-harm reflects the basic conceptual struggle underlying both ethical and legal aspects of the clinical management of suicidal persons.

In this chapter, we will first explore the ethical principles and ambiguities that underlie society's response to suicidal behavior. We will then examine suicide from the perspective of the law, including a review of civil commitment, malpractice, and guidelines for managing suicidal patients in the context of the American legal system. We conclude with a discussion of forensic issues that may arise after a suicide or suicide attempt.

Ethics And Suicide

Two questions emerge in reviewing the ethics of suicide. First, does the patient have a moral right to commit suicide? Second, what is the moral obligation of others, particularly the clinician, to intervene to prevent the suicide? The prevailing traditional approach to suicide, the scientific "determinist" view, permits and even mandates aggressive suicide prevention. But this scientific view may be debated based on religious, social, or "value-of-life" grounds. Two alternative approaches challenge the scientific view of suicide: an approach based on autonomy, and one based on a consideration of rational suicide. Overall, ethical principles form the foundation of the practitioner's moral authority in making treatment decisions for the suicidal patient. A more thorough analysis on ethics and suicide, on which some of the following discussion is based, may be found in a work by Battin (1982).

The Traditional Determinist View

The traditional view of suicide, sometimes called "determinist," holds that suicidal behavior is caused by factors beyond the individual's control (Battin 1982). Consequently, the patient's decision to commit suicide is not rational or autonomous. Because the patient's behavior is otherwise determined, the patient is not responsible and is therefore not faced with a moral decision. Society, however, has a moral obligation to intervene and save the patient, provided the intervention does not incur undue countervailing social costs. To a large extent, our current laws and mental health system are based on the determinist view.

Three variations of the determinist view have been advanced. In the medical model approach, suicide is seen as the result of a mental disorder. Increasingly, the medical model approach is being supported by empirical evidence. For example, researchers have correlated neurobiological factors, such as neurochemical function, endocrinology, and genetics, with suicide (Blumenthal and Kupfer 1986; Mann and Stanley 1986; Maris 1986). A causal relationship between mental disorder and suicide is, however, difficult to establish. Furthermore, although psychiatric disorder may be a risk factor for suicide, at least some people commit suicide without evidence of a mental disorder. The claim that every suicidal person suffers from a mental disorder, even if true, does not establish that the mental disorder alone causes the suicidal behavior.

In a second variation to the determinist view, suicide is considered an adaptive behavior aimed at mobilizing support from the patient's environment. The patient wants to die, but also wants to live. According to this viewpoint, the clinician attempts to ally with the patient's truer desire, presumed to be the will to live. But there is the real possibility, perhaps even realized through psychotherapy, that the patient genuinely wants to die. In such a system, one can question whether the therapist is justified in imposing his or her own values rather than permitting the patient to achieve the result he or she wishes. Under this model, psychosocial supports would be mobilized as a means of treatment intervention, to respond to the patient's cry for help.

A third variation to the determinist view considers suicide as the result of social forces beyond the patient's control (Durkheim 1951). Under this model, suicide prevention consists of altering aspects of a culture's social organization.

Although the determinist view of suicide is prevalent in society today, the validity of this scientific view may be debated on several grounds. For example, the Judeo-Christian tradition is usually thought to prohibit suicide. But persuasive arguments can be advanced that the Judeo-Christian tradition does not absolutely prohibit suicide, and there are alternative theological traditions that permit suicide, such as release of the soul, self-sacrifice, avoidance of sin, and attainment of a higher spiritual state (Battin 1982).

Social arguments have also been advanced on both sides of the suicide issue. On the one hand, suicide hurts society by harming family and friends, depriving society of that person's contribution, and undermining society's system of laws. Yet suicide as either martyrdom or as a way of removing social burdens, as might occur with a dying or comatose patient, may be construed as benefiting society.

The ethical theory of utilitarianism, based on evaluating the consequences of an action, is useful when weighing benefits and burdens in deciding whether to prevent suicide. This theory holds that decisions should be based on achieving the greatest good for the greatest number of people. Utilitarianism is difficult to operationalize, however, in the case of suicide. Suicide has varied and often unexpected effects on others that cannot be adequately measured and compared. The utilitarian view may not take into account the consequences to the victim of the suicide. If others gain enough, or if the misery of the patient is ended, a utilitarian approach would argue that suicide may be the only morally appropriate choice, even if it goes against the will of the patient. The politically powerful could use such arguments to advocate suicide for certain supposedly burdensome populations. In short, the utilitarian approach can lead to disturbing results.

Finally, we may consider whether suicide is morally wrong because of the absolute value society places on life itself. Under the deontological theory of ethics, suicide is always morally wrong. But the taking of life is considered morally acceptable in at least some situations in our society, as in self-defense, martyrdom, and war. In medicine, decisions to forgo life-sustaining treatment are gaining acceptance. These decisions reflect a willingness to end life, or at least to allow a person to die, based on that person's assessment of the quality of his or her life. As a society, we have not yet fully embraced the principle that life must always be preserved regardless of the costs.

To summarize, the clinician's response to a patient's suicidal behavior may be understood from a variety of ethical, religious, and social viewpoints. In the mental health setting, the clinician's decision-making process usually reflects a determinist approach in which suicide is viewed as involuntary behavior by a victim of a mental disorder, ambivalence that leads to eliciting help, social forces, or some combination of these factors. At least when a mental disorder is present, the clinician is believed to have a moral and professional obligation to intervene; however, this traditional determinist view has been challenged. Some have contended that there are situations in which suicide is acceptable. Two alternative views argue that it is morally wrong to stop someone from committing suicide.

The Autonomy View: The Right to Suicide

Some have argued that there is a fundamental right to commit suicide (Szasz 1986). The right to commit suicide may derive from the increasingly valued principle of autonomy; a legally competent individual has the right to control his or her own life (Beauchamp and Childress 1983). In a related view, the right to commit suicide may derive from a libertarian philosophy; a competent individual has the right to do as he or she freely chooses provided others are not harmed. The right to commit suicide would not necessarily mean that suicide was morally correct. Rather, the right would override other arguments about the morality of suicide.

Recognizing the right to commit suicide would dramatically alter society's approach to suicidal behavior. Under the determinist view, suicide should be prevented, with rare exceptions. If a fundamental right to commit suicide is recognized, the situation is reversed; suicide would normally be permitted, and suicide prevention would become the exception.

This approach has significant implications for the mental health professional. Although the clinician may treat the patient, the clinician would not be empowered to prevent the suicide act. This is analogous to a physician's treating a medical illness where the patient exercises autonomy by rejecting life-saving treatments.

The mental health community generally rejects the notion that persons with mental disorders have a right to commit suicide. The existence of a fundamental right to take one's own life may be disputed. But perhaps more significantly, the mental disorder represents the very exception under which the right to commit suicide may be overridden; the mentally disordered are not as capable of exercising autonomy. Taking refuge in the scientific determinist view, most practitioners would argue that suicidal behavior by a mentally disordered patient represents a manifestation of the mental disorder, not the exercise of a fundamental right.

Rational Suicide

The concept of "rational suicide" further challenges the traditional view of suicide (Kjervik 1984; Siegel 1986). By definition, rational suicide is not the product of mental disorder and may therefore be permissible even under a scientific determinist view. The problem with this approach is defining and identifying suicides that are truly rational.

The ability to reason requires logic and understanding of the consequences of one's decision. Arguably, one can find distorted reasoning in anyone with suicide ideation, particularly in a psychiatric patient with abnormal perceptions or thinking. Even with an intact ability to reason, rational suicide would require decision making based on adequate information. The suicidal patient may be misinformed or otherwise limited in his or her thinking about what options are available to improve the patient's life situation. Depressed mood or other emotional states may compromise a patient's ability to process information. Further, it may be impossible to understand truly the meaning of one's own death. For example, Freud (1915/1953) claimed that "it is indeed impossible to imagine our own death. . . . in the unconscious every one of us is convinced of his own immortality " (p. 289).

Some argue it is always irrational to choose the certainty of death, knowing that there is uncertainty about the future. But there may be a high price to pay. In terminal medical illnesses, for example, there is always hope for a miracle cure. But to insist on keeping such patients alive may result in significant suffering. With strong evidence for future harm, suffering, or a painful death, permitting an earlier death may not be unreasonable. The medical and legal communities have struggled with this issue in a series of so-called right-to-die cases (Ruark et al. 1988). Forgoing life-sustaining treatment is not considered suicide by the courts, but each right-to-die case raises the ethical issues involved in suicide. This raises the further question of whether it is proper to assist a suicide, particularly when a medically ill patient requests assistance to hasten death.

Assisting Suicide and Euthanasia

While suicide and attempted suicide are not crimes under any state statutes, assisting suicide is a crime in more than one-third of the states, although the laws governing assisted suicide are often inflexible and inconsistently enforced (Shaffer 1986).

In the health care setting, requests to assist a suicide will increase due to the expanding elderly population with debilitating illnesses, the spread of fatal diseases such as acquired immune deficiency syndrome (AIDS), and the ability of new medical technologies to sustain life despite terminal illnesses. Some patients request assistance to end their lives after being diagnosed with a terminal medical illness. Others, anticipating terminal illness at some time in the future, express a wish to be allowed to die rather than be artificially maintained. These wishes may be expressed through advanced directives, such as oral statements or the increasingly common practice of written "living wills" (Society for the Right to Die 1986). A growing number of states have enacted natural death acts, which recognize the right of competent adults to refuse life-sustaining treatment, give legal weight to living wills, and may absolve health care professionals of criminal liability if a living will is followed (Shaffer 1986). Advanced directives and living wills do not, however, authorize assisted suicide.

Assisted suicide and the broader issue of euthanasia raise additional ethical quandaries. In particular, what are the moral distinctions between self-administered euthanasia and euthanasia administered by others, between active euthanasia (i.e., by an act of commission such as lethal injection) and passive euthanasia (i.e., "letting die" by withholding medical intervention), and between voluntary euthanasia (i.e., the person directly or indirectly takes his or her own life) and nonvoluntary euthanasia (i.e., the decision about death is not made by the person who is to die) (Munson 1979)? Deliberately killing another person, except in special circumstances, is considered morally wrong and is legally proscribed. But allowing a person to die is not illegal. Specific cases may fall between these two extremes (It's over, Debbie 1988; Letters: It's over, Debbie 1988). In short, the ethical and legal parameters for justifying assisted suicide, especially in the medical setting, have yet to be worked out.

Ethics and the Clinician

The ethical issues presented by suicidal behavior are complex and require at least two levels of analysis. One level of analysis addresses the moral right of the patient to act. Society currently avoids this issue by considering a suicidal patient incapable of a moral choice because the patient suffers from a mental disorder. The other level of analysis addresses the moral right and professional obligation of the clinician to intervene when a mental disorder is clearly present. Important arguments challenge the presumption of preventing suicide in all cases. Nevertheless, once the clinician has assumed the professional responsibility for treating a patient, society imposes both a moral and a legal obligation on the clinician to act responsibly in treating that patient. In the remainder of this chapter, we will examine these legal ramifications.

SUICIDE AND THE LAW

Many mental health practitioners perceive the law as intruding into the clinical domain. Despite this tension between the legal and mental health systems, the law strives to serve a variety of societal functions, including protecting patient rights, redressing wrongs, and enhancing the quality of patient care. As in the area of ethics, the law fundamentally seeks to balance society's interest in fostering a person's freedom and autonomy with the competing need to protect a person from self-injury. The more knowledgeable the clinician becomes about the law regarding suicidal patients, the more able the clinician will be to provide professional care within the law's purview.

In this section we will focus on civil commitment and malpractice, two prominent legal issues confronting the clinician who treats suicidal patients. We will then review principles in the management of suicidal patients from a clinical-legal perspective. Finally, we will briefly discuss several forensic issues that may arise following a suicide or suicide attempt.

Civil Commitment

All forms of psychiatric intervention are subject to legal scrutiny. The rules, regulations, and procedures governing psychiatric hospitalization and treatment are, to some extent, unique to each state, and are contained in the mental health code for that jurisdiction (American Psychiatric Association 1983b). Voluntary treatment modalities are less subject to legal regulation than involuntary treatment, because civil liberties are less at stake. Yet, according to the law, even patients who voluntarily enter a psychiatric hospital must have the ability to make this choice competently, free from coercion. But voluntary patients are frequently unable to decide whether to be hospitalized and appear to be induced into agreeing to hospitalization by mental health professionals, relatives, or friends (Appelbaum et al. 1981; Gilboy and Schmidt 1971). In some jurisdictions, patients who agree to enter the hospital voluntarily may not be committed (*In the Matter of Blair* 1986). In many jurisdictions, voluntary patients can be at least briefly detained in the hospital after they ask to leave whether or not they meet commitment criteria.

In contrast, civil commitment to a hospital deprives a person of the freedom to live in the community. It may also entail restrictions on the patient's ability to refuse psychotropic medication or to refuse certain medical and psychiatric evaluation procedures. In contrast to earlier law, a patient civilly committed under contemporary legal procedures loses few legal rights (Brakel et al. 1985). Nevertheless, brief periods of involuntary emergency hospitalization can be obtained by mental health professionals without court notice or approval in many jurisdictions; longer detention, or formal commitment, requires formal court petition and hearings. Involuntary hospitalization is proper only when it is the least restrictive intervention consistent with the patient's treatment needs.

After reviewing the threshold issue of meeting legal definitions for mental illness and suicide risk, we will consider "parens patriae" and "police" powers, the legal authority for civil commitment. This will be followed by a consideration of the newer practice of outpatient civil commitment.

Legal Definitions of Mental Illness. Civil commitment statutes universally require that a person be mentally disordered upon commitment; this threshold commitment criterion may be variously stated as mental "disease," "defect," "illness," or "disorder." For the purpose of commitment, mental disorder is defined by statute or regulation. Clinical and legal definitions of mental disorder often differ widely from one another. DSM-III-R cautions that psychiatric disorders found within its classification system may not meet legal criteria for mental illness or mental disorder (American Psychiatric Association 1987a). Just as there has been considerable controversy in the definition and nosology of mental illness or mental disorder within the mental health professions, legal definitions also vary widely.

In defining mental disorder for the purpose of civil commitment, the law fulfills social as well as medical purposes (Gerard 1987). The law attempts to specify what kinds of disorders justify invoking civil commitment, to what degree of severity they must be present, and for what period of time. Statutory language may be either vague or explicit, may include certain psychiatric conditions while excluding others, and may or may not use diagnoses currently accepted within the psychiatric profession. As one example, the current civil commitment statute in Pennsylvania excludes persons who are exclusively "mentally retarded, senile, alcoholic, or drug dependent" (Mental Health Procedures Act 1976). Statutes in other jurisdictions bar commitment on the basis of a personality disorder (Brakel et al. 1985; Huber et al. 1982). The clinician must therefore be aware of how mental disorder and dangerousness to self are legally defined for the purpose of commitment within his or her jurisdiction.

Parens Patriae Powers. *Parens patriae* refers to the state's power to act in a citizen's presumed best interest much as a parent would act on behalf of a child. Parens patriae powers are invoked when a patient is involuntarily hospitalized because of a "need for treatment," or an inability to care for oneself, sometimes referred to as "gravely disabled." It is sometimes difficult, however, to define these terms operationally. Some states restrict commitment based on parens patriae powers to those who would suffer from physical rather than emotional harm to themselves, particularly when self-neglect is involved. In parens patriae situations, the state intervenes to provide treatment that the patient is unable to obtain on his or her own (Roth 1979). The legal system tends to defer to the clinician's expertise in a parens patriae and medical model approach to civil commitment.

In the 1960s and 1970s, parens patriae authority for commitment fell into disfavor, and many procedural protections for patients subject to commitment were enacted. Past abuses of patients in psychiatric hospitals, constitutional objections (Developments in the Law 1974), and society's increasing respect for patient autonomy eroded the legitimacy of parens patriae powers. During these years, commitments were largely limited to police power situations. Given the failures of deinstitutionalization, however, some states have recently moved to returning some parens patriae authority to the state for commitment of the chronically and severely mentally ill (Durham and La Fond 1985).

Police Powers. *Police power* refers to the state's authority to ensure safety for the community. Police powers are commonly invoked when a patient is involuntarily hospitalized because the patient represents a physical danger to him- or herself or to others. This "danger-to-self" criterion for commitment of a suicidal patient actually encompasses both parens patriae and police powers; the state provides treatment to the patient, protects the patient from self-harm, and protects others from harm inflicted by a suicide. In some jurisdictions, commitments based on danger to self are procedurally distinct from those based on danger to others; commitment duration may also be different for the two criteria.

As with other legal standards, the danger-to-self criterion requires further definition. Many factors may come into play in establishing the requisite extent of danger-to-self prior to commitment.

First, the law requires a threshold degree and type of predicted self-harm before commitment can be authorized. The risk of future suicidal thoughts or even nonlethal suicide attempts may not be sufficient for commitment. In some states, a predicted self-mutilation, or a predicted serious suicide attempt, may be required.

Second, the law defines the nature of the evidence required to demonstrate present danger to self. For example, evidence of prior self-injurious behavior may be required before permitting commitment. By requiring rigorous evidence of prior suicidal behavior, the law seeks to improve the accuracy of suicide prediction, and thereby limits commitment to those patients who are more likely to be truly suicidal. However, evidence of past suicidal behavior may not sufficiently improve the accuracy of suicide prediction for the purpose of avoiding unnecessary deprivation of liberty (Greenberg 1974). Further, such restrictions could bar the commitment of a person who has never made a suicide attempt but who is presently believed to be extremely suicidal.

Third, commitment laws apply various time limitations. One type of time limitation addresses the imminence of the future suicidal behavior. Statutory language, for example, may require the suicidal behavior to be "imminent," "in the near future," or predicted to occur "in the next 30 days." Another time limitation pertains to how recently in the past the person showed self-destructive behavior. For example, suicidal behavior that occurred 6 months prior to the current evaluation may have no relevance to a commitment law that requires that such behavior occur within the preceding 30 days.

In addition to the problems of operationalizing the danger-to-self criterion, there are conceptual problems in hospitalizing patients based on police powers. With regard to the danger to others, for example, investigators have questioned the presumption that clinicians have special expertise in predicting dangerousness, particularly over a long period of time (Huber et al. 1982; Monahan 1981). On purely statistical grounds, it is difficult to predict an infrequent event such as suicide to meet a legal standard of reasonable medical probability (Livermore et al. 1968; Murphy 1972; Rosen 1954). Empirical work has demonstrated the failures of our current predictive efforts with regard to suicide (Pokorny 1983). Notwithstanding this evidence, courts continue to admit psychiatric testimony about future danger to self or others for the purpose of civil commitment (*Lyle G. v. Harlem Valley Psychiatric Center* 1987).

The evolution of commitment statutes over time reflects concerns about the proper exercise of police powers by the state. Many states have attempted to protect patients' rights by more precisely defining the circumstances under which police powers may be invoked as well as by adding elaborate procedural safeguards. Recently, as state legislatures continue to struggle to strike the proper balance between protecting individual liberty and protecting the safety of citizens, the pendulum appears to be swinging from the dangerousness standard toward a parens patriae approach.

Outpatient Civil Commitment. Over the past two decades, outpatient civil commitment has been advanced as an alternative to involuntary hospitalization for providing mental health care (Mulvey et al. 1987). The availability of outpatient commitment reflects a need to treat those chronic mentally ill persons who are noncompliant with psychiatric care, who are usually dangerous to themselves or others because of their noncompliance, and who frequently require rehospitalization. Under this approach, a patient who meets outpatient commitment criteria may be compelled by court order to attend outpatient treatment. Noncompliance may result in commitment to an inpatient setting, sometimes without additional procedural due process protections such as a formal hearing.

Outpatient commitment presents many dilemmas to mental health professionals as well as to society at large. Among potential problems represented by outpatient commitment are the definition and threshold of dangerousness before which intervention can occur, the logistics in enforcement, the threat of excessively infringing on patients' civil rights, and the implications for altering the role of the health care professional to include a police function. Approximately half the states currently permit some form of outpatient commitment, whether expressly by statute or otherwise, but the procedure is infrequently used except in a few jurisdictions (Miller 1988).

Civil Commitment and the Clinician. Civil commitment raises ethical and legal issues for the clinician. From an ethical perspective, the decision to commit a patient requires that the clinician balance factors favoring commitment (i.e., patient welfare and safety, treatment to relieve suffering, and the welfare and safety of others) and factors opposing commitment (i.e., individual liberty, patient privacy, and the uncertainty of predicting future self-harm) (Hundert 1987). From a legal perspective, clinicians who manage suicidal patients need to know the standards and procedures for civil commitment, whether inpatient or outpatient, within their state. When commitment laws are strict and commitment is difficult to obtain, other management options must be pursued to obtain adequate treatment for a patient and to reduce the patient's danger to self. Because courts, however, are immune from "wrong" decisions whereas clinicians may be found liable for such, the clinician, when in doubt, should seek judicial review about the commitability of a potentially dangerous-to-self patient. This leads to the subject of malpractice and the suicidal patient.

Malpractice

Overview. In our increasingly litigious society, clinical decision making has tended to assume a defensive posture designed to avoid professional liability, sometimes at the expense of the patient. Attempted and completed suicide, in particular, are leading causes of malpractice litigation against mental health professionals and mental health care facilities (Besharov 1985; Slawson 1984). An understanding of the basis for malpractice demonstrates that providing quality care is, in fact, the best overall strategy for minimizing liability risks.

Professional liability in the form of malpractice is classified under the legal category of a tort. A *tort* is defined as a civil wrong, as opposed to a criminal wrong. More specifically, malpractice in the form of negligence is an unintentional tort. When suing for malpractice, an injured party seeks compensation from the professional who allegedly caused an injury. Malpractice claims for suicide and attempted suicide are unusual in that the patient or the patient's estate seeks compensation for an injury that is self-inflicted; in other malpractice situations, the patient is assumed to have little or no responsibility for the resulting injury.

Many parties may be found liable for a patient's suicide. These include the health care providers, consultants, employers, clinics, and hospitals. Architects who design hospital bathrooms and bedrooms or jails and prisons can also be named as defendants. Strict liability and common law negligence claims have been brought against the manufacturers of safety windows, as well as the contractors who install them (*Gilbertson v. Rolscreen* 1986; *Honey v. Barnes Hospital et al.* 1986).

The Four Elements of Proof in Malpractice. To prevail in a malpractice suit, the injured party must prove four elements, sometimes known as the "four D's": duty, dereliction of duty, damages, and direct causation.

First, the plaintiff must prove that the clinician had a legal duty to care for the patient. Ordinarily, there is no duty for one person to care for another. But once a professional relationship has been established between the clinician and the patient, the clinician assumes the legal duty to provide care. In medicine, the existence of a duty is created by the establishment of the doctor-patient relationship. The duty may be explicitly assumed by agreeing to treat the patient or implicitly assumed by evaluating a patient in a psychiatric emergency room. The duty to provide care may end by appropriately discharging the patient or by arranging for alternate care. Without proper follow-up, the clinician who unilaterally discontinues treatment may be found liable under the legal theory of abandonment.

Second, the plaintiff must prove that there was a dereliction or breach of the legal duty, referred to as negligence. The key issue in proving breach of duty is demonstrating that the professional failed to meet the applicable standard of care, whether by omission or commission (Murphy 1975a, 1975b). Many jurisdictions have abandoned the locality rule, which defined the standard of care based on the particular practice in a local region. Today, the standard of care is established according to the practices of similarly trained professionals in the same or similar circumstances as the defendant. Expert witnesses will be called on by the plaintiff to establish the standard of care as well as the existence of negligence. In addition, the plaintiff can use hospital policies, government regulations, professional literature, and accreditation standards to prove its case.

Third, the plaintiff must prove that there was an injury or damages. A completed suicide, or an attempted suicide resulting in a substantial physical injury, is clearly a harm, not only to the patient but perhaps to others as well. But negligent treatment without a completed suicide or other injury may not result in damages. A negligent act or omission without a harm would not sustain a malpractice claim. Emotional and physical injuries can be legally claimed as damages, although emotional injuries are more difficult to quantify and prove.

Fourth, the plaintiff must prove causation between the defendant's negligence and the injury or damages. Depending on the applicable jurisdiction, such proximate causation can be established by proving that the defendant's negligence was a substantial factor in the injury. The law recognizes that events may in fact be multiply determined, and there may be more than one proximate or legal cause in a given case. As noted above, suicide presents a particular paradox regarding causation. Although the patient is the agent of his or her own death, courts can nevertheless hold clinicians responsible for the suicide. Expert witness testimony will be used at trial to establish or reject causation.

Assuming liability is found, damages may be compensatory or punitive. Compensatory damages provide monetary compensation for the injury and include, for example, loss of wages, funeral expenses, health care expenses following a suicide attempt prior to the person's death, and loss of companionship and consortium by family members. Ironically, damages in the case of an unsuccessful suicide attempt resulting in a serious chronic injury may exceed those in a suicide. Punitive damages impose an additional monetary penalty on the negligent practitioner. Punitive damages are usually not awarded unless there was gross negligence or intentional harm. Damages awarded may be in the millions of dollars, although very large sums are uncommon.

Examples of Alleged Psychiatric Malpractice. *Legal Allegations.* Professional liability for the suicidal behavior of patients is frequently decided by determining whether there was a breach of duty, as defined by failing to meet the standard of ordinary and reasonable care. Mental health professionals and treatment facilities cannot guarantee a patient's safety; the law does not require prevention of self-harm beyond what is expected by the standard of care. Allegations of breach of duty may be divided into two types: failure to diagnose or assess suicide potential, and failure to treat a patient already assessed as suicidal. In either case, the clinician will be held liable only if the patient's suicidal behavior was, or should have been, foreseeable by the clinician.

Specific allegations of negligent failure to diagnose or assess suicide potential include failure to take an adequate history (e.g., by failing to evaluate depression, past and present suicide ideation, or suicidal intent and behavior); failure to obtain a patient's past psychiatric records; and failure to perform an evaluation or testing, whether of suicidal behavior or a condition associated to it. The emphasis in these allegations is on performing adequate suicide assessment rather than making a prediction of suicide per se.

For example, in *Bell v. New York City* (1982), a man who set himself on fire 1 week after discharge from a psychiatric hospital recovered damages against the hospital. The plaintiff also alleged inadequate suicide assessment because the treating psychiatrist had failed to ask the patient about delusions and hallucinations. The plaintiff was awarded $564,225.

In *Szimonisz v. United States* (1982), the defendant failed to order diagnostic tests to detect a meningioma that was found at autopsy after the patient's suicide. The patient had reported signs and symptoms of a central nervous system lesion, including headaches, nystagmus, lethargy, and gait disorder. The court held that the negligent failure of the Veterans Administration to order testing was a proximate cause of the patient's suicide. The plaintiff was awarded $358,889.

Specific allegations of negligent failure to treat a patient already assessed as suicidal, whether by omission or commission, include failure to treat the patient's psychiatric disorder; failure to restrain (e.g., by failing to provide seclusion, restraint, a secure hospital unit, or a secure window); negligent release (e.g., when providing a pass) or negligent discharge; failure to design and maintain a safe facility; failure to monitor the patient (e.g., by providing inadequate suicide precautions); failure to remove dangerous instruments from the patient; failure to supervise other professionals; failure to obtain previous treatment records; and failure to communicate among hospital staff. In general, the law tends to believe that suicide can be prevented once it has been foreseen. Given the limitations of influencing and controlling a patient's behavior in the community, however, professional responsibility to control the patient is greater for an inpatient than for an outpatient.

Several cases illustrate allegations of negligent failure to treat. For example, in *Pisel v. Stamford Hospital et al.* (1980), a hospitalized patient with command hallucinations to injure herself wedged her head between the side rail of her bed and the mattress while in seclusion. At trial, evidence was presented that she had been inadequately monitored and treated. She survived and was awarded $3.6 million. In *Huntley v. State of New York* (1984), one day before her attempted suicide, a psychiatric inpatient communicated her specific suicide plan involving an off-premises location to a hospital staff member. This information was not transmitted to the staff psychiatrist who controlled her off-grounds privileges. Judgment was entered for the plaintiff and upheld on appeal. In *De Sanchez v. Genoves-Andrews et al.* (1987), the plaintiffs recovered damages based on the allegation of failure to design and maintain a safe facility. In that case, an inpatient hanged himself from an overhead dividing bar inside a toilet stall.

Legal Defenses. In responding to the allegation of malpractice, the clinician or treatment facility may offer a number of defenses. These include compliance with the standard of care; patient concealment of suicidal intent; reasonable errors in clinician judgment; proper assessment of the patient despite the adverse outcome; impossibility of suicide prediction, or the patient was not foreseeably suicidal; release consistent with the least-restrictive alternative while still meeting the patient's clinical needs; that clinical restrictions were antitherapeutic;

the occurrence of injury regardless of whether the clinician was negligent; governmental immunity for decision makers; and that the patient's suicidal behavior was competent and volitional.

Several cases illustrate the successful use of some of these defenses. In *Johnson v. United States* (1976), for example, a court rejected the claim of the patient's widow that the psychiatrist had negligently released her husband from the hospital. The court ruled that:

> Modern psychiatric practice does not require a patient to be isolated from normal human activities until every possible danger has passed. Because of the virtual impossibility of predicting dangerousness, such an approach would necessarily lead to prolonged incarceration for many patients who could become useful members of society . . . constant supervision and restriction will often tend to promote the very disorders which they are designed to control. (p. 1293)

In *Topel v. Long Island Jewish Medical Center* (1981), the court found for the defendant using the defenses of reasonable errors in judgment, proper assessment of the patient despite the adverse outcome, and choosing the least-restrictive, and clinically appropriate alternative. The court ruled, contrary to the plaintiff's contention, that it was a matter of professional judgment whether to conduct observation of a suicidal patient at 15-minute intervals or on a continuous basis. The court further stated that it was proper for the clinician to consider the patient's reaction to constant observation and the benefits of less restrictive treatment in the decision making about monitoring.

In *Speer v. United States* (1981), the defendant prevailed based on compliance with the standard of care. The court rejected the widow's claim that the standard of care was breached when a psychiatrist prescribed a month's supply of amitriptyline and perphenazine to an outpatient who fatally overdosed on the medication. The court stated that "in the absence of any persuasive indicia that a known risk existed that [the decedent] might use the Etrafon to commit suicide, the Court is unwilling to say that [the defendant] had a responsibility to limit each prescription" (p. 678). The court also held that, since the suicide was not reasonably foreseeable, the defendant's negligence, even if any existed, was not the proximate cause of the patient's death.

Clinical-Legal Issues in Managing Suicidal Patients

Issues Common to Both Inpatient and Outpatient Settings. Clinical *Evaluation of Suicide Risk.* Evaluation of suicide risk is the cornerstone for the clinical-legal management of suicidal patients. Proper assessment and treatment of potentially suicidal patients requires familiarity with the risk factors for suicide and attempted suicide, including biological, cognitive, affective, and external factors (Blumenthal, Chapter 26, this volume). Specifically, one should consider the patient's demographic profile, stressful life events, history of suicide attempts, family psychiatric history, family dynamics, social supports, religious beliefs, drug or alcohol use, medical disease, depressed mood, hopelessness, psychosis (including command hallucinations), organic deficits, personality traits, and relationships with treatment staff (including transference issues). The results of the clinician's inquiry may identify some factors that raise the patient's suicide risk and factors that lower the patient's suicide risk. Risk factors should be considered in the context of the individual under evaluation.

Therapeutic Alliance. Proper assessment and use of the patient's therapeutic alliance with the treatment staff or therapist is useful in managing chronically suicidal patients, especially when the clinician knows the patient well. The clinician should assess the patient's ability to report any suicidal ideation and intention, to manage his or her own suicidal impulses, and to participate in his or her own treatment planning (Bursztajn et al. 1983; Hendren, Chapter 10; Kahn, Chapter 16, this volume). The treatment alliance may be further enhanced when the clinician begins to share the inherent uncertainty of any clinical outcome with the suicidal patient. This provides the patient with a sense of control, hope, and, together with the therapist, a mutual acceptance of uncertainty (Gutheil et al. 1984).

Written or informal "contracts" between patient and therapist in which the patient promises not to attempt suicide are without legal effect. After the suicide, depressed and suicidal patients are often seen by the courts as functionally impaired, childlike, unable to "contract," and unable to control self-destructive impulses because of their mental disorder. At times, however, such devices will have therapeutic use.

Confidentiality. Dilemmas regarding confidentiality may confront the clinician treating a suicidal patient. As a general rule, the mental health professional has both an ethical and a legal duty to maintain confidentiality with the patient (American Psychiatric Association 1987b). A breach of confidentiality can provide grounds for litigation based on negligence, breach of statutory duty, slander and libel, or defamation, or may result in sanction by ethical and professional licensing boards (*Martino v. Family Service Agency of Adams County* 1983; *State Board v. Hosford* 1987). The need to maintain confidentiality should not, however, be used to avoid working with relatives involved with the patient's care or to avoid maintaining proper records. Further, the law defines situations in which confidentiality can be breached. These usually consist of emergency situations (e.g., emergency detention or commitment evaluations), in which serious harm would ensue in the absence of information disclosure. In non-emergent situations, the patient's right to confidential treatment must be carefully weighed against other treatment goals and the patient's safety. If the clinician determines that contact with family members or significant others is crucial to a patient's care, the clinician may be compelled to breach confidentiality. Preferably, the patient should be informed of the limits of confidentiality when beginning treatment and told when confidences are about to be breached. *Tarasoff v. Regents of the University of California* (1976) provided a situation in which confidentiality may be breached to protect purported victims from a patient who is dangerous to others. Yet there is no analogous legal duty to warn the patient's family members of the patient's need for treatment or potential suicide (*Bellah v. Greenson* 1978; *Brandt v. Grubin* 1974).

Questions about the confidentiality of the patient's treatment also arise after a patient's death. Issues concerning life insurance benefits, income and estate taxes, testamentary capacity, and malpractice litigation can arise at this time. From a legal and ethical viewpoint, clinicians must nevertheless continue to maintain the confidentiality of the treatment even after death. Some state statutes authorize release of information by executors or administrators of the patient's estate. As in any release of psychiatric information, only that information responsive to the purpose stated in the request should be disclosed. This sometimes presents problems to clinicians who wish to meet with family members after a patient's suicide, whether at a funeral or in bereavement counseling.

Documentation. Documentation facilitates communication among clinicians; promotes systematic assessment, treatment planning, and implementation; and provides a clinical record for future reference. Furthermore, psychiatric malpractice cases can rise or fall on the adequacy of clinical documentation.

Significant aspects of the patient's care must be documented in the medical record in a contemporaneous, rather than post hoc, manner. This includes pertinent factors in the patient's history, mental status examination, diagnosis, suicide assessment, and treatment plan. The usual tendency to avoid recording pertinent negative findings should be resisted, and these should be recorded explicitly (e.g., "the patient denies suicide ideation, intention, or plan"). Documentation in the record provides proof of the clinician's observations, judgment, and thinking at the time of the patient's care. The absence of such information permits a trier of fact to conclude later that the clinician failed to perform a critical element of the examination, even though the clinician testifies that he or she in fact did so (Perr 1985). Documentation of clinical decision making is particularly important when the clinician makes decisions regarding hospital admission, transfer, discharge, or privileges. Presentation of a risk-benefit assessment in the record presents evidence that the clinician considered the relevant factors in the decision. In such cases, for example, the clinician would acknowledge the existence of a suicide risk for a patient but then would explain the rationale for an alternative intervention (Gutheil 1980).

Consultation. Obtaining a consultation from a colleague may be both clinically and legally useful, particularly with a difficult or unusual patient (Gutheil and Appelbaum 1982). Clinically, the consultant can assist the treating clinician in assessing and managing suicide risk. Legally, agreement between the primary clinician and the consultant provides evidence that the clinician's judgment conformed to the standard of care of a reasonable practitioner and thus helps support a defense to a malpractice claim. A consultation may be either formal or informal; the consultant need not necessarily examine the patient personally, although this is often useful in difficult cases.

Inpatient Treatment. Inpatient management of suicidal patients presents a basic conflict. On the one hand, treatment goals may require increasing a patient's responsibility and freedoms (*Meier v. Ross General Hospital* 1968). On the other hand, restrictive measures may be required to ensure a patient's safety from self-injury (Margolis et al. 1965). In resolving this conflict, a variety of management strategies are possible. No hospital is expected to be suicide-proof. From the legal perspective, the psychiatric hospital and its staff need only meet the standard of ordinary and reasonable care in assessing and managing the hospitalized suicidal patient.

From the administrative viewpoint, written policies and procedures should be formulated to ensure uniformity of patient management and compliance with treatment standards. Such policies should provide guidelines for specific levels of supervision of potentially suicidal patients, including seclusion, restraint, one-to-one observation, and transfer to other units (American Psychiatric Association 1984; Tardiff 1984). These policies should define the restrictive measure, identify how the decision to implement the practice should be made, and delineate who has the authority to make the decision. The policies should also require that the rationale for these decisions be clearly documented. Use of such terms as *close observation* or *suicide watch* in physician orders or as a description of nursing practices, when the meaning of these terms is not clearly defined, does not promote uniform care and should be avoided (Benensohn and Resnik 1973).

Clinically, proper care is likely to be obtained by anticipating methods of suicide by inpatients and by taking appropriate precautions. Hanging is one of the most common means of suicide in hospitals, and suicidal patients should therefore not have access to ropes, belts, exposed plumbing, or nonbreakaway bars in bathrooms. Patients should not have access to windows from which they could jump or objects with which they could injure themselves. Such restrictions also need to be communicated with the patient's visitors. Hospitalized patients should also be prevented from hoarding medications. Without warning, patients may act on their suicidal impulses when given the means or opportunity to do so.

Communication among hospital staff members, through the written chart as well as orally, is an important element in inpatient psychiatric treatment of suicidal patients. Staff must have a means of communicating relevant clinical information between shifts, as well as across disciplines. Unit administration should ensure accurate and complete communication of relevant clinical information regarding the suicidal patient through regular treatment planning meetings as well as crisis situations.

Another example of good practice is the frequent reevaluations of suicide risk among inpatients during the course of treatment, especially for patients explicitly admitted because of suicide risk. Suicide potential will be modified by the response to treatment, as well as by changes in external precipitants. No suicide attempt, whether in the hospital or the community, should be readily dismissed or labeled as "manipulative" without clear evidence that such is the case.

If a suicide occurs, a "psychological autopsy" conducted with the treatment team may contribute to improving the quality of care for other patients (Ebert 1987). In a psychological autopsy, the staff reviews the patient's history, clinical presentation, and response to treatment, as well as their clinical decision making for a patient who committed suicide or made a serious suicide attempt. Hospitals may be reluctant to conduct such peer review, fearing that it may be subsequently used against them in a lawsuit. Indeed, under certain circumstances, informal discussions may be used against a defendant in a lawsuit. Psychological autopsies and other forms of peer review, however, when not recorded in the patient's chart, are legally protected from discovery by plaintiffs in a lawsuit (Ruben, Chapter 23, this volume).

Finally, upon hospitalization, psychiatric patients often have the right to refuse treatment, particularly psychotropic medication. In nonemergencies, a growing number of states require administrative or judicial review to override the treatment refusal of a committed patient (Appelbaum 1988). Others require review of the patient's refusal and overall care by an independent psychiatrist before treatment can proceed. In these cases, questions about the patient's competency to refuse treatment must be addressed. In emergency situations, however, the suicidal patient may be forced to accept treatment, including medication, for the duration of the emergency. Voluntarily hospitalized patients generally have the right to refuse treatment in nonemergency situations. Nevertheless, failure to initiate procedures to override a patient's treatment refusal, if available, may open the clinician to allegations of failure to treat.

Outpatient Treatment. Since clinicians are more limited in their ability to control outpatients, outpatient treatment requires different strategies for meeting the standard of care with regard to suicide and attempted suicide. For example, the clinician should consider how likely the patient is to abuse medication. A paradox in treating suicidal patients is that the medications most needed for treatment may also be the most lethal if abused, particularly tricyclic antidepressants for a suicidal patient. The clinician can choose to prescribe a limited number of pills to a depressed patient, perhaps only enough until the patient's next visit. Further precautions may include more frequent outpatient prescriptions or enforcing compliance by testing medication blood levels. Medication refills without clinical examination should be provided only after considering the potential for misuse. Unit dosing, when available, also reduces the potential misuse of medication (Murphy 1975a).

The clinician must also properly communicate information about treatment to the patient. Patient safety is usually promoted by informing the patient about the proper use and risks of medication. Without such information, what was perhaps intended as a nonlethal suicide attempt could result in an accidental death if the patient naively takes too many pills, mixes medications, or combines medication with alcohol. The clinician must consider the possibility, however, that a patient may use information to calculate a more lethal suicide attempt.

Aside from medication, the clinician should assess the presence of other risks of self-injury, such as access to weapons. In the outpatient situation, the clinician cannot enforce restricted access to such weapons. Based on an assessment of the risk, however, the clinician could insist that the patient or a family member remove weapons from the patient's home as a prerequisite to continuing outpatient treatment. The clinician could also insist on contacting a family member to confirm that such weapons were removed.

FORENSIC ISSUES FOLLOWING A SUICIDE OR SUICIDE ATTEMPT

Mental health professionals are sometimes asked to respond to legal questions about a person's death. These questions are answered by those who had previously evaluated or treated the person, as well as those who had never previously met the person. The issues that are raised at this time include manner of death, eligibility for insurance benefits, and workers' compensation awards.

Medical-legal certifications of the manner, mechanism, and cause of death are ordinarily made by coroners and medical examiners, typically without the assistance of mental health experts. Questions have been raised about the reliability and validity of these determinations (Jobes et al. 1987), particularly the manner of death (e.g., natural, accident, suicide, homicide, undetermined). Distinguishing accident from suicide in many cases such as drug and alcohol intoxication, single-car fatality, and drowning is often problematic. Litman (1980) proposed that expert mental health witnesses, when asked to render an opinion about the manner of death, state the respective probabilities of accident and suicide. Such certifications have substantial implications for life insurance benefits, professional liability, public policy, and research in suicide.

Life insurance policies sometimes exclude suicide from coverage, in which case the beneficiary is entitled only to a refund of premiums paid. Litigation about whether the decedent was legally "sane" or "insane" at the time of death or injury can then ensue (Nolan 1988). Difficulties performing retrospective forensic mental health determinations of legal insanity in this civil context parallel those of legal sanity determinations in the criminal context (American Psychiatric Association 1983a). Given the limited experience of most jurisdictions with this issue, even the legal standard of responsibility for the forensic mental health expert to use in the case of suicide is unclear (see Appendixes V and VI). As well, evidence from pathology, toxicology, police, survivors, and witnesses is often insufficient for the forensic expert to render an opinion with reasonable certainty about the decedent's intent, cognitive capacity, or volitional capacity. Life insurance policies that exclude from coverage "suicide sane or insane" or injury from intentional acts by the insured reduce but do not eliminate the likelihood of litigation over this issue. The majority of courts have ruled that the insurer is not liable for suicide under "suicide sane or insane" life insurance clauses "regardless of whether the insured decedent realized or was capable of realizing that such act would cause his death or whether he was capable of entertaining an intention to kill himself" (*Atkinson v. Life Insurance Company of Virginia* 1976, p. 120). On the other hand, a minority of courts have ruled that the insurer is liable for death benefits when the deceased did not understand the physical nature and consequences of the suicidal act (*Searle v. Allstate Life Insurance Company* 1985).

Work-related suicides and suicide attempts are often compensable under workers' compensation and private disability insurance policies, depending on state law (Batt and Bastien 1984). In some workers' compensation programs, a work-related physical injury must precede the suicide for it to be compensable (*Lather v. Huron College* 1987). In others, an emotional injury caused by the emotional stress of the claimant's working conditions may be compensable. In many jurisdictions, compensation is denied if the claimant's self-inflicted injury was caused by intoxication or intentional injury (*Harvey v. Raleigh Police Department* 1987); in such cases, suicide constitutes an independent, intervening cause of the patient's death. The presence of a mental disorder at the time of the suicide or attempted suicide, however, can render the act nonvoluntary or not willful and permit recovery of damages. Forensic mental health experts are asked to render an opinion about whether the decedent was mentally disordered at the time of the self-injury, and the effect of the mental disorder or nonwork-related factors on the decedent's intention, cognition, and volition.

CONCLUSION

Ethics and the law struggle to balance individual freedom with protecting a person from self-injury. The clinician's responsibility for treating the suicidal patient reflects an underlying determinist ethical principle, which has been challenged in certain situations. Civil commitment and involuntary treatment provide a means of preventing suicide through parens patriae or police powers, but the benefits of suicide prevention must be balanced against the deprivation of individual liberties. Suicides will occur despite the use of ordinary and reasonable care required by the law; liability risks can be reduced but not eliminated. Clinical assessment and management will help ensure quality patient care, thereby also minimizing liability risks when caring for suicidal patients. Armed with a deeper understanding of ethical and legal aspects of suicide, clinicians will be better able to practice their clinical craft.

REFERENCES

American Psychiatric Association, Insanity Defense Work Group: American Psychiatric Association statement on the insanity defense. Am J Psychiatry 140:681–688, 1983a

American Psychiatric Association: Guidelines for legislation on the psychiatric hospitalization of adults. Am J Psychiatry 140:672–679, 1983b

American Psychiatric Association, Task Force: Seclusion and restraint: the psychiatric uses (Task Force Report 22). Washington, DC, American Psychiatric Association, 1984

American Psychiatric Association: Diagnostic and Statistical Manual of Mental Disorders, 3rd Edition, Revised. Washington, DC, American Psychiatric Association, 1987a

American Psychiatric Association, Committee on Confidentiality: Guidelines on confidentiality. Am J Psychiatry 144:1522–1526, 1987b

Appelbaum PS: The right to refuse treatment with antipsychotic medications: retrospect and prospect. Am J Psychiatry 145:413–419, 1988

Appelbaum PS, Mirkin SA, Bateman AL: Empirical assessment of competency to consent to psychiatric hospitalization. Am J Psychiatry 138:1170–1176, 1981

Atkinson v Life Insurance Company of Virginia, 228 SE2d 117 (Va 1976)

Batt J, Bastien CP: Suicide as a compensable claim under workers' compensation statutes: a guide for the lawyer and the psychiatrist. West Virginia Law Review 86:369–392, 1984

Battin MP: Ethical Issues in Suicide. Englewood Cliffs, NJ, Prentice-Hall, 1982

Beauchamp TL, Childress JF: Principles of Biomedical Ethics, 2nd Edition. New York, Oxford University Press, 1983

Bell v New York City, 456 NYS2d 787 (1982)

Bellah v Greenson, 146 Cal Rptr 535 (1978)

Benensohn HS, Resnik HLP: Guidelines for "suicide-proofing" a psychiatric unit. Am J Psychotherapy 27:204–212, 1973

Besharov DJ: The Vulnerable Social Worker: Liability for Serving Children and Families. Silver Spring, MD, National Association of Social Workers, 1985

Blumenthal SJ, Kupfer DJ: Generalizable treatment strategies for suicidal behavior. Ann NY Acad Sci 487:327–340, 1986

Brakel SJ, Parry J, Weiner BA: The Mentally Disabled and the Law, 3rd Edition. Chicago, IL, American Bar Foundation, 1985

Brandt v Grubin, 329 A2d 82 (NJ 1974)

Bursztajn H, Gutheil TG, Hamm RM, et al: Subjective data and suicide assessment in the light of recent legal developments. Part II: Clinical uses of legal standards in the interpretation of subjective data. Int J Law Psychiatry 6:331–350, 1983

De Sanchez v Genoves-Andrews et al, 410 NW2d 803 (Mich 1987)

Developments in the Law: Civil commitment of the mentally ill. Harvard Law Review 87:1190–1406, 1974

Durham ML, La Fond JQ: The empirical consequences and policy implications of broadening the statutory criteria for civil commitment. Yale Law Policy Review 3:395–446, 1985

Durkheim E: Suicide: A Study in Sociology. Translated by Spaulding JA, Simpson G. Glencoe, IL, Free Press, 1951

Ebert BW: Guide to conducting a psychological autopsy. Professional Psychology Research and Practice 18:52–56, 1987

Freud S: Thoughts for the times on war and death: Our Attitudes Towards Death (1915), in The Standard Edition of the Complete Psychological Works of Sigmund Freud, Vol 14. Translated and edited by Strachey J. London, Hogarth Press, 1953, p 289–300

Gerard JB: The usefulness of the medical model to the legal system. Rutgers Law Review 39:377–423, 1987

Gilbertson v Rolscreen, 501 NE2d 954 (Ill 1986)

Gilboy JA, Schmidt RJ: "Voluntary" hospitalization of the mentally ill. Northwestern University Law Review 66:429–453, 1971

Greenberg DF: Involuntary psychiatric commitments to prevent suicide. New York University Law Review 49:227–269, 1974

Gutheil TG: Paranoia and progress notes: a guide to forensically informed psychiatric recordkeeping. Hosp Community Psychiatry 31:479–482, 1980

Gutheil TG, Appelbaum PS: Clinical Handbook of Psychiatry and the Law. New York, McGraw-Hill, 1982

Gutheil TG, Bursztajn H, Brodsky A: Malpractice prevention through the sharing of uncertainty: informed consent and the therapeutic alliance. N Engl J Med 311:49–51, 1984

Harvey v Raleigh Police Department, 355 SE2d 147 (NC 1987)

Honey v Barnes Hospital et al, 708 SW2d 686 (Mo 1986)

Huber GA, Roth LH, Appelbaum PS, et al: Hospitalization, arrest, or discharge: important legal and clinical issues in the emergency evaluation of persons believed dangerous to others. Law and Contemporary Problems 45:99–123, 1982

Hundert EM: A model for ethical problem solving in medicine, with practical applications. Am J Psychiatry 144:839–846, 1987

Huntley v State of New York, 464 NE2d 467 (1984)

In the Matter of Blair, 510 A2d 1048 (DC 1986)

"It's over, Debbie," A Piece of My Mind. JAMA 259:272, 1988

Jobes DA, Berman AL, Josselson AR: Improving the validity and reliability of medical-legal certifications of suicide. Suicide Life Threat Behav 17:310–325, 1987

Johnson v United States, 409 F Supp 1283 (Fla 1976)

Kjervik DK: The psychotherapist's duty to act reasonably to prevent suicide: a proposal to allow rational suicide. Behavioral Sciences and the Law 2:207–218, 1984

Lather v Huron College, 413 NW2d 369 (SD 1987)

"Letters: It's over, Debbie." JAMA 259:2094–2098, 1988

Litman RE: Psycholegal aspects of suicide, in Modern Legal Medicine, Psychiatry, and Forensic Science. Edited by Curran W, McGarry AL, Petty CS. Philadelphia, Pa, FA Davis, 1980, pp 841–853

Livermore JM, Malmquist CP, Meehl PE: On the justifications for civil commitment. University of Pennsylvania Law Review 117:75–96, 1968

Lyle G v Harlem Valley Psychiatric Center, 521 NYS2d 94 (1987)

Mann J, Stanley M (eds): Psychobiology of suicidal behavior. Ann NY Acad Sci, Vol 487 (whole issue), 1986

Margolis PM, Meyer GG, Louw JC: Suicidal precautions: a dilemma in the therapeutic community. Arch Gen Psychiatry 13:224–231, 1965

Maris R (ed): Biology of Suicide. New York, Guilford, 1986

Martino v Family Service Agency of Adams County, 445 NE2d 6 (Ill 1983)

Meier v Ross General Hospital, 71 Cal Rptr 903 (1968)

Mental Health Procedures Act, Title 50, Section 7102, Purdon's Pennsylvania Statutes Annotated, 1976

Miller RD: Outpatient civil commitment of the mentally ill: an overview and an update. Behavioral Sciences and the Law 6:99–118, 1988

Monahan J: The Clinical Prediction of Violent Behavior. Rockville, MD, National Institute of Mental Health, 1981

Mulvey EP, Geller JL, Roth LH: The promise and peril of involuntary outpatient commitment. Am Psychol 42:571–584, 1987

Munson R: Intervention and Reflection: Basic Issues in Medical Ethics. Belmont, CA, Wadsworth, 1979

Murphy GE: Clinical identification of suicidal risk. Arch Gen Psychiatry 27:356–359, 1972

Murphy GE: The physician's responsibility for suicide. I: An error of commission. Ann Intern Med 82:301–304, 1975a

Murphy GE: The physician's responsibility for suicide. II: Errors of omission. Ann Intern Med 82:305–309, 1975b

Nolan JL (ed): The Suicide Case: Investigation and Trial of Insurance Claims. Chicago, IL, American Bar Association, 1988

Perr IN: Suicide litigation and risk management: a review of 32 cases. Bull Am Acad Psychiatry Law 13:209–219, 1985

Pisel v Stamford Hospital et al, 430 A2d 1 (Conn 1980)

Pokorny AD: Prediction of suicide in psychiatric patients. Arch Gen Psychiatry 40:249–257, 1983

Rosen A: Detection of suicidal patients: an example of some limitations in the prediction of infrequent events. Journal of Consulting Psychology 18:397–403, 1954

Roth LH: A commitment law for patients, doctors and lawyers. Am J Psychiatry 136:1121–1127, 1979

Ruark JE, Raffin TA, Stanford University Medical Center Committee on Ethics: Initiating and withdrawing life support: principles and practice in adult medicine. N Engl J Med 318:25–30, 1988

Shaffer CD: Criminal liability for assisting suicide. Columbia Law Review 86:348–376, 1986

Searle v Allstate Life Insurance Company, 696 P2d 1308 (Cal 1985)

Siegel K: Psychosocial aspects of rational suicide. Am J Psychother 40:405–418, 1986

Slawson PF: The clinical dimension of psychiatric malpractice. Psychiatric Annals 14:358–364, 1984

Society for the Right to Die: Handbook of 1985 Living Will Laws. New York, Society for the Right to Die, 1986

Speer v United States, 512 F Supp 670 (ND Tex 1981)

State Board v Hosford, 508 So2d 1049 (Miss 1987)

Szasz T: The case against suicide prevention. Am Psychol 41:806–812, 1986

Szimonisz v United States, 537 F Suppl 147 (Or 1982)

Tardiff K: The Psychiatric Uses of Seclusion and Restraint. Washington, DC, American Psychiatric Press, 1984

Tarasoff v Regents of the University of California, 551 P2d 340 (Cal 1976)

Topel v Long Island Jewish Medical Center, 431 NE2d 293 (NY 1981)

Chapter 25

Youth Suicide: Public Policy and Research Issues

Herbert Pardes, M.D.
Susan J. Blumenthal, M.D., M.P.A.

INTEREST IN THE DEVELOPMENT and implementation of public policy recommendations for suicide has intensified as our nation has experienced an extraordinary rise in youth suicide over the past 30 years. While the suicide rates for other age groups of the population have remained relatively stable over this time period, the epidemic of teenage suicide has precipitated a burst of public attention and has raised a panoply of policy and research questions. The public wants to know why young people are killing themselves at an increased rate and what can be done to prevent these tragedies. Unfortunately, few systematic research studies have been undertaken to determine the risk factors for suicide in this age group, and interventions have not been well tested for their efficacy. It is also unclear whether conclusions drawn from research on adult suicide can be applied to understanding this phenomenon in young people. In this chapter, we will focus on public policy issues relevant to youth suicide, with particular emphasis on nosologic and diagnostic concerns, using this age group as a model for the types of recommendations needed generally in suicide research, training, and prevention over the life cycle.

In 1959, searching for papers on youth suicide, Motto (1984) found only one report of four cases of suicide attempts by young people. Although there was an increase in the number of reports on adolescent suicide in the 1960s, these were mostly theoretical papers or clinical case studies focusing on suicidal ideation and attempts rather than on completed suicide. From 1960 to 1980, only two data-based investigations of the characteristics of youth suicide completers were undertaken (Shaffer et al. 1988; Shafii et al. 1985, 1988). Shafii and Shafii (1982) attributed this underreporting of completed suicides in children and adolescents to an insensitivity to the "world of children and youth." In the 1980s, new studies were undertaken to determine the risk factors for suicide in this age group. Brent and Kolko (Chapter 11, this volume) provide a thorough review of childhood and adolescent suicide, as do Schwartz and Whitaker (Chapter 12, this volume) on college student suicide.

Paralleling an increased awareness about rising rates of teenage suicide has been the resurgence and virtual revolution in psychiatric research over the past decade. This research excitement has clearly benefited the field of suicidology. In recent years, systematic research studies have been undertaken to study this problem. Indeed, the breadth of approaches characterizing contemporary suicide research described in the chapters of this volume parallels the breadth of approaches in psychiatric research generally.

Additionally, several major policy groups were formed to respond to this public health crisis among our nation's youth. In 1984, the leadership of the National Institute of Mental Health worked with the Secretary of Health and Human Services to appoint a Department of Health and Human Services Task Force that identified the main issues and secured the best advice for appropriate societal and research responses to youth suicide. This Task Force on Youth Suicide held several conferences and developed a comprehensive set of recommendations for research, intervention, and prevention (Alcohol, Drug Abuse, and Mental Health Administration 1989). Additionally, states like New York instituted their own Commissions on Youth Suicide; in the private sector, groups such as the National Committee for Youth Suicide were established. The work of all these groups has resulted in a consensus: The study of youth suicide demands a multifaceted, multidisciplinary approach to its etiology, treatment, and prevention, one that incorporates diverse public and health care professional input from both the public and private sectors. Several major policy and research issues, which are described in the remainder of this chapter, have emerged from the deliberations of these groups.

RESEARCH ISSUES

Nosology

A major issue in suicide research involves the use of specific and uniform criteria to describe and classify the range of self-destructive behaviors. Suicide is underreported in this country, in part due to a lack of uniform reporting criteria. Social stigma and personal considerations (e.g., loss of insurance benefits) may also be factors. Statistically based investigations of suicide have been hampered by many methodological problems, such as this underreporting and the lack of control groups in studies. Additionally, there has not been adequate agreement nor clarity in past studies about distinguishing the population who attempt suicide from those who complete suicide (Robins 1985). The way in which these two population groups of suicide attempters and suicide completers are conceptualized has important research, educational, and prevention implications.

Robins (1985) pointed out that attempted suicides and completed suicides are distinct phenomena that occur in "overlapping, but different populations." Annually, 1% to 2% of attempters go on to complete suicide. Attempts, which occur in far greater numbers than completed suicides, may often be symptoms of other problems rather than necessarily representing precursors to future suicide (Robins 1985). Shafii et al. (1985) saw much greater connectiveness between these two phenomena, particularly among youth, stating that "in our study a large majority of children and adolescents who have committed suicide had previously verbalized their wish to die or threatened suicide. Only a small number of victims had not expressed the wish to die or threatened suicide." In this study, frequently the "talkers" became the "doers." Likewise, Brent et al.'s (1988) findings support a continuum of suicidality from ideation to completion. While acknowledging that suicide attempters and completers have different demographic characteristics, Shaffer et al. (1988) underscored the importance of a prior suicide attempt as a powerful risk factor for later suicide in adolescents. These investigators found a high frequency of discussed, threatened, or attempted suicide in those youth with current suicidal behavior. These researchers emphasized the possibility of interactive effects (e.g., implying that in some instances the attempts may be more significant than in others). In contrast, Motto (1984) found no significant differences between those adults who committed suicide, those who reported previous suicide attempts, and those who reported never having made a previous suicide attempt. He also emphasized other studies of completed suicides that revealed little evidence of prior suicide attempts.

Our review of research findings on the relationship of suicide attempters and completers suggests that 1) attempters should be considered as a distinct high-risk population; 2) the relationship between attempters and completers must be more carefully refined, looking for particular subgroups that may be at the highest risk; and 3) greater attention must be paid both clinically and scientifically to youth suicide attempters, since there appears to be considerable overlap between the attempter and completer populations.

Diagnostic Issues

The evolution of research on suicide has occurred in the context of a changing conceptual framework for psychiatric diagnosis. In their review, Black and Winokur (Chapter 6, this volume) found that the number of suicide victims across studies with psychiatric illness ranged from 73% to 100%. In a large, retrospective study of completed suicide (Robins 1981), 94% of the 134 cases of adult suicides had a diagnosable psychiatric disorder: 67% had an affective disorder and 25% had alcoholism.

However, the diagnostic issue for youth suicide has been less clear. Lack of systematic research studies about adolescent suicide has created controversy in the field, with diverse opinions being expressed about the explanation for the increasing rates of youth suicide. Is suicide a behavioral response of normal adolescents to life stresses, an adverse effect of broad social trends, a result of a psychiatrically ill youngster attempting to end his or her pain, or a phenomenon dependent largely on teenagers' propensities for imitating or copying other people's actions? The answer to this question has implications for all of the involved sectors concerned with suicide, including researchers and community and health care organizations, and affects the nature of preventive and intervention efforts. As the number of systematic data-based studies increases, the answer may soon become clear. From recent research evidence, it appears that a far greater number of youth suicides have diagnosable psychiatric illnesses than had been thought in earlier years (Brent and Kolko, Chapter 11, this volume; Shaffer et al. 1988; Shafii et al. 1988). Shafii et al. (1988), noting the results of Robins' (1981) earlier study, highlighted the methodological weaknesses in previous research on teen suicide (Stearns 1953) that found youth suicide to occur "in the midst of what usually seems to be a well-adjusted life." In their study of 23 youth suicides, Shafii et al. found that 95% of the suicide victims as compared to 48% of the matched pair controls had at least one serious diagnosable psychiatric disorder. Further, 81% of the suicide victims had two or more mental disorders as compared with 29% of the control group. Additionally, 76% of the suicide victims as compared to 24% of the controls had a primary or secondary diagnosis of major depression and/or dysthymia. In this study, the youth suicide victims had a greater frequency of major depressive disorder and a primary or secondary diagnosis of alcohol and/or drug abuse. The investigators concluded that "completed suicide in children and adolescents does not occur on the spur of the moment or as an impulsive act of an otherwise healthy child as a reaction to a personal crisis. In almost all of our cases suicide was the final outcome of serious emotional disorders" (p. 232). Further, they emphasized that psychiatric disorders in these children were often not recognized. The authors underscored the need to educate health care professionals and the general public about the early detection and treatment of these illnesses.

In a larger study using the psychological autopsy method, Shaffer et al. (1988) also found a strong association between psychiatric disorder and youth suicide. Symptoms of major depressive disorder were found in approximately one-quarter of the youngsters, drug and alcohol abuse in about one-third of the sample, and a history of aggressive and antisocial behavior in almost one-half of the victims. Learning disorders were also noted to be common. Other groups found to be at risk were youngsters with perfectionistic characteristics who become excessively anxious in the face of certain kinds of stresses, and who can usually meet the diagnostic criteria for overanxious disorder. In another study, Cohen-Sandler et al. (1982) suggested three subgroups of young people who commit suicide: 1) adolescents with conduct disorders complicated by drug abuse; 2) depressed adolescents; and 3) perfectionists who feel threatened by certain academic or social challenges.

Comparisons of the association between psychiatric diagnosis and suicide in teenagers and adults reveal similarities but also important differences. For example, alcohol dependence plays a far greater role in adults, but alcohol abuse is associated with a very large percentage of youth suicides (Shaffer et al. 1988; Shafii et al. 1988). Although major affective disorder is an important risk factor in adult suicides, it is not necessarily the major risk factor in young people. In part, this may be attributable to the increasing incidence of depression with age (Klerman and Weissman 1989; Shaffer et al. 1988; Vaillant and Blumenthal, Chapter 1, this volume). Blumenthal and Kupfer (1988) suggest a continuum between psychiatric disorders associated with suicide in adolescence and adulthood. For example, conduct disorders, impulsivity, and aggressivity are important risk factors in youth suicide, and antisocial personality disorder along with these aforementioned personality traits are contributory factors in adulthood. Furthermore, the phenomenon of suicide among the ostensibly "well" may, in fact, represent patients suffering from psychiatric illness who did not manifest symptoms of the disorder in a typical form (Robins 1985).

Shaffer et al. (1988) also stressed the critical role of precipitants, demonstrating that most teenage suicide victims had a disciplinary confrontation only a short time before their death and feared unknown consequences of that trouble. Blumenthal (1988) pointed out that this precipitating life event is generally humiliating in nature, with the young person being unable to face the shame, guilt, or ramifications of the event.

Conclusions derived from these research findings have important implications for health policy related to youth suicide. The first is to underscore that more research is needed to clarify precisely the number and characteristics of youngsters who are vulnerable to suicidal behavior. Given the numerous risk factors for youth suicide, the stresses affecting youth, and the different environmental settings in which young people may become suicidal, education is needed for those people in a position to detect vulnerable teenagers in a range of settings. As a health policy recommendation, it is necessary for pediatricians, school health officials, teachers, and family members to be knowledgeable about the warning signs of suicidal behavior. Additionally, prevention strategies must be devised that are targeted to various high-risk settings.

RESEARCH FRONTIERS

Increased public and health care professional awareness about suicide has broadened research approaches to the problem. This growth in suicide research has occurred in the increasingly fertile arena of psychiatric research generally. The contemporary study of suicide is consistent with another trend in today's psychiatric research, the finer-tuned disaggregation of psychiatric phenomena. Investigators are steadily enhancing our capacity to refine psychiatric disorders into more discrete subtypes. This work is likely to be enhanced further by current work on genetics, brain imaging, and the identification of biologic markers and trait factors in psychiatric disorders. In light of recent research discoveries, scientists may soon be able to examine whether suicidal risk is greater in people with particular chromosomal abnormalities. There may, in fact, be a genetic factor contributing to suicidal behavior independent of psychiatric diagnosis. This topic is explored by Kety (Chapter 5, this volume). Research is now under way to determine whether the abnormally low level of metabolites of the neurotransmitter serotonin found in violent suicide attempters and completers is also found in teenagers (see Winchel et al., Chapter 4, this volume). Scientists are examining the extent to which this biologic variable is a meaningful measure in individual suicides across psychiatric disorders.

Additionally, epidemiologic studies have been sharpened to examine suicide in both adults and children. The psychological autopsy method has been used with renewed vigor in studies of teenage suicide. In cases of youth suicide, there are greater opportunities than with adults to interview the entire family, friends, teachers, and health care professionals. Thus the possibility for reconstruction of the events leading to the suicide is increased and makes psychological autopsy in this population a particularly fruitful diagnostic tool. Research studies have also helped identify high-risk groups of young people, including children of parents who have made suicide attempts, runaway youth, young women undergoing an unwanted pregnancy, truants, and teenagers in trouble with the law (Blumenthal and Kupfer 1988). Investigators have focused more closely on determining the particular risk factors for each of these groups and on targeting intervention strategies specifically for these high-risk populations.

Of particular importance to the problem of teenage suicide is the issue of "copycat" or imitative phenomena (see Gould, Chapter 19, this volume). The adolescent period is well described as a time when young people are in the process of self-definition and individuation and often choose role models from their peers. This increases the likelihood of emulating peer behavior, whether it be constructive or destructive. Conflicting reports about the impact of fictional suicide portrayals on television increasing the youth suicide rate have motivated investigators to examine this phenomenon further. Gould and Shaffer (1986) concluded that current evidence strongly supports the existence of imitative suicides following media coverage of nonfictional suicides and that in some instances media presentations and fictional suicide stories may also increase the incidence of attempted and completed suicides. They suggest that either an interaction effect with geographic location or some dose-response effect explains what at first seem like contradictory findings (i.e., the excess of suicides following broadcast of fictional suicide television films in the New York and Cleveland region, but not in the Dallas or Los Angeles areas) (Gould et al. 1988). A recent report (Davidson et al. 1989), however, did not find that exposure to suicide was a significant risk factor in two adolescent suicide clusters.

Another important aspect of a comprehensive approach to teenage suicide is the need to evaluate current suicide prevention efforts for their effectiveness. This should be considered both under the overall research agenda and as a part of any institutional, clinical, or educational intervention strategy.

STRATEGIES FOR SUICIDE PREVENTION

Most suicide research is designed to enhance our ability to predict who will actually commit suicide. Pokorny (1983) emphasized the difficulty of prediction due to the large numbers of false positives identified by certain risk factors (i.e., gender, marital status). He focused on the differences between prediction in clinical practice and that based on prospective research. For example, Pokorny stressed the need for clinicians to pay greater attention to suicide as a clinical phenomenon and to integrate their evaluations of patients with knowledge of risk factors from the research literature. The clinician should conceptualize the subsequent assessment process as a search for additional warning signs to determine what course of action is warranted. This type of approach to suicidal patients needs to be emphasized in clinical training and in continuing medical education programs as well. Pokorny also provided an important message to lawyers, judges, the courts, and to the general public: it is unrealistic to assume that clinicians can predict with complete certainty who will eventually suicide. However, research findings do suggest certain factors, settings, and conditions when the likelihood of suicide is increased (Blumenthal, Chapter 26, this volume). For example, alcoholic patients who suffer rejection and interpersonal loss are at higher risk for suicide (Robins 1985) as are boys who have made a previous suicide attempt serious enough to be admitted to a psychiatric inpatient facility (Shaffer et al. 1988). By assessing factors from several risk domains using our current best knowledge about psychological, genetic, and biochemical correlates of suicide, an enhanced predictive capacity should be achieved (Blumenthal, Chapter 26, this volume). Studies that integrate these various streams of research and test interventions that target all of the risk domains must be encouraged.

One problem facing planners of suicide prevention programs is the lack of substantial and convincing data about the efficacy of existing programs. In the past, little systematic research has been undertaken to compare and test different interventions (Bridge et al. 1977; Hirsch 1981; Shaffer et al. 1988). Evaluation studies of suicide prevention centers have generally not found much of an impact on preventing suicide (Shaffer et al. 1988). In a review of the literature, Shaffer et al. documented the existence of 1,000 suicide prevention programs operating in the United States in 1976, reaching about 150,000 teenagers. The greatest numbers of calls received by these hotlines dealt with matters other than suicide. Findings from studies evaluating these programs suggest that most callers were not acutely suicidal and may have been better served by more individualized treatment approaches. Efforts to conduct evaluation research have also been complicated by the underreporting of suicides, the geographic mobility of people being studied, difficulties in measuring the delayed effects of programs, the lack of comparable measures and methods across research studies, problems in the follow-up of anonymous hotline callers, the rarity of suicide, and ethical problems in withholding interventions from high-risk individuals. Before costly broad-based suicide prevention programs are undertaken, model preventive and treatment interventions in communities should be evaluated and tested.

One possible focus for prevention is community-based suicide prevention programs closely tied to the educational system. Shaffer et al. (1988) concluded that a large problem with school-based programs is that they are not targeted to high-risk groups because they are based on the assumption that any normal adolescent may commit suicide. Therefore, all teenagers are targeted for the preventive intervention. For example, given the adolescent suicide rate of 12.5 per 100,000, 100 high-school-based suicide prevention programs that reach 150,000 young people would prevent 18 of the 2,000 youth suicides (if maximally successful) reported annually in the United States. One can see the weakness in this approach, since at best only 18 of the 2,000 potential suicides could be saved. Further, the notion that suicide can affect any adolescent creates a nondiscriminating mental health focus, ignoring data that demonstrate that most teenagers who commit suicide have some psychiatric problem.

More extensive and refined evaluation of suicide prevention programs is needed to shed light on their efficacy and on what components of the intervention are most helpful. The results of these studies should be used to modify the nature of extant programs. Increased focus on high-risk groups to enhance the productivity of prevention efforts should be a prime target of such studies.

Additionally, collaborative efforts are needed between researchers, clinicians, media experts, and policymakers to explore methods to modify the portrayal of suicide in the media to eliminate the potential role of imitation as a contributory factor. Deromanticizing stories about suicide in the press, minimizing the coverage of suicide stories, accompanying media presentations with information about available sources of help, and avoiding the details of the suicide method all have been suggested (Gould, Chapter 19, this volume) as ways of preventing potential tragedies.

Other policy issues for suicide prevention relate to environmental and societal contributions to suicidal behavior. For example, the availability of firearms has been noted to be an important factor. Boyd and Moscicki (1986) reported that the dramatic increase in the teenage suicide rate is paralleled by an increase in the availability of firearms. Moreover, the use of firearms as a means of suicide has been associated with intoxication of the victim at the time of death. In fact, the proportion of youth who suicide having blood levels of alcohol indicative of intoxication has increased nearly fourfold since 1960 (Brent et al. 1987).

Public Policy Recommendations

Suicide prevention efforts should benefit immensely from today's increased attention by researchers, educators, and policymakers. The following research and policy recommendations represent a compilation of the recommendations *taken directly* from the Youth Suicide Task Force Report (Alcohol, Drug Abuse, and Mental Health Administration 1989) and the National Institute of Mental Health's (1988) program announcement on suicide and suicidal behavior. The reader is advised to consult these documents for a more in-depth discussion of these excellent recommendations. Greater public, health care professional, and societal attention to these recommendations should contribute to reducing this public health problem.

Research

There is an urgent need to increase our knowledge about suicidal behavior and suicide through enhanced systematic research efforts, including further attention to the following issues:

Suicide Surveillance Data. The collection of accurate data on suicide is essential to research, services, and educational programs. Uniform and consistent standards for classifying suicidal behavior should be developed and utilized. Surveillance systems must be improved to identify and report attempted and completed suicides at the local, state, and national levels. Collaborative efforts need to be established between mental health professionals and the medical examiner's office to conduct systematic psychological autopsy studies on suicidal deaths.

Definitions of Suicidal Behavior. Most studies of suicide have employed different terms and definitions, which complicates the comparison of research findings across studies. Careful attention must be paid to ensure the validity and reliability of instrumentation and methodologies used to assess and classify suicidal behavior in research studies (i.e., suicidal ideation needs to be differentiated from a carefully planned suicidal act) (NIMH 1988).

Instrumentation and Methodology. In studies of suicidal behavior where psychopathology will be assessed, standardized diagnostic methods should be employed. Interdisciplinary research that broadens perspectives and methods from other fields of study should be applied to suicide research. Studies that incorporate biological and psychosocial approaches to the study of risk factors and treatment should also be encouraged. This includes clinical investigations of psychosocial, psychiatric, and biological factors (including genetic, familial, and biochemical approaches) with a broad array of psychometric instruments (including standardized questionnaires, self-reports, clinical interviews, and postmortem assessments). New valid and reliable research instruments for assessing suicidal behavior and its epidemiology over the life cycle must be developed. Attention must be paid to the selection of cases for studies and the representativeness of appropriate control or comparison groups (NIMH 1988).

Multidisciplinary Research. Broad-based, multidisciplinary research efforts on suicide are needed. More research should be undertaken on the epidemiology of suicide, on its short- and long-term risk factors, and on protective factors. In this regard, population-based, prospective longitudinal studies are needed. Researchers should be encouraged to "piggyback" questions about suicide onto ongoing, longitudinal data sets originally collected for other purposes.

Risk Factor Definition and Assessment. Attention must be paid to the reliability and validity of risk factor assessment, particularly to data obtained from retrospective studies where poor recall, selective nonreporting, and bias may influence outcome. Research is needed to determine the contribution of significant risk factors, such as human immunodeficiency virus (HIV) infection, substance abuse, previous suicide attempts, and humiliating life events, in increasing the risk of suicidal behavior over the life cycle. Investigations of the relative contribution of particular risk factors at different stages of the life span and protective factors that may operate at each stage to modify risk are needed. In this regard, research on the developmental precursors, predictors, and correlates differentiating child and adolescent suicidal behavior from these behaviors in adults and elderly populations should be undertaken (NIMH 1988).

Basic Biological Mechanisms. Studies are needed "to increase our understanding of the underlying brain systems and mechanisms hypothesized to be related to suicidal behavior, including the role of serotonin in the brain, the mechanism of action of psychotropic drugs used to treat psychiatric disorders associated with suicide, neuroendocrine studies examining systems implicated in depression, and suicide, and basic brain studies in animal models of self-destructive behavior. In postmortem biological studies, attention must be paid to the quality of the case and control specimens, the handling procedures, and the quality of the available clinical information"(NIMH 1988, p. 6).

Genetic Factors. Research is needed on the biochemical and molecular genetic determinants of suicide and their phenotypic expression to improve diagnostic classification of the psychiatric disorders. Studies should be undertaken of the genetic epidemiology of suicidal behavior and suicide, including the elucidation of the contributions and interactions of environmental factors and individual biological vulnerability (NIMH 1988).

Psychosocial Studies. Studies of the psychosocial correlates of suicidality at different stages of the life cycle should be encouraged, including exploration of vulnerability to emotional separation, early loss of parents and/or significant others, and premorbid character configuration. Recent stressful life events further require examination.

Association With Psychiatric and Personality Disorders. More research is needed on the relationship of antecedent conditions to suicidal behavior and suicide, including mood, conduct, substance abuse, and personality disorders as well as schizophrenia. Studies on the contribution of traits and/or behavior patterns (e.g., aggressivity, impulsivity, aggression, excessive perfectionism) to suicidal behaviors are needed.

Association With Medical Illnesses. Studies of the association of medical illnesses (e.g., AIDS, epilepsy, cancer, diabetes) and suicidal behavior are needed. Variables to be examined include the contribution of neurological and neurochemical predictors of suicide (i.e., neurotransmitters, neuroendocrine modulators, and neuropathological correlates) and immunological variables. The mechanisms by which mood and behavioral changes are affected in medical illnesses require further examination. Additionally, the role of specific protective factors in people with medical illnesses, including the strength of social supports and specific personality traits, must be studied. Research on the interaction of these variables and the mechanisms by which suicidal behavior is precipitated in medically ill persons over the life cycle is needed.

Comorbidity. Studies of diagnostic comorbidity predictive of suicidal behavior throughout the life span and the mechanisms underlying the production of self-destructive behavior are needed (e.g., mood and personality disorders; substance abuse, depression, and medical illness).

Protective Factors. Studies must be encouraged of protective factors that buffer the risk of suicidal behavior, including the role of social supports and receiving appropriate treatment.

Suicide Clusters.   Studies are needed of suicide clusters and the mechanisms of contagion, including the role of the media.

Treatment Research.   Research on the full range of short- and long-term treatments, including psychosocial, psychopharmacological, and environmental interventions and their combinations at different stages of the life cycle should be undertaken.

Research Advocacy.   Policymakers, health care professionals, and the general public must be encouraged to advocate for suicide research in both the public and private sectors.

Prevention and Interventions

Establishment of a Suicide Prevention Data Bank.   The full range of suicide prevention methods, including information about their efficacy, should be coalesced into an authoritative document to communicate to the general public and to the health, regulatory, and legal systems the facts regarding the scope of the problem and intervention and prevention strategies. Uniform procedures and protocols should be developed and tested for detecting, assessing, and treating suicidal people (Alcohol, Drug Abuse, and Mental Health Administration 1989).

Studies of Preclinical Preventive Interventions.   Studies of preventive interventions that precede clinical diagnosis are needed. Research is also needed on "promotive interventions that aim to develop, maintain, and enhance healthy psychosocial functioning." Such interventions should be based on empirically derived theoretical models, with a research design and procedures appropriate to the developmental and sociodemographic characteristics of the target group. Studies should have a sufficiently long duration to determine the efficacy of the intervention (National Institute of Mental Health 1988).

High School Education Prevention Programs.   Mental health information regarding self and peer recognition of psychiatric symptoms, coping strategies, stress management, and the value of appropriate mental health treatment should be incorporated into high school education programs.

Evaluation Studies. Comprehensive evaluation of prevention efforts should be undertaken to ensure that prevention programs are effective and to enable refinement and modification as new information is gathered. "Interventions should particularly focus on high-risk groups for suicide, including middle-aged and elderly white males, male youth, and persons with chronic medical illnesses. Types of preventive interventions include interpersonal cognitive problem solving, group skills training, life skills training, social competence promotion, stress management, and assertiveness training. Such interventions can be implemented in a range of settings, including the workplace, family, and educational, health services, and community institutions." The efficacy of multiple interventions to prevent suicidal behavior requires testing (National Institute of Mental Health 1988).

Preventive Interventions in Primary Health Care Settings. Studies of the effectiveness of primary care practitioners (i.e., physicians, nurses) in detecting patients across the life cycle who are at high risk for suicide are needed. In this regard, systematically designed research interventions aimed at enhancing the identification and management of these patients in primary care settings should be encouraged (National Institute of Mental Health 1988).

Service Utilization Research. Studies of service utilization and the follow-up care received by suicide attempters in health and mental health settings are needed (NIMH 1988).

Development of Community Suicide Response Plans. Communities should develop a response plan to deal with the problem of suicide both before tragedies occur and to employ when suicides take place in the community. Suicide attempt and completion clusters must be quickly identified so that this plan can be rapidly implemented. This involves developing an early warning surveillance system for unusual patterns of suicide attempts and completions (O'Carroll, Chapter 18, this volume). Particular attention should be given to special high-risk groups and/or situations including children of parents who have made a suicide attempt, runaway youth, pregnant teenagers, teenage males who are hospitalized for a serious suicide attempt, and others. A composite of these various high-risk individuals and situations should be formulated and distributed to those persons who are in positions to detect these situations and to intervene. State and local health organizations should collaborate to develop pilot intervention programs for these groups. Comprehensive mental health services linked to crisis hotlines should be developed and publicized (ADAMHA 1989; O'Carroll, Chapter 18, this volume).

Suicide Prevention Advocacy. Advocacy is needed to limit the availability of firearms, the number one method for suicide in the United States.

Education and Training

Clinical Training Curricula. Directors of training programs for health and mental health care professionals must ensure that the educational curricula contain state-of-the-art knowledge about risk factors, assessment, and treatment of suicidal behavior.

Broad-Based Training Programs. Education and training programs on suicide should be developed for medical examiners, coroners, and other public health state officials to help facilitate more accurate reporting. Persons who have frequent contact with teenagers (e.g., teachers, pediatricians, counselors) should be educated regarding the warning signs of suicidal behavior and referral practices (ADAMHA 1989).

Media Education. Concerted efforts should be made to bring together scientists, clinicians, policymakers, and media specialists to develop guidelines about effective ways to minimize the potentially adverse effects of both nonfictional and fictional media coverage of suicide.

Enhanced Awareness and Coalition Building. Educational efforts are needed to promote awareness among policymakers, civic leaders, health care professionals, and the general public, that they all play a key role in the prevention of suicide and can form coalitions to enhance support of suicide research and prevention programs.

CONCLUSION

The problem of suicide, like other issues of concern to the mental health field, is benefiting from new research technologies, advances in the neurosciences and clinical psychiatry, and our society's increased attention and readiness to deal more openly with mental illness. Research to date has identified specific risk factors for suicide that can serve as a basis for carefully designed prevention efforts. There is strong epidemiologic and clinical evidence that the diagnosis of a psychiatric disorder is a powerful risk factor for suicidal behavior across the life cycle. Other important risk factors include gender, age, lower socioeconomic status, substance abuse, a family history of suicidal behavior, exposure to suicide, certain biological factors, specific personality traits, lack of social supports, and access to lethal methods.

As has been emphasized throughout this volume, suicide is a complex, multifaceted behavior: there is no one reason why a person ends his or her life. The trend toward disaggregation of psychiatric phenomena into subtypes (in more refined and differentiated ways) is contributing to our increased knowledge about suicide. Strikingly, suicide is the most serious complication of psychiatric illness. Most assuredly, enhanced research efforts and greater clinical and educational attention to this public health problem and to psychiatric disorders generally will benefit the health of our nation. It is unfortunate that we have to wait until public health problems such as youth suicide take on epidemic proportions before our society takes notice. While this has been too often true of other major social problems, the good news is that we now appear ready to intervene decisively. For policymakers, the richness of the research menu outlined in this chapter should be understood: increased support in fiscal, person power, and other resources is needed to mount a full-fledged attack on this public health problem. This will lead us to more intensive examinations of suicide over the life cycle, built on the strong foundation and excitement in psychiatric research occurring in our country today.

REFERENCES

Alcohol, Drug Abuse, and Mental Health Administration: Report of the Secretary's Task Force on Youth Suicide, Vol 1–4. (DHHS Pub No ADM-89-1623). Washington, DC, U.S. Government Printing Office, 1989

Blumenthal SJ: Suicide: a guide to risk factors, assessment, and treatment of suicidal patients. Med Clin North Am 72:937–971, 1988

Blumenthal SJ, Kupfer DJ: Overview of early detection and treatment strategies for suicidal behavior in young people. Journal of Youth and Adolescence 17:1–23, 1988

Boyd JH, Moscicki EK: Firearms and youth suicide. Am J Public Health Soc 76:1240–1242, 1986

Brent DA, Perper JA, Allman CJ: Alcohol, firearms, and suicide among youth. JAMA 257:3369–3372, 1987

Brent DA, Perper JA, Goldstein CT, et al: Risk factors for adolescent suicide: a comparison of adolescent suicide victims with suicidal inpatients. Arch Gen Psychiatry 45:581–588, 1988

Bridge TP, Potkin SG, Zung WW, et al: Suicide prevention centers. J Nerv Ment Dis 164:18–24, 1977

Cohen-Sandler R, Berman L, King RA: Life stress and symptomatology: determinants of suicidal behavior in children. Journal of the American Academy of Child Psychiatry 21:178–186, 1982

Davidson LE, Rosenberg ML, Mercy JA, et al: An epidemiologic study of risk factors in two teenage suicide clusters. JAMA 261:2687–2692, 1989

Gould MS, Shaffer D: The impact of suicide in television movies: evidence of imitation. N Engl J Med 315:690–694, 1986

Gould MS, Shaffer, D, Kleinman, M: The impact of suicide in television movies: replication and commentary. Suicide Life Threat Behav 18:90–99, 1988

Hirsch S: A critique of volunteer-staffed suicide prevention centers. Can J Psychiatry 26:406–410, 1981

Klerman GL, Weissman MN: Increasing rates of depression. JAMA 261:2229–2235, 1989

Motto JA: Suicide in male adolescents, in Suicide in the Young. Edited by Sudak HS, Ford AB, Rushforth NA. Boston, MA, John Wright PSG, 1984

National Institute of Mental Health: Studies of Suicide and Suicidal Behavior Program Announcement (Catalog of Federal Domestic Assistance No 13242). Rockville, MD, Department of Health and Human Services, 1988

Pokorny AD: Prediction of suicide in psychiatric patients. Arch Gen Psychiatry 40:249–257, 1983

Robins E (ed): The Final Months: A Study of the Lives of 134 Persons Who Committed Suicide. New York, Oxford University Press, 1981

Robins E: Suicide, in Comprehensive Textbook of Psychiatry IV. Edited by Kaplan H, Sadock B. Baltimore, MD, Williams & Wilkins, 1985, pp 1311–1315

Shaffer D, Garland A, Gould M, et al: Preventing teenage suicide: a critical review. J Am Acad Child Adolesc Psychiatry 27:675–687, 1988

Shafii M, Shafii SL: Pathways of human development, normal growth, and emotional disorders, in Infancy, Childhood, and Adolescence. New York, Thieme-Stratton, 1982

Shafii M, Carrigan S, Whittinghill JR, et al: Psychological autopsy of completed suicide in children and adolescents. Am J Psychiatry 149:1061–1064, 1985

Shafii M, Steltz-Lenarsky J, McCue Derrick A, et al: Comorbidity of mental disorders in the post-mortem diagnosis of completed suicide in children and adolescents. J Affective Disord 15:227–233, 1988

Stearns AW: Cases of probable suicide in young persons without obvious motivation. Journal of the Maine Medical Association 44:16–23, 1953

Section 4

Synopsis and Epilogue

Chapter 26

An Overview and Synopsis of Risk Factors, Assessment, and Treatment of Suicidal Patients Over the Life Cycle

Susan J. Blumenthal, M.D., M.P.A.

O NE OF THE most difficult clinical problems facing the health care professional is the prediction and prevention of suicide. Most general physicians see at least six seriously suicidal patients each year and will encounter many more patients in their practices who have suicidal thoughts and feelings. Between 50% to 80% of people who commit suicide have seen a doctor in the weeks to month prior to their death and often use medications prescribed by their physician to end their lives (Barraclough et al. 1974; Dorpat and Ripley 1960; Hagnell et al. 1981; Robins 1981; Robins et al. 1959). This disturbing fact can change through increased health care professional education about suicide. This chapter underscores the message of other chapters in this volume, namely that prevention of completed suicide depends on the medical and mental health practitioner's early detection and intervention with patients at risk for suicidal behavior.

Another goal of this chapter is to provide the reader with a comprehensive summary of *Suicide Over the Life Cycle* by presenting several theoretical models for understanding suicidal behavior across the life cycle, distilling what we know from the research literature about risk factors, including sociodemographic, psychiatric, psycho-

This chapter has been adapted from Blumenthal SJ: Suicide: A Guide to Risk Factors, Assessment, and Treatment of Suicidal Patients. Med Clin North Am 72:937–971, 1988, with permission from W. B. Saunders.

social, genetic, and biological variables, and translating this information into clinical assessment and intervention strategies for suicidal patients. This review is meant to be an *overview* and *condensation* of the excellent chapters in this volume that precede it, where the reader should turn for more complete and detailed discussions of the topics raised in this chapter. The reader should use this chapter as a synopsis of the salient points emphasized in this volume when time does not permit more in-depth study. The important points to remember in the assessment of suicidal patients are emphasized here. This chapter is meant to provide the clinician with a framework for carrying out rigorous diagnostic evaluations and formulating rational and effective treatment plans.

One of the most important facts to remember is that most suicidal patients are suffering from a psychiatric disorder. In fact, suicide is one of the most common complications of mental illness, carrying with it a 10 times greater risk than in the general population (see Black and Winokur, Chapter 6, this volume; Barraclough et al. 1974; Dorpat and Ripley 1960; Goldberg 1981; Guze and Robins 1970; Hillard et al. 1983; Miles 1977; Morrison 1982; Pokorny 1964). Importantly, more psychiatric patients are treated by primary-care physicians than by psychiatrists, with more than 88% of patients experiencing a first psychiatric crisis seeking medical rather than psychiatric treatment. It has also been estimated that 25% to 30% of ambulatory patients in general medical practices have a diagnosable psychiatric condition (Blumenthal 1984). In addition, 10% to 15% of people suffering from major psychiatric illnesses such as affective disorder, schizophrenia, and alcoholism will end their lives by suicide (Miles 1977). Unfortunately, physicians detect only one of six patients who go on to kill themselves, even though information about warning signs may have been available from others (Barraclough et al. 1974; Murphy 1972). For many of these patients, the physician has missed the psychiatric diagnosis or, if recognized, has undertreated the illness. Therefore, attempts at targeting efforts to prevent successful suicide—that is, to detect all behavior that leads to a final common pathway, which is suicide completion—is best done if there is an understanding of the various risk-factor domains through which suicidal behavior emerges. Since these domains can be detected and manipulated, they represent important opportunities for the clinician to intervene. The clinician, then, has a critical role to play in the early detection and clinical diagnosis of mental illness, which is a cornerstone to prevention, effective intervention, and treatment of suicidal behavior.

EPIDEMIOLOGY OF SUICIDE

Suicide is the eighth leading cause of death in the United States today and the third leading killer of young people. In 1987, 30,796 suicides were recorded in our country, 4,924 of these by young people, ages 15 to 24 (see Buda and Tsuang, Chapter 2, this volume). The rate of suicide for our nation's youth has tripled over the past 30 years (Blumenthal 1984; Centers for Disease Control 1987b). The actual number of suicides may be two to three times higher because of the underreporting that occurs. In addition, many single motor car accidents and many homicides are, in fact, suicides. In the world at least 1,000 suicides occur each day; 645,680 years of productive life are lost each year alone in the United States due to deaths by suicide. Of these productive years lost attributable to suicide, 71% occurred among white males; white females accounted for another 19% (Centers for Disease Control 1987a).

Suicide cuts across all age, racial, occupational, religious, and social groups (see Buda and Tsuang, Chapter 2; Diekstra, Chapter 20, this volume). Considerable research efforts have been made to determine specific demographic risk factors for suicide over the life cycle. Important differences have been found in sociodemographic variables, including age, race, and sex. The most pronounced shifts in suicide rates are occurring for particular age groups. Suicide rates are known to increase steadily with age, but current rates for young adults, ages 25 to 34, are rivaling those in older age groups. While the overall base rate of suicide (12.7/100,000) has remained about the same over the past 20 years, the rate has soared for young people ages 15 to 24 and has increased by 25% for the elderly from 1981 to 1986 (Centers for Disease Control 1987a, 1987b). However, although the rates for young people have plateaued since 1980, it is not yet clear if they have begun to decline. Nonetheless, the United States now has one of the highest suicide rates for young men in the world, surpassing Japan and Sweden, countries long identified with high rates of suicide. One group of youth at lower risk for suicide are college students, with rates about half that of their nonstudent age-mates (see Schwartz and Whitaker, Chapter 12, this volume). Reports of suicide among very young children are rare, but suicidal behavior is not. As many as 12,000 children, ages 5 to 14, may be hospitalized in this country every year for deliberate self-destructive acts (Department of Health and Human Services 1986; Pfeffer 1981).

Why has this increase in youth suicide over the past 20 years occurred? A number of explanations have been proposed to account for the rise in the youth suicide rate. Increasing rates of suicide appear to parallel the rise in risk factors associated with suicide in young people, including depression, conduct disorders, and substance abuse (Klerman 1989; Robins 1986; see Vaillant and Blumenthal, Chapter 1, this volume). Holinger and Offer (1982) suggest that the increase in youth suicide is related to population effects. They hypothesize that when the proportion of youth in the society is high, then a rise in suicide will occur. These authors propose that large numbers of young people in a society result in increased competition for desirable opportunities such as jobs and educational experiences that in turn may lead to failure to achieve goals. This may result in hopelessness, despair, and suicidal ideation and behavior for some youth (see Brent and Kolko, Chapter 11, this volume). A similar pattern of high youth suicide rates occurred at the beginning of the 20th century when young people also comprised a higher proportion of the total population (Goldney and Katsikitas 1983; Hendin 1986; Holinger et al. 1987). Other theories link the dramatic rise in youth suicide rates to the increase in violent behavior and access to violent methods (Boyd and Moscicki 1986). Some researchers postulate that the increased rates of both depression and suicide shifting to younger age groups in recent years may be due to certain social influences such as the increased divorce rate, geographic mobility (with its loss of attachments), changes in family structure, increased urbanization, and decreased religious affiliation, interacting with individual genetic vulnerability (see Vaillant and Blumenthal, Chapter 1, this volume; Klerman and Weissman 1989).

Despite the rapid increase in youth suicide, the highest suicide rates and greatest number of suicides are in older people. Although this group comprises 26% of the total United States population, it accounts for approximately 39% of deaths by suicide. White males over the age of 50 represent the preponderance of these deaths (Department of Health and Human Services 1986). Epidemiologic research has shown that large birth cohorts demonstrate higher suicide rates at every age level (Blumenthal 1984; Goldney and Katsikitas 1983). As the post-World War II generations move into the older age groups, suicide is likely to become an even more significant problem for these birth cohorts (Goldney and Katsikitas 1983; Hendin 1986).

The overwhelming majority of completed suicides across the life cycle are males. They comprise approximately three-fourths of the total, with white males accounting for about 70%. Well over half of male suicides shoot themselves, and the use of guns is increasing rapidly. Women attempt suicide three times as frequently as men, using potentially less lethal means, including medications and wrist slashing. However, one-third of women who complete suicide and over half of the 15- to 29-year-old group use guns. This has been an alarming trend since the 1970s, when the use of firearms became the primary method of suicide for younger people (Blumenthal 1988; Boyd 1983; Boyd and Moscicki 1986; Brent et al. 1987; Centers for Disease Control 1987a, 1987b).

College students, who have a 50% lower suicide rate than their nonuniversity-attending peers, use guns less frequently as a method of suicide (see Schwartz and Whitaker, Chapter 12, this volume). Among racial groups, whites commit suicide twice as frequently as blacks. However, sharp increases in the suicide rate among young black men have been reported. Native American youth also have a very high rate of suicide, with the highest rate being for young people in those tribes that are undergoing faster cultural assimilation (see Brent and Kolko, Chapter 11, this volume). While Hispanics have a lower suicide rate than whites, more than one in three Hispanic men and more than one in four Hispanic women who commit suicide are under the age of 25 (Smith et al. 1985). Religious groups with the highest rates of suicide are Protestants followed by Jews and Catholics. Other important sociodemographic factors include being separated or divorced, losing a job, living alone, and being recently bereaved (see Adam, Chapter 3, this volume; Blumenthal 1988).

Research findings provide evidence for the delineation of two separate but overlapping groups of people who engage in suicidal behavior at different points in the life cycle: those who attempt suicide and those who complete suicide (Blumenthal 1988; Brown et al. 1982a; Linehan 1986). Attempters tend to be younger and more often women, and their attempts tend to be more impulsive and ambivalent. Completers are most often male, tend to be older, and use more lethal methods for self-destruction (Blumenthal 1988; Frances 1986; Department of Health and Human Services 1986). A history of a previous suicide attempt is one of the most powerful predictors of suicide (Linehan 1986; Tuckman and Youngman 1968). About 1% of suicide attempters will go on to kill themselves each year; 10% to 20% of suicide attempters eventually end their lives by suicide (Avery and Winokur 1978). Additionally, persons who threaten suicide have higher rates of completed suicide (Fowler et al. 1979; Pokorny 1966).

Research has also suggested that different psychiatric disorders are associated with suicide attempts and completions across the life cycle. Nonfatal attempters are more likely to have personality disorders, chemical dependence, and situational disorders. Weissman et al. (1989) found that 20% of patients with the diagnosis of panic disorder had made a suicide attempt, a finding that could not be explained by the comorbidity of substance abuse and/or affective disorder. Those who actually kill themselves have shown a predominance of major affective disorders, alcoholism, schizophrenia, and, in young people, conduct disorders and depression. The co-occurrence of one of these illnesses with certain personality disorders, including antisocial and borderline personalities, appears to increase suicidal risk significantly (Blumenthal 1984; Blumenthal and Kupfer 1986a, 1988; Frances 1986; Frances and Blumenthal 1989; Department of

Health and Human Services 1986).

However, there are limitations in trying to predict suicide based on these demographic variables (Motto 1977). In trying to do so, Pokorny (1983) found many false positives, that is, people who had a number of risk factors but who did not go on to kill themselves. Nonetheless, despite the low base rate of suicide in the general population, the clinician and patient are best served when all symptoms and clues of suicidal behavior are assessed and when rapid intervention is undertaken.

SOCIOCULTURAL AND PSYCHOLOGICAL EXPLANATIONS OF SUICIDE

The physician is no stranger to death. Clearly, one goal of the practice of medicine is to avert untimely mortality. Therefore, the clinician may be particularly perplexed by patients who want to end their lives. There is *no one reason* why people decide to kill themselves. Suicide is a complex human behavior and is the final common pathway for many human problems. This self-destructive act can reflect many motivational determinants across the life cycle: personal and interpersonal, biological, familial, and cultural. For many, it is a response to loss, separation, and abandonment. For some, it may represent a release from the despair of what seems to be a barren future or the hopelessness of old age. For others, it may be an impulsive act, experienced as revenge for rejection. For yet others, it may symbolize the desire to be reunited with a lost loved one. Suicide can also be a response to the disordered thinking of psychoses, a toxic state such as drug use, or the cognitive distortions that occur with depressive illness or schizophrenia (Blumenthal 1984; 1988).

Suicides have been reported throughout history with several biblical references to self-destructive acts. Reports of suicidal behavior have been found in most ancient literary texts, but the root of the religious prohibition against suicide comes from the Judeo-Christian tradition (Hankoff and Einsidler 1979). As the frequency of suicide among early Christians began to increase, the Church introduced the concept that suicide was both a sin and a crime. In the fourth century, St. Augustine rejected suicide as an option. He reasoned that suicide precluded the possibility of individual repentance and violated the Fifth Commandment relating to killing (Schneidman 1979).

The contemporary study of suicide began around the turn of the century with the contributions of two major streams of thought: sociological and psychological (see Adam, Chapter 3, this volume; Schneidman 1979). In 1897, Durkheim examined society's effects on individual behavior and posited that suicide was the result of society's influences and control over the individual. In his book *Le Suicide*, Durkheim (1951) formulated four types of suicide. The first, the "altruistic" suicide, occurs as a result of society's expectations of the individual. An example of this would be hara-kiri, where the society's customs dictate that the honorable action for the individual is to end one's own life. In the United States, the most frequent form of suicide would be the "egoistic" type. In this case, the individual has poor social supports and poor ties to the society. An example of this type of suicide is that of the older man without children who is recently divorced. The third category of suicide according to Durkheim's theory is the "anomic" suicide, where the individual's relationship to society is suddenly disrupted, such as when a person unexpectedly loses a job. "Fatalistic" suicides, the fourth type described by Durkheim, occur when individuals lose control over their own destiny, such as the mass suicide that occurred on Masada (Schneidman 1979).

Psychological explanations of suicide were first developed by Freud. Whereas Durkheim conceptualized the explanation of suicide in terms of societies' influences on the individual, Freud (1917) postulated that the reasons for suicide were intrapsychic. In his work *Mourning and Melancholia*, Freud (1917) theorized that suicide represents unconscious hostility aimed at the introjected (ambivalently viewed) love object. For Freud, suicide was viewed as "murder in the 180th degree" (Schneidman 1979).

In 1936, Zilboorg proposed a cultural-ethnological model that suggested that people at highest risk for suicide unconsciously identified with a dead person and wished to be reunited with him or her. Bender and Schilder (1937) hypothesized that suicidal behavior in children represented an attempt to escape unbearable family situations, such as being the victim of child abuse. Other psychoanalysts have extended Freud's perspective. In his book *Man Against Himself*, Menninger (1938) described the psychodynamics of hostility, formulating that the hostile drive in suicide had three components: 1) the wish to kill, 2) the wish to be killed, and 3) the wish to die (Schneidman 1979). Interpersonal theorists, including Sullivan, Horney, and Fromm, rejected Freud's drive theory and stressed the importance of the social and cultural context affecting the individual in understanding suicidal behavior. Object-relations theorists further extended the psychoanalytic formulation of suicidal behavior, suggesting that suicidal acts represent a developmental failure to negotiate the transition from the symbiotic phase of attachment to mother to the separation/individuation phase (Kohut 1977). Kohut (1977) suggests that self-destructiveness is often precipitated by failures that elicit intense feelings of shame. The suffering ego attempts to do away with the self in order to erase the disappointing reality of failure. The products of narcissistic injury (i.e., fragmentation and narcissistic rage) lead to self-destructive acts. Kernberg (1984) describes three types of self-destructive patients: the borderline whose self-mutilation is a means of control over inner chaos; the pathological narcissistic who is at extremely high risk because of grandiosity that is particularly vulnerable to trauma and heightened by aggression; and the patient with psychotic features whose suicide attempt corresponds to autistic fantasies about bodily or psychological transformation.

Other contemporary theorists have examined the role of additional emotional states, such as hopelessness (Beck 1986; Beck et al. 1974a, 1974b, 1975a, 1975b, 1979, 1985) and helplessness (Seligman 1975), in the pathogenesis of depression and suicide. Beck related the "negative triad" of depression to suicide in that the individual's thinking when depressed becomes distorted: the person has a negative view of him- or herself, the future, and the world (Beck 1986; Beck et al. 1974a, 1974b, 1975a, 1975b, 1979, 1985).

Asch (1980) has stressed the dyadic nature of suicides; that is, the suicidal act often occurs in relationship to another person and often times transfers the pain to the survivor. Adam (see Chapter 3, this volume) has proposed an attachment model for understanding suicidal behavior that posits that suicidal people are more sensitive to threats of separation and abandonment. He suggests that early deficiencies in parental care are predisposing factors to suicidal behavior; that current threats to attachment figures are precipitating factors; and that associated mental illness and alcohol/drug abuse are contributing factors that allow pathological attachments to be unmasked.

Another way of explaining suicidal behavior has been the philosophical or existential. Camus (1959) wrote in *The Myth of Sisyphus* that the most important task of man was to respond to life's apparent absurdity, meaninglessness, and despair. Other philosophers, including Hume, Sartre, Heidegger, Kant, and Nietzsche, have considered suicide to be a primary ethical problem for man (Schneidman 1979).

Over the past two decades, another model for understanding suicide has emerged: one that focuses on the biomedical aspects of self-destruction, emphasizing its relationship to psychiatric illness, familial and genetic factors, and biological abnormalities. It is my view that an overlap model incorporating the psychobiological contributions of all of these explanatory models and factors is the most comprehensive and useful framework for understanding suicidal behavior over the life cycle.

THE OVERLAP MODEL: RISK FACTOR DOMAINS FOR SUICIDAL BEHAVIOR

Five domains of risk factors—psychiatric diagnosis, personality traits and disorders, psychosocial and environmental factors, genetic and familial variables, and biochemical factors—comprise a theoretical overlap model for understanding suicidal behavior over the life cycle (Blumenthal and Kupfer 1986a). It is suggested that these five domains, organized as a matrix or multiaxial approach, provide a simple model for considering risk factors for suicide that can assist the health care professional in formulating clinical interventions as well as benefit researchers.

This overlap model of risk, shown graphically in Figure 1 as a series of interlocking Venn diagrams, represents an important alternative to notions of final common pathways or single explanatory schemas (Blumenthal and Kupfer 1986a). These risk-factor domains for suicide appear to operate across the life cycle for all age groups (see Vaillant and Blumenthal, Chapter 1, this volume). They represent not just risk factors, but also spheres of vulnerability. The overlap model posits that the presence of contributory factors from each of these domains increases the risk for suicide and helps explain why only certain patients suffering from particular psychiatric disorders at-

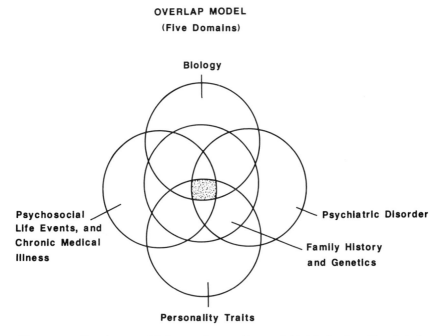

Figure 1. Overlap model for understanding suicidal behavior. Reprinted from Blumenthal SJ, Kupfer DJ: Generalizable treatment strategies for suicidal behavior. *Annals of the New York Academy of Sciences* 487:327–340, 1986, with permission from the New York Academy of Sciences.

tempt or complete suicide. For example, in applying this model, the loss of a job might be a final humiliating experience that triggers a depressive episode in a person with a family history of affective disorder. Such an individual may also be very impulsive, have poor social supports, and abuse alcohol. These factors then interact with the other identified risk factors to increase the individual's vulnerability for suicide. However, what remains to be determined is at what level and in what degree do each of these factors contribute to suicide potential. Is it the degree of overlap of all of the factors that is most significant? It is known, for example, that 15% of people who suffer from an affective disorder end their lives by suicide, but this of course means that the other 85% do not. The reasons for this phenomenon might be explained by application of the overlap model. Using this model, what may emerge, for example, is that the subgroup of patients with affective disorder who commit suicide have a greater overlap of other risk domains, such as increased hopelessness, impulsivity, decreased social supports, certain biological abnormalities, a recent humiliating life experience, and/or an increased family history of affective disorder or suicidal behavior (Blumenthal and Kupfer 1986a).

As mentioned previously, there are five domains that comprise this risk factor model. The first is a *careful clinical description according to psychiatric diagnosis*. More than 90% of adults who end their lives by suicide have an associated psychiatric illness (Barraclough et al. 1974; Black and Winokur, Chapter 6, this volume; Dorpat and Ripley 1960; Hagnell and Rorsman 1980; Robins 1981; Robins et al. 1959). The few studies on adolescent suicide suggest high percentages as well (Crumley 1982b; Shaffer 1974; Shaffer et al. 1985; Shafii et al. 1985, 1988). Current research shows that affective disorders and substance abuse in adults and conduct disorders and depression in young people are the most highly associated psychiatric diagnoses with suicide. Second, *personality traits* relating to suicide, such as aggression, impulsivity, and hopelessness, are important in and of themselves in characterizing suicide since they may represent personality styles that cross diagnostic groupings. In addition, this domain includes certain *personality disorders*, such as borderline personality and antisocial personality disorders, which are more highly correlated with suicidal behavior and represent risk factors. The comorbidity (or co-occurrence) of antisocial and depressive symptoms appears to be a particularly lethal combination in both adults and young people (Blumenthal and Kupfer 1986b, 1988; Frances 1986; Frances and Blumenthal 1986; Goldsmith et al., Chapter 7, this volume). The third domain is concerned with *psychosocial factors, social supports, life events, and chronic medical illness*. For example, early loss, increased negative life events, the presence of a chronic medical illness, exposure to suicide (both intra- and extrafamilial), and decreased social supports increase the risk for suicide. (see Adam, Chapter 3; Mackenzie and Popkin, Chapter 9, this volume). In addition, most people who end their lives have had a recent humiliating life experience (Blumenthal 1988; Blumenthal and Kupfer 1986a; Hirschfeld and Blumenthal 1986). The fourth area is the identification of both *genetic and familial factors* that predispose an individual to suicide. Investigators have suggested that the genetics of suicide may be independent of the genetics of having a family history relating to specific psychiatric disorders, such as affective disorder or alcoholism (Kety 1986; Kety, Chapter 5, this volume; Roy 1983, 1986a; Schulsinger et al. 1979; Tsuang 1977). The final domain in the overlap model are the *neurochemical and biochemical variables* currently under active investigation in an attempt to identify either a biological abnormality or a vulnerability state for suicide. In particular, a deficiency in the neurotransmitter serotonin appears to be associated with aggressive, violent suicidal behavior across psychiatric diagnoses (Ågren 1980; Åsberg et al. 1976, 1981, 1984, 1986a, 1986b; Brown and Goodwin 1986; Brown et al. 1982a, 1982b; Mann et al. 1986; Ninan et al. 1984; Oreland et al. 1981; Stanley et al. 1986; Traskman et al. 1981; Winchel et al., Chapter 4, this volume).

In summary, the following discussion of the five risk-factor domains for completed suicide over the life cycle should provide the clinician with a rubric for the early detection of suicidal behaviors. Other chapters in this volume provide the reader with an in-depth exploration of the issues raised here. The clinician, knowledgeable of the factors in these domains, will be well equipped to assess suicidal patients of all age groups and to intervene and treat these patients in his or her clinical practice.

Psychiatric Diagnosis

The risk for suicidal behavior and suicide is increased with almost every major psychiatric disorder (Barraclough et al. 1974; Black and Winokur, Chapter 6, this volume; Blumenthal 1988; Borg and Stahl 1982; Dorpat and Ripley 1960; Hagnell and Rorsman 1980; Khuri and Akiskal 1983; Miles 1977; Morrison 1982; Pokorny 1964; Robins 1981; Robins et al. 1959). Evidence from psychological autopsy studies of adult suicides (Barraclough et al. 1974; Dorpat and Ripley 1960; Hagnell et al. 1981; Robins 1981; Robins et al. 1959) and adolescent suicides (Brent and Kolko, Chapter 11, this volume; Crumley 1982b; Shaffer 1974; Shaffer and Fisher 1981; Shaffer et al. 1985, 1988; Shafii et al. 1985, 1988) reveal that most people who commit suicide were suffering from a major psychiatric illness at the time of their death, although only a small percentage were being treated (Robins 1981; Robins et al. 1959; Shaffer et al. 1985; Shafii et al. 1985). As mentioned earlier in this chapter, these studies reveal that more than 90% of people who end their lives by suicide suffered from a psychiatric disorder; less than 10% of people who kill themselves have no documentable psychiatric illness (Barraclough et al. 1974; Blumenthal 1988; Dorpat and Ripley 1960; Hagnell and Rorsman 1980; Robins et al. 1959). Affective disorders followed by alcoholism are the major psychiatric diagnoses associated with suicide in adults (Barraclough et al. 1974; Dorpat and Ripley 1960; Hagnell et al. 1981; Robins 1981; Robins et al. 1959; Winokur and Black 1987).

Suicide is the most serious and tragic complication of affective disorders, with 15% of those suffering from these illnesses ending their lives by suicide (Black and Winokur 1986; Guze and Robins 1970; Kerr et al. 1969; Miles 1977). More than 10 million Americans suffer from depressive disorders. One-quarter of all women and 10% of men in the United States will suffer from a clinical depression at some time in their life. Suicidal thoughts and plans are often symptoms of major depression, and treatment of the illness should be associated with remission of suicidal ideation in most people (see Brent and Kolko, Chapter 11; Goldblatt and Schatzberg, Chapter 15, this volume). Other symptoms include a sad mood and the persistence and clustering of several other complaints for greater than a 2-week period, including appetite changes, sleep disturbance, psychomotor agitation or retardation, loss of interest or pleasure in usual activities, loss of energy and fatigue, feelings of worthlessness, self-reproach, or excessive or inappropriate guilt, difficulty concentrating, and hopelessness. In children and adolescents, the symptoms of depression are quite similar, but, in addition, young people often have vague somatic complaints, school problems, low self-esteem, and "acting out" of aggressive behaviors. In elderly patients, depression may present with memory changes, confusion, and profound social withdrawal.

The clinician should be aware that specific subtypes of affective disorder have differential influences on prognosis and treatment (Blumenthal 1988; Brent et al. 1988a; Fawcett et al. 1987; Jamison 1986). Patients of all ages who suffer from hypomania or mania are at particularly high risk for suicide and suicidal behavior (Avery and Winokur 1978; Brent et al. 1988a; Jamison 1986; Johnson and Hunt 1979; Stallone et al. 1980) as are those patients with a mixed state (cycling between depression and mania), particularly at the time of the switch (Fawcett et al. 1987; Jamison 1986). One study of adolescent suicides found that one-fifth of the victims had a diagnosis of bipolar disorder (Brent et al. 1988b). Brent et al. (1988a) suggested that the association between suicide and bipolar affective disorder may contribute to the seasonality of suicide rates (highest in April-May and

September-October) (Lester 1971; Nayha 1983; Parker and Walter 1982; Zung and Green 1974), perhaps corresponding to the seasonal patterns of bipolar illness (Brent et al. 1988; Parker and Walter 1982). They further hypothesized that the seasonality of suicide rates may also be related to another type of affective disorder known as seasonal affective disorder (Rosenthal et al. 1984), which is characterized by hypersomnia, hyperphagia, and a depressive syndrome in the winter months, which can be treated by phototherapy. The clinician is advised to take a careful menstrual history, since it has been reported that affective disorder is exacerbated premenstrually (Abramowitz et al. 1982; Blumenthal 1988; Halbreich and Endicott 1983; Osofsky and Blumenthal 1985) and that suicidal behavior in women is increased during this period (Brent et al. 1988; Fourestié et al. 1986; Osofsky and Blumenthal 1985). Furthermore, patients who suffer from psychotic depression have a five times greater risk for completed suicide than nonpsychotic depressed patients (Roose et al. 1983). Studies have suggested that the risk for suicide may be related to the delusional component of the illness in these patients as well as to the affective state (Roose et al. 1983).

Additionally, the comorbidity (co-occurrence) of affective disorders with other psychiatric disorders, especially antisocial personality and substance abuse, are particularly lethal combinations in both adults and young people (Blumenthal 1984; Blumenthal and Kupfer 1986a, 1986b, 1988; Frances 1986; Frances and Blumenthal 1989; Rich et al. 1986; Shafii et al. 1985). These patients are especially difficult to treat and have a greater incidence of relapse (Akiskal 1982; Clayton and Lewis 1981; Weissman et al. 1981).

Therefore, the early detection and treatment of affective disorders represents a major prevention strategy for completed suicide (Blumenthal 1984, 1988; Blumenthal and Kupfer 1988; Griest and Griest 1979; Khuri and Akiskal 1983). Treatment of affective disorders includes 1) psychotherapeutic approaches, consisting of psychodynamic, cognitive/behavioral, and interpersonal therapies aimed at decreasing hopelessness and altering the cognitive distortions that may occur; and/or 2) medications, including tricyclic antidepressants, monoamine oxidase inhibitors, lithium, and other somatic treatments such as electroconvulsive shock therapy (Barraclough 1972; Bellack et al. 1981; Blackburn et al. 1981; Brent et al. 1988b; DiMascio et al. 1979; Janicak et al. 1985; Kovacs et al. 1981; Murphy et al. 1984; Rush et al. 1977). Additionally, strengthening social supports, promoting better interpersonal relationships, and providing patient and family education are also important elements of the treatment of depression (Blumenthal 1984, 1988; Blumenthal and Kupfer 1986a; Frank and Kupfer 1986).

Alcohol and substance abuse also represent major risk factors for

suicide across the life cycle in both alcoholic and nonalcoholic populations (see Flavin et al., Chapter 8, this volume). Alcohol use is associated with 25% to 50% of suicides (Barraclough et al. 1974; Dorpat
and Ripley 1960; Frances et al. 1986; Hagnell et al. 1981; Robins 1981;
Robins et al. 1959), and its contribution is second only to that made by
affective disorders. Between 5% and 27% of all deaths of alcoholics are
caused by suicide (Frances et al. 1986; Murphy 1986), with the lifetime
risk for suicide estimated to be 15% (Frances et al. 1986; Guze and
Robins 1970; Miles 1977; Murphy 1986). The relationship of suicide
and substance abuse in young people is also very significant. Substance abuse has been diagnosed in over one-third of youthful suicide
victims both alone and in combination with affective disorder (Brent et
al. 1988b; Rich et al. 1986). A recent study of adolescent suicide found
that 70% of the victims suffered from alcohol or substance abuse
problems (Shafii et al. 1985, 1988). In a study examining differences
among 133 consecutive suicide victims under the age of 30 and 150
consecutive suicides over the age of 30, 67% of the younger group
were identified as substance abusers as compared to 46% of the older
group (Rich et al. 1988). When patients are suffering from alcohol
dependence, suicide frequently occurs late in the disease and is often
related to rejection or some interpersonal loss as well as to the onset of
medical complications of the illness (Barraclough et al. 1974; Frances
et al. 1986; Miles 1977; Murphy 1986; Rich et al. 1988; Robins 1981;
Robins et al. 1959). This is in contrast to affective disorders, where
suicide often occurs earlier in the course of the illness (Khuri and
Akiskal 1983).

Alcohol and drug abuse can be a complication of other psychiatric
disorders, including affective and anxiety disorders, schizophrenia,
and certain personality disorders (Brent et al. 1988a). In fact, it is
estimated that 60% to 70% of alcoholic patients have an additional
psychiatric diagnosis (Frances et al. 1986; Murphy 1986). Additionally, it is likely that substance abuse exacerbates the course of psychiatric illnesses (Brent et al. 1988a; Frances et al. 1986; Murphy 1986;
Schuckit 1979) and may predispose to depressive symptomatology.
Many patients use alcohol and other drugs to self-medicate. Alcohol
may also potentiate other methods of suicide, such as drug overdose.
Many victims of single motor car accidents, thought to be suicides,
have been drinking. Additionally, chronic alcohol abuse may contribute to the disruption of social relationships, which may increase social
isolation (Murphy 1986). Furthermore, the biological effects of chronic
alcohol consumption include depression and central serotonergic depletion, both of which are risk factors for suicide (Frances et al. 1986;
Murphy 1986; Schuckit 1979).

For drug abusers, where the incidence of suicide is 20 times greater than that for the general population, the increased incidence of suicide may be related to a depressive reaction to the individual's dismal life circumstances, to certain vulnerable personality traits, to the lack of social supports, or to certain biological factors related to drug use (see Flavin et al., Chapter 8, this volume; Frances et al. 1986). The clinician's ability to prevent suicide in chemically dependent persons is associated with accurate diagnosis and appropriate treatment of the substance abuse and any other concurrent psychiatric disorder as well as mobilizing and strengthening the social supports of these patients (Frances et al. 1986; Murphy 1986; Schuckit 1979).

Schizophrenia, a disease that afflicts 1% of the population, carries with it a high incidence of suicide; 15% of schizophrenic patients end their life by suicide (Johns et al. 1986; Roy 1982b, 1986b). The risk is greatest for those patients who feel hopeless, are suicidal, fear mental disintegration, have made previous suicide attempts, have a chronic relapsing course to their illness, and are not compliant with treatment (Brent et al. 1988a; Drake et al. 1984; Johns et al. 1986; Roy 1986b; Virkkunen 1976). Most schizophrenic suicides are by young males who are unemployed and who had been functioning at a high level prior to the onset of the illness. Many have been suffering from symptoms of akathisia (Brent et al. 1988a; Drake and Ehrlich 1985; Shear et al. 1983). The co-occurrence of alcohol or drug abuse in these patients also contributes to suicidal risk (Alterman et al. 1984; Drake and Cotton 1986; Drake and Ehrlich 1985; Drake et al. 1984; Johns et al. 1986; Negrete et al. 1986). Additionally, there is a high incidence of nonpsychotic depression in schizophrenic patients at the time of suicidal behavior (Drake and Cotton 1986; Johnson 1980; McGlashan and Carpenter 1976; Roy 1986b). Some clinicians report that the addition of antidepressant medication to the treatment regimen may help eliminate suicidal ideation in these patients (Prusoff et al. 1979; Roy 1986b; Siris et al. 1985). It should be emphasized that early intervention and appropriate psychotherapeutic and psychopharmacological treatment are critical to the prevention of suicide in schizophrenic patients. Importantly, attention must also be paid to community interventions that link the patient to treatment and social services as well as to occupational and recreational activities.

For suicides occurring in young people, the diagnostic picture is less clear but bears resemblance to what has been found for adults (see Brent and Kolko, Chapter 11, this volume). A study by Shafii et al. (1985) found that 95% of the adolescent suicide victims had an associated psychiatric disorder. A high percentage of these young people had an affective disorder: 76% had major affective disorder or dysthymia as compared to 28% in the control group. This research also demonstrated that 70% of youngsters who end their lives by suicide have associated substance abuse, 70% have a history of anti-social behaviors, 65% have "inhibited" personality traits, and 50% have made a previous suicide attempt. Preliminary data from a large ongoing psychological autopsy study of adolescents (Shaffer et al. 1985) suggest that at least one-third of the young people in the study who ended their lives by suicide had an associated conduct disorder and that one-quarter of the sample population were suffering from a depressive disorder. In addition, a high percentage of these youth abused alcohol or drugs. Approximately 50% of these young people had a family history of suicidal behavior. Furthermore, suicide attempts in this age group have likewise been linked to depressive symptoms (Carlson and Cantwell 1982; Chiles et al. 1980; Crumley 1982a, 1982b). Many of these youngsters are angry, impulsive, and recently stressed and have problems with low self-esteem.

The high rates of suicide in older people may reflect an accumulation of risk factors as the individual ages (Vaillant and Blumenthal, Chapter 1, this volume). The actual numbers of suicides in this age group are probably underestimated because older people sometimes end their lives surreptitiously by not eating or by taking prescribed medication in overdose amounts. Depression is prevalent among the elderly as old age may bring with it an accumulation of losses, including loss of spouse, friends, health, status, and a meaningful role in society. Depression may be confused with dementia in this age group with the result that older people may not receive appropriate treatment for their illness. With advances in medical technology, there have been steady increases in longevity; this is sometimes at the cost of maintaining personal dignity, however, with "rational" suicide gaining increased acceptance in some quarters. Additionally, low-cost preventive and treatment services that may have provided the needed interventions to avert premature death may not be readily available to older people.

In summary, certain psychiatric illnesses are strongly associated with an increased risk for suicide across the life span. Almost all persons who commit suicide are suffering from a psychiatric disorder. Additionally, the triad of aggressivity, impulsivity, and depressive symptomatology represents a major contribution to risk for suicide over the life cycle (Blumenthal 1984, 1988; Blumenthal and Kupfer 1986a, 1986b, 1988). The clinician's early detection and treatment of these behaviors and illnesses in patients is an important suicide prevention strategy throughout the life span.

Personality Traits and Disorders

Personality traits and disorders have been found to be important contributory risk factors to suicide across all age groups (see Goldsmith et al., Chapter 7, this volume). Research studies suggest that antisocial and borderline personality disorders are particularly associated with suicidal behavior in adults (Frances 1986; Frances and Blumenthal 1989). This is true for adolescent suicide as well, where conduct disorders and borderline personality features are highly associated with suicide (Crumley 1981; Frances and Blumenthal 1989; Shaffer 1974; Shaffer and Fisher 1981; Shaffer et al. 1985). Additionally, the co-occurrence of depression with conduct disorder, antisocial personality disorder, or borderline personality disorder across all age groups represents an extremely lethal combination of factors (Blumenthal 1988; Blumenthal and Kupfer 1986a, 1986b, 1988; Frances 1986; Frances and Blumenthal 1989).

Although patients with borderline personality disorder often engage in self-destructive behavior without lethal intent, a substantial number (at least 5% to 10%) do eventually commit suicide (Frances 1986; Frances and Blumenthal 1989). The presence of concurrent major affective disorder and/or substance abuse increases the risk of suicide in these patients (Frances 1986). An estimated 5% of patients with antisocial personality disorder die by suicide, and as many as 46% make suicide attempts (Frances 1986; Miles 1977). Antisocial personality disorder and criminality have been reported as predictors of recurrent suicide attempts (Frances 1986). One-half of these attempts are preceded by a crisis in a significant relationship, involve a nonviolent method, and can be seen as an effort to change other people's behavior. It may be that the 5% of persons with this disorder who complete suicide also have concurrent affective disorder, substance abuse, and/or other personality traits or environmental stressors that increase risk for suicide (Frances 1986).

Research studies of young people who end their lives by suicide point to specific associated personality traits, including the tendencies to be withdrawn, perfectionistic, impulsive, or aloof (Shaffer 1974). Preliminary findings from an ongoing large psychological autopsy study of adolescents (Shaffer et al. 1985) suggest that at least one-third of the young people in the study who committed suicide had an associated conduct disorder, a disorder characterized by and thought to be associated with the development of antisocial personality disorder later in life. In fact, there appears to be a continuum of certain personality traits and disorders associated with suicidal behavior in adolescence, with such behavior in adulthood suggesting stability in some personality characteristic, such as impulsivity and aggressivity, over the life cycle (Frances 1986; Frances and Blumenthal 1989; Robins 1986).

The importance of the relationship of suicide and aggression must be underscored. The study of this association stems originally from psychodynamic formulations of depression and suicide that emphasize hostility and murderous impulses turned against the self (Frances 1986; Freud 1917). In addition, the personality variables of impulsivity and aggressivity appear to have biological correlates, including evidence of a serotonin deficiency (Ågren 1980; Åsberg et al. 1984; 1986b; Brown et al. 1982a, 1982b; Mann et al. 1986; Ninan et al. 1984; Oreland et al. 1981; Stanley et al. 1986; Traskman et al. 1981).

Other studies of the relationship of specific personality traits and suicide have found suicidal people to be more socially withdrawn, to have more interpersonal difficulties, to exhibit lower self-esteem, and to be less trusting than nonsuicidal individuals (Hirschfeld and Blumenthal 1986). Negativity and the expectation of undesirable events have been repeatedly associated with suicide attempts (Frances 1986). Excessive risk-taking behaviors have also been found in some suicidal persons (Weissman et al. 1973).

The relationship of personality variables to cognitive style has been another focus of suicide research (see Weishaar and Beck, Chapter 17, this volume). In one study (Patsiokas et al. 1979), cognitive characteristics of rigidity, impulsivity, and field dependence characterized a group of suicide attempters as compared to a group of nonsuicidal psychiatric controls, supporting the hypothesis of a cognitive predisposition to attempting suicide. Other research (Neuringer 1974) suggests that cognitively rigid individuals faced with naturally occurring life stress are unable to generate or imagine alternative solutions to their problems; as a result, they are inclined to develop feelings of helplessness and hopelessness, which, in turn, heighten the risk of suicidal ideation and/or behavior. Powerlessness and an external locus of control have also been identified in suicidal populations (Frances 1986). Studies of hysterical traits in people who suicide have yielded conflicting results. To date, there is little evidence to support increased histrionic characteristics in suicide completers (Frances 1986; Frances and Blumenthal 1986).

Another important factor in suicide is *hopelessness*. A study of hospitalized patients with suicidal ideation found that after a 5- to 10-year follow-up period, 14 of the 207 patients in the study committed suicide. Of all the data collected at the time of hospitalization, only results of the Hopelessness Scale (Beck et al. 1974a) and the pessimism item of the Beck Depression Inventory correctly identified 91% of the completed suicides. Taken in conjunction with previous studies showing the relationship between hopelessness and suicidal intent, these findings indicate the importance of the degree of hopelessness as an indicator of long-term suicidal risk across psychiatric diagnoses (Beck 1986; Beck et al. 1973, 1974a, 1974b, 1975a, 1975b, 1979, 1985; Dyer and Kreitman 1984; Wetzel 1976).

In summary, there are specific personality disorders, including antisocial and borderline personality disorders, that are more highly associated with suicide. However, it is most likely the combination of certain personality traits that cut across traditional diagnostic categories (i.e., impulsivity, hopelessness, cognitive rigidity) that are better predictors of suicidal behavior and completed suicide than specific personality disorders (Frances 1986; Frances and Blumenthal 1989).

Psychosocial and Environmental Factors

In addition to the important role of psychiatric diagnosis, personality variables, family history, and biological factors associated with suicidal behavior, it is important for the clinician to consider the critical role of psychosocial, environmental, and specific life events in understanding and preventing suicidal behavior (see Adam, Chapter 3, this volume). Recent bereavement, separation or divorce, early loss, and decreased social supports are all potentially important factors that can affect the lethality of a suicide attempt (Blumenthal 1984, 1988; Blumenthal and Kupfer 1986a, 1986b, 1988; Borg and Stahl 1982; Hirschfeld and Blumenthal 1986; Paykel et al. 1975; Petzel and Riddle 1981). Precipitants of suicidal behavior are generally humiliating life events such as interpersonal discord (particularly the breakup of an important relationship), loss of a job, impending disciplinary crisis, or the threat of incarceration (Blumenthal 1984; Blumenthal and Kupfer 1986a, 1986b, 1988; Cohen-Sandler et al. 1982; Hirschfeld and Blumenthal 1986; Murphy et al. 1979; Paykel 1986; Shaffer 1974). The shame and humiliation for the individual associated with these events is of particular importance in understanding suicide attempts and completions. Situational factors such as a chaotic family life or being the victim of physical abuse also increase the likelihood of suicidal acts if the individual is not removed from these stressors (Hirschfeld and Blumenthal 1986). For older people, who comprise the largest number of deaths by suicide, crises such as death of loved ones, retirement, and one's own physical decline are contributory factors (see Osgood and Thielman, Chapter 13, this volume; Blumenthal 1988). However, the vast majority of older people who are bereaved, depressed, or suffering from medical illness do not end their life by suicide. A history of poor adaptation to life stress, vulnerability to loss and disruptions, loss of mastery and control, and cognitive impairment caused by organic mental disorders are important risk factors that have been identified in suicidal older people (Klerman and Hirschfeld 1979).

Additionally, there is evidence that knowing someone who committed or attempted suicide or exposure to suicide through the media may render some people, particularly adolescents, more vulnerable to suicidal behavior (Blumenthal 1984, 1988; Bollen and Phillips 1982; Gould, Chapter 19, this volume; Gould and Shaffer 1986; Phillips and Carstensen 1986; Robbins and Conroy 1983; Shaffer et al. 1985; Shafii et al. 1985). This appears to be a particularly important factor in cluster suicides (Robbins and Conroy 1983). Studies have demonstrated that the reporting of a suicide on the front page of newspapers and on multiple television channels increases the rate of suicide for a 9-day period (Phillips and Carstensen 1986). Additionally, television movies about suicide have been associated with an increased rate of suicide shortly after the movies were shown (Gould and Shaffer 1986). However, a recent report analyzing two suicide clusters (Davidson et al. 1989) did not find evidence of direct or indirect exposure to suicide as a significant factor. Risk factors found to be associated with adolescent suicide in these clusters were previous suicide attempts, a previous history of self-mutilatory acts, knowing someone who died violently, violence or antisocial behavior, a history of substance abuse, and recently having broken up with a boyfriend or girlfriend. Interventions aimed at deromanticizing portrayals of suicide in the media so that the likelihood of identification is decreased should help prevent imitation.

The strength of social supports is also an important area to assess in suicidal persons. It has been well documented that the strength and quality of these supports are important in the etiology of psychiatric problems, compliance with treatment (Frank and Kupfer 1986; Haas et al. 1986), and response to treatment regimens (Hogarty et al. 1986; Khuri and Akiskal 1983). Individuals suffering from psychiatric illnesses may be more vulnerable to environmental stressors or to a loss of social support systems. Conversely, recent losses, a humiliating life event, or recent exposure to suicide may precipitate psychiatric vulnerability (Blumenthal 1984, 1988; Blumenthal and Kupfer 1986a, 1986b, 1988; Hirschfeld and Blumenthal 1986).

Although the data base is limited, there is considerable convergence of findings in the area of family and environmental factors in relation to youth suicidal behavior (see Brent and Kolko, Chapter 11, this volume; Hirschfeld and Blumenthal 1986). Adolescents who make suicide attempts are characterized by considerably increased life stress and have had many losses (particularly early loss) and significant changes within the nuclear family as compared with other psychiatrically disturbed youngsters, depressed adolescents, and the general population (Hirschfeld and Blumenthal 1986). They have also had both physical and psychiatric illnesses. Precipitating events are often humiliating and are almost invariably interpersonal problems between the adolescent and his or her parents or peers (Blumenthal

1984, 1988; Blumenthal and Kupfer 1986a, 1986b, 1988; Hirschfeld and Blumenthal 1986). The social and familial background of these adolescents is marked by parental death, divorce, or separation. Adolescents who attempt suicide have a greater number of negative life events; fewer social supports; higher incidence of being abused, running away from home, and having unwanted pregnancies; and fewer personal resources than adolescents who do not (Blumenthal and Kupfer 1986b, 1988; Shaffer et al. 1985, 1988; Shafii et al. 1985, 1988).

Medical Illness. Another important risk factor for suicide across all age groups is the presence of a chronic medical illness (see Mackenzie and Popkin, Chapter 9, this volume). In particular, diseases with chronic debilitating courses are frequent "stimuli" to suicidal behavior (Barraclough et al. 1974; Blumenthal 1984, 1988; Blumenthal and Kupfer 1986a, 1986b, 1988; Brent et al. 1988b; Dorpat et al. 1968; Hirschfeld and Blumenthal 1986; Luscomb et al. 1980; Mackenzie and Popkin 1987; Paykel et al. 1974; Robins 1981; Robins et al. 1959; Whitlock 1986). The prevalence of physical illness in suicides varies from 25% to 70% of cases and appears to be an important contributory cause in 11% to 51% (Barraclough et al. 1974; Dorpat et al. 1968; Mackenzie and Popkin 1987; Robins 1981; Robins et al. 1959; Whitlock 1986). Among those disorders most frequently associated with suicide are cancer, Huntington's chorea, epilepsy, musculoskeletal disorders, peptic ulcer disease, and AIDS (Dorpat et al. 1968; Mackenzie and Popkin 1987; Marzuk et al. 1988; Whitlock 1986; Winokur and Black 1987).

Medical illnesses appear to contribute to suicidal behavior in several ways, including 1) precipitating severe depression and/or initiating or exacerbating a psychiatric illness, or 2) producing an organic mental disorder (e.g., delirium), which leads to perceptual, cognitive, and mood changes that may predispose to impaired judgment, impulsivity, and suicidal behavior. In some cases, the choice to die by suicide may be a rational act where the prospect of suffering and loss of dignity is intolerable. However, research evidence suggests that suicide in the physically ill rarely occurs in the absence of psychiatric disorder (Dorpat et al. 1968; Mackenzie and Popkin 1987; Robins 1981; Robins et al. 1959). Therefore, the physician must carefully evaluate suicidal risk in patients suffering from these medical illnesses in his or her practice. Since the physician will treat many patients suffering from these diseases, a more detailed exploration of the association of these illnesses with suicide will be provided.

The suicide rate in epileptic patients is about four times that of normal controls (Matthews and Barabas 1981). Among patients with temporal lobe epilepsy, the rate is 25 times greater than would be expected. Epilepsy appears to be one of the medical illnesses capable of causing suicidal behavior without the patient first experiencing a period of severe depression and may be related to a sudden urge to suicide as part of an ictus (Hawton et al. 1980). Conversely, depression may occur postictally, causing some patients to become suicidal. Also, mood-impairing side effects of treatment with phenobarbital may predispose to suicidal behavior in both adults and children (Brent et al. 1988a; Mackenzie and Popkin 1987). Other characteristics of the illness, such as the unpredictable nature of the attacks and certain social restrictions and occupational limitations, may also be contributory factors (Brent et al. 1988a; Hawton et al. 1980; Mackenzie and Popkin 1987; Matthews and Barabas 1981).

Cancer has been associated with increased rates of suicide in several reports (Campbell 1966; Dorpat et al. 1968; Louhivuori and Hakama 1979; Mackenzie and Popkin 1987; Whitlock 1986). The cancer prevalence in suicide victims has been shown to be several times higher than in the general population (Campbell 1966; Dorpat et al. 1968; Louhivuori and Hakama 1979; Mackenzie and Popkin 1987; Whitlock 1986). The risk appears to be highest immediately following diagnosis and in those people receiving chemotherapy (Fox et al. 1982; Louhivuori and Hakama 1979; Mackenzie and Popkin 1987; Whitlock 1986). While suicide in people suffering from malignancies may in part be related to having a potentially terminal, painful illness requiring prolonged and difficult treatment (Siegel and Tuckel 1984-85), there may also be additional explanations, including the association of other risk factors for suicide with specific types of cancer (e.g., the association of alcohol abuse with gastrointestinal carcinoma) (Brent et al. 1988a; Louhivuori and Hakama 1979; Whitlock 1986). Some cancers, such as pancreatic tumors, are associated with depressive symptoms before overt signs of the medical disease are apparent (Brent et al. 1988a). Additionally, people with a severe and morbid fear of cancer are also at increased risk (Dorpat et al. 1968; Mackenzie and Popkin 1987; Whitlock 1986).

Other medical illnesses also are associated with an increased risk of suicide. The high rates of peptic ulceration among people who commit suicide are probably related to the prevalence of alcoholism as a cause of ulceration and gastritis (Knop and Fisher 1981; Viskum 1985; Whitlock 1986). Patients who have had surgery for their illness have higher rates of suicide (Mackenzie and Popkin 1987; Whitlock 1986). Additionally, there is a sixfold increase in the rate of suicide among people suffering from Huntington's chorea and in family members who do not yet have overt symptoms of the disease as compared to the general population (Dewhurst et al. 1970; Mackenzie and Popkin 1987; Whitlock 1986). Patients undergoing renal dialysis often experience depression, and reports have shown a 10- to 100-times greater incidence of suicide in these patients as compared to rates for the general population (Mackenzie and Popkin 1987; Whitlock 1986). This may be explained in part by the loss of pleasure experienced by some patients on renal dialysis, the diminished quality of life, the dependency on a machine for survival, the associated depression, and the higher age of patients receiving the treatment (Brent et al. 1988b). There is also evidence of increased rates of suicide in people who have suffered spinal cord injuries and in patients who have multiple sclerosis (Mackenzie and Popkin 1987). Cushing's disease, thyroid disorders, and hyperparathyroidism are endocrinopathies that may be complicated by severe depression and, if not diagnosed and treated, may result in suicidal behavior.

Acquired immune deficiency syndrome (AIDS) is a fatal and incurable illness characterized by a profound disturbance in the immune system. There is evidence that suicide may be increased in people suffering from this illness. A study revealed a 36 times greater incidence of suicide in AIDS victims than in the general population (Marzuk et al. 1988). To date, there have been more than 100,000 deaths from AIDS, and it is estimated that 1.5 to 2.0 million persons in the United States are infected with the human immunodeficiency virus (HIV). Depression frequently accompanies the disease, and, in some cases, psychiatric symptomatology and cognitive disturbances are the first signs of illness. Evidence exists that AIDS directly invades the brain. AIDS dementia complex, a syndrome characterized by progressive cognitive and motor impairment, occurs in more than half of AIDS patients and, for 10% to 20% of the patients, may be the presenting manifestation of the disease. Given the high incidence of depression, dementia, and extreme debilitation associated with AIDS along with the disruption in social supports that may accompany the illness, it can be understood why patients suffering from this illness are at increased risk for suicide.

The clinician should also be alert for the onset of depressive symptoms with possible suicidal behavior in medically ill patients being treated with certain medications. Antihypertensive medications such as propranolol and reserpine have been associated with depression. Steroids also can produce depressive or manic symptoms (Mackenzie and Popkin 1987; Whitlock 1986). Other drugs that may produce severe mood changes include antiparkinsonian agents such as levadopa, exogenous hormones, anticancer drugs, and antituberculin agents. The clinician should administer doses of these medications that keep psychiatric side effects to a minimum and be sure to change drugs if severe symptomatology persists.

Studies of the relationship of medical illness and suicide suggest that severe or incapacitating medical status when associated with depression, alcoholism, organicity, and neurological impairment are important contributing factors leading to diminished judgment and increased impulsivity in medically ill patients (Mackenzie and Popkin 1987).

As mentioned earlier in this chapter, most people who commit suicide have seen a health care professional shortly before their death. It must be assumed in these cases that the psychiatric state of the patient was not adequately assessed or the impact of the illness not fully appreciated. The clinician then must carefully evaluate suicidal risk in chronically ill patients and be aware of the psychiatric side effects of medications prescribed. Attention to these factors will help prevent patient suicides.

In summary, there are a number of important psychosocial factors, including suffering from a medical illness, that operate as contributory weights in the overlap model of suicidal behavior, helping to explain individual differences across high-risk groups.

Family History and Genetics

A family history of suicide is a significant risk factor for suicide (see Kety, Chapter 5, this volume). Explanations for this association include identification with and imitation of a family member who has committed suicide, family stress or contagion, transmission of genetic factors for suicide, and transmission of genetic factors for psychiatric disorders such as affective disorders (Blumenthal 1984, 1988; Blumenthal and Kupfer 1988; Kety 1986; Murphy and Wetzel 1982; Roy 1983, 1986a; Schulsinger et al. 1979; Tsuang 1977, 1983; Zaw 1981). Lines of evidence for these findings come from several types of research, including twin and adoption studies, studies of familial risk, and epidemiologic research. For example, a study of psychiatric inpatients revealed that 1) half of the persons with a family history of suicide had attempted suicide themselves, and 2) more than half of all patients in this study with a family history of suicide had a primary diagnosis of affective disorder (Roy 1982a, 1983). In another study, a greater incidence of suicide was found in the relatives of psychiatric patients who committed suicide than in the relatives of the control group (Zaw 1981). An investigation of suicide in the general population found that 6 of 100 suicide completers also had a parent who committed suicide. This rate was 88 times higher than predicted (Farberow and Simon 1969). A study of the Amish, a religious group with a 100-year history of nonviolence, no alcohol or drug abuse, a high degree of social cohesion, no divorce or family dissolution, and a philosophy of suicide as the ultimate sin, has demonstrated, quite unexpectedly, that suicides do occur among this group (Egeland and Sussex 1985). Between 1880 and 1980, 26 suicides were documented among the Amish of southeastern Pennsylvania; 24 of the 26 individuals who committed suicide were diagnosed with a major affective disorder, with the suicides occurring in four primary pedigrees. This research further suggests possible genetic factors in both the transmission of affective disorders and suicide.

Other investigations have suggested a high concordance rate for suicide in twins. A Danish study of monozygotic twins found that in 20% of the cases in which one twin was a suicide, the other twin had also died by suicide (Hendin 1986). Additionally, a review of 149 twin pairs, of whom 60 were identical and 98 were fraternal, found that nine sets of identical twin pairs were concordant for suicide, whereas none of the fraternal twins both died by suicide, again suggesting a genetic component to suicidal behavior (Haberlandt 1965, 1967). In a major Danish adoption study comparing the incidence of suicide in the biological and adoptive relations of adoptees who killed themselves, a six times greater incidence of suicide was found in the biological relatives of adoptees who committed suicide than in their adoptive relatives as compared to adoptee controls (Schulsinger et al. 1979).

These studies suggest that we may be able to separate out the contribution of a family history of suicide and a family history of affective disorder to isolate high-risk groups for both research and clinical purposes. Issues of family history and genetic factors are complicated not only by concordance for psychiatric diagnoses in families but also by the environment in terms of identification and imitation of suicidal behavior by family members over long periods of time (Blumenthal and Kupfer 1986a).

Biochemical Factors

Recent biochemical investigations of suicidal behavior have shown that some suicide victims and violent suicide attempters have a deficit in the functioning of a brain neurotransmitter, serotonin (see Winchel et al., Chapter 4, this volume). There have been a number of studies measuring 5-hydroxyindoleacetic acid (5-HIAA), a serotonin metabolite, in the cerebrospinal fluid (CSF) and serotonin and imipramine binding in the brains of suicide victims, which appear to confirm this finding (Ågren 1980, 1983; Åsberg et al. 1976, 1981, 1984, 1986a, 1986b; Banki et al. 1985; Brown et al. 1982a, 1982b, Lidberg et al. 1985; Linnoila et al. 1983; Mann et al. 1986; Ninan et al. 1984; Oreland et al. 1981; Stanley et al. 1986; Traskman et al. 1981). Much of this research has emphasized the close association between suicide and the propensity toward violence, attempting to identify behavioral and biological factors related to suicide that are not specific to any one psychiatric diagnosis. These studies have found a common biochemical association among aggression, impulsivity, and reduced serotonergic function. Furthermore, reduced central serotonergic activity is associated with suicidal behavior, not only when there is a diagnosis of unipolar depressive disorder but also in association with a range of other psychiatric disorders (Brown and Goodwin 1986; Brown et al. 1982a, 1982b). Some studies suggest that the finding of decreased serotonin in violent suicide attempters may increase the risk of completed suicide 10-fold at 1-year follow-up (Åsberg et al. 1976, 1986b). Interestingly, murderers have a suicide rate several hundred times greater than individuals the same age who have not killed anyone (West 1966). Similarly, arsonists, a group with high degrees of aggressivity and impulsivity and low serotonin levels, show a very high incidence of violent suicide attempts (Linnoila et al. 1983).

It should be noted that while low 5-HIAA levels are associated with violent suicide attempts and completions, low 5-HIAA levels are found in patients with diverse psychiatric illnesses and also in groups of normal controls (Banki et al. 1981; Brown and Goodwin 1986; Brown et al. 1982a, 1982b). Also, an increased incidence of depressive illness has been found in the relatives of both patients and normals with decreased CSF 5-HIAA levels (Roy-Byrne et al. 1983; Sedvall et al. 1980; van Praag 1982). Although the serotonergic data represent the most compelling current evidence for a biological correlate of suicidal behavior, other biological factors (i.e., neuroendocrine and neurophysiologic) are also being actively investigated (Koscis et al. 1986; Meltzer and Arora 1986). One recent study found reduced binding of corticotropin-releasing factor (CRF) in the frontal cortex of suicide victms (Nemeroff et al. 1988). This finding is consistent with the hypothesis that CRF is hypersecreted in depression, with resultant receptor down-regulation. Some studies have also indicated a relationship between specific maternal and perinatal factors such as hypoxia at birth and eventual adolescent suicide (Salk et al. 1985). These biological findings offer the promise of new pharmacological detection and treatment methods for suicidal behavior.

ASSESSMENT AND TREATMENT OF THE SUICIDAL PATIENT

In the assessment and treatment of the suicidal patient, the clinician will translate knowledge about the risk factors for suicide into a coherent plan for the careful evaluation and clinical management of suicidal patients over the life cycle. The health care professional will then target interventions to the various risk domains he or she has identified to be operating in a particular patient (Blumenthal 1984, 1988; Blumenthal and Kupfer 1986a, 1986b, 1988).

Assessment of the Suicidal Patient

The suicidal patient may present with many different clinical signs and symptoms. Mood disturbances are frequently present and so are somatic complaints. These may take many forms, from a request for a physical exam, complaints of fatigue, weight loss, and insomnia, to specific physical symptoms, including persistent headaches and gastric problems. Oftentimes a suicidal person may present to the doctor with physical complaints for which there is no apparent medical cause. Warning signs of suicide include sudden changes in behavior, including a dramatic brightening of mood after a period of despondency, social withdrawal, impulsivity, excessive risk taking, having multiple "accidents," changes in appetite, sleep disturbances, a humiliating life experience, persistent feelings of guilt, self-reproach and hopelessness, alcohol or drug abuse, loss of interest in usual activities (such as work, school, social, or sports activities), decreased concentration, suicide "talk," making a will, and giving away prized possessions (Blumenthal 1984, 1988). When several of these warning signs persist and cluster, the clinician should be alert to a risk of suicidal behavior in his or her patient.

The health care professional should take a careful medical and psychiatric history, paying specific attention to the mental status exam and the psychosocial history, evaluating the patient for any recent humiliation, losses, life stresses, and substance use or abuse (Table 1). The clinician's interviewing approach will vary depending on whether the patient is a child, adolescent, adult, or person in late life. (Hendren, Chapter 10, this volume).

As in any medical examination, the clinician begins with an exploration of the chief complaint and a review of the present illness, including what brought the patient to the physician's office or to the emergency room. Attention should be paid to any medical problems and medications used. The clinician should perform a physical examination and order any pertinent laboratory tests to rule out medical causes for psychiatric complaints. Empathic, attentive listening on the part of the health care professional is a key element of the assessment.

In performing a mental status examination, the clinician should determine the quality of the patient's mood, the content of his or her thoughts (e.g., whether hallucinations or delusions are present) and whether the patient's speech is pressured or slow. Other areas of inquiry include asking about a history of previous psychiatric problems and the clinical course and treatment of these disorders and

Table 1.   Assessing the emotionally troubled patient

Chief complaint

History of present illness

History of past emotional illness

Family history of psychiatric disorder and/or substance abuse

Nonpsychiatric medical history

Evaluation of social support system

Mental status examination
   Appearance and behavior
   Mood and affect
   Speech
   Content of thoughts
   Mental function
   Insight
   Judgment

Physical examination

Laboratory tests

---

determining whether a family history of affective disorders, substance abuse, and suicidal behavior is present. Contrary to popular lore, directly questioning the patient about suicidal thoughts and plans will not result in the patient taking suicidal actions. Rather, most people who have come to the doctor thinking about suicide wish to be rescued and stopped from carrying out their self-destruction. Most patients will experience relief when the clinician inquires about these feelings. Explicit questions about suicidal ideation, plans, attempts, suicide notes, putting one's business affairs in order, and giving away prized possessions must be asked in a direct and compassionate manner. One of the most important questions to be asked is whether the patient feels that he or she can promise to control his or her behavior and not act on impulses. If the patient cannot do this, immediate psychiatric hospitalization is indicated (Waltzer 1979).

Specific questions aimed at eliciting information about risk factors for suicidal behavior are a critical part of the health care professional's evaluation of the patient (Hawton and Catalan 1982; Kreitman 1986). The clinician may find the SADS Person Scale useful to evaluate risk (Patterson et al. 1983). Factors the clinician must consider in the assessment of the suicidal patient are listed in Table 2.

Clinical Management of Suicidal Patients

Once the clinician has determined that serious suicidal ideation and/ or plans are present, there are several essential components of good

Table 2. Assessment of the suicidal person: Factors the physician must consider in evaluating the patient

Assessing circumstances of an attempt
  Precipitating humiliating life event
  Preparatory actions—acquiring a method; putting affairs in order; suicide
    "talk"; giving away prized possessions; suicide note
  Use of violent method or more lethal drugs/poisons
  Understanding of lethality of chosen method
  Precautions taken against discovery

Presenting symptoms
  Hopelessness
  Self-reproach; feelings of failing and unworthiness
  Depressed mood
  Agitation and restlessness
  Persistent insomnia
  Weight loss
  Slowed speech, fatigue, social withdrawal
  Suicidal thoughts and plans

Psychiatric illness
  Previous suicide attempt
  Affective disorders
  Alcoholism and/or substance abuse
  Conduct disorders and depression in adolescents
  Early dementia and confusional states in the elderly
  Combinations of the above

Psychosocial history
  Recently separated, divorced, or bereaved
  Lives alone
  Unemployed; recent job change or loss
  Multiple life stresses (move; early loss; breakup of important relationship;
    school problems; threat of disciplinary crisis)
  Chronic medical illness
  Excessive drinking or substance abuse

Personality factors
  Impulsivity, aggressivity, hostility
  Cognitive rigidity and negativity
  Hopelessness
  Low self-esteem
  Borderline or antisocial personality disorder

Family history
  Family history of suicidal behavior
  Family history of affective disorder and/or alcoholism

clinical management, which will be discussed in greater detail. Interventions should be targeted at the entire system in which suicidal behavior occurs—that is, for the individual patient, the family, and the community, where possible. They include psychological and/or medical components as well as environmental interventions, including detoxification of the home, community support, and public health measures (Table 3). The clinician should consider life-cycle issues that impact on the patient and design interventions consistent with these developmental concerns (see Brent and Kolko, Chapter 11; Hendren, Chapter 10; Osgood and Thielman, Chapter 13; Schwartz and Whitaker, Chapter 12, this volume). Most importantly, the clinician must determine if the patient is suffering from a psychiatric illness and is receiving adequate treatment for the disorder that has been diagnosed (see Goldblatt and Schatzberg, Chapter 15; Kahn, Chapter 16; Weishaar and Beck, Chapter 17, this volume). This is a cornerstone to the prevention of suicide.

Table 3. Clinical management of suicidal patients

General points
    Inquire about suicidal thoughts and plans at every visit
    Set up frequent appointments and contact by telephone
    Follow-up missed appointments
    Document positive and negative findings in the chart
    Seek psychiatric consultation when necessary

Psychological aspects
    Establish therapeutic relationship (alliance)
    Allow expression of painful feelings
    Use a flexible, empathic, and supportive therapeutic style
    Provide reassurance and hope
    Rectify cognitive distortions
    Strengthen social supports and interpersonal relationships
    Form a no-suicide contract
    Develop and administer follow-up plan

Medical components
    Importance of symptomatic relief
    Adequate doses
    No refills
    Supervision by a relative when possible
    Assess patient compliance
    Obtain serum levels when appropriate
    Pay attention to side effects

Environmental interventions
    Detoxification of the home
    Close supervision
    Family therapy
    Community support
    Work/school interventions

The psychological aspects of clinical management of the suicidal patient are crucial (see Table 3) (see Kahn, Chapter 16; Weishaar and Beck, Chapter 17, this volume). One of the most important factors in the management of the patient is the doctor-patient relationship. The clinician will provide supportive care by allowing the patient to ventilate painful feelings through discussions that help the patient to discover alternatives, to improve interpersonal relationships, and to change negative thinking, refocusing on the future. This can be achieved by listening intently and empathically to what the patient says, by asking pertinent questions that help the patient to share suicidal feelings, and by the provision of hope. The clinician's therapeutic style must be flexible and supportive during this time, providing the patient with reassurance. This is *not* the time for a more distant approach. The health care professional must communicate to the patient that he or she cares. The medical practitioner or designated substitute should be available around the clock to maintain frequent contact with the patient, through office visits and by telephone. This provides an important lifeline to a source of help for the patient. Through repeated telephone contacts at moments of crisis when the patient fears loss of control, the clinician helps the patient recognize the difference between the experiencing of an impulse and the carrying out of an act (Waltzer 1979). Psychosocial interventions during this crisis period should focus on ameliorating the cognitive distortions that accompany depressive illness, helping the patient to become more flexible and hopeful, and improving interpersonal relationships. Many patients are experiencing a state of hopelessness and cannot imagine any other alternative but suicide. The physician helps the patient to problem solve to find alternative resolutions to the crisis, apart from suicide (see Weishaar and Beck, Chapter 17, this volume).

Additionally, medication can relieve some of the initial suffering that accompanies the biological symptoms of psychiatric illness (e.g., the weight loss, sleep disturbance, cognitive distortions, agitation, and loss of pleasure), giving the patient more energy to explore feelings and to problem solve. The type of medication will be determined by the symptoms and clinical diagnosis (see Goldblatt and Schatzberg, Chapter 15, this volume). When prescribing psychopharmacologic agents, the physician must pay careful attention to 1) providing the patient with information about the drugs and their side effects; 2) making sure that doses are adequate; 3) entrusting the medication to a relative where possible; and 4) prescribing medicine only in small quantities to prevent overdose (i.e., no more than a 5-day supply) and *not* permitting refills without writing another prescription. Careful attention to these details helps prevent tragedies, keeping in mind that many suicidal people end their lives with medicine prescribed by their doctors. Additionally, attending to these details gives the patient the feeling that the clinician cares, that he or she is taking precautions to keep the patient alive. However, if the situation is extremely precarious, psychiatric consultation or immediate hospitalization may be more appropriate.

The clinician must also pay attention to his or her own feelings and attitudes (countertransference) that can arise in the treatment of suicidal persons (see Kahn, Chapter 16, this volume). Suicidal patients are often difficult to treat and their families can be quite demanding. Initially, the clinician may be seen as the person who can immediately solve *all* problems; when this does not happen, a great deal of anger may come his or her way. Also, families may resist the treatment recommendations. These factors can combine to make the health care professional feel helpless, and when this happens, many clinicians retreat from active involvement or convey negative messages to their patients. Therefore, it is very important that the clinician manage his or her own feelings, reactions, and anxiety generated by working with suicidal patients to ensure the delivery of effective treatment to suicidal patients and their families.

Disposition and Clinical Interventions

There are several options available to the clinician in the management of the suicidal person (see Doyle, Chapter 14, this volume; Smith and Bope 1986). First, the patient presents in crisis. The clinician must gather all the information discussed earlier in this volume in the Section on assessment, formulate a differential diagnosis, and develop a plan for management of the patient's suicidal behavior. Given all of the information gathered from the diagnostic evaluation, the health care professional must decide whether the crisis can be managed in an outpatient setting or whether the patient will need to be hospitalized.

For most acutely suicidal patients (those who have made an attempt or have a serious plan), an inpatient psychiatric hospital unit is the best place to manage the patient. It provides a safe environment, immediate removal from environmental stressors often related to family interactions, and an opportunity for a careful diagnostic workup and intensive psychotherapeutic and psychopharmacologic interventions. Additionally, compliance to the medication regimen can be assessed, the strength of social supports and interpersonal relationships evaluated, and a follow-up plan after discharge constructed. These are all critical reasons to hospitalize a patient on a psychiatric inpatient unit. Sometimes when the patient is acutely suicidal and refuses hospitalization, involuntary commitment may be necessary.

When suicidal patients are hospitalized on a general medical or surgical ward where there is less supervision, it is crucial that the patient be protected from jumping from upper-story windows and from falling down open stairwells, since jumping from heights is the most common method of suicide by hospitalized general medical patients (Mackenzie and Popkin 1987; Waltzer 1979). Scissors, razors, and other potentially lethal objects should also be removed and plastic utensils used. Suicidal patients may be quite impulsive, and therefore constant staff supervision is required (Appendix II). The patient's bed should be located close to the nursing station within easy view. Flagging the beds and charts of these patients might help to alert ward personnel (Waltzer 1979). Consultations with the hospital staff and family should be held to deal with their reactions and feelings about the suicidal person and to ensure a consistent approach to the patient (Mackenzie and Popkin 1987; Waltzer 1979). The clinician should pay particular attention to the nurses' notes, which often report the patient's talk of wanting to die or symptoms of depression manifested by crying spells, anorexia, apathy, insomnia, and social withdrawal (Waltzer 1979). When the patient's suicidal risk poses a greater threat than the medical condition, transfer to an inpatient psychiatric unit is indicated (Waltzer 1979).

Some suicidal patients can be managed in an outpatient setting. The clinician will make this decision based on evaluation of the person's absolute risk of suicide, the strength of social support available from family and friends, the patient's wishes, an appraisal of the patient's ability to comply with a treatment plan, the strength of the therapeutic relationship (alliance) between patient and physician, how quickly the patient is responding to treatment, and how available the clinician is for consultation with the patient.

However, management of the suicidal patient almost *always* requires the assistance of a psychiatric consultant and is clearly indicated for all patients who have a serious plan for suicide or who have made an attempt. In the outpatient setting, a psychiatric consultant can be very helpful in refining the psychiatric diagnosis, developing a treatment plan, and providing more intensive psychiatric management of the patient. If necessary, this colleague can also help facilitate hospitalization of the patient. Additionally, the psychiatric consultant provides the patient with essential psychiatric treatment necessary during hospitalization and may also continue to provide psychiatric follow-up after the patient has been discharged from the hospital.

There are some general points that are helpful to remember in managing suicidal patients over the life cycle, and they should be underscored (see Table 3). First, *accurate diagnosis and appropriate treatment for associated psychiatric disorders* is a major prevention strategy for suicidal behavior. Rapid and intensive treatment is particularly important. Second, the clinician should always *inquire about suicidal thoughts and plans* as a routine part of every diagnostic evaluation and in every visit with a suicidal or depressed person. Third, the clinician should *document in the chart* both positive and negative findings. If the health care professional does not feel comfortable or does not wish, for whatever reason, to explore suicidal risk or to treat the patient, he or she still has the moral and legal obligation to *refer the patient* for psychiatric treatment (Waltzer 1979). When suicides do occur in practice, clinicians may encounter medicolegal difficulties if they have not documented their clinical management of the patient or if they have failed to take action in the presence of clear-cut suicidal intent (see Amchin et al., Chapter 24; Ruben, Chapter 23, this volume). Waltzer (1979) remarked that "failure to take an EKG [electrocardiogram] in the presence of chest pain would be considered an inadequate medical work-up, below the standard of care in medical practice. Similarly, sending a patient home without exploring immediate suicidal potential, and/or making a psychiatric referral for that purpose, would be considered inadequate treatment, below standard acceptable medical care." Fourth, the clinician must strive to *establish a therapeutic relationship* (alliance) with the patient. The strength of this alliance is an important "lifeline" for the patient. Some doctors find the use of a "no-suicide contract" to be helpful. This contract involves an exchange of the patient's agreement to refrain from suicidal actions and a promise that if suicidal thoughts or plans are contemplated, the patient will call the health care professional, for the assurance that the clinician or designated replacement will be available at all times to consult with the patient. Fifth, the clinician must instruct the family to *remove all potentially lethal objects* from the house, including guns, knives, and medications. This removal of a method from the immediate access of an impulsive patient conveys the important message that steps have been taken to help keep the patient alive. Sixth, the clinician should always inquire about the patient's *compliance with medications* and use serum levels when necessary to monitor. Seventh, the clinician should always immediately *follow up missed appointments* with an acutely suicidal person. Clinical experience reveals that suicides often occur during this missed office visit or therapy session. Finally, *consultation* with a psychiatric colleague who has specialty training in the diagnosis and treatment of mental illness is essential and may be particularly helpful in the assessment and management of acutely suicidal persons.

The clinician should also be aware of several important public health interventions that may help prevent suicide (Table 4) (see O'Carroll, Chapter 18; Pardes and Blumenthal, Chapter 25, this volume).

Table 4. Suicide prevention: Public health interventions

Gun control and decreased availability of lethal weapons

Educational campaigns to decrease alcohol and substance abuse

Educational campaigns to increase public awareness about depression and suicide

Deromanticization of the reporting and portrayal of suicides in the media

Community at-risk clinics combining expert clinical assessment and treatment with strong community supports

Development of community response plans

Increased health care professional education through training programs and continuing medical education about diagnosis and treatment of depression and suicidal behavior

Increased insurance benefits for psychiatric disorders and substance abuse

---

Studies have shown that states that have strict gun control laws have lower suicide rates (Boyd 1983; Boyd and Moscicki 1986; Brent et al. 1987, 1988a; Lester and Murrell 1980, 1982; Markush and Bortolucci 1984). Restricting availability of these weapons and other lethal methods becomes an important suicide prevention strategy (Kreitman 1976). Similarly, alcohol and drug use are associated with as many as 80% of suicides and are particularly important factors in youth suicide (Shaffer et al. 1988; Shafii et al. 1988). Efforts to restrict access to alcohol and other substances of abuse are additional important prevention methods. Intervention strategies including educational campaigns and community involvement to decrease substance abuse are indicated. Additionally, the media have an important role to play in suicide prevention given the evidence that exposure to a suicide through newspapers and television enhances risk (see Gould, Chapter 19, this volume; Gould and Shaffer 1986; Phillips and Carstensen 1986). Portrayals of suicide in television movies must be devoid of romanticization, and reports of suicides in newspapers may best be relegated to back-page news. These interventions should help prevent identification with the victims by vulnerable people. Additionally, the media can make valuable educational contributions through increasing public and health care professional awareness about this major public health problem.

Educational measures and curricula on suicide in the schools require further development and evaluation (Bromet et al. 1985; Shaffer et al. 1988; Pardes and Blumenthal, Chapter 25, this volume). Currently, there is a paucity of knowledge about the effects of school-based education on suicidal behavior (Shaffer et al. 1988). Perhaps the most sensible approach to suicide education is to integrate teaching about suicide into curricula on general mental health topics, focusing on increasing self-esteem in adolescents and strengthening their coping skills. The development of "at-risk clinics" in communities may also be helpful in preventing suicide. Such clinics might offer expert clinical assessment and treatment combined with strong community links, increased social supports, family education, and hotlines staffed by mental health professionals. Additionally, the development and implementation of a community response plan to suicide is strongly advised before these tragedies occur (see O'Carroll, Chapter 18, this volume). Finally, education of the public and health care professionals is needed to increase knowledge about the warning signs of suicide and intervention strategies. The health care professional has an important role to play in spearheading some of these efforts in his or her community.

CONCLUSION

In this chapter, the risk factors for suicide over the life cycle have been reviewed, providing the reader with a synopsis of the chapters in Section 1 of this volume. Five overlapping spheres of vulnerability for suicidal behavior have been described: psychiatric disorders, personality traits and disorders, psychosocial and environmental factors, genetic and familial variables, and biochemical factors. The point has been underscored that the presence and interaction of several of these domains increase the risk of suicide over the life cycle. Assessment and treatment strategies for suicidal behavior targeted at these risk domains have been discussed. Figure 2 provides a way of applying the overlap model (Figure 1) to a framework the clinician can use for the early detection and treatment of suicidal patients.

In this threshold model for suicidal behavior, certain predisposing factors such as a family history of suicide and biological vulnerability interact with risk factors developed later in life, including having a psychiatric illness (e.g., depression or substance abuse) or exposure to a suicide. When a person with these risk factors undergoes a humiliating life experience and when there is an available method for suicide, the threshold for suicidal behavior may be lowered. However, the presence of certain protective factors, including cognitive flexibility, hopefulness, strong social supports, and receiving appropriate treatment for an associated psychiatric disorder, contribute to maintaining a barrier to suicidal behavior, helping to explain why some people do not become suicidal given certain conditions and why others do. The clinician has an important role to play in the early detection of risk factors for suicidal behavior and in strengthening

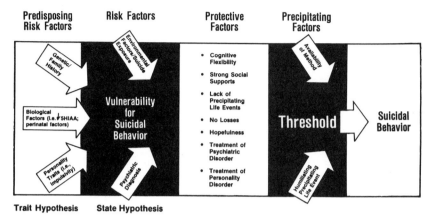

Figure 2. Threshold model for suicidal behavior. Reprinted from Blumenthal SJ, Kupfer DJ: Clinical assessment and treatment of youth suicide. *Journal of Youth and Adolescence* 17:1–24, 1988, with permission from Plenum Publishing Corporation.

these protective factors in his or her patients. Interventions that target as many risk factor domains as possible, including family treatment, environmental modification, and treatment of the associated psychiatric disorder, will maximize prevention of suicidal behavior by heightening the barriers to suicide.

Clinicians need to be certain that treatment for suicidal patients in their practice includes state-of-the-art psychotherapeutic and psychopharmacologic techniques geared to the treatment of specific psychiatric disorders as well as to suicidal behaviors. This is critical insofar as many psychiatrically ill suicide victims never receive proper treatment. Therefore, the proper identification, assessment, and treatment of psychiatric disorders is a key element in the prevention of suicide. It was mentioned earlier in this chapter that many health and mental health care professsionals will evaluate suicidal people in their offices during the weeks when these patients are deciding whether to live or to die. Alarmingly, many of these patients' suicidal thoughts have gone undetected because clinicians have not known or wanted to ask the necessary questions. Waltzer (1979) emphasized that "it is incumbent upon us as clinicians, whenever and wherever possible, to try to avert the patient's carrying out of a suicidal act. If one is to err, then let it be on the safe side, since it is impossible to predict with absolute certainty which individuals will end their lives by suicide. Tragically, mistakes in prediction are irreversible."

Other important components in the clinical management of patients at high risk for suicide over the life cycle include 1) providing the patient with support and hope; 2) helping the patient to problem solve; 3) actively involving the family to enhance compliance with treatment and to decrease the chance of relapse; 4) using psychiatric consultation and hospitalization appropriately; and 5) restricting the availability of lethal methods (Blumenthal 1984, 1988; Blumenthal and Kupfer 1986a, 1986b, 1988; Brent et al. 1988a; Waltzer 1979). Careful attention must be paid to the patient's environment and support systems. In this regard, a comprehensive follow-up plan is critical to preventing suicide—creating a lifeline and meaningful link for the patient to people who care and who can help in both the treatment and community settings. A final point: it is crucial that curricula in health and mental health care professional training and in continuing education programs contain information about the diagnosis and treatment of psychiatric disorders and complex human behaviors such as suicide.

It is hoped that this review of risk factors for suicide and strategies for assessment and treatment of suicidal behavior over the life cycle will serve as a useful summary of the more detailed chapters in this volume, providing you, the concerned health care professional, with a guiding framework for your efforts to prevent this tragic loss of human life in clinical practice.

References

Abramowitz ES, Baker AH, Fleischer S: Onset of depressive psychiatric crises and the menstrual cycle. Am J Psychiatry 139:475–478, 1982

Ågren H: Symptom patterns in unipolar and bipolar depression correlating with monoamine metabolites in the cerebrospinal fluid. II: Suicide. Psychiatry Res 3:225–236, 1980

Ågren H: Life at risk: markers of suicidality in depression. Psychiatric Developments 1:87–103, 1983

Akiskal HS: Factors associated with incomplete recovery in primary depressive illness. J Clin Psychiatry 43:266–271, 1982

Alterman AI, Ayre FR, Williford WO: Diagnostic validation of conjoint schizophrenia and alcoholism. J Clin Psychiatry 45:300–303, 1984

Åsberg M, Traskman L, Thoren P: 5-HIAA in the cerebrospinal fluid: a biochemical suicide predictor. Arch Gen Psychiatry 33:1193–1197, 1976

Åsberg M, Bertilsson L, Rydin E, et al: Monoamine metabolites in CSF in relation to depressive illness, suicidal behavior and personality, in Recent Advances in Neuropsychopharmacology. Edited by Angrist B, Burrows GD, Lader M, et al. Elmsford, NY, Pergamon, 1981, pp 257–271

Åsberg M. Bertilsson L, Martensson B: CSF monoamine metabolites, depression and suicide, in Frontiers in Biochemical and Pharmacological Research in Depression. Edited by Usdin E, Åsberg M, Bertilsson L, et al. New York, Raven, 1984, pp 87–97

Åsberg M, Nordstrom P, Traskman-Bendz L: Biological factors in suicide, in Suicide. Edited by Roy A. Baltimore, MD, Williams & Wilkins, 1986a, pp 47–72

Åsberg M, Nordstrom P, Traskman-Bendz L: Cerebrospinal fluid studies in suicide: an overview. Annals of the American Academy of Science 487:243–255, 1986b

Asch SS: Suicide and the hidden executioner. International Review of Psychoanalysis 7:51–61, 1980

Avery D, Winokur G: Suicide, attempted suicide, and relapse rates in depression. Arch Gen Psychiatry 35:749–753, 1978

Banki CM, Vojnik M, Molnar G: Cerebrospinal fluid amine metabolites, tryptophan and clinical parameters in depression. I: Background variables. J Affective Disord 3:81–89, 1981

Banki CM, Voynik M, Papp Z, et al: Cerebrospinal fluid magnesium and calcium related to amine metabolites, diagnosis, and suicide attempts. Biol Psychiatry 20:163–171, 1985

Barraclough B: Suicide prevention, recurrent affective disorder and lithium. Br J Psychiatry 121:391–392, 1972

Barraclough B, Bunch J, Nelson B, et al: A hundred cases of suicide: clinical aspects. Br J Psychiatry 125:355–373, 1974

Beck AT: Hopelessness as a predictor of eventual suicide. Ann NY Acad Sci 487:90–96, 1986

Beck AT, Davis JH, Frederick CJ, et al: Classifications and nomenclature, in Suicide Prevention in the 70s. Edited by Resnik HLP, Hawthorne BC. Rockville, MD, National Institute of Mental Health, 1973

Beck AT, Weissman A, Lester D, et al: The measurement of pessimism: the Hopelessness Scale. J Consult Clin Psychol 42:861–865, 1974a

Beck AT, Resnik HLP, Lettieri DJ (eds): The Prediction of Suicide. Bowie, MD, Charles Press, 1974b

Beck AT, Beck R, Kovacs M: Classification of suicidal behaviors. I: Quantifying intent and medical lethality. Am J Psychiatry 132:285–287, 1975a

Beck AT, Kovacs M, Weissman A: Hopelessness and suicidal behavior: an overview. JAMA 234:1146–1149, 1975b

Beck AT, Kovacs M, Weissman A: Assessment of suicidal intention: the Scale for Suicidal Ideation. J Consult Clin Psychol 47:343–352, 1979

Beck AT, Steer R, Kovacs M, et al: Hopelessness and eventual suicide: a 10-year prospective study of patients hospitalized with suicidal ideation. Am J Psychiatry 142:559–563, 1985

Bellack AS, Hersen M, Himmelhoch J: Social skills training compared with pharmacotherapy and psychotherapy in the treatment of unipolar depression. Am J Psychiatry 138:1562–1567, 1981

Bender L, Schilder P: Suicidal preoccupations and attempts in children. Am J Psychiatry 7:225–235, 1937

Black DW, Winokur G: Prospective studies of suicide and mortality in psychiatric patients. Ann NY Acad Sci 487:106–113, 1986

Blackburn I, Bishop S, Glen A, et al: The efficacy of cognitive therapy in depression: a treatment trial using cognitive therapy and pharmacotherapy, each alone and in combination. Br J Psychiatry 139:181–189, 1981

Blumenthal SJ: An overview of suicide risk factor research. Presented at the annual meeting of the American Psychiatric Association, Los Angeles, May 1984

Blumenthal SJ: Suicide: a guide to risk factors, assessment, and treatment of suicidal patients. Med Clin North Am 72:937–971, 1988

Blumenthal SJ, Kupfer DJ: Generalizable treatment strategies for suicidal behavior. Ann NY Acad Sci 487:327–340, 1986a

Blumenthal SJ, Kupfer DJ: Overview of early detection and treatment strategies for suicidal behavior in young people, in Alcohol, Drug Abuse, and Mental Health Administration. Report of the Secretary's Task Force on Youth Suicide, Vol 2, Risk Factors for Youth Suicide (DHHS Publ No ADM-89-1622). Washington, DC, U.S. Government Printing Office, 1989

Blumenthal SJ, Kupfer DJ: Overview of early detection and treatment strategies for suicidal behavior in young people. Journal of Youth and Adolscence 17:1–24, 1988

Bollen KA, Phillips DA: Imitative suicides: a national study of the effects of television news stories. American Social Review 47:802–809, 1982

Borg ES, Stahl M: Prediction of suicide: a prospective study of suicides and controls among psychiatric patients. Acta Psychiatr Scand 65:221–232, 1982

Boyd JH: The increasing rate of suicide by firearms. N Engl J Med 308:872–874, 1983

Boyd JH, Moscicki EK: Firearms and youth suicide. Am J Public Health 76:1240–1242, 1986

Brent DA, Perper JA, Allman CJ: Alcohol, firearms, and suicide among youth. JAMA 257:3369–3372, 1987

Brent DA, Kupfer DJ, Bromet EJ, et al: The assessment and treatment of patients at risk for suicide, in Psychiatry Update: American Psychiatric Association Annual Review, Vol 7. Edited by Frances AJ, Hales RE. Washington, DC, American Psychiatric Press, 1988a, pp 353–385

Brent DA, Perper JA, Goldstein CE, et al: Risk factors for adolescent suicide. Arch Gen Psychiatry 45:581–588, 1988b

Bromet EJ, Dew MA, Brent D: Suicide Prevention: A Review (Contract No 85M059146401S). Rockville, MD, National Institute of Mental Health, Suicide Research Unit, Center for the Study of Affective Disorders, 1985

Brown GL, Goodwin FK: Cerebrospinal fluid correlates of suicide attempts and aggression. Ann NY Acad Sci 487:175–188, 1986

Brown G, Ebert M, Goyen P, et al: Aggression, suicide, and serotonin: relationships of CSF amine metabolites. Am J Psychiatry 139:741–746, 1982a

Brown GL, Goodwin FK, Bunney WE: Human aggression and suicide: their relationship to neuropsychiatric diagnosis and serotonin metabolism, in

Serotonin in Biological Psychiatry. Edited by Ho BT, Schooler JC, Usdin E. New York, Raven, 1982b, pp 287–307

Campbell PC: Suicide among cancer patients. Connecticut Health Bulletin 80:207–212, 1966

Camus A: The Myth of Sisyphus. New York, Vintage, 1959

Carlson G, Cantwell D: Suicidal behavior and depression in children and adolescents. Journal of the American Academy of Child Psychiatry 21:361–368, 1982

Centers for Disease Control: Morbidity and Mortality Weekly Report 36:531–534, 1987

Centers for Disease Control: 1987 Suicide Surveillance. Atlanta, GA, U.S. Department of Health and Human Services, Public Health Service, 1987b

Chiles JA, Miller ML, Cox GB: Depression in an adolescent delinquent population. Arch Gen Psychiatry 37:1179–1184, 1980

Clayton PJ, Lewis CE: The significance of secondary depression. J Affective Disord 3:25–35, 1981

Cohen-Sandler R, Berman AL, King RA: Life stress and symptomatology: determinants of suicidal behavior in children. Journal of the American Academy of Child Psychiatry 21:178–186, 1982

Crumley F: Adolescent suicide attempts and borderline personality disorder: clinical features. Southwest Medical Journal 74:546–549, 1981

Crumley FE: The adolescent suicide attempt: a cardinal symptom of a serious psychiatric disorder. Am J Psychother 36;158–165, 1982a

Crumley F: Adolescent suicide attempts and melancholia. Tex Med 78:62–65, 1982b

Davidson LE, Rosenberg ML, Mercy JA, et al: An epidemiologic study of risk factors in two teenage suicide clusters. JAMA 261:2687–2692, 1989

Department of Health and Human Services: Suicide (Publ No ADM-86-1489). Washington, DC, U.S. Department of Health and Human Services, 1986

Dewhurst K, Oliver JE, McKnight AL: Socio-psychiatric consequences of Huntington's disease. Br J Psychiatry 116:255–258, 1970

DiMascio A, Weissman MM, Prusoff BA, et al: Differential symptom reduction by drugs and psychotherapy in acute depression. Arch Gen Psychiatry 36:1450–1456, 1979

Dorpat T, Ripley H: A study of suicide in the Seattle area. Compr Psychiatry 1:349–359, 1960

Dorpat TL, Anderson WF, Ripley HS: The relationship of physical illness to suicide, in Suicidal Behaviors. Edited by Resnick LP. Boston, Little, Brown, 1968

Drake RE, Cotton PG: Depression, hopelessness and suicide in chronic schizophrenia. Br J Psychiatry 148:554–559, 1986

Drake RE, Ehrlich J: Suicide attempts associated with akathisia. Am J Psychiatry 142:499–501, 1985

Drake RE, Gates C, Cotton PG, et al: Suicide among schizophrenics: who is at risk? J Nerv Ment Dis 172:613–617, 1984

Durkheim E: Suicide: A Study in Sociology. Translated by Spaulding JA, Simpson G. New York, Free Press, 1951

Dyer JAT, Kreitman N: Hopelessness, depression and suicidal intent in parasuicide. Br J Psychiatry 144:127–133, 1984

Egeland J, Sussex J: Suicide and family loading for affective disorders. JAMA 254:915–918, 1985

Farberow N, Simon M: Suicides in Los Angeles and Vienna: an intercultural study of two cities. Public Health Rep 84:389–403, 1969

Fawcett J, Sheftner W, Clark D, et al: Clinical predictors of suicide in patients with major affective disorders: a controlled prospective study. Am J Psychiatry 144:35–40, 1987

Fourestié V, de Lignieres B, Roudot-Thoraval F, et al: Suicide attempts in hypo-estrogenic phases of the menstrual cycle. Lancet 2:1357–1360, 1986

Fowler RC, Tsuang MT, Kronfol Z: Communication of suicidal intent and suicide in unipolar depression: a forty year follow-up. J Affective Disord 1:219–225, 1979

Fox BH, Stanek EJ, Boyd SC, et al: Suicide rates among cancer patients in Connecticut. J Chronic Dis 35:89–100, 1982

Frances A: Personality and suicide. Ann NY Acad Sci 487:281–293, 1986

Frances A, Blumenthal SJ: Personality disorders and characteristics in youth suicide, in Alcohol, Drug Abuse, and Mental Health Administration. Report of the Secretary's Task Force on Youth Suicide, Vol 2, Risk Factors for Youth Suicide (DHHS Publ No ADM-89-1622). Washington, DC, U.S. Government Printing Office, 1989, pp 172–183

Frances R, Franklin J, Flavin D: Suicide and alcoholism. Ann NY Acad Sci 487:316–326, 1986

Frank E, Kupfer DJ: Psychotherapeutic approaches to treatment of recurrent unipolar depression: work in progress. Psychopharmacol Bull 22:558–563, 1986

Freud S: Mourning and melancholia (1917), in The Standard Edition of the Complete Psychological Works of Sigmund Freud, Vol 14. Translated and edited by Strachey J. London, Hogarth Press, 1957

Friedman IM: Alcohol and unnatural deaths in San Francisco youths. Pediatrics 76:191–193, 1985

Goldberg EL: Depression and suicide ideation in the young adult. Am J Psychiatry 138:35–40, 1981

Goldney RD, Katsikitas M: Cohort analysis of suicide rates in Australia. Arch Gen Psychiatry 40:71–74, 1983

Gould MS, Shaffer D: The impact of suicide in television movies: evidence imitation. N Engl J Med 315:690–694, 1986

Griest J, Griest T: Antidepressant Treatment: The Essentials. Baltimore, MD, Williams & Wilkins, 1979

Guze SB, Robins E: Suicide and primary affective disorder. Br J Psychiatry 117:437–438, 1970

Haas GL, Glick ID, Spencer JH, et al: The patient, the family, and compliance with posthospital treatment for affective disorders. Psychopharmacol Bull 22:999–1005, 1986

Haberlandt W: Der suizid als genetisches problem (zwillingsand familier analyse). Anthrop Anz 29:65–89, 1965

Haberlandt W: Aportacion a la genetica del suicidio. Folia Clin Int 17:319–322, 1967

Hagnell O, Rorsman B: Suicide in the Lundby study: a controlled prospective investigation of stressful life events. Neuropsychobiology 6:319–332, 1980

Hagnell O, Lanke J, Rorsman B: Suicide rates in the Lundby study: mental illness as a risk factor for suicide. Neuropsychobiology 7:248–253, 1981

Halbreich U, Endicott J: Premenstrual depressive changes. Arch Gen Psychiatry 40:535–542, 1983

Hankoff LD, Einsidler B: Suicide: Theory and Clinical Aspects. Littleton, MA, PSG Publishing, 1979

Hawton K, Catalan J: Attempted Suicide: A Practical Guide to its Nature and Management. New York, Oxford University Press, 1982

Hawton K, Fagg J, Marsack P: Association between epilepsy and attempted suicide. J Neurol Neurosurg Psychiatry 43:168–170, 1980

Hendin H: Suicide: a review of new directions in research. Hosp Community Psychiatry 37:148–154, 1986

Hillard JR, Ramm D, Zung WWK, et al: Suicide in a psychiatric emergency room population. Am J Psychiatry 140:459–462, 1983

Hirschfeld R, Blumenthal S: Personality, life events, and other psychosocial factors in adolescent depression and suicide, in Suicide and Depression Among Adolescents and Young Adults. Edited by Klerman GL. Washington, DC, American Psychiatric Press, 1986, pp 213–253

Hogarty GE, Anderson CM, Reiss DJ, et al: Family psychoeducation, social skills training, and maintenance chemotherapy in the aftercare treatment of schizophrenia. I: One-year effects of a controlled study on relapse and expressed emotion. Arch Gen Psychiatry 43:633–642, 1986

Holinger PC, Offer D: Prediction of adolescent suicide: a population model. Am J Psychiatry 139:302–307, 1982

Holinger PC, Offer D, Ostrov E: Suicide and homicide in the United States: an epidemiologic study of violent death, population changes, and the potential for prediction. Am J Psychiatry 144:215–219, 1987

Hume D: On Suicide, in The Philosophical Works of David Hume, Vol 4. Edinburgh, Black & Tait, 1826

Jamison KR: Suicide and bipolar disorders. Ann NY Acad Sci 487:301–315, 1986

Janicak P, Davis J, Gibbons R, et al: Efficacy of ECT: a meta-analysis. Am J Psychiatry 142:297–302, 1985

Johns C, Stanley M, Stanley B: Suicide in schizophrenia. Ann NY Acad Sci 487:294–300, 1986

Johnson DA: Studies of depressive symptoms in schizophrenia, I: the prevalence of depression and its possible causes. Br J Psychiatry 138:89–101, 1980

Johnson GF, Hunt G: Suicidal behavior in bipolar manic-depressive patients and their families. Compr Psychiatry 20:159–164, 1979

Kernberg O: Severe Personality Disorders. New Haven, CT, Yale University Press, 1984

Kerr, TA, Schapira K, Roth M: The relationship between premature death and affective disorders. Br J Psychiatry 115:1277–1282, 1969

Kety SS: Genetic factors in suicide, in Suicide. Edited by Roy A. Baltimore, MD, Williams & Wilkins, 1986, pp 41–45

Khuri, R, Akiskal HS: Suicide prevention: the necessity of treating contributory psychiatric disorders. Psychiatr Clin North Am 6:193–207, 1983

Klerman GL, Hirschfeld RM: Treatment of depression in the elderly. Geriatrics 34:51–57, 1979

Klerman GL, Weissman MM: Increasing rates of depression. JAMA 261:2229–2235, 1989

Knop J, Fisher A: Duodenal ulcer, suicide, psychopathology and alcoholism. Acta Psychiatr Scand 63:346–355, 1981

Kohut H: The Restoration of the Self. New York, International Universities Press, 1977

Koscis TH, Kennedy S, Brown, RP, et al: Neuroendocrine studies in depression: relationship to suicidal behavior. Ann NY Acad Sci 487: 256–262, 1986

Kovacs M, Rush A, Beck A, et al: Depressed outpatients treated with cognitive therapy or pharmacotherapy: a one year follow-up. Arch Gen Psychiatry 38:33–39, 1981

Kreitman N: The coal gas story: United Kingdom suicide rates, 1960–1971. Br J Soc Prev Med 30:86–93, 1976

Kreitman N: The clinical assessment and management of the suicidal patient, in Suicide. Edited by Roy A. Baltimore, MD, Williams & Wilkins, 1986, pp 181–197

Lester D: Seasonal variation in suicidal deaths. Br J Psychiatry 118:627–628, 1971

Lester D, Murrell ME: The influence of gun control laws on suicidal behavior. Am J Psychiatry 137:121–122, 1980

Lester D, Murrell ME: The preventive effect of strict gun control laws on suicide and homicide. Suicide Life Threat Behav 12:131–140, 1982

Lidberg L, Tuck JR, Asburg GP, et al: Homicide, suicide and CSF 5-HIAA. Acta Psychiatr Scand 71:230–236, 1985

Linehan MM: Suicidal people: one population or two? Ann NY Acad Sci 487:16–33, 1986

Linnoila M, Virkkunen M, Scheinin M, et al: Low cerebrospinal fluid 5-hydroxyindoleacetic acid concentration differentiates impulsive from nonimpulsive violent behavior. Life Sci 33:2609–2614, 1983

Louhivuori KA, Hakama M: Risk of suicide among cancer patients. Am J Epidemiol 109:59–65, 1979

Luscomb RL, Clum GA, Patsiokas AT: Mediating factors in the relationship between life stress and suicide attempting. J Nerv Ment Dis 168:644–650, 1980

Mackenzie TB, Popkin MK: Suicide in the medical patient. Int J Psychiatry Med 17:3–22, 1987

Mann T, McBride A, Stanley M: Postmortem monamine receptor and enzyme studies in suicide. Ann NY Acad Sci 487:114–121, 1986

Markush RE, Bortolucci AA: Firearms and suicide in the United States. Am J Public Health 74:123–127, 1984

Marzuk DM, Tierney M, Tardiff K, et al: Increased risk of suicide in persons with AIDS. JAMA 259:1333–1337, 1988

Matthews W, Barabas G: Suicide and epilepsy: a review of the literature. Psychosomatics 22:515–524, 1981

McGlashan TH, Carpenter T: Postpsychotic depression in schizophrenia. Arch Gen Psychiatry 33:231–239, 1976

Meltzer HY, Arora RC: Platelet markers and suicide. Ann NY Acad Sci 487:271–280, 1986

Menninger KA: Man Against Himself. New York, Harcourt, Brace, 1938

Miles C: Conditions predisposing to suicide: a review. J Nerv Ment Dis 164:231–246, 1977

Morrison JR: Suicide in a psychiatric practice population. J Clin Psychiatry 43:348–352, 1982

Motto JA: Estimation of suicide risk by the use of clinical models. Suicide Life Threat Behav 7:236–245, 1977

Murphy GE: Clinical identification of suicidal risk. Arch Gen Psychiatry 27:356–359, 1972

Murphy GE: Suicide in alcoholism, in Suicide. Edited by Roy A. Baltimore, MD, Williams & Wilkins, 1986, pp 89–96

Murphy GE, Wetzel RD: Family history of suicidal behavior among suicide attempters. J Nerv Ment Dis 170:86–90, 1982

Murphy GE, Armstrong JW, Hermele SL, et al: Suicide and alcoholism: interpersonal loss confirmed as a predictor. Arch Gen Psychiatry 36:65–69, 1979

Murphy GE, Simons AD, Wetzel RD, et al: Cognitive therapy and pharmacotherapy: singly and together in the treatment of depression. Arch Gen Psychiatry 41:33–41, 1984

Nayha S: The bi-seasonal incidence of some suicides: experience from Finland by marital status, 1961–1976. Acta Psychiatr Scand 67:32–42, 1983

Negrete JC, Knapp WP, Douglas DE, et al: Cannabis affects the severity of schizophrenic symptoms: results of a clinical survey. Psychol Med 16:515–520, 1986

Nemeroff CB, Owens MJ, Bissette G, et al: Reduced corticotropin releasing factor binding sites in the frontal cortex of suicide victims. Arch Gen Psychiatry 45:577–592, 1988

Neuringer C (ed): Psychological Assessment of Suicidal Risk. Springfield, IL, Charles C Thomas, 1974

Ninan PT, van Kammen DP, Scheinin M, et al: CSF 5-hydroxyindoleacetic acid levels in suicidal schizophrenic patients. Am J Psychiatry 141: 566–569, 1984

Oreland L, Wiberg A, Åsberg M, et al: Platelet MAO activity and monoamine metabolites in cerebrospinal fluid in depressed and suicidal patients and in healthy controls. Psychiatry Res 4:21–29, 1981

Osofsky H, Blumenthal SJ: Premenstrual Syndrome: Current Findings and Future Directions. Washington, DC, American Psychiatric Press, 1985

Parker G, Walter S: Seasonal variation in depressive disorders and suicidal deaths in New South Wales. Br J Psychiatry 140:626–632, 1982

Patsiokas AT, Clum GA, Luscomb RL: Cognitive characteristics of suicide attempters. J Consult Clin Psychol 47:478–484, 1979

Patterson WM, Dohn HH, Bird J, et al: Evaluation of suicidal patients: the SAD Persons Scale. Psychosomatics 24:343–349, 1983

Paykel ES: Stress and life events, in Alcohol, Drug Abuse, and Mental Health Administration. Report of the Secretary's Task Force on Youth Suicide, Vol 2, Risk Factors for Youth Suicide (DHHS Publ No ADM-89-1662). Washington DC, U.S. Government Printing Office, 1989

Paykel ES, Myers JK, Lindenthal JJ, et al: Suicidal feelings in the general population: a prevalence study. Br J Psychiatry 124:460–469, 1974

Paykel ES, Prusoff BA, Myers JR: Suicide attempts and recent life events: a controlled comparison. Arch Gen Psychiatry 32:327–333, 1975

Petzel SV, Riddle M: Adolescent suicide: psychosocial and cognitive aspects. Adolesc Psychiatry 9:343–398, 1981

Pfeffer CR: Suicidal behavior in children: a review with implications for research and practice. Am J Psychiatry 138:154–159, 1981

Pfeffer CR: The Suicidal Child. New York, Guilford, 1986

Pfeffer CR: Suicidal behavior among children and adolescents: risk identification and intervention, in American Psychiatric Press Review of Psychiatry, Vol. 7. Edited by Frances AJ, Hales RE. Washington, DC, American Psychiatric Press, 1988, pp 386–402

Pfeffer CR (ed): Suicide Among Youth: Perspectives on Risk and Prevention. Washington, DC, American Psychiatric Press, 1989

Phillips DP, Carstensen LL: Clustering of teenage suicides after television news stories about suicide. N Engl J Med 315:685–689, 1986

Pokorny AD: Suicide rates in various psychiatric disorders. J Nerv Ment Dis 139:499–506, 1964

Pokorny AD: A follow-up of 618 suicidal patients. Am J Psychiatry 22:1109–1116, 1966

Pokorny AD: Prediction of suicide in psychiatric patients. Arch Gen Psychiatry 40:249–257, 1983

Prusoff BA, Williams DH, Weissman MM, et al: Treatment of secondary depression in schizophrenia: a double-blind, placebo-controlled trial of amitriptyline added to perphenazine. Arch Gen Psychiatry 36:569–575, 1979

Rich CL, Young D, Fowler RC: San Diego Suicide Study. I: Young vs. old subjects. Arch Gen Psychiatry 43:577–582, 1986

Rich CL, Fowler RC, Fogarty LA, et al: San Diego Suicide Study. III. Relationships between diagnoses and stressors. Arch Gen Psychiatry 45:589–592, 1988

Robbins D, Conroy R: A cluster of adolescent suicide attempts: is suicide contagious? J Adolesc Health Care 364:253–255, 1983

Robins E: The Final Months: A Study of the Lives of 134 Persons Who Committed Suicide. New York, Oxford University Press, 1981

Robins E, Murphy GE, Wilkinson RM, et al: Some clinical considerations in the prevention of suicide based on a study of 134 successful suicides. Am J Public Health 49:888–898, 1959

Robins LN: Changes in conduct disorder over time, in Risk in Intellectual and Psychosocial Development. Edited by Farran DC, McKinney JD. Orlando, FL, Academic, 1986, pp 227–259

Roose SP, Glassman AH, Walsh T, et al: Depression, delusions, and suicide. Am J Psychiatry 140:1159–1162, 1983

Rosenthal NE, Sack DA, Gillin JC, et al: Seasonal affective disorder: a description of the syndrome and preliminary findings with light therapy. Arch Gen Psychiatry 41:72–80, 1984

Rounsaville BJ, Kosten TR, Weissman MM, et al: Prognostic significance of psychopathology in treated opiate addicts: a 25 year follow-up study. Arch Gen Psychiatry 43:739–745, 1986

Roy A: Risk factors for suicide in psychiatric patients. Arch Gen Psychiatry 39:1089–1095, 1982a

Roy A: Suicide in chronic schizophrenia. Br J Psychiatry 141:171–177, 1982b

Roy A: Family history of suicide. Arch Gen Psychiatry 40:971–974, 1983

Roy A: Genetics of suicide. Ann NY Acad Sci 487:97–105, 1986a

Roy A: Suicide in schizophrenia, in Suicide. Edited by Roy A. Baltimore, MD, Williams & Wilkins, 1986b, pp 97–112

Roy-Byrne P, Post RM, Rubinow DR, et al: CSF 5HIAA and personal and family history of suicide in affectively ill patients: a negative study. Psychiatry Res 10:263–274, 1983

Rush A, Beck A, Kovacs M, et al: Comparative efficacy of cognitive therapy and pharmacotherapy in the treatment of depressed outpatients. Cognitive Therapy Research 1:17–37, 1977

Salk L, Lipsitt LP, Sturner WQ, et al: Relationship of maternal and perinatal conditions to eventual adolescent suicide. Lancet 1:624–627, 1985

Schneidman ES: An overview: personality, motivation, and behavior theories, in Suicide: Theory and Clinical Aspects. Edited by Hankoff LD, Einsidler B. Littleton, MA, PSG Publishing, 1979

Schuckit MA: Alcoholism and affective disorder: diagnostic confusion, in Alcoholism and Affective Disorders. Clinical, Genetic, and Biochemical Studies. Edited by Goodwin DW, Erickson CF. New York, SP Medical & Scientific Books, 1979

Schulsinger R, Kety S, Rosenthal D, et al: A family study of suicide, in Origin, Prevention, and Treatment of Affective Disorders. Edited by Schou M, Stromgren E. New York, Academic, 1979

Sedvall G, Fyro B, Gullberg B, et al: Relationships in healthy volunteers between concentrations of monoamine metabolites in cerebrospinal fluid and family history of psychiatric morbidity. Br J Psychiatry 136:366–374, 1980

Seligman MEP: Helplessness: On Depression, Development and Death. San Francisco, WH Freeman, 1975

Shaffer D: Suicide in childhood and early adolescence. J Child Psychol Psychiatry 15:275–291, 1974

Shaffer D, Fisher P: The epidemiology of suicide in children and young adolescents. Journal of the American Academy of Child Psychiatry 20:545–565, 1981

Shaffer D, Gould M, Trautman P: Suicidal behavior in children and young adults. Paper presented at the New York Academy of Sciences NIMH Conference on the Psychobiology of Suicidal Behavior, New York, September 1985

Shaffer D, Garland A, Gould M, et al: Preventing teenage suicide: a critical review. J Am Acad Child Adolesc Psychiatry 27:675–687, 1988

Shafii M, Carrigen S, Whittinghill JR, et al: Psychological autopsy of completed suicide in children and adolescents. Am J Psychiatry 142:1061–1064, 1985

Shafii M, Steltz-Lenarsky J, Denick AM, et al: Co-morbidity of mental disorders in the post-mortem diagnosis of completed suicide in children and adolescents. J Affective Disord 15:227–233, 1988

Shear MK, Frances A, Weiden P: Suicide associated with akathisia and depot fluphenazine treatment. J Clin Psychopharmacol 3:235–236, 1983

Siegel K, Tuckel P: Rational suicide and the terminally ill cancer patient. Omega 15:263–269, 1984-85

Siris SG, Rifkin A, Reardon GT, et al: A trial of adjunctive imipramine in postpsychotic depression. Psychopharmacol Bull 21:114–116, 1985

Smith CW, Bope ET: The suicidal patient: the primary care physician's role in evaluation and treatment. Postgrad Med 79:195–202, 1986

Smith JC, Mercy JA, Warren CW: Comparison of suicides among Anglos and Hispanics in five southwestern states. Suicide Life Threat Behav 15:14–26, 1985

Stallone F, Dunner DL, Ahean J, et al: Statistical predictions of suicide in depressives. Compr Psychiatry 21:381–387, 1980

Stanley M, Mann JJ, Cohen LS: Serotonin and serotonergic receptors. Ann NY Acad Sci 487:122–127, 1986

Traskman L, Åsberg M, Bertilsson L, et al: Monoamine metabolites in CSF and suicidal behavior. Arch Gen Psychiatry 38:631–636, 1981

Tsuang MT: Genetic factors in suicide. J Clin Psychiatry 38:498–501, 1977

Tsuang MT: Risk of suicide in the relatives of schizophrenics, manics, depressives, and controls. J Clin Psychiatry 44:396–400, 1983

Tuckman J, Youngman WF: A scale for assessing suicide risk for attempted suicide. J Clin Psychol 24:17–19, 1968

van Praag HM: Depression, suicide and the metabolism of serotonin in the brain. J Affective Disord 4:275–290, 1982

Virkkunen M: Attitude to psychiatric treatment before suicide in schizophrenia and paranoid psychoses. Br J Psychiatry 128:47–49, 1976

Viskum K: Ulcer, attempted suicide and suicide. Acta Psychiatr Scand 51:221–227, 1975

Waltzer H: The medical practitioner, in Suicide. Edited by Hankoff LD and Einsidler B. Littleton, MA, PSG Publishing, 1979, pp 353–361

Weissman MM, Fox K, Klerman GL: Hostility and depression associated with suicide attempts. Am J Psychiatry 130:450–455, 1973

Weissman MM, Klerman GL, Prusoff BA, et al: Depressed outpatients: results one year after treatment with drugs and/or interpersonal psychotherapy. Arch Gen Psychiatry 38:51–55, 1981

Weissman MM, Klerman GL, Markowitz JS, et al: Suicidal ideation and suicide attempts in panic disorder and attacks. N Engl J Med 321:1209–1213, 1989

West J: Murder Followed by Suicide: An Inquiry Carried Out for the Institute of Criminology, Cambridge. Cambridge, MA, Harvard University Press, 1966

Wetzel RD: Hopelessness, depression, and suicide intent. Arch Gen Psychiatry 33:1069–1073, 1976

Whitlock FA: Suicide and physical illness, in Suicide. Edited by Roy A. Baltimore, MD, Williams & Wilkins, 1986, pp 151–170

Winokur G, Black DW: Psychiatric and medical diagnoses as risk factors for mortality in psychiatric patients: a case-control study. Am J Psychiatry 144:208–211, 1987

Zaw K: A suicidal family. Br J Psychiatry 139:68–69, 1981

Zilboorg G: Considerations on suicide, with particular reference to that of the young. Am J Orthopsychiatry 7:15–31, 1937

Zung WW, Green RL: Seasonal variation of suicide and depression. Arch Gen Psychiatry 30:89–91, 1974

Chapter 27

Epilogue

Susan J. Blumenthal, M.D., M.P.A.
David J. Kupfer, M.D.

The man, who in a fit of melancholy, kills himself today,
would have wished to live had he waited a week.
—Voltaire, *Philosophical Dictionary*, "Cato"

T HIS VOLUME HAS attempted to bridge current knowledge from the scientific research literature on epidemiologic, psychosocial, diagnostic, genetic, and biological risk factors for suicide with practical intervention strategies that the clinician can use in treating suicidal patients over the life cycle. The point has been repeatedly underscored that the presence and interaction of several of these variables increases risk for suicide. A precise understanding of suicidal behavior implies incorporating knowledge about these factors into the design of interventions targeted at the various domains of risk described in Section 1 of this volume. The reader's integration of this information into clinical practice will ensure that treatment is multimodal and addresses all of the contributory variables discussed in this book.

It is hoped that *Suicide Over the Life Cycle* has provided you, the reader, with answers about the etiology of this complex human behavior and presented useful strategies for evaluating suicidal patients and for intervening in crisis, outpatient, and inpatient settings. In this regard, Section 2 has provided principles for formulating a rational treatment plan including state-of-the-art psychotherapeutic, psychopharmacologic, and environmental interventions. Section 3 reviewed special issues about suicide, including cluster suicides, international perspectives, suicide in minority groups, suicide among physicians, how to survive a suicide in your own clinical practice, legal and ethical concerns, and public policy considerations. Armed with this information, the clinician should have a comprehensive view of the determinants and deterrents of suicidal behavior and be better equipped to deal effectively with suicidal patients in clinical practice.

An important conclusion of this volume is that both the early identification and the proper assessment and treatment of the psychiatric disorders associated with suicidal behavior are cornerstones to the prevention of suicide. Other critical aspects of the clinical management of patients at high risk for suicide include strategies to give the patient increased hope and help with problem-solving capabilities. Careful attention must be given to the patient's environment and support systems. For example, families and other significant others need to be involved in the treatment plan, and alliances between patients and clinicians must be strengthened to help prevent further suicidal behavior. Consultation and hospitalization must be used when necessary. In addition, a comprehensive and systematic follow-up plan is mandatory if suicide is to be prevented.

Suicide is a complex human behavior that represents the confluence of psychological, biological, and environmental vulnerabilities. The overlap of multiple contributory risk factors explored in this volume influences the expression of suicidal behavior in particular individuals and helps explain why only the minority of people suffering from specific psychiatric disorders (who will have several of these risk factors operating) will end their lives by suicide. Self-destruction is a behavior. The suicidal individual—often feeling humiliated, suffering from a psychiatric disorder that has not been well treated, and having few social supports—can no longer imagine any other possibility than to end the pain and despair of living. In this way, hopelessness appears to be a key mediating factor in suicidal behavior. As clinicians, it is our role and obligation to use our knowledge and skills to try to avert the patient's carrying out of a suicidal act. If we are to err with respect to prediction, then it should be on the safe side, because we can never predict with complete certainty who among our patients will end their life by suicide. Tragically, mistakes in this regard are irreversible.

Further research is needed to determine who is at risk for suicide and to elucidate the mechanisms underlying the complex interactions between psychological, biological, and environmental influences in self-destructive behavior. Exciting investigations are under way to determine biological and psychosocial factors that characterize subgroups of suicide attempters and completers. New pharmacologic treatment strategies are being tested that build on this knowledge and offer promise to help prevent these tragedies. While we are waiting for these answers, clinicians must become trained in the lifesaving aspects of assessing suicide risk in their patients, must become more vigilant in recognizing the warning signs of suicide, and must become more actively involved by providing support, alternative choices, and appropriate treatment to their suicidal patients.

Suicide Over the Life Cycle has underscored that suicidal patients can be helped. As Voltaire recognized many years ago, time is a critical factor for the suicidal patient. Pain, hopelessness, and despair can be replaced with renewed hope and purpose with the proper treatment. This volume has attempted to demonstrate how this goal can be achieved. It is hoped that the in-depth review and life-cycle approach to risk factors for suicide and strategies for assessment and treatment of suicidal behavior provided here will be a useful guide for health care professionals in your efforts to prevent this tragic loss of human life in clinical practice.

> Where there's life, there's hope.
> —Terence, *Heauton Timoroumenos*

Appendixes

Child Suicide Potential Scales

Name of child _____ Sex __

Age _____ Date of birth _____ Race/ethnicity _____ Religion _____

Sample population: Hospital _____ Outpatient _____ Comparison _____

Date of admission _____

Address _____ Phone _____ Business phone _____

Mother's name _____ Race/ethnicity _____ Religion _____

Occupation _____ Highest school grade completed _____

Date of birth _____

Father's name _____ Race/ethnicity _____ Religion _____

Occupation _____ Highest school grade completed _____

Date of birth _____

Siblings or others at home:

	Name	Relationship	Date of birth
1.	_____	_____	_____
2.	_____	_____	_____
3.	_____	_____	_____
4.	_____	_____	_____
5.	_____	_____	_____

Reprinted from Pfeffer CR: *The Suicidal Child*. New York, Guilford Press 1986, with permission from Guilford Press.

Siblings not home:

	Name	Relationship	Date of birth
1.	_____	_____	_____
2.	_____	_____	_____
3.	_____	_____	_____
4.	_____	_____	_____
5.	_____	_____	_____

SPECTRUM OF SUICIDAL BEHAVIOR

Listed below are definitions and some examples of the suicidal behavior spectrum. Please consider them when rating the severity of this child's suicidal behavior during the past 6 months.

1. *Nonsuicidal*—No evidence of any self-destructive or suicidal thoughts or actions.

2. *Suicidal ideation*—Thoughts or verbalization of suicidal intention.
   Examples:
   a. "I want to kill myself."
   b. Auditory hallucination to commit suicide.

3. *Suicidal threat*—Verbalization of impending suicidal action and/or a precursor action which, if fully carried out, could have led to harm.
   Examples:
   a. "I am going to run in front of a car."
   b. Child puts a knife under his or her pillow.
   c. Child stands near an open window and threatens to jump out.

4. *Mild attempt*—Actual self-destructive action which realistically would not have endangered life and did not necessitate intensive medical attention.
   Example:
   a. Ingestion of a few nonlethal pills; child's stomach pumped.

5. *Serious attempt*—Actual self-destructive action which realistically could have led to the child's death and may have necessitated intensive medical care.
   Example:
   a. Child jumped out of fourth-floor window.

Describe suicidal ideas or acts: _____

_____

SPECTRUM OF ASSAULTIVE BEHAVIOR

Listed below are definitions of some examples of the assaultive behavior spectrum. Please consider them when rating the severity of the child's assaultive behavior. Circle as many types of behavior as are appropriate.

During the last 6 months, which forms of assaultive behavior were most applicable?

1. *Nonassaultive behavior*—No evidence of assaultive ideas and/or behavior which could have injured someone.

2. *Assaultive ideation*—Thoughts of wanting to harm or kill someone.
   Examples:
   a. "I wish you were dead." "Drop dead."
   b. Hallucinations of commanding to hurt or kill someone.

3. *Assaultive threats*—Ideas and/or a precursor assaultive act toward someone.
   Examples:
   a. Child holds knife, planning to hurt or kill someone.
   b. Child tells someone he or she will hurt or kill someone.

4. *Mild assaultive action*—Assaultive actions which may have injured someone but would not have resulted in injury requiring extensive medical care.
   Examples:
   a. Hitting, pushing, burning, kicking, throwing objects at someone.
   b. Child scratches another but no stitches required.

5. *Serious assaultive action*—Assaultive actions toward others which may have resulted in serious injury requiring extensive medical care.
   Examples:
   a. Child pushes mother downstairs.
   b. Child burns another.
   c. Child cuts another with a knife.
   d. Child sets fires.
   e. Child rapes or sexually molests someone.

6. *Homicide*—An action which caused the death of a victim.
   Examples:
   a. Child beat infant sibling until dead.
   b. Child drowned another.
   c. Child pushed another out window.

Describe specific type of assaultive behavior: _____

PRECIPITATING EVENTS

During the last 6 months, have any of the following things happened?

	Yes	No
1. Has the child expected to do poorly at school?	____	____
2. Has the child expressed fears of being punished for doing poorly at school?	____	____
3. Did the child do poorly at school?	____	____
4. Was the child punished for doing poorly at school?	____	____

	Yes	No
5. Has the child changed schools?	⎯⎯	⎯⎯
6. Did the child tend to stay by himself or herself?	⎯⎯	⎯⎯
7. Did the child have no friends to play with outside of school?	⎯⎯	⎯⎯
8. Has the child been worried about losing a good friend?	⎯⎯	⎯⎯
9. Did the child break up with a good friend?	⎯⎯	⎯⎯
10. Did the child tend to be bullied or teased?	⎯⎯	⎯⎯
11. Has the child had many physical illnesses?	⎯⎯	⎯⎯
12. Has the child had a serious illness?	⎯⎯	⎯⎯
13. Has the child been hospitalized?	⎯⎯	⎯⎯
14. Has the child been punished more than usual?	⎯⎯	⎯⎯
15. Has the child moved to a new home?	⎯⎯	⎯⎯
16. Has someone joined the household?	⎯⎯	⎯⎯
17. Has someone left the household?	⎯⎯	⎯⎯
18. Did the child blame himself or herself as the cause of family problems?	⎯⎯	⎯⎯
19. Has the child lost a pet?	⎯⎯	⎯⎯
20. Has the child been separated from mother for more than 1 week?	⎯⎯	⎯⎯
21. Has the child been separated from father for more than 1 week?	⎯⎯	⎯⎯
22. Has someone emotionally important to the child been seriously ill?	⎯⎯	⎯⎯
23. Has someone emotionally important to the child been hospitalized?	⎯⎯	⎯⎯
24. Has someone emotionally important to the child died?	⎯⎯	⎯⎯
25. Has a child been born into the family?	⎯⎯	⎯⎯

GENERAL PSYCHOPATHOLOGY (RECENT)

During the last 6 months, have any of the following things happened?

	Yes	No
1. Has the child become more nervous or anxious?	⎯⎯	⎯⎯
2. Has the child become more fearful?	⎯⎯	⎯⎯
3. Has the child become more quiet?	⎯⎯	⎯⎯
4. Has the child become more withdrawn?	⎯⎯	⎯⎯
5. Does the child seem more sad or depressed?	⎯⎯	⎯⎯
6. Has the child cried more frequently?	⎯⎯	⎯⎯
7. Has the child expressed feelings of hopelessness?	⎯⎯	⎯⎯
8. Has the child expressed feelings of being worthless?	⎯⎯	⎯⎯
9. Does the child blame himself or herself for bad things that have happened?	⎯⎯	⎯⎯
10. Does the child never seem proud of the things he or she does?	⎯⎯	⎯⎯
11. Has the child said that he or she wanted to die?	⎯⎯	⎯⎯
12. Has the child exhibited more nail biting?	⎯⎯	⎯⎯
13. Has the child changed eating pattern?	⎯⎯	⎯⎯

	Yes	No

14. Has the child complained more about aches and pains? ____ ____
15. Has the child had more difficulty sleeping? ____ ____
16. Has the child shown an increase in nighttime bed wetting? ____ ____
17. Has the child shown an increase in his or her tendency to ignore danger? ____ ____
18. Has the child become more irritable or belligerent? ____ ____
19. Has the child become more defiant? ____ ____
20. Has the child become more argumentative? ____ ____
21. Has the child had more fights? ____ ____
22. Has the child had more temper tantrums? ____ ____
23. Has the child shown more restless, hyperactive movements? ____ ____
24. Has the child been more easily frustrated? ____ ____
25. Has the child been more destructive of objects? ____ ____
26. Has the child more often tried to hurt other children? ____ ____
27. Has the child shown evidence of stealing? ____ ____
28. Has the child set fires? ____ ____
29. Has the child shown an increase in truancy? ____ ____
30. Has the child run away? ____ ____
31. Has the child ingested any harmful materials? ____ ____
32. Has the child had any accidents requiring a physician's attention? ____ ____
33. Has the child shown greater difficulty in learning? ____ ____

GENERAL PSYCHOPATHOLOGY (PAST)

Prior to the last 6 months, did any of the following things happen?

	Yes	No

1. Was the child nervous or anxious? ____ ____
2. Was the child fearful? ____ ____
3. Was the child quiet? ____ ____
4. Was the child withdrawn? ____ ____
5. Was the child depressed? ____ ____
6. Did the child cry frequently? ____ ____
7. Did the child express feelings of hopelessness? ____ ____
8. Did the child express feelings of being worthless? ____ ____
9. Did the child blame himself or herself for bad things that had happened? ____ ____
10. Was the child never proud of the things he or she did? ____ ____
11. Did the child exhibit nail biting? ____ ____
12. Did the child say he or she wanted to die? ____ ____
13. Did the child expect to do poorly at school? ____ ____
14. Did the child express fears of being punished for doing poorly at school? ____ ____
15. Did the child tend to be bullied or teased? ____ ____
16. Did the child blame himself or herself as the cause of family problems? ____ ____

	Yes	No
17. Has the child had more difficulty sleeping?	____	____
18. Did the child have problems eating?	____	____
19. Has the child shown an increase in nighttime bed wet-ting?	____	____
20. Has the child been irritable or belligerent?	____	____
21. Was the child defiant?	____	____
22. Was the child argumentative?	____	____
23. Did the child get into fights?	____	____
24. Did the child show restlessness, hyperactive move-ments?	____	____
25. Was the child easily frustrated?	____	____
26. Was the child destructive of objects?	____	____
27. Did the child try to hurt other children?	____	____
28. Was the child a head banger?	____	____
29. Did the child have temper tantrums?	____	____
30. Has the child been frequently punished?	____	____
31. Has the child shown evidence of stealing?	____	____
32. Has the child set fires?	____	____
33. Has the child shown an increase in truancy?	____	____
34. Has the child run away?	____	____
35. Has the child shown an increase in his or her tendency to ignore danger?	____	____
36. Was the child's speech delayed?	____	____
37. Did the child have poor coordination?	____	____
38. Did the child ingest harmful materials?	____	____
39. Did the child have accidents requiring a physician's attention?	____	____
40. Did the child show difficulty in learning?	____	____
41. Did the child do poorly at school?	____	____
42. Did the child have serious physical illnesses?	____	____

FAMILY BACKGROUND

Note: The word "mother" refers to the child's natural mother or to a surrogate. The same applies to the word "father."

	Yes	No
1. Are the child's parents currently separated?	____	____
2. Were the child's parents ever separated?	____	____
If "yes," how old was the child at first separation? ____		
3. Are the child's parents divorced?	____	____
If "yes," how old was the child at divorce? ____		
4. Have there been several parental separations?	____	____
5. Has a father figure always been absent in the child's household?	____	____
6. Has the child had multiple father figures?	____	____
7. Has the child had multiple mother figures?	____	____
8. Is the child's mother dead?	____	____
If "yes," how old was the child at her death? ____		
If "no," go to Item #9.		

	Yes	No
a. Did the mother's death result from an accident?	___	___
b. Did the mother's death result from illness?	___	___
c. Did the mother's death result from suicide?	___	___
d. Did the mother's death result from homicide?	___	___

9. Is the child's father dead? ___ ___
   If "yes," how old was the child at his death? ___
   If "no," go to Item #10.
   a. Did the father's death result from an accident? ___ ___
   b. Did the father's death result from illness? ___ ___
   c. Did the father's death result from suicide? ___ ___
   d. Did the father's death result from homicide? ___ ___
10. Has any other person who lived in the child's household died? ___ ___
    If "no," go to Item #11.
    a. Did this person's death result from an accident? ___ ___
    b. Did this person's death result from illness? ___ ___
    c. Did this person's death result from suicide? ___ ___
    d. Did this person's death result from homicide? ___ ___
11. Does the mother hit or beat the child frequently? ___ ___
12. Does the father hit or beat the child frequently? ___ ___
13. Has the child witnessed frequent arguments or violence between his or her parents? ___ ___
14. Is the child frequently blamed for family problems? ___ ___
15. Does the child frequently hear parental arguments about the child? ___ ___
16. Is the child frequently picked on by siblings? ___ ___
17. Do the child's parents frequently not speak with each other? ___ ___

For the following items, please place a checkmark where applicable.

	Mother	Father	Other family member
18. Chronic medical illness?	___	___	___
19. Severe depression?	___	___	___
20. Hospitalization for psychiatric illness?	___	___	___
21. Problems with alcohol and/or drug abuse?	___	___	___
22. Extensive use of over-the-counter medications?	___	___	___
23. Suicide attempt(s)?	___	___	___
24. Verbal expression of suicidal thoughts?	___	___	___
25. Assaultive ideation (thoughts of wanting to harm or kill someone)?	___	___	___
26. Assaultive threats (ideas and/or a precursor assaultive act toward someone)?	___	___	___

	Mother	Father	Other family member

27. Mild assaultive attempt (assaultive action that may have injured someone but did not result in injury requiring extensive medical care)?

28. Serious assaultive attempt (assaultive action toward others that may have resulted in serious injury requiring medical care)?

29. Homicide (an action that caused the death of a victim)?

CONCEPT OF DEATH SCALE

Please ask the child the following:

	Never	Sometimes	Often

1. Have you ever thought about dying?
2. Have you ever thought about people in your family dying?
3. Do you ever dream about people dying?
4. Do you dream that you are dying?
5. Do you dream about dead relatives?
6. Have you ever thought about the death of someone you liked a lot?

	Yes	No

7. Have you ever seen a dead person?
8. Have you ever been to a funeral home?
9. Have you ever been to a funeral?
10. Do you think people come back to life after they die?
11. Do you think animals come back to life after they die?
12. Do you think a person goes to a better place after death?
13. Do you think a person goes to a terrible place after death?

Interviewer's rating of child's concept of death

(Please circle appropriate number.)

Does the child think of death as pleasant or unpleasant?

Unpleasant 1 2 3 4 5 Pleasant

Does the child think of death as final or
temporary? Final 1 2 3 4 5 Temporary

ASSESSMENT OF CURRENT EGO FUNCTIONS

1. *IQ*
   If tested: Verbal _____ Performance _____ Full scale _____
   If not tested: Dull normal _____ Normal _____ Above normal _____

2. *Achievement*
   Reading score _____ at or above grade level _____ below grade level _____
   Spelling score _____ at or above grade level _____ below grade level _____
   Math score _____ at or above grade level _____ below grade level _____

3. *Affects* How frequently does the child show these affects?	Never	Sometimes	Often	All the time
a. Irritability, aggression, anger	___	___	___	___
b. Depression, sadness, crying	___	___	___	___
c. Anxiety, fearfulness	___	___	___	___
d. Passivity, dependency, timidity	___	___	___	___
e. Cheerfulness, humor	___	___	___	___

How often does the child shift affects?
Seldom ____ Sometimes ____ Often ____
Is the child's affect appropriate to the situations that arise?
Seldom ____ Sometimes ____ Often ____

4. *Impulse control*	Low	Average	High
a. Degree of frustration tolerance	___	___	___
b. Ability to delay actions	___	___	___
c. Ability to plan for future events	___	___	___
d. Ability to tolerate deprivations	___	___	___
e. Ability to handle restlessness resulting from restrictions	___	___	___
f. Ability to make a decision when faced with alternatives	___	___	___
g. Tendency to retreat into fantasy in face of a choice problem	___	___	___
h. Persistent tendency to daydream	___	___	___

5. *Reality testing*
   a. Knowledge of present place
      Yes ____ No ____
   b. Knowledge of time
      Yes ____ No ____

c. Knowledge of identity
Yes ____ No ____
d. Child answers questions logically
Never ____ Sometimes ____ Often ____ All the time ____
e. Child perceives situations appropriately
Never ____ Sometimes ____ Often ____ All the time ____
f. Child appears to understand the consequences of his or her behavior
Never ____ Sometimes ____ Often ____ All the time ____

6. *Object relations*
a. Does the child relate to the interviewer in an appropriate way?
Seldom ____ Sometimes ____ Often ____
b. Does the child relate to other people in an appropriate way?
Seldom ____ Sometimes ____ Often ____

EGO DEFENSES

To what extent does the child use each of the defense mechanisms defined below?

	Never	Sometimes	Often
1. *Regression* (manifestation of a return to an earlier level of ego development) Examples: Biting, sucking fingers and objects, autistic behavior, smearing and dirtying, use of baby talk or more primitive language, refusal of child to do tasks when he or she is capable of them	____	____	____
2. *Denial* (will include mechanisms of isolation and splitting, the tendency to deny painful sensations and facts) Examples: a. Child's parent deserted the family, and the child believes parent will return soon. b. Child says he or she has many friends, but has none. c. Child's parents are severely punishing, and the child says that this does not happen. d. Child tells a frightening story in a calm way without manifestation of frightened feelings (isolation). e. Child shows love to one person and to another person only hate (splitting).	____	____	____

	Never	Sometimes	Often

3. *Projection* (emotions and ideas which the ego tried to ward off are attributed to someone else)
   Examples:
   a. Child whose anger is intense believes that others are angry at the child.
   b. Child who has difficulty controlling his or her impulses thinks that others will harm the child.
   c. "All teachers are stupid."   _____   _____   _____

4. *Introjection* (taking in of characteristics, ideas, and feelings of another person)
   Examples:
   a. Child's aggressive behavior is an identification of a parent's aggressive behavior.
   b. Child's mother or father is depressed, and child becomes depressed.
   c. Parent is punitive, and child acts similarly to peers.   _____   _____   _____

5. *Reaction formation* (manifestation of a reverse of the repressed instinctual impulses)
   Examples:
   a. Child cannot tolerate dirt or messy things.
   b. Child feels disgusted by certain foods.
   c. Child too intensely dislikes showing off.   _____   _____   _____

6. *Undoing* (something is done or thought and is immediately undone by an act or thought that negates it)
   Examples:
   a. Child buys toys and usually changes his or her mind and returns them.
   b. Child is friendly and then immediately becomes angry.   _____   _____   _____

7. *Displacement* (channelling instinctual feelings, actions, and ideas into a new object or situation)

	Never	Sometimes	Often

Examples:
    a. Child afraid of parent and
       becomes afraid of dogs.
    b. Child scapegoats other children.
    c. Child kicks pet when angry.   ————   ————   ————

8. *Intellectualization* (child discusses
   ideas rather than expressing feelings
   in situation where feelings should be
   discussed)
   Examples:
     a. Child reads, in contrast to
       playing with others.
     b. Child says little about his or her
       feelings but becomes
       enthusiastic when discussing
       intellectual ideas.   ————   ————   ————

9. *Compensation* (child experiences
   inadequacy or inability and
   overdevelops in another area)
   Examples:
     a. Child tries to be group clown.
     b. Child tries to be superstrong.
     c. Child is a risk taker.   ————   ————   ————

10. *Sublimation* (under the influence of
   the ego, unacceptable feelings are
   changed into a socially useful
   modality without blocking an
   adequate discharge)
   Examples:
     a. Child enjoys hobbies.
     b. Child has strong aggressive
       feelings and collects soldiers.
     c. Child likes to paint.
     d. Child likes to model clay.   ————   ————   ————

11. *Repression* (unconsciously
   purposefully forgetting or not
   becoming aware of internal impulses
   or external events)
   Examples:
     a. Child has difficulty describing
       events of childhood, and child
       says he or she does not
       remember.
     b. Child does not remember
       feelings when first entered
       school.

	Never	Sometimes	Often
c. Child does not remember feelings when siblings were born.			
d. Child does not remember dreams.	____	____	____

DIAGNOSTIC IMPRESSION(S)

Check all that apply.

1. Mental retardation ____
2. Attention deficit disorder ____
   a. With hyperactivity ____
3. Conduct disorder ____
   a. Undersocialized, aggressive ____
   b. Undersocialized, nonaggressive ____
   c. Socialized, aggressive ____
   d. Socialized, nonaggressive ____
4. Anxiety disorder ____
   a. Separation anxiety disorder ____
   b. Avoidant disorder ____
   c. Overanxious disorder ____
5. Other disorders of childhood ____
   a. Oppositional disorder ____
   b. Identity disorder ____
6. Eating disorders ____
7. Stereotyped movement disorders ____
8. Other disorders with physical manifestations (stuttering, functional enuresis, functional encopresis, sleep walking, sleep terror) ____
9. Pervasive developmental disorders (infantile autism, childhood onset, atypical, etc.) ____
10. Specific developmental disorder ____
    a. Developmental language disorder ____
11. Organic brain syndrome (delirium, dementia, amnesic syndrome, organic delusional, etc.) ____
12. Epilepsy ____
13. Schizophrenic disorder ____
14. Psychotic disorders, other (schizophreniform, brief reactive, psychosis, schizoaffective, atypical) ____
15. Neurotic disorders ____
16. Affective disorders ____
    a. Major depression ____
    b. Dysthymic disorder ____
    c. Cyclothymic disorder ____
17. Adjustment disorder ____
18. Personality disorders ____
    a. Borderline personality ____
    b. Schizotypal ____
    c. Other (specify) _____ ____
19. No psychopathology ____

Administrative Policy Regarding Suicide and Homicide

I. **PURPOSE:** To keep a suspected or confirmed suicidal and/or homicidal patient from harming himself and others.

II. **SCOPE:** This policy affects the physicians and all staff personnel involved in providing patient services.

III. **RESPONSIBILITY:** The attending physician or his designee and the nursing staff are responsible for carrying out this policy and procedure.

IV. **PROCEDURE**

   A. Admitting
   1. Patients who are suicidal/homicidal may be admitted to any nursing division and remain if:
       a) no bed is available on the psychiatric unit;
       b) the patient is cleared medically by a physician for transfer to the psychiatric unit; or
       c) the responsibility for the care of the patient has not been accepted by a designated psychiatrist.
   2. Admit the patient to a room as close as possible to the nurses' station and block the other bed. Assign to a private room if available.
   3. Contact psychiatric division personnel for consultation.
   4. The physician's admission note and nursing staff observations

must state presence and indicate the relative severity of suicide/homicide risk.

5. The physician must state on the order sheet that suicidal and/or homicidal precautions shall be taken in relation to the estimated degree of risk.

B. **Care of the patient: Once the patient is admitted and while waiting for a psychiatric consult and disposition, the following steps should be taken:**

1. Request a family member or friend to stay with the patient or make arrangements for a sitter, unless otherwise ordered by the psychiatrist.

2. If family member/friend is not available, arrangements shall be made to obtain a sitter unless otherwise ordered by the psychiatrist. Note: A sitter shall be responsible for observing the patient at all times, under the supervision of the nursing staff, but the presence of a sitter *does not* release nurses from full responsibility.

3. If none of the above arrangements can be made, obtain an order from the attending physician and/or designee or the psychiatrist for restraints.

C. **Nursing responsibilities**

1. Restrict patient to his room.

2. A member of the nursing staff must observe patient at least every 30 minutes—more often if alone and in restraints. Documentation shall be noted on the chart on a separate sheet and also on the inside of the patient's closet door.

3. Free room of objects potentially dangerous to the patient:

   a) Two (2) staff members check room for restricted items. See Restricted Items list.

   b) Remove overbed stand.

   c) Remove light cords and eliminate hazards from electrical sources.

   d) Remove signal cord and replace with tap bell.

   e) Have housekeeping remove blinds and drapes with cords.

   f) Remove radio pillow speaker.

   g) Remove telephone and table or support bracket.

RESTRICTED ITEMS

Glass vases	Glass items
Nail files	All spray containers
Nail clippers	Mirrors
Nail polish	Crochet hooks
Nail polish remover	Knitting hooks
Perfume	Electric equipment (except
Picture frames	battery-powered radio)
Matches	Alcoholic beverages
Scissors	Pins
Needles	Pop cans
Knives	Hangers
Guns	Plastic bags
Tweezers	Lighters
Electric razor	Razor blades

4. Place patient's belongings in personal belongings bag, label, and keep at the nursing station.
5. Take only rectal or axillary temperatures. Keep thermometers locked in bathroom out of patient's reach.
6. Meal trays
    a) Mark or stamp diet sheet *Special Precautions*
    b) When serving meal to patient, assure that paper or styrofoam service and plastic utensils are on the tray *before* and *after* the meal. Document on the chart. *Report any missing items to the charge nurse STAT.*
7. When administering oral medications, observe that patient swallows the drugs. Do mouth check if necessary. Do not leave ointments and lotions in the patient's room.
8. Maintain side rails and restraints as needed.
9. Remain with patient until completion of *any* routine procedure.
10. Document relevant conversations and observations accurately in nurses' notes. Any statement about intention to do violence must be accurately stated.

V. **IDENTIFIED SUICIDAL/HOMICIDAL PATIENTS:** Potentially violent patients should be reported immediately to attending physician or designee. Implementation of suicidal/homicidal precautions is to be initiated with the least possible delay.

If the physician is not available and/or refuses to acknowledge the risk, the charge nurse shall notify the nursing supervisor. The chief of staff shall then be notified of the special hazard.

If the threat is recognized:

A. **8:00 a.m.–4:30 p.m.: Nursing supervisor also shall notify department head, the chief executive officer, and the president of the executive committee.**
B. **4:00 p.m.–12:30 a.m.; 12:00 p.m.–8:30 a.m.; weekends and holidays: Nursing supervisor shall notify the administrator on call.**

VI. **ELOPEMENT OF SUSPECTED SUICIDAL/HOMICIDAL PATIENT**

A. **Staff member shall immediately notify the nurse in charge.**
B. **Nurse in charge:**
    1. Requires the ward clerk to notify security and the information desk with a description of the patient.
    2. Notifies the nursing supervisor.
    3. Notifies the attending physician and/or designee.
    4. Assigns staff members to search within the hospital grounds.
        a) If unable to locate the patient within thirty (30) minutes, staff members return to the nursing division and inform the charge nurse.
        b) If the patient is found, the staff member should attempt to persuade him to return to the ward voluntarily. Physical effort to detain, restrain, or return the patient to the hospital against his will is not permitted unless legal sanction for involuntary status has been previously established.
    5. Notifies the family of the facts regarding the situation.

C. If the patient has committed an act of violence against himself or others, resulting in injury or damage to property in the act of elopement, or if the patient has been admitted by a legal restraining order, the police are to be called by the nursing supervisor and/or security and asked to assist in the search for and apprehension of the patient.
1. The attending physician will be notified of this action.
2. The nursing supervisor will decide if and when the hospital administrator will be called.
3. The immediate family is to be notified of developments as they occur.
4. Disposition of the patient to be determined, depending on condition and prevailing circumstances, by attending physician in consultation with the administrator.

D. The nurse in charge is to complete incident reports and submit them to the nursing service office and ensure that accurate documentation has been completed on the patient's chart.

VII. SUICIDE/HOMICIDE RISK LABEL

A. The chart of any patient deemed to be suicidal, homicidal, or potentially violent is to be identified with a special chart label.
B. The label is an informal signal that alerts all personnel that the patient may be violent or dangerous to self and others.
C. Label may be applied by a nurse with approval of a supervisor or by a physician.
1. No physician's written order is required.
2. Physician should be notified within 24 hours of application of label.
3. Label is automatically instituted when suicidal precautions are ordered by a physician.
4. The reason for instituting the label will be documented in either the nurses' notes or the physician's progress note.
5. Label will be removed by physician's order only.
6. Label will be affixed to the front of the chart for as long as it is in effect and will read in capital letters ADMINISTRATIVE POLICY IN EFFECT. No other wording is to be used.

VIII. SUICIDE/HOMICIDE PRECAUTIONS
A. Suicide/homicide precautions are protective procedures to be instituted for any patient who may be considered a potential threat to himself or others. This will include suicidal, assaultive, or homicidal patients.
B. The procedure is divided into three categories:
1. Grade I—suspected suicide/homicide risk,
2. Grade II—serious suicide/homicide risk, and
3. Grade III—extreme suicide/homicide risk.
C. A nurse may institute this procedure at any time, if deemed necessary.
1. The physician must be notified, and a written order is to be obtained.
2. Procedures remain in effect until discontinued by a written order of the physician.

D. The names of all patients on suicide/homicide precautions are written in red ink on the observation list.
E. The Kardex care plan of these patients carries a green tag with written specification of Grade I, Grade II, or Grade III.
F. The status of these patients shall be discussed daily by the treatment team.
G. The patient should receive an explanation of the procedures and should be advised what to expect in regard to day-to-day care.

IX. **GRADE I—SUSPECTED SUICIDE/HOMICIDE RISK:** The patient whose ideational trend and verbal content suggests rumination and consideration of death by suicide or of other violent acts.

A. **The patient is ambivalent about wanting to live or die, but has no definite plan to commit suicide or other act of violence, and there has been no suicide attempt or overt act of violence. The patient acknowledges he is fearful of his thought content and impulse control.**
B. **The following policies relate to this level of suicide precaution:**
   1. The patient must be seen by a nurse (RN), licensed practical nurse (LPN), or nurse attendant (NA) no less often than every half-hour.
   2. Nurses' notes on the patient's chart will include a resumé of the patient's behavior and activities and a statement that the patient was seen every half-hour. This shall be instituted on each shift.
   3. Some items on the Restricted List may be used. However, the RN, LPN, or NA must make checks while the patient is using any restricted item and must assure that the item is returned to the nurses' station immediately after use. The patient's assigned RN, LPN, or NA will be responsible to issue the restricted item and assure control and supervision.
   4. The patient may go off the ward, accompanied by an RN, LPN, or NA, if:
      a) the RN, LPN, or NA judges the patient is under control and compliant, and
      b) the patient indicates to the RN, LPN, or NA that he feels in control of his thought processes and will be compliant.
   5. The patient may go on therapeutic home visits, accompanied by a person specifically requested by the physician, if the person responsible for the patient understands and accepts the need for protecting the patient away from the hospital and agrees not to leave the patient alone at any time while away from the hospital.
   6. The patient may have visitors.
   7. The patient may participate in general ward activities.
   8. The patient may have regular dishes and utensils.
   9. The patient may wear his/her own clothing.
   10. A room search is to be done by two (2) staff members whenever it is suspected that the patient may have a dangerous item in his possession.

X. **GRADE II—SERIOUS SUICIDE/HOMICIDE RISK:** The patient whose thought content is primarily and admittedly suicidal.

A. **The patient is no longer ambivalent about wanting to live or die, but has arranged a plan of action. The patient's actions are directed toward self-destruction (e.g., saving medications, attempting to hide silverware, failure or refusal to return razor to RN, LPN, or NA after use and then denying it).**

B. **The following policies relate to this level of suicide precaution:**
   1. The patient must be seen by the RN, LPN, or NA every quarter-hour or less.
   2. Nurses' notes on the patient's chart will include a resumé of the patient's behavior and activities, with a statement that the patient has been seen every quarter-hour. This shall be instituted on each shift.
   3. Restricted items may be used but only in the presence of the patient's RN, LPN, or NA. For example, the RN, LPN, or NA must remain with the patient who is shaving with a razor.
   4. The patient may go off the ward for procedures and treatments ordered by the physician, such as X-rays, scans, EEGs, consultations, only if accompanied by one or more staff members.
   5. The patient may not go home on therapeutic home visits.
   6. The patient may have visitors. However, the assigned caregiver should check with the visitors to make certain they understand that they are not to give the patient any items on the Restricted List. It should be determined that the visitor is welcome by the patient and is not upsetting to him/her.
   7. The patient may participate in general ward activities unless ordered otherwise by the physician.
   8. The patient may wear his/her own clothing.
   9. Regular dishes and utensils may be used. However, they may not be left unattended with the patient. A utensil count should be done before and after the meal.
   10. The patient should be assigned to a room close to the nurses' station and the intercom turned on at all times while the patient is in the room.
   11. A room search is to be done by two (2) staff members at least once a day and whenever it is suspected that the patient may have a dangerous item in his/her possession.

XI. **GRADE III—EXTREME SUICIDE/HOMICIDE RISK:** The patient whose behavior, both verbally and nonverbally, is almost totally in the direction of self-destruction.

A. **The patient must have constant nursing attendance or constant attendance by a family member or close friend under close supervision of the nurse. There shall be documentation to this effect in the nurses' notes on the patient's chart for each shift.**
B. **No restricted items may be used unless specifically ordered in writing by the physician.**
C. **The patient may not go off the ward except when specially**

ordered by the physician. When he leaves the ward at least two competent attendants shall accompany the patient.

D. No visitors shall be permitted except as sitters, as noted in A. above.

E. Paper dishes and plastic utensils shall be used. If necessary, plastic utensils may be restricted and finger foods ordered for the patient.

F. The patient is to wear a hospital gown at all times.

G. The patient is to be placed in a seclusion room with reduced environmental stimuli.
   1. All extra furniture and other articles should be removed from the room.
   2. If necessary, the mattress may be removed from the bedframe and placed on the floor.
   3. Restraints should be used for further protection, if necessary, by order of the physician.
   4. The intercom is to be turned on and monitored at all times.

Scale for Suicide Ideation (for Ideators)

Name _____ Date _____

Day of Interview		*Time of Crisis/Most Severe Point of Illness*

I. *Characteristics of Attitude Toward Living/Dying*

( )   1. Wish to Live   ( )
   - 0. Moderate to strong
   - 1. Weak
   - 2. None

( )   2. Wish to Die   ( )
   - 0. None
   - 1. Weak
   - 2. Moderate to strong

( )   3. Reasons for Living/Dying   ( )
   - 0. For living outweigh for dying
   - 1. About equal
   - 2. For dying outweigh for living

Day of Interview			*Time of Crisis/Most Severe Point of Illness*
( )	4. Desire to Make Active Suicide Attempt 0. None 1. Weak 2. Moderate to strong		( )
( )	5. Passive Suicidal Attempt 0. Would take precautions to save life 1. Would leave life/death to chance (e.g., carelessly crossing a busy street) 2. Would avoid steps necessary to save or maintain life (e.g., diabetic ceasing to take insulin)		( )

If all four code entries for Items 4 and 5 are "0," skip sections II, III, and IV, and enter "8"—"Not Applicable" in each of the blank code spaces.

II. *Characteristics of Suicide Ideation/Wish*

( )	6. Time Dimension: Duration 0. Brief, fleeting periods 1. Longer periods 2. Continuous (chronic), or almost continuous		( )
( )	7. Time Dimension: Frequency 0. Rare, occasional 1. Intermittent 2. Persistent or continuous		( )
( )	8. Attitude toward Ideation/Wish 0. Rejecting 1. Ambivalent; indifferent 2. Accepting		( )
( )	9. Control over Suicidal Action/Acting-out Wish 0. Has sense of control 1. Unsure of control 2. Has no sense of control		( )
( )	10. Deterrents to Active Attempt (e.g., family, religion; possibility of serious injury if unsuccessful; irreversibility) 0. Would not attempt suicide		( )

because of a deterrent
1. Some concern about
   deterrents
2. Minimal or no concern
   about deterrents

(Indicate deterrents, if any: _____

_____

( ) 11. Reason for Contemplated
     Attempt   ( )
     0. To manipulate the
        environment; get
        attention, revenge
     1. Combination of "0" and
        "2"
     2. Escape, surcease, solve
        problems

III. *Characteristics of Contemplated Attempt*

( ) 12. Method: Specificity/Planning   ( )
     0. Not considered
     1. Considered, but details
        not worked out
     2. Details worked out/well
        formulated

( ) 13. Method: Availability/
     Opportunity   ( )
     0. Method not available; no
        opportunity
     1. Method would take time/
        effort; opportunity not
        readily available
     2a. Method and opportunity
         available
     2b. Future opportunity or
         availability of method
         anticipated

( ) 14. Sense of "Capability" to Carry
     out Attempt   ( )
     0. No courage, too weak,
        afraid, incompetent
     1. Unsure of courage,
        competence
     2. Sure of competence,
        courage

Day of Interview				Time of Crisis/Most Severe Point of Illness

( )   15. Expectancy/Anticipation of
Actual Attempt   ( )
0. No
1. Uncertain, not sure
2. Yes

IV. *Actualization of Contemplated Attempt*

( )   16. Actual Preparation   ( )
0. None
1. Partial (e.g., starting to
collect pills)
2. Complete (e.g., had pills,
razor, loaded gun)

( )   17. Suicide Note   ( )
0. None
1. Started but not completed;
only thought about
2. Completed

( )   18. Final Acts in Anticipation of
Death (e.g., insurance, will,
gifts)   ( )
0. None
1. Thought about or made
some arrangements
2. Made definite plans or
completed arrangements

( )   19. Deception/Concealment of
Contemplated Attempt
(Refers to communication of
ideation to interviewing
clinician)   ( )
0. Revealed ideas openly
1. Held back on revealing
2. Attempted to deceive,
conceal, lie

V. *Background Factors*

Items 20 and 21 are not included in total score.

( )   20. Previous Suicide Attempts   ( )
0. None
1. One
2. More than one

| *Day of* | | *Time of Crisis/Most* |
| *Interview* | | *Severe Point of Illness* |

(   )   21. Intent to Die Associated with
Last Attempt   (   )
(if N/A enter "8")
0. Low
1. Moderate; ambivalent,
   unsure
2. High

Suicide Intent Scale (for Attempters)

Name _____ Date _____

For all items in this scale, use code number "8" for "Not applicable." "8's" are *not* counted when calculating the total score.

I. *Objective Circumstances Related to Suicide Attempt*

1. Isolation
   0. Somebody present
   1. Somebody nearby, or in visual or vocal contact
   2. No one nearby or in visual or vocal contact

2. Timing
   0. Intervention is probable
   1. Intervention is not likely
   2. Intervention is highly unlikely

3. Precautions against Discovery/Intervention
   0. No precautions
   1. Passive precautions (as avoiding others but doing nothing to prevent their intervention; alone in room with unlocked door)
   2. Active precautions (as locked door)

4. Acting to Get Help During/After Attempt
   0. Notified potential helper regarding attempt
   1. Contacted but did not specifically notify potential helper regarding attempt
   2. Did not contact or notify potential helper

5. Final Acts in Anticipation of Death (e.g., will, gifts, insurance)
   0. None
   1. Thought about or made some arrangements
   2. Made definite plans or completed arrangements

6. Active Preparation for Attempt
   0. None
   1. Minimal to moderate
   2. Extensive

7. Suicide Note
   0. Absence of note
   1. Note written, but torn up; note thought about
   2. Presence of note

8. Overt Communication of Intent Before the Attempt
   0. None
   1. Equivocal communication
   2. Unequivocal communication

II. *Self Report*

9. Alleged Purpose of Attempt
   0. To manipulate environment, get attention, revenge
   1. Components of "0" and "2"
   2. To escape, surcease, solve problems

10. Expectations of Fatality
    0. Thought that death was unlikely
    1. Thought that death was possible but not probable
    2. Thought that death was probable or certain

11. Conception of Method's Lethality
    0. Did less to self than he thought would be lethal
    1. Wasn't sure if what he did would be lethal
    2. Equaled or exceeded what he thought would be lethal

12. Seriousness of Attempt
    0. Did not seriously attempt to end life
    1. Uncertain about seriousness to end life
    2. Seriously attempted to end life

13. Attitude Toward Living/Dying
    0. Did not want to die
    1. Components of "0" and "2"
    2. Wanted to die

14. Conception of Medical Rescuability
    0. Thought that death would be unlikely if he received medical attention
    1. Was uncertain whether death could be averted by medical attention
    2. Was certain of death even if he received medical attention

15. Degree of Premeditation
    0. None; impulsive
    1. Suicide contemplated for three hours or less prior to attempt
    2. Suicide contemplated for more than three hours prior to attempt

III. *Other Aspects (Not Included in Total Score)*

16. Reaction to Attempt
    0. Sorry that he made attempt; feels foolish, ashamed (circle which one)
    1. Accepts both attempt and its failure
    2. Regrets failure of attempt

17. Visualization of Death
    0. Life-after-death, reunion with decedents
    1. Never ending sleep, darkness, end-of-things
    2. No conceptions of, or thoughts about death

18. Number of Previous Attempts
    0. None
    1. One or two
    2. Three or more

19. Relationship between Alcohol Intake and Attempt
    0. Some alcohol intake prior to but not related to attempt, reportedly not enough to impair judgment, reality testing
    1. Enough alcohol intake to impair judgment, reality testing and diminish responsibility
    2. Intentional intake of alcohol in order to facilitate implementation of attempt

20. Relationship between Drug Intake and Attempt (narcotics, hallucinogens, etc., when drug is *not* the method used to suicide)
    0. Some drug intake prior to but not related to attempt, reportedly not enough to impair judgment, reality testing
    1. Enough drug intake to impair judgment, reality testing and diminish responsibility
    2. Intentional drug intake in order to facilitate implementation of attempt

CLINICIAN'S ESTIMATE OF RELIABILITY

Estimated reliability of patient
    0. Uncertain
    1. Poor
    2. Fair
    3. Good

VARIABLES INFLUENCING RELIABILITY OF PATIENT

Confusion as a medical consequence of attempt
    0. None   1. Some   2. Moderate   3. Severe

Disorientation at time of attempt due to alcohol or drug abuse
    0. None   1. Some   2. Moderate   3. Severe

Disorientation at time of attempt due to emotional state
    0. None   1. Some   2. Moderate   3. Severe

Lack of truthfulness or reluctance to disclose information
    0. None   1. Some   2. Moderate   3. Severe

Current memory impairment, amnesia, "blocking" regarding attempt
    0. None   1. Some   2. Moderate   3. Severe

Current withdrawal, partial mutism, inability to verbalize
    0. None   1. Some   2. Moderate   3. Severe

"Objective" items that patient didn't explicitly answer (list by **#**):

_____

Clinician's confidence in his inferences about above questions:
    0. N/A   1. Low   2. Moderate   3. High

"Self-report" items that patient didn't explicitly answer (list by **#**):

_____

Clinician's confidence in his inference about above questions:
    0. N/A   1. Low   2. Moderate   3. High

Clinician's overall estimate of the Scale's validity as a measure of suicidality, in view of all above factors.
    0. Low   1. Moderate   2. High

SUPPLEMENT TO INTENT SCALE

Why did the patient choose this particular method? (Enter patient's verbatim response and then enter appropriate category)

Patient's Response: _____

_____

_____

0. Most immediately accessible.
1. Believed to be most lethal.
2. Least painful.
3. Method suggested by another person.

4. Imitation of suicide attempt by another person.
5. Method suggested or demanded by voices.
6. Method has particular psychological or symbolic significance to this patient.
7. Other.

If the patient took a drug overdose and had ingested alcohol, was he or she aware of the fact that the combined effects of alcohol and certain drugs are greater than the total of their separate effects?

0. Yes, patient was aware of it.
1. No, he (she) was not aware of it.
2. Question is not applicable to this case.

What is the relationship between alcohol ingestion and the attempt?

0. No alcohol ingestion.
1. Alcohol ingestion was normal for this patient, and unrelated to the suicide attempt.
2. Alcohol ingestion was excessive and may have impaired judgment, but patient did not drink in order to facilitate the attempt.
3. Patient drank excessively to gain courage for the attempt.
4. Patient drank in order to add to the effects of an overdose.
5. Patient took alcohol in combination with a drug overdose, knowing that this would produce an extra lethal effect.
6. Alcohol ingestion was related to the attempt in another way. (Specify) _____

_____

_____

Suicide, Suicidal Intent, Irresistible Impulse, and Statutes Limiting Suicide Defense— Summary of Jurisdictions

I. Suicide, Sane or Insane
   A. All Nonaccidental Self-destruction Excluded Regardless of Mental State

Idaho	*Nielsen v. Provident Life & Accid. Ins. Co.*, 100 Idaho 223, 596 P.2d 95 (1979).
Illinois	*Seitzinger v. Modern Woodmen*, 204 Ill. 58, 68 N.E. 478 (1903) *but cf. Maddox v. MFA Life Ins. Co.*, 132 Ill. App. 2d 109 (1971) [appears to adopt "suicidal intent" standard], citing Supreme Lodge v. Gelbke, 198 Ill. 365, 64 N.E. 1058 (1902).
Indiana	*Kunse v. Knights of Modern McCabees*, 45 Ind. App. 30, 90 N.E. 89 (1909).
Iowa	*Scarth v. Security Mutual Life Society*, 75 Iowa 346, 39 N.W. 658 (1888).
Massachusetts	*Moore v. Northwestern Mutual Life*, 192 Mass. 468, 78 N.E. 488 (1906).
Minnesota	*Cotter v. Royal Neighbors of Am.*, 76 Minn. 518, 79 N.W. 542, 543 (1899).
Mississippi	*Sovereign Camp, W.O.W. v. Hunt*, 136 Miss. 156, 98 So. 62 (1924).
Nebraska	*Scherar v. Prudential Ins. Co.*, 63 Neb. 530, 88 N.W. 687 (1902).

New Mexico	*Galloway v. Guaranty Income Life Ins. Co.*, 104 N.M. 627, 725 P.2d 827 (N.M. 1986) [appears to adopt majority position].
New York	*Franklin v. John Hancock Mutual Life Ins. Co.*, 298 N.Y. 81, 80 N.E.2d 746 (1948); *De Gogorza v. Knickerbocker Life Ins. Co.*, 65 N.Y. 232 (1875).
North Carolina	*Spruill v. Northwestern Mutual Life Ins. Co.*, 120 N.C. 141, 27 S.E. 39 (1897).
North Dakota	*Clemens v. Royal Neighbors of Am.*, 14 N.D. 116, 103 N.W. 402 (1905).
Pennsylvania	*Tritschler v. Keystone Mutual Ben. Assoc.*, 180 Pa. 205, 36 A. 734 (1897).
South Carolina	*Latimer v. Sovereign Camp, W.W.*, 62 S.C. 145, 40 S.E. 155 (1901). *Hartin v. Sovereign Camp. W.O.W.*, 124 S.C. 397, 117 S.E. 409 (1923). *But see Gibson v. Reliance Life Ins. Co.*, 172 S.C. 94, 172, S.E. 772 (1934).
Texas	*Aetna Life Ins. Co. v. McLaughlin*, 380 S.W.2d 101, 9 A.L.R.3d 1005 (Tex. 1964); *Southern Farm Bureau Life Ins. Co. v. Dettle*, 707 S.W.2d 271 (Tex. App. 1986).
Vermont	*Billings v. Accident Ins. Co.*, 64 Vt. 78, 24 A. 656 (1892).
Virginia	*Atkinson v. Life Ins. Co. of Va.*, 217 Va. 208, 228 S.E.2d 117 (1976).
Washington	*Campbell v. Order of Washington*, 53 Wash. 398, 102 P. 410, 413 (1909).

B. Proof of Suicidal Intent Required

California	*Searle v. Allstate Life Ins. Co.*, 38 Cal. 3d 425, 212 Cal. Rptr. 466, 696 P.2d 1308 (1985).
Florida	*Charney v. Illinois Mutual Life Cas. Co.*, 764 F.2d 1441 (11th Cir. 1985) [Florida law requires the intent to achieve self-destruction for suicidal intent to be found].
Georgia	*Christensen v. New England Mut. Life Ins. Co.*, 197 Ga. 807, 30 S.E.2d 471 (1944); *Metropolitan Life Ins. Co. v. Plumstead*, 111 Ga. App. 630, 142 S.E.2d 429 (Ga. App. 1965), *citing id.*
Kansas	*Muzenich v. Grand Carniolian Slovenian Catholic Union*, 154 Kan. 537, 119 P.2d 504 (1941).
Kentucky	*New York Life v. Dean*, 226 Ky. 597, 11 S.W.2d 417 (1928).
Michigan	Courtemanche v. Supreme Court of Independent Order of Foresters, 136 Mich. 30, 98 N.W. 749 (1904). *But see Ann Arbor Trust Co. v. North American Co. for L. & H. Ins.*, 527 F.2d 526 (6th Cir.), *cert. denied*, 425 U.S. 993 (1976).
Ohio	*Hartenstein v. New York Life Ins. Co.*, 93 Ohio App. 413, 113 N.E.2d 712 (Ohio App. 1947); *Paganhardt v. Metropolitan Life Ins. Co.*, 4 Ohio N.P. 169, 6 Ohio Dec. 190 (1897).

Oklahoma	*Metropolitan Life Ins. Co. v. Plunkett,* 129 Okla. 292, 264 P.827 (1928).
Tennessee	*Metropolitan Life Ins. Co. v. Staples,* 5 Tenn. App. 436 (1927).
Wisconsin	*Ladwig v. National Guardian Life Ins. Co.,* 211 Wis. 56,247 N.W. 312 (1933).

II. Irresistible Impulse
   A. Irresistible Impulse Does Not Negate Suicide or Suicidal Intent

California	*Searle v. Allstate Life Ins. Co., supra.*
Indiana	*Kunse v. Knights of Modern MacCabees, supra.*
Kentucky	*National Life Ins. Co. v. Watson,* 194 Ky. 355, 239 S.W. 35 (1922).
Massachusetts	*Moore v. Northwestern Mutual Life Ins. Co., supra.*
Vermont	*Billings v. Accident Ins. Co., supra.*

   B. Irresistible Impulse May Negate Suicide or Suicidal Intent
      1. "Suicide, sane or insane" clause

New York	*Strasberg v. Equitable Life Assoc. Soc. of U.S.,* 117 N.Y.S.2d 236, 281 App. Div. 9 (1952).
Pennsylvania	*Tritschler v. Keystone Mutual Ben. Assoc., supra.*

      2. No "sane or insane" clause

Missouri	*Garmon v. General American Life Insurance Co.,* 624 S.W.2d 42 (1981). [In Missouri, suicide while insane is unintentional as a matter of law. . . . an irresistible impulse, therefore, is "a form of insanity." Id. at 47.]
Maine	*Eastabrook v. Union Mutual Life Ins. Co.,* 54 Me. 224, 89 Am. Dec. 743 (1866). [Insanity defeats exclusion and a blind or irresistible impulse equaled insanity.]
New Hampshire	*Cole v. Combined Ins. Co. of Am.,*125 N.H. 395, 480 A.2d 178 (1984). [Insanity defeats exclusion. Insanity was defined as 1) mental incapacity to understand the physical consequences of one's act or 2) mental incapacity to resist the influence to cause one's own death.]

III. Statutes Limiting Suicide Defense

Colorado	COLO. REV. STAT. § 10-7-109—one year.
Mississippi	MISS. CODE ANN. § 83-37-13—one year.
Missouri	MO. REV. STAT. § 376.620—must show insured contemplated suicide at time applied for policy.
North Dakota	N.D. CENT. CODE § 26-03-24—one year.
Virginia	VA. CODE §38.2-3106—two years.

Jurisdictions That Employ Some Form of Presumption Against Suicide in the Context of Recovery for Accidental Death on Life Insurance Policies

Alabama	*Jefferson Standard of Life Ins. Co. v. Pate*, 290 Ala. 110, 274 So. 2d 291 (1973).
Arizona	*Pacific Mutual Life Ins. Co. of California v. Young*, 40 Ariz. 1, 9 P.2d 188 (1932).
Arkansas	*Security Life & Trust Co. v. First National Bank*, 249 Ark. 572, 460 S.W.2d 94 (1970).
Colorado	*National Farmers Union Life Ins. Co. v. Norwood*, 147 Colo. 283, 363 P.2d 681 (1961).
Florida	*Mutual Life Ins. Co.v. Bell*, 147 Fla. 734, 3 So. 2d 487 (1941).
Georgia	*Security Life & Trust Co. v. Smith*, 220 Ga. 744, 141 S.E.2d 405 (1965).
Idaho	*Haman v. Prudential Ins. Co. of America*, 91 Idaho 19, 415 P.2d 305 (1966).
Illinois	*Kettlewell v. Prudential Ins. Co. of America*, 4 Ill. 2d 383, 122 N.E.2d 817 (1954).
Iowa	*Bill v. Farm Bureau Life Ins. Co.*, 254 Iowa 1215, 119 N.W.2d 768 (1963).
Kentucky	*Commonwealth Life Ins. Co. v. Hall*, 517 S.W.2d 488 (1974).
Louisiana	*Siracusa v. Prudential Life Ins. Co. of America*, 211 La. 1066, 31 So. 2d 213 (1947).
Maine	*Hinds v. John Hancock Mutual Life Ins. Co.* 155 Me. 349, 155 A.2d 721 (1959).

Massachusetts	*Krantz v. John Hancock Mutual Life Ins. Co.*, 335 Mass. 703, 141 N.E.2d 719 (1957).
Michigan	*Cummins v. John Hancock Mutual Life Ins. Co.*, 337 Mich. 629, 60 N.W.2d 490 (1953).
Minnesota	*Hestad v. Pennsylvania Life Ins. Co.*, 295 Minn. 306, 204 N.W.2d 433 (1973).
Missouri	*Griffith v. Continental Casualty Co.*, 299 Mo. 426, 253 S.W. 1043 (1923).
Nebraska	*Mustard v. St. Paul Fire and Marine Ins. Co.*, 183 Neb. 15, 157 N.W.2d 865 (1968).
New Jersey	*Kirschbaum v. Metropolitan Life Ins. Co.*, 133 N.J.L. 5, 42 A.2d 257 (1945).
New York	*Begley v. Prudential Life Ins. Co.*, 1 N.Y.2d 530, 136 N.E.2d 839 (1956).
North Carolina	*Barnes v. Home Beneficial Life Ins. Co.*, 271 N.C. 217, 155 S.E.2d 492 (1967).
Ohio	*Evans v. National Life and Accident Ins. Co.*, 22 Ohio St.3d 87, 488 N.E.2d 1247 (1986).
Oregon	*Wyckoff v. Mutual Life Ins. Co.*, 173 Ore. 592, 147 P.2d 227 (1944).
Pennsylvania	*Watkins v. Prudential Ins. Co.*, 315 Pa. 497, 173 A. 644 (1934).
South Carolina	*Clements v. Metropolitan Life Ins. Co.*, 266 S.C. 488, 224 S.E.2d 309 (1976).
Texas	*Combined American Insurance Co. v. Blanton*, 163 Tex. 225, 353 S.W.2d 847 (1962).
Virginia	*Atkinson v. Life Ins. Co. of Virginia*, 217 Va. 208, 228 S.E.2d 117 (1976).
Washington	*Gould v. Mutual Life Ins. Co.*, 95 Wash. 772, 629 P.2d 1331 (1981).

Index

781

Schizophrenia
  alcohol use, abuse, and
    dependence, 699
  children and adolescents, 148,
    281–282, 699
  clinical population studies, 138
  college students, 326
  dexamethasone suppression test,
    119
  elderly, 344
  general population studies,
    136–137
  hallucinated commands factor, 74
  hebephrenic, 145
  high level of education role, 145
  independent treatment for
    suicide, 112
  low 5-hydroxyindoleacetic acid
    levels, 101–102
  paranoid, 145
  physicians, 606, 609
  risk factors for suicide, 144–146
  social and interpersonal variables
    role in suicide, 74–75
  somatic therapy, 433–435
  substance abuse, 699
  suicide as early mortality cause,
    144
  and suicide rate, 30–31
School-based programs, 673, 677,
  719–720
Secondary countertransferences,
  465–466
Selective abstraction, 471, 489–490
Self-control training, 287–288
Separation, from spouse. *See*
  Marital status
Serotonergic system manipulation
  fenfluramine, 116
  5-hydroxytryptophan, 115
  monoamine oxidase inhibition,
    116
  postsynaptic receptors, 116
  presynaptic autoreceptors, 116
  serotonin reuptake blockers, 115
  tricyclic antidepressants, 115
  tryptophan, 114–115
  See also Serotonin
Serotonin
  aggressive behavior regulation,
    192
  and aggressive impulsivity, 165

alcoholism, association with,
  192, 435–436
children and adolescents, 670
clinical implications, 110–111
deficiency, genetic factor role,
  130–131, 709
neuroendocrine challenge tests,
  118–119
predicting suicide risk, 116–117,
  119–120
reuptake blockers, 115
suicide relation studies, 100–110
tests of serotonergic activity,
  116–119
treatment implications, 111–114
Sex differences. *See* Gender
  differences
SMRs. *See* Standard mortality ratios
Social ecology, 366
Social isolation, 47, 64, 82, 326, 342
Social learning theory role, 526
Social skills problems, 267
Social support networks, 193–196,
  238, 326–328, 704
Sociological studies
  definition, 39–40
  economic depression, 40–41, 42
  social change dynamics, 42
  societal integration, 41
Socratic dialogue, 485
Sodium amytal, 403
Somatic therapy
  aims, 430
  alcohol use, abuse, and
    dependence, 435–436
  balancing dosage and duration,
    430
  borderline personality disorder,
    436–437
  depression, 431
  schizophrenia, 433–435
  See also names of specific drugs
Somatization disorder, 139, 146
Standard mortality ratios (SMRs),
  305–307
Substance abuse
  children and adolescents, 258,
    280–281, 698–699
  drug use patterns, 185
  elderly, 348–349
  general population studies,
    136–137, 147